# Practical Guide to Reproductive Medicine

# Dedication

The Editors dedicate this book to their families, relatives and friends.

# Practical Guide to Reproductive Medicine

Edited by

Paul A. Rainsbury, MA, FRCOG
and
David A. Viniker, MD, FRCOG

BUPA Roding Hospital
and
Whipps Cross Hospital,
London, UK

The Parthenon Publishing Group
International Publishers in Medicine, Science & Technology

NEW YORK LONDON

Published in the USA by
The Parthenon Publishing Group Inc.
One Blue Hill Plaza
PO Box 1564, Pearl River,
New York 10965, USA

Published in the UK and Europe by
The Parthenon Publishing Group Limited
Casterton Hall, Carnforth,
Lancs. LA6 2LA, England



**Library of Congress Cataloging-in-Publication Data**
Practical guide to reproductive medicine/edited by P. A. Rainsbury and D. A. Viniker
p. cm.
Includes bibliographical references and index.
ISBN 1-85070-727-8
1. Generative organs–Diseases. 2. Infertility. 3. Endocrine gynecology.
I. Rainsbury, Paul A. II. Viniker, D. A.
[DNLM: 1. Reproductive Medicine. 2. Reproduction Techniques.
3. Infertility–physiopathology. 4. Infertility–therapy. WQ 205 P895 1997]
RC875.P73 1997
616.6′5–dc20
DNLM/DLC 96-38763
for Library of Congress CIP

**British Library Cataloguing in Publication Data**
Practical guide to reproductive medicine
1. Gynecology. 2. Reproduction.
I. Rainsbury, Paul A. II. Viniker, D. A.
618.1
ISBN 1-85070-727-8



Cook UK Ltd. has kindly given permission for the use of the illustration on the cover
Typeset by AMA Graphics, Preston, Lancashire
Printed and bound by Butler & Tanner Ltd., Frome and London

# Contents

# List of contributors

**Tim Appleton**
IFC Resource Centre
44 Eversden Road
Harlton
Cambridge CB3 7ET
UK

**Susan M. Avery**
Bourn Hall Clinic
Infertility & Assisted Conception
Bourn
Cambridge CB3 7TR
UK

**Adam H. Balen**
Leeds General Infirmary
Clarendon Wing
Leeds LS2 9NS
UK

**Peter R. Brinsden**
Bourn Hall Clinic
Infertility & Assisted Conception
Bourn
Cambridge CB3 7TR
UK

**Charles G. D. Brook**
The Middlesex Hospital
Mortimer Street
London W1N 8AA
UK

**Howard J. A. Carp**
Department of Obstetrics & Gynecology
Sheba Medical Center
Tel Hashomer 52621
Israel

**Margaret Clark**
Linscott House
Russell Road
Buckhurst Hill
Essex IG9 5QE
UK

**Willem de Boer**
NV Organon
PO Box 20
5340 BH Oss
The Netherlands

**Ruth Deech**
The Human Fertilisation and Embryology Authority (HFEA)
Paxton House
30 Artillery Lane
London E1 7LS
UK

**James O. Drife**
Academic Department of Obstetrics and Gynaecology
University of Leeds
D Floor, Clarendon Wing (LGI)
Belmont Grove
Leeds LS2 9NS
UK

**Robert G. Edwards**
Human Reproduction Office
Manor Barns Farm House
Madingley Road
Coton
Cambridge
UK

**T. B. Paul Geurts**
NV Organon
PO Box 20
5340 BH Oss
The Netherlands

**Deborah J. Harrington**
Nuffield Department of Obstetrics and Gynaecology
John Radcliffe Hospital
Headington
Oxford OC3 9DU
UK

**Roger Hart**
Minimally Invasive Therapy Unit & Endoscopy Training Centre
University Department of Obstetrics & Gynaecology
The Royal Free Hospital
Pond Street
Hampstead
London NW3 2QG
UK

**Marie Hayes**
BUPA Roding Hospital
Roding Lane South
Ilford
Essex IG4 5PZ
UK

**Anthony V. Hirsh**
Department of Andrology
Whipps Cross Hospital
Whipps Cross Road
Leytonstone
London E11 1NR
UK
*and*
The BUPA Roding Hospital Fertility Unit
Roding Lane South
Redbridge
Ilford
Essex IG4 5PZ
UK

**Parameswaran Kishore**
Public Health Medicine
Lambeth
Southwark and Lewisham Health Authority
1 Lower Marsh Street
London SE1 7NT, UK

**Terry Leonard**
Laboratory Services
Northamptonshire Fertility Service
The Cliftonville Suite
Three Shires Hospital
The Avenue
Cliftonville
Northampton NN1 5DR, UK
*formerly*
IVF Laboratories
Assisted Conception Unit
Lister Hospital
London SW1W 8RH, UK

**Adam Magos**
Minimally Invasive Therapy Unit & Endoscopy Training Centre
University Department of Obstetrics & Gynaecology
The Royal Free Hospital
Pond Street
Hampstead
London NW3 2QG
UK

**Terry Matthews**
Oldchurch Hospital
Romford
Essex, UK

**P. M. Shaughn O'Brien**
Department of Obstetrics & Gynaecology
Maternity Department
City General
North Staffordshire NHS Trust
Newcastle Road
Stoke-on-Trent, Staffordshire ST4 6QG
UK
*and*
School of Postgraduate Medicine
Keele University
UK

**Dana A. Ohl**
Department of Surgery
Section of Urology
University of Michigan Medical Center
Ann Arbor
Michigan
USA

**Henry Okuson**
Whipps Cross Hospital
Whipps Cross Road
Leytonstone
London E11 1NR
UK

**Henk-Yan Out**
NV Organon
PO Box 20
5340 BH Oss
The Netherlands

**Marjo J. H. Peters**
NV Organon
PO Box 20
5340 BH Oss
The Netherlands

**Elliot E. Philipp**
166 Rivermead Court
Ranelagh Gardens
London SW6 3SF
UK

**Frances Plowman**
BUPA Roding Hospital
Roding Lane South
Ilford
Essex IG4 5PZ
UK

**Andrew Prentice**
Department of Obstetrics & Gynaecology
The University of Cambridge School of Clinical Medicine
The Rosie Maternity Hospital
Robinson Way
Cambridge CB2 2SW
UK

**Paul A. Rainsbury**
Department of Obstetrics & Gynaecology
Whipps Cross Hospital
Whipps Cross Road
Leytonstone
London E11 1NR
UK
*and*
IVF Unit
BUPA Roding Hospital
Roding Lane South
Ilford
Essex IG4 5PZ
UK

**Timothy C. Rowe**
Department of Gynaecology
Division of Reproductive Endocrinology and Infertility
The University of British Columbia
Vancouver Hospital and Health Sciences Center
Room 211-805 West 12th Avenue
Vancouver, BC V5Z 1N1
Canada

**Satha M. Sathanandan**
Department of Obstetrics & Gynaecology
5th Floor, Maternity Block
Harold Wood Hospital
Gubbins Lane
Harold Wood
Essex RM3 0BE
UK

**Stephen W. J. Seager**
National Rehabilitation Hospital
Washington DC
USA

**Stephen K. Smith**
Department of Obstetrics & Gynaecology
University of Cambridge School of Clinical Medicine
The Rosie Maternity Hospital
Robinson Way
Cambridge CB2 2SW
UK

**Jens Sønksen**
Department of Urology
Rigshospitalet
University of Copenhagen
9 Blegdamsvej
DK 2100 Copenhagen
Denmark

**Patrick J. Taylor**
Department of Gynaecology
Division of Reproductive Endocrinology and Infertility
The University of British Columbia
Vancouver Hospital and Health Sciences Center
Room 211-805 West 12th Avenue
Vancouver, BC V5Z 1N1
Canada

**Pat Thurley**
Whipps Cross Hospital
Whipps Cross Road
Leytonstone
London E11 1NR
UK

**Andrew Vallance-Owen**
BUPA Health Services
Provident House
15 Essex Street
London WC2R 3AU
UK

**Hans G. C. van Bruggen**
NV Organon
PO Box 20
5340 BH Oss
The Netherlands

**David A. Viniker**
Department of Obstetrics & Gynaecology
Whipps Cross Hospital
Whipps Cross Road
Leytonstone
London E11 1NR, UK
*and*
The BUPA Roding Hospital Fertility Unit
Roding Lane South
Redbridge
Ilford
Essex IG4 5PZ, UK

# About the Editors

## Paul A. Rainsbury

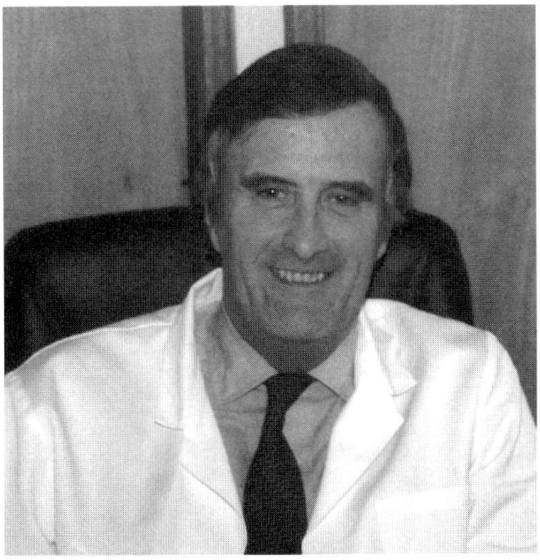

Paul Rainsbury qualified from Trinity College, Dublin in 1969. He practised as an obstetrician and gynaecologist in Ireland until 1981 and then went to Saudi Arabia for 5 years.

Following 5 years with the Bourn Hallam Group, the last year as Medical Director of the Hallam Medical Centre in London, he subsequently joined BUPA in 1992 as Medical Director of what is now the BUPA Regional Centre for Assisted Reproductive Medicine in South Eastern England.

## David A. Viniker

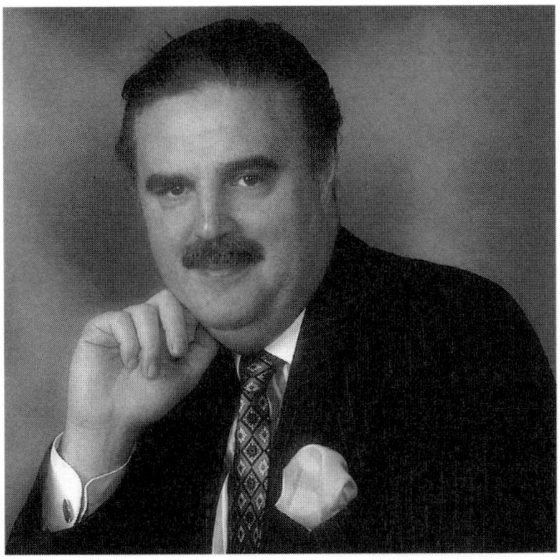

David Viniker qualified from University College Hospital, London. His postgraduate training hospitals have included University College Hospital, The Royal Postgraduate Teaching Hospital, Hammersmith, The London Hospital and the Leicester Hospitals. He is currently Consultant Obstetrician and Gynaecologist at Whipps Cross Hospital, London, Honorary Senior Lecturer in The University of London, and Associate Medical Director to The BUPA Roding Hospital Fertility Unit.

His research interests have included perinatal cerebral function monitoring, and this culminated in an MD from the University of London and The Blair-Bell Memorial Lecture at The Royal College of Obstetricians and Gynaecologists. Although primarily a clinical obstetrician and gynaecologist with special interests in infertility and reproductive endocrinology, he continues to enjoy undergraduate and postgraduate teaching and research.

This book has been published with the support of an educational grant from BUPA.

The views expressed by the contributors do not necessarily reflect those of BUPA.

# Foreword

*Robert G. Edwards*

A book such as this will be welcomed by many investigators working on assisted human conception. We have seen many publications on the advanced scientific and clinical aspects of the field, which have provided excellent insights into the details of current knowledge and new advances. *Practical Guide to Reproductive Medicine* is targeted at a different topic and a different audience. It is concerned with the steps needed to maintain high standards of care in day-to-day situations that face the clinician, embryologist, ethicist and nurse. It also provides an easy access to many details of the complexities of today's reproductive medicine. This advantage should ensure that it is widely read by those professionals working at the day-to-day forefront care of the infertile patient where new techniques and methods have to be introduced safely into clinical care.

The book is well designed to achieve its aims. There are tables and illustrative material in every chapter, designed for easy understanding and informative presentation. There is a total of 30 chapters, each dealing with a single topic. Each chapter is informative, clearly written, with well-constructed diagrams and illustrations. In short, this book is highly user-friendly for those facing the considerable variety of methods of assisted conception that are now available. Indeed, the numbers seem to increase year on year. At the same time, there are enough data on new advances to give a lead into more advanced aspects of the field.

It is impossible to discuss each of the chapters in turn. My initial selection of some of them for discussion is intended to illustrate the breadth of the topics covered in the book, and does not imply that the others are no less valuable and well presented. Pat Thurley discusses the use of ultrasound for several indications in assisted conception. The topics include the assessment of the female pelvis, and monitoring natural and induced cycles. Methods of oocyte retrieval were revolutionized by ultrasound, and so too was the analysis of early pregnancy and of fetal abnormalities. Her chapter is highly illustrated with excellent pictures. Terry Leonard writes very clearly about intracytoplasmic injection of spermatozoa into oocytes. He describes the conditions when this treatment is needed, especially the quality of semen parameters. Full details of the equipment and the various techniques, including sperm preparation and the making of pipettes for micromanipulation, are given. Treatments of the spermatozoon, including immobilization, its pick-up in the injection pipette and the injection pipette are well documented. He also illustrates data handling and has time to discuss the future of such treatments. Adam Balen covers the topics of amenorrhoea and anovulation. He gives detailed analyses on the investigation of endocrine and ovarian systems. Causes are discussed, including developmental anomalies such as Turner's and Müllerian duct anomalies. The hypothalamic causes of these conditions are presented, with secondary amenorrhoea being assessed in detail. He also describes ovarian causes of these conditions, to conclude a chapter full of information. He joins with Deborah Harrington to write another endocrine chapter on polycystic ovarian disease and hirsutism. The aetiology and heterogeneity of polycystic ovarian disease are described in some detail. The causes and problems arising from luteinizing hormone hypersecretion are well covered, including management. The origins and effects of androgens, the issue of menstrual irregularity and infertility are analysed.

Shaughn O'Brien discusses the premenstrual syndrome. This widespread condition is assessed in relation to the physiology of the reproductive tract, the aetiology of the condition and the role of neurotransmitters. Old and new theories are covered, the symptoms of the condition are assessed, and a computerised questionnaire is included. Goserelin tests are recommended to separate ovarian versus noncyclic disorders, and management is divided into three parts. Non-medical treatments include counselling and stress management, with hypnotherapy. Medical treatments include nonhormonal therapy with psychotic drugs and diuretics, and hormonal treatment using oral contraceptives, various hormones such as gonadotrophin releasing hormone analogues, and even surgery. Peter Brinsden and Sue Avery discuss IVF, its history and methods, including freezing. They indicate the excellent results that can be gained, and add a section on the Human Fertilisation and Embryology Authority (HFEA). This latter topic is covered well by Ruth Deech, who must surely be very high among those people who really understand the opportunities for an acceptable ethical standard offered by the HFEA.

Some contributors have provided more than one chapter. One of the Editors, David Viniker, writes several of the chapters including a description of the basic concepts in reproductive medicine. He covers infertility management in one of them, and discusses ovulatory dysfunction, endometriosis, tubal factor, cervical problems and trials. Two chapters deal with infertility treatment including ovarian stimulation, IVF, intracytoplasmic sperm injection and the treatment of common disorders. He also provides a most useful chapter on computer technology, with extensive comments on hardware, software, databases and methods of analysis. His final contributions include discussions of menorrhagia and dysfunctional bleeding, the climacteric and hormone replacement therapy, and a down-to-earth guide on hormone production and action, follicle growth, steroids and pharmacology. Conditions such as puberty, anaemia, hirsutism and anovulatory infertility are assessed, together with a comment on communication between patient and physician. Paul Rainsbury also contributes several chapters, especially on assisted conception. He is concerned about the state of the art, obstetric outcome and surrogacy, three diverse topics that encompass the complex clinical and ethical nature of the field.

Practical clinical and laboratory techniques are well covered by several authors. In those chapters on conditions affecting the female is one by Timothy Rowe and Patrick Taylor who discuss tubal surgery, including the use of laparoscopy, and comment on the pitfalls of the treatment and, I was glad to see, the numerous causes of this condition. Stephen Smith provides an analysis of fibroids, together with their pathophysiology, clinical treatments, and surgery, and Andrew Prentice discusses the complexities of endometriosis. Minimal access surgery, a development arising from early pioneering work on laparoscopy, has now entered several surgical disciplines and is well described by Roger Hart and Adam Magos. Howard Carp draws attention to the difficulty in classifying recurrent pregnancy loss as he gives ten causes and a concluding table on treatment.

Male infertility is covered in several chapters. Tony Hirsh deals with andrology in the 1990s, with descriptions of classic anatomy from its early origins to modern genetics, with liberally illustrated tables and figures. Jens Sønksen and his colleagues continue the topic in their description of vibratory ejaculation, the underlying physiology, technique and sperm quality. Laboratory methods and inventions are not overlooked. Marie Hayes describes techniques in the embryology laboratory, including oocyte recovery and culture, the oocyte complex, embryo grading and transfer, cryopreservation, semenology and the actions of reactive oxygen species. Paul Guerts and colleagues give details of the introduction of recombinant follicle stimulating hormone (FSH), in this case Puregon. They describe FSH receptors and their properties, pharmacokinetics, clinical trials and results.

I was also glad to see that support services are covered in several chapters. Francis Plowman describes the nurse's role, now that IVF is a clinical nursing specialty, with especial attention to the insistence of the HFEA on proper counselling, and to a practical guide to ovarian stimulation and IVF. I was glad to see that Tim Appleton discusses counselling in this book, surely one of the most essential of topics with an importance that is at last being recognized as fundamental to the whole process of assisted reproduction. Satha Sathanandan and Parameswaran Kishore assess NHS services for subfertility, with detailed analyses of service provisions – including a section on infertility – and debate whether infertility service is a luxury. Wider issues are not neglected, as shown by Charles Brook's analysis of puberty, physiology and their disorders, while James Drife describes hormonal contraception, discussing oral contraception in detail, including long-acting methods, new hormonal treatments, and contraception for men.

This book will find a place on the shelves of many IVF clinics and laboratories. Assisted conception has spread worldwide and the number of clinics continues to grow almost exponentially. There is also an enthusiasm to keep pace with the most recent advances, an aspect which is partly driven by the interest and knowledge of so many patients attending for treatment. The worldwide spread of intracytoplasmic sperm injection from discovery to widespread clinical application within 5 years has shown what can be achieved with the existing talent in so many clinics in so many countries. IVF has always demanded careful attention to detail, as shown by the strict control of sterility in handling media and embryos, and the current arguments on overstrong ovarian stimulation. Molecular methods are now increasing in number and variety, and once again a whole new technology will have to be mastered by those working in assisted human reproduction. There is always a need for new books giving details of existing and novel methods in every branch of the subject. This book will help immensely to fill this need for knowledge at every level.

# Preface

*Andrew Vallance-Owen*

Many people have suggested that the half-life of scientific knowledge is in the region of 10 years, but this may be an under-statement in the field of reproductive medicine. There have been huge advances and changes in thinking in the last 10 years, just as there were in the 10 before that. This book aims to cover much of that ground, both for the benefit of the specialist, who wishes to keep up-to-date with advances in other areas of the specialty, and for the benefit of the generalist who wishes to gain a comprehensive and systematic review of developments in the field.

The book concentrates primarily on the problems of infertility for which there are an increasing diversity of treatments available. These range from the surgical aspiration of sperm, for instance in cases of failed vasectomy reversal, to exciting developments in *in vitro* fertilization, including the management of the male factor. The book also covers difficult issues ranging from the possibilities of research activity, such as embryo biopsy, to the practical and ethical implications of surrogacy.

The Editors have brought together contributions from many acknowledged experts in the field of reproductive medicine and have done so in the context of growing public awareness and demand for wider availability of treatments for infertility. There has, in fact, been a significant increase in accessibility to treatment over the last few years, as evidenced by the growth in treatment cycles from 11 500 in 1990 to over 25 000 in 1995. In that time, there has also been an increase not only in the number of HFEA licensed clinics, but also in the number of procedures for which licences have been granted – 42 for intracytoplasmic sperm injection, 10 for subzonal sperm insertion, 53 for egg donation and 37 for sperm donation, all new categories of licence since 1991 (HFEA data).

Much of this development work is conducted in NHS units but, because of the need to set priorities within funding constraints, there has been increasing difficulty in obtaining treatment for infertility within the NHS in some parts of the country. A greater proportion of treatment, therefore, is now being provided by the independent sector and it is because of BUPA's commitment to the treatment of infertility that we have supported this book.

Ten of BUPA's network of hospitals currently offer fertility treatment of varying types; these hospitals completed over 2500 treatment cycles in 1995 and are respected for the range of treatments made available and their success rates. The BUPA Roding Hospital accounts for 300 of these treatment cycles annually and is one of the network's regional centres for reproductive medicine. The Editors, Paul Rainsbury and David Viniker, have pioneered the introduction of advanced techniques there and have made the unit one of our most successful. Their experience qualifies them to assemble this practical and comprehensive guide.

I hope that this book will stimulate thought and broaden the minds of those new to the subject matter, and prove to be a refreshing update to those already established in this field at the cutting edge of modern medicine.

*Medical Director, BUPA*

# A short history of infertility, its investigations and treatment

# 1

*Elliot E. Philipp*

## INTRODUCTION

The urge to reproduce is virtually universal. When a man and a woman who come together to satisfy that urge have failed to do so, they are infertile. Throughout the ages, they have sought ways and means to overcome their infertility.

It is not easy to be certain when the first references to infertility appeared in the literature or in art. The Venus of Willendorf, an infertility icon, a little statue, about five and a half inches tall, was unearthed in Willendorf, a village on the Danube, in Austria in 1928. The statue is reliably said to come from the middle Aurignacian period of the Old Stone Age, some time between 40 000 and 16 000 BC[1].

In the Bible in *Genesis* Chapter 1, verse 28, the commandment is given to increase, to be fruitful, to multiply and to replenish the Earth. In the same book of the Bible in Chapter 18, verse 12, Sarah was the first person in history to be recorded as laughing; but she 'laughed within herself, saying, after I am waxed old shall I have pleasure, my Lord being old also'. In that verse in *Genesis*, Abraham and Sarah were promised that they would have a son. He, the future father, was 100 years old and Sarah the mother 90, when that promise was made. She knew that her periods had stopped. She said she was 'out of her time and her husband was old', but she did conceive and had a son, and she said 'God has given me good reason to laugh. Everybody who hears will laugh with me'. Abraham had taken Sarah's maid Hagar as a 'licensed' concubine because of Sarah's failure to have a child; so Hagar was the first surrogate mother. Her and Abraham's child was called Ishmael.

Sarah is not the only infertile patient in the Bible to be cured. Rachel, married to Sarah's grandson Jacob, said to him in *Genesis* Chapter 30, verse 22, 'give me children or else I die'. She was given children but not until her sister Leah had proved that Jacob was fertile by presenting him with six children without any preceding infertility. Jacob had managed to make two concubines pregnant as well.

The story is told in the first chapter of the first book of *Samuel* of how Hannah, who was childless, prayed silently and tearfully in the House of the Lord for the gift of a child. There, the priest Eli thought she was drunk. She explained to him her great need and she vowed that, if she would have a child, she would give the child to the Lord to serve him all its life. If it was a boy, she would see to it that 'no razor should ever touch his head'.

Eli told her to 'go in peace', and asked the God of Israel to answer her prayer. He did and Hannah bore a son Samuel, who did devote his life as a priest to the Lord. As a prophet, he advised King Saul and later Kind David wisely.

In the second book of *Samuel* in Chapter 6, verse 23, Saul's daughter Michal was reported to be infertile; and there was no cure for her.

We leave the Bible to go to classical Greek mythology. We are told that the Greeks worshipped Hermes, who was the son of Zeus and Maia. Hermes became the god of fertility, as did Eros who combined the role with that of being god of passion. Aphrodite, the goddess of sexual love, was a busy lady because she not only is said to have produced Eros but also Hermaphroditus, a beautiful youth who was fathered by Hermes. Hermaphroditus grew to maturity with the nymph Salmacis. He spurned her love, and, as a revenge while he was swimming in her pool one day, Salmacis merged with him physically so he grew long hair and female breasts and thus combined male and female characteristics[2].

## FROM MYTHOLOGY TO FACTUAL HISTORY

The great Hippocrates (460–377 BC), in paragraph 59 of his *Aphorisms*, wrote 'If a woman do not conceive, and wish to ascertain whether she can conceive, having wrapped her up in blankets, fumigate below, and if it appear that the scent passes through the body to the nostrils and mouth, know that of herself she is not unfruitful.'

In paragraph 62 of Section *Aphorisms*, he wrote 'Women who have the uterus cold and dense do not conceive; and those also who have the uterus humid, do not conceive, for the semen is extinguished, and in women whose uterus is very dry and very hot the semen is lost for the want of food; but women whose uterus is in an intermediate state between these temperatures, prove fertile'.

One paragraph later, he wrote, 'And in like manner with respect to males; for either, owing to the laxity of the body, the pneuma is dissipated outwardly, so as not to propel the semen, or, owing to its density, the fluid will not pass outwardly; or owing to coldness, it is not heated so as to collect in its proper place, or owing to its heat the very same thing happens'[3].

Hippocrates, therefore, well understood that semen was essential for reproduction and that female infertility existed and could be tested for, albeit in a somewhat unscientific way.

Aristotle (384–332 BC) (Figure 1) followed Hippocrates and wrote 'Of animals otherwise, a great many have . . . an organ for excretion of the sperm: and of animals capable of generation one secretes into another, and the other into itself. The latter is termed "female" and the former "male"'. He also wrote 'In the human species, the male is generative at the longest, up to 70 years, and the female up to 50; but such extended periods are rare. As a rule, the male is generative up to the age of 65 and, to the age of 45, the female is capable of conception'[4].

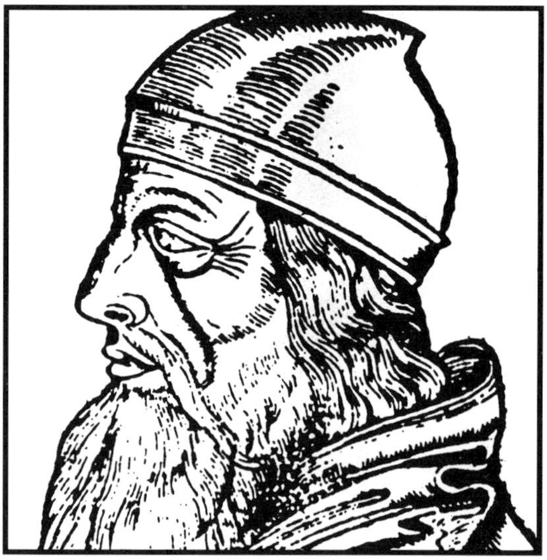

**Figure 1** Aristotle – the first known Greek writer to mention contraceptive methods. Reproduced with kind permission from the IPPF

Soranus (*c.* AD 98–138) was born in Ephesus, a city in Asia Minor. He studied in Alexandria, and then in Rome at the time of Trajan (98–117) and Hadrian (117–138), which was just about the time when Galen was born. What is the best time for fruitful intercourse? It is 'When menstruation is abating, when urge and appetite for coitus are present, when the body is neither in want, nor too congested and heavy from drunkenness and indigestion . . . The time before menstruation is not suitable. The uterus has already been overburdened . . . because of the ingress of material to be discharged at menstruation' (Figure 2). Soranus said that the seed could not unite during menstruation . . . 'when it is repelled by the bloody substance'. The rest of his chapter gives six reasons for his choosing the day he does, but of course there was no mention yet of ovulation, nor of spermatozoa. Yet, we are beginning to find mention of a fertile period[5].

Rufus of Ephesus (*c.* AD 110–180) was one of the first to describe both the male and female reproductive organs including the oviducts (in animals) and the various parts of the vulva. He

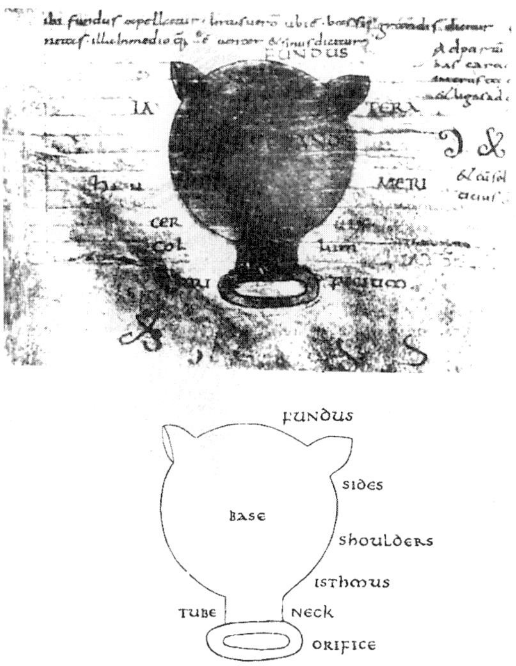

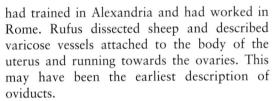

**Figure 2** Earliest known representation of the anatomy of the uterus. It embodies Soranus' conception of the organ and appears in a Muscio text of the ninth century. From Weindler (1908). Courtesy of the National Library of Medicine, Bethesda, Maryland, USA

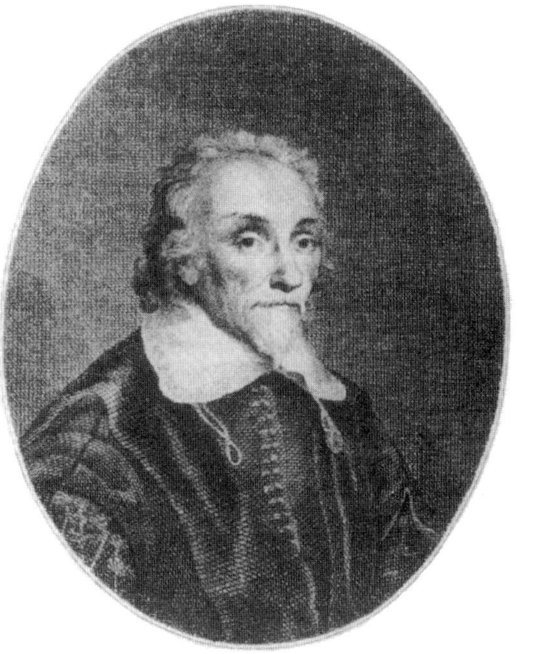

**Figure 3** William Harvey (1578–1657). The discoverer of the circulation of blood and a founder of the science of embryology. Reproduced with kind permission from the Wellcome Institute Library, London

had trained in Alexandria and had worked in Rome. Rufus dissected sheep and described varicose vessels attached to the body of the uterus and running towards the ovaries. This may have been the earliest description of oviducts.

Galen (*c.* AD 130–200) wrote 'The canal of the uterus affords an entrance to the semen and an exit to the fetus. But in this latter case, again, were the eliminative faculty evident, the attractive faculty is not so obvious to most people'.

It was long known that ejaculation of semen into the vagina or at least on to the vulva was necessary for pregnancy to result, but nobody knew for a very long time what element in the semen was needed. In 1674 and again in 1677, Anton van Leeuwenhoek (1632–1723) of Delft, who was a linen draper, described, with a Dutch student Hamen, the microscopic appearances of sperm. van Leeuwenhoek carried on a lively correspondence with Henry Oldenburg (1615–77) who was the first Secretary of The Royal Society of London. In all, 300 letters were exchanged. van Leeuwenhoek must have realized that the spermatozoa which he was seeing down the microscope were very important for fertilization[6].

Some philosophers thought that the baby was preformed and that the early embryo was a miniature version of the adult. William Harvey (1578–1657) (Figure 3) wrote, in his most important book *Exercitationes de Generatione Animalium*[7], that he did not believe the doctrine of 'preformation' of the fetus. His book on reproduction contains much original anatomical material, as well as a chapter on midwifery. His more famous contribution on the circulation of blood was published in Frankfurt, Germany in 1628 and is probably the most important book in the history of medicine.

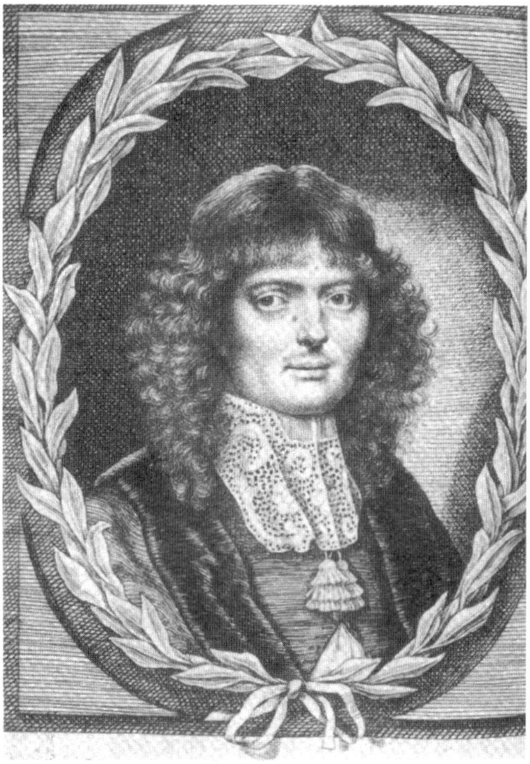

**Figure 4** Regnier de Graaf (1641–1673). Portrait (1966) from the first edition (1668) of his *Virorum Organis Generationi*

Regnier de Graaf (1641–73) (Figure 4) first described in detail and with illustrations what we now call gamete production. de Graaf was born in Holland and, after studying in France and Delft, had his first book published in 1668, entitled *De Virorum Organis Generationi In Serventibus, De Clysteribus Et De Usu Siphonis In Anatomia*[8]. This book gave the first exact and detailed account of the male reproductive system. His second book published in 1672 and entitled *De Mulierum Organis Generationi Inservientibus*[9] described fully the internal female genital organs and had a plate showing a ruptured Fallopian tube containing a fairly advanced pregnancy. de Graaf demonstrated anatomically, pathologically and experimentally. He recognized that gonorrhoea could cause salpingitis and could also damage the prostate gland, of which he was the first to describe the anatomy, together with that of the seminal vesicles, in great detail[8].

The stage had now been reached when scientists knew that semen, and particularly the sperm that it contained, fertilized eggs that were produced in the ovaries. But they were still not certain of the mechanisms by which the spermatozoa reached the eggs nor how the spermatozoa penetrated the eggs, or where in the female body this penetration occurred, but they knew enough to start treating some male infertility by artificial insemination from the husband.

In 1766, John Hunter inseminated a woman with the semen of her husband who had hypospadias. The man ejaculated into a warmed jar and Hunter, using a quill, successfully inseminated the wife with the semen. This was a 'one-off' success. He tried several other times but failed. Because of the attitude towards sex in those days, Hunter did not report his case until 1785 – 20 years after he had carried out the procedure.

John Hunter (1728–93) made many contributions towards knowledge of infertility, including removing one ovary from a sow and showing that, with only one remaining ovary, the sow could reproduce but would do so only over a shorter period of time. He concluded that 'one ovary uses its number in a less time than would probably have been the case if both ovaria had been preserved'. Hunter knew nothing about the date when ovulation occurred in the cycle. He did know enough to be the first man to transplant a testis from one part of an animal's body to another, and note that it carried out some of its functions successfully at the new site.

About 50 years later in 1849, Arnold Adolf Berthold, a physiologist from Göttingen, carried out experiments with testicular transplantation. He discovered that removal with subsequent regrafting of the testicle to another part of the body prevented atrophy of the castrated cock's (capon) comb[10]. He interpreted the results of his transplantations by holding that the testis might influence the male secondary sex characteristics through their action on the blood, and so he was probably the first man to describe hormonal actions.

A great thinker and experimenter, Abbé Lazzaro Spallanzani (1729–99), investigated whether frog sperm had any action. He chose frogs because the eggs are fertilized outside the body, by the male spraying his semen on to eggs released by the female into water. Spallanzani made pairs of tight-fitting taffeta pants for frogs to contain their semen. Frogs that kept their trousers on were unable to fertilize the eggs. He then took semen directly from the male frogs and painted it on to unfertilized eggs, again stimulating fertilization. Finally, he demonstrated that the liquid portion of the semen would not fertilize eggs and that it was the cellular fraction, containing the sperm, that was effective.

Meanwhile, Spallanzani had also shown that, if the fluid caught in the taffeta pants placed on the frogs was mixed with the eggs, the eggs became fertilized. In other words, he carried out artificial insemination from semen caught in a container, namely taffeta waterproof pants. Spallanzani wrote a paper on artificial insemination. So scientists were moving towards the discovery of how spermatozoa function in fertilization[11,12]. But still the true significance of sexual reproduction became really apparent only in the 19th century.

At the beginning of the 19th century, Alfred Donné (1801–78), who had been a lawyer, changed profession and became a doctor of medicine. He was the first to discover *Trichomonas vaginalis* in vaginal secretions and the first to show that these secretions were acid, while the cervical mucus was alkaline. He found spermatozoa on microscopic examination of the cervical mucus of a patient who had been admitted the night before, and later described how sperm could be found sometimes in vaginal fluids. He was the first man to publish an atlas with photomicrographs using a Daguerreotype, an early form of photography. Between 1831 and 1845, he wrote four impressive books on his microscopic findings[13].

Donné was not the only one to realize that spermatozoa were happier in the cervical mucus than in the vaginal fluids. James Marion Sims (1813–83) wrote his wonderful book *Clinical Notes on Uterine Surgery with Special Reference to the Management of the Sterile Condition* which appeared simultaneously in London and New York in 1866. On page 385, Sims wrote 'I can safely say that spermatozoa never live more than 12 hours in the vaginal mucus. But in the mucus of the cervix they live much longer . . . 36–48 hours after coition. We shall ordinarily find as many spermatozoa dead as alive.' Live spermatozoa were found in the cervical mucus 6 days after the flow ceased and 10 days after it began, and Sims concluded 'The proper time for conception (is) about one week more or less after the cessation of the flow.' So, Sims accurately predicted the time of maximum fertility in a cycle. He tried intrauterine insemination but his results were very poor, with only one pregnancy after 27 trials and that one miscarried, 'but all these attempts were made in women with anatomical abnormalities'.

Sims wrote a lecture on 'The microscope as an aid in the diagnosis and treatment for sterility'. He wrote to the New York County Medical Society in 1868 that doctors should look for spermatozoa under the microscope in fluid taken from the cervix and the vagina[14].

In 1913, Max Hühner (1873–1947), who was born in Berlin, Germany, and who was taken as a child to America, wrote a major work *Sterility in the Male and Female and its Treatment*[15]. He described an up-to-date postcoital test and found a few lively sperm in the cervical mucus as long as 5½ days after coitus, but there were no sperm present 8 days after coitus. It was his observations that made it quite clear that the cervix was a much better receptacle for the semen than the posterior fornix of the vagina.

A still better postcoital test was described by Kroeks and Kremer in 1975, and they included in their test migration rates, velocity, direction and duration of movements.

Earlier in the 20th century, Ogino of Japan in 1930[16], and Knaus of Austria in 1933[17] observed a relatively constant relationship between ovulation and succeeding menstruation, and, from this, the calendar method was evolved. They differed in that Ogino thought that the fertile span lasted 8 days in the cycle, while Knaus thought the fertile interval was just 5 days.

Microscopic examination of the changes in the endometrium after curettage was described for the first time by Hitschmann and Adler in 1907 and 1908[18].

What had not been achieved until the 20th century was a proper scientific approach to the investigation and treatment of infertility. Patency of the Fallopian tubes could not be accurately determined until X-rays were used for this diagnostic purpose.

Isidore Clinton Rubin (1883–1958), like Hühner 10 years earlier, was born in Germany but taken to New York when he was an infant. He was an important founder of the modern approach. He injected Collargol solution into a uterus to diagnose whether a fibroid was present in the cavity[19]. This classic paper was published in 1914 at the time that he, and in the same year W. H. Cary, demonstrated patency of the Fallopian tubes using a radio-opaque dye. He injected a 15% solution of Collargol into a patient in the gynaecological service of the Beth Israel Hospital in New York and in other patients in 1914. By 1926, he was able, together with A. J. Benbick, to demonstrate peristalsis of the Fallopian tubes using Lipiodol. Lipiodol had the disadvantage of not being completely absorbable, but Collargol had the disadvantage of causing peritoneal irritation. It was only later that water-soluble radio-opaque dyes and, in particular, iodide dyes were discovered. Rubin also determined the patency of the Fallopian tubes by insufflating them with oxygen. He described the procedure in a classic paper[20]. The first clinical application of this technique had been carried out on November 3rd 1919. In a talk to the American Medical Association in New Orleans, he showed radiologically on film that a pneumoperitoneum had been achieved.

## HORMONAL ACTION

Brown-Sequart (1817–94), born in Mauritius, the son of an American sea captain and a French mother, was one of the first to discover 'the internal secretions' and, in 1890, published an article on the effects of injecting fluid obtained from animal ovaries into women[21]. In the beginning of the 20th century, other authors started to write that the ovaries produced a substance which was essential for the development and maintenance of the genital organs and the mammary glands and that the ovary was an organ of 'internal secretion which induced menstruation and heat in animals'. Soon the search was on to produce an active principle from the ovaries and this was carried out in Europe and in America, with the first indication of an ovarian extract being by Henry Iscovesco (1912) in France[22].

One of the most important advances was made by Edgar Allen and Edward Doisy in 1923. They believed that they had found an ovarian hormone which they extracted[23]. This was only one of many papers written by Allen between 1923 and 1934 on the ovarian hormones.

At the same time in Germany and in Austria, researchers were working on the other ovarian hormone, progesterone.

### The pituitary gland

Vesalius had already in 1543 described the presence of the pituitary gland at the base of the skull. By 1900, extracts were being made from it and were found to have vasopressor effects as well as effects on uterine muscle, particularly immediately after labour. It was only when the pituitary was extirpated experimentally at the beginning of the 20th century that the effects of this mutilation were elucidated. The search was on for pituitary extracts. By the beginning of the 1930s, it was realized that there were two important hormones, namely the follicle stimulating hormone (FSH) and the luteinizing hormone (LH) accurately described by Gemzell and his colleagues in 1958[24]. These pituitary hormones acted on the ovaries.

### The hypothalamus

It had for quite a long time been thought that the hypothalamus contained releasing factors to control the function of the anterior pituitary gland. Harris in Oxford and others worked intensively on hypothalamic function and made the suggestion that the initiation of puberty was caused by maturation of the *nervous system* and not by the pituitary alone.

In 1955, two separate groups, one under Andrew Victor Schally, a Polish scientist working in New Orleans, and the other under Roger Guillemin, a French scientist born in Dijon but working in the Salk Institute, La Jolla, California, raced one another to discover the active hypothalamic substance. In 1971, Schally was able to isolate the FSH- and LH-releasing hormone (GnRH)[25]. He used in all 5 tons of hypothalamic tissue taken from abattoirs before he could work out the chemistry of the hormone, and soon after analogues were synthesized. Both Schally and Guillemin received the Nobel Prize in 1977 for this discovery.

### Extracted hormones

It was a tedious and very expensive process to obtain hormones from the hypothalamic or the pituitary glands. By 1960, Lunenfeld and others were investigating the clinical effects of gonadotrophins obtained from human postmenopausal urine.

In 1961, Greenblatt and others[26] found that clomiphene citrate, which is structurally related to diethylstilboestrol, stimulated ovulation. The story of this discovery is a good demonstration of serendipity. The manufacturers had sent Greenblatt some clomiphene to try out as a contraceptive and he, the acute observer that he was, noted that more of these patients became pregnant than was to be expected from untreated cycles, so the 'contraceptive' was really the first discovered fertility drug. New fertility drugs led to the ability to stimulate ovulation, which is now the basis of much therapy and is used, in particular, to obtain several oocytes at a time in order to carry out *in vitro* fertilization, but the process is by 'down regulation' followed by pituitary hormone stimulation.

## *IN VITRO* FERTILIZATION

In 1968, Patrick Steptoe, a gynaecologist working in Oldham, England, met, at the Royal Society of Medicine, Robert Edwards, an animal physiologist working in Cambridge, England. This meeting started a collaboration between the two which was to result in the birth of the first *in vitro* fertilization baby – Louise Brown on 25th July 1978 in Oldham.

Experimental work had already been carried out on *in vitro* fertilization in small mammals and Edwards had long been working on oocytes in mice, as is recounted in their fascinating book[27].

Already Alan Beatty and M. C. Chang separately had performed some *in vitro* fertilization work. Beatty had taken the fertilized egg from the uterus of one mouse and injected it into the uterus of another mouse, resulting in the delivery of a healthy baby mouse.

Edwards and his wife Ruth Fowler worked on stimulating mouse ovaries to produce eggs for fertilization and, in fact, they managed to induce mice to produce so many eggs at one time that the resulting embryos burst out of their wombs into the peritoneal cavities. Edwards was one of the first people to superovulate mammals and was the first to fertilize a human egg outside the body. This egg had been taken from the ovary of a patient who was undergoing hysterectomy, and it was fertilized by human semen. He was the first to determine the 36-h interval taken by the egg to ripen after the luteinizing hormone surge in the human ovary. In 1965, he first published a paper in the *Lancet* about ripening ova and fertilization, possibly outside the human body. He was the first to foresee that certain inherited human diseases, particularly those that were sex-linked, could be eliminated. Patrick Christopher Steptoe (1913–1988), a consultant gynaecologist working in Oldham, Lancashire, saw Raoul Palmer, the great French gynaecologist, demonstrate his laparoscope techniques and, as a result, Steptoe introduced laparoscopy in England and later in the USA for diagnosis and soon for operative treatment. He was the first in England to practise a form of 'key-hole' surgery.

Edwards and Steptoe had met shortly after Steptoe had shown at the Royal Society of Medicine the first laparoscopic pictures taken in England. At the very beginning of their research, they realized that there would be many difficulties and ethical problems connected with *in vitro* fertilization, but they painstakingly persisted until Louise Brown was born. The women they selected for work on *in vitro* fertilization all had blocked Fallopian tubes and it was in order to bypass this block that this procedure was adopted. When Steptoe and Edwards talked at the Royal College of Obstetricians and Gynaecologists in London about their success at the end of January 1979, they had already had two live babies born, namely Louise Brown and a little boy in Scotland. Other centres followed very quickly so that a child was born in Melbourne, Australia in June 1980 and later one in Norfolk, Virginia, USA in December 1981. By 1982, Rene Frydman had delivered a French baby.

During their experimental work, Steptoe and Edwards found that oocytes were released during a period of 24–27 h after the natural surge of LH was detectable in urine. Before Steptoe died in early 1988, he was able to supervise oocyte recovery using ultrasound instead of the laparoscope and this was a tremendous advance.

It is ironical that in 1995 much of the funding for gynaecological and obstetric research is devoted to developments coming from Steptoe and Edwards' original work. They themselves had the most tremendous difficulty in obtaining funding and were refused twice by the Medical Research Council, yet theirs was the most important of all the pioneering work in *in vitro* fertilization.

## SCIENTISTS TACKLE MALE INFERTILITY

It must be clear by now that most of the work had been carried out to overcome infertility only in women. The old superstitions that an infertile couple was infertile because of the barrenness of the female partner held sway for a very long time, although, as has been seen, male dysfunction had been tackled as early as the time of John Hunter. It was only in the last quarter of the twentieth century that much started to be done for male infertility.

### Gamete donation, freezing and surrogacy

It is true that Hunter had artificially inseminated a woman with her husband's sperm and Spallanzani had inseminated large numbers of female animals with semen taken from the same species. Spallanzani had even suggested that semen might be frozen and later thawed, but until cryopreservation it was not possible to store sperm. The wives of some infertile men are inseminated by freshly donated semen from donors with similar physical characteristics to their husbands. It was much more difficult to donate eggs to women who have normal genitalia but whose stock of oocytes had been used up by menopause which may have occurred at a young age.

In 1949, Christopher Polge and a team in Cambridge first described cryopreservation using glycerol as a sperm preservative agent in animals[28]. This enabled sperm banks to be set up using the semen of prize bulls to inseminate large numbers of cows, many of them from inferior herds. Human sperm banks followed.

Until the late 1990s, no method had been found to freeze human eggs, but embryos produced by *in vitro* fertilization could be frozen and almost every reputable *in vitro* fertilization unit now has facilities for freezing and storing embryos.

Infertile women were resorting to the services of surrogate mothers to produce children for them, sometimes just by acting as an incubator for their own and their husband's embryos in cases where their own uteri were not suitable for carrying pregnancies. Various combinations of gamete and embryo transfers have been worked out, giving rise to ethical problems that have been debated widely.

### Treating male infertility

More and more sophisticated methods of counting spermatozoa and assessing their concentrations and motility developed and much had been done to determine the percentages of normal spermatozoa found in various ejaculates. Even in August 1995, there was a report by Barenbaum and Carmeli from St. Louis, Missouri, showing that there was still discrimination against men in infertility treatment in spite of the fact that there had been very great advances to make it possible for fertilization to take place in most infertile partnerships where the fault lay with the man[29].

It became fairly clear that *in vitro* fertilization could also help when there were only small numbers of spermatozoa and motility was not very good, but where the female partner was 'normal'.

Putting an egg that had been retrieved from the female directly into a medium that contained as many spermatozoa as could be obtained from a man with low fertility overcame the problem of the sperm having to journey up through the cervix, the body of the uterus, and the Fallopian tubes, and indeed some couples with primary male factor infertility were helped by *in vitro* fertilization.

In normal intercourse, the sperm traverse the physical barriers present in the female reproductive tract, but they must also penetrate the cumulus cells and bind to specific receptors on the surface of the zona pellucida. They must then penetrate the zona by acrosome-mediated enzymatic digestion accompanied by vigorous tail movement, and finally the sperm plasma membrane must fuse with the oocyte membrane to begin the process of fertilization[30].

Cohen and his colleagues developed techniques to carry out subzonal insertion of spermatozoa into the perivitelline space surrounding the oocyte (SUZI)[31]. In this technique, the authors used mechanical force. The cumulus and corona of oocytes were removed and the cytoplasm was shrunk to 50–75% of its usual volume. The oocytes were then held by suction and the spermatozoa pushed underneath the zona.

The next step was to carry out partial zone section (PZD) for introducing spermatozoa. This was carried out by the Reproductive Pathology Association and the Department of Gynaecology and Obstetrics in the Emory Unit, Atlanta, Georgia[32].

The real breakthrough came with the development in 1992 of techniques leading to pregnancies after intracytoplasmic injection of a single spermatozoan into an oocyte (ICSI). Work was carried out in van Steirteghem's laboratory at the Centre for Reproductive Medicine in Brussels, Belgium. Using his technique, the sperm were obtained from semen samples 1 day before oocyte recovery and also on the day of oocyte retrieval. They held the oocyte by gentle suction against the end of a pipette and introduced the spermatozoan directly into the cytoplasm of the oocyte using a finer, sharper pipette[32]. It was soon clear that, even in men with badly blocked vasa, spermatozoa could be obtained either from the epididymis or even from the testis itself. This tremendous advance has, as a result, meant that very few infertile men need to be denied the boon of having a child. It is true that there was a price to pay in that there was a definite increase to nearly 3% in the number of abnormal babies born, but this figure will probably be decreased before very long. In 1992, van Steirteghem's team was able to report that they had obtained six pregnancies from treating 47 metaphase II oocytes, with the delivery of four singletons and one twin birth. One patient aborted. All the consorts had very low semen counts. ICSI is now used in many laboratories throughout the world.

We have come a long, long way.

## REFERENCES


1. Speert, H. (1993). *Iconographia Gyniatrica*, p. 409 (Philadelphia: F. A. Davis)
2. Cotterell, A. (1989). *The Illustrated Encyclopaedia of Myths and Legends*, p. 205. (London: Castle Publishers Ltd)
3. Great Books of the Western World (1952). Hippocratic writings, Volume 10, p. 139. (Chicago: Encyclopedia Britannica Inc., William Benton)
4. Great Books of the Western World (1952). Vol. 9, Aristotle II, Book I, Chapter 3, p. 10 and Book 7, Chapter 6, p. 110. *History of Animals*. (Berlin No 489A)

5. Soranus. *Gynecology*, Book 1, p. 34, translated by Temkin, O. (SWEI) 1956. (Autumn John Hopkins Press)
6. van Leeuwenhoek, A. (1678). De natis e semine genitali animalicules. *Phil. Trans. R. Soc. London*, **12**, 1040
7. Harvey, W. (1651). *Exercitationes de Generatione Animalium*. (London: O. Pulleyn)
8. De Graaf, R. (1668). *De Virorum Organis Generationi Inserventibus, De Clysteribus Et De Usu Siphonis In Anatomis*. Lugd. Batan et Roterod. *ex off.* Hackiana
9. De Graaf, R. (1672). *De Mulierum Organis Generationi Inservientibus*. Lugd. Batan et Roterod. *ex off.* Hackiana
10. Berthold, A. (1849). Transplantation der Hoden. *Arch. Anat. Physiol. Wissen. Med.*, 42–46. The transplantation of testis. Translation by Quiring, D. P. (1944). *Bull. Hist. Med.*, **16**, 399–401
11. Weatherall, D. (1995). *Science and the Quiet Art*, p. 230. (Oxford: Oxford University Press)
12. Medvei, V. C. (1993). *The History of Clinico-Endocrinology*, 2nd edn., pp. 100–4. (Carnforth, UK: Parthenon)
13. Donné, A. (1845). *Atlas Executé d'apres Nature au Microscope-Daguerreotype*. (Paris: Baillière)
14. Sims, J. M. (1866). *Clinical Notes on Uterine Surgery with Special Reference to the Management of the Sterile Condition*, p. 385. (London: Hardwicke Publishers)
15. Hühner, M. (1913). *Sterility in the Male and Female and its Treatment*. (New York: Rebman)
16. Ogino, K. (1930). Ovulations termin und Konzeptionstermin. *Zentbl. Gynakol.*, **54**, 464–79
17. Knaus, H. (1933). Die periodische Frucht und Unfruchbarkeit des Weibes. *Zentralbl. Gynakol.* **57**, 1393
18. Hitschmann, F. and Adler, L. (1907). Die lehre von der Endometritis. *Z. Geburt. Gynaekol.*, **60**, 63–86
19. Rubin, I. C. (1914). *Zentralbl. Gynakol.*, **18**
20. Rubin, I. C. (1920). Non-operative determination of patency of fallopian tubes in sterility: intrauterine inflation with oxygen and production of a sub-phrenic pneumoperitoneum. Preliminary Report. *J. Am. Med. Assoc.*, **74** (15), 1017
21. Brown-Sequard, C. E. (1890). Remarques sur les effets produits sur la femme par des injections sous-cutanées d'un liquide retire d'ovaires d'animaux. *Arch. Physiol. Norm. Pathol.*, **2**, 456–7
22. Iscovesco, H. (1912). Les lipoides de l'ovaire. *C. R. Soc., Biol. Paris*, **63**, 16–18, 104–6
23. Allen, E. and Doisy, E. A. (1923). An ovarian hormone: preliminary report on its localization, extraction and partial purification, and action in test animals. *J. Am. Med. Assoc.*, **81**, 819–21
24. Gemzell, C. A., Diczfalusy, E. and Tillinger, K. G. (1958). Clinical effect of human pituitary follicle stimulating hormone. *J. Clin. Endocrinol.*, **29**, 1333
25. Schally, A. V., Arimura, A., Baba, Y., Nair, R. M. G., Matsuo, A., Redding, T. W., Debeljuk, L. and White, W. P. (1971). Isolation and properties of the FSH and LH releasing hormone. *Biochem. Biophys. Res. Commun.*, **43**, 393–9
26. Greenblatt, R. E., Barfield, W. E. and Jung, C. K. (1961). Induction of ovulation with MRL-41: preliminary report. *J. Am. Med. Assoc.*, **178**, 101
27. Edwards, R. and Steptoe, P. (1980). *A Matter of Life*. (London: Hutchison)
28. Polge, C., Smith, A. V. and Parkes, A. S. (1949). Survival of spermatozoa after vitrification and dehydration at low temperature. *Nature (London)*, **164**, 666
29. Barenbaum, D., Carmeli, Y. S. and Caspar, R. F. (1995). Discrimination against men in infertility treatment. *J. Reprod. Med.*, **40**, 595–8
30. Talansky, B. E., Malter, A. V., Adler, A., Alikani, M., Bercley, A., Davis, O., Graf, M., Reing, A., Rosenwaks, Z. and Cohen, J. (1990). In Matson, P. L. and Lieberman, B. A. (eds.) *Limitations of Zona Pellucida Micromanipulation in the Human Clinical IVF Forum*. (Manchester, UK: Manchester University Press)
31. Cohen, J., Malter, H., Fehil, T. Y. C., Wright, G., Elsner, C., Kort, H. and Massey, J. (1988). Implantation of embryos after partial opening of oocyte zone pellucida to facilitate sperm penetration (PZD). *Lancet*, **2**, 162
32. Palermo, G., Joris, H., Devroey, P. and van Steirteghem, A. C. (1992). Pregnancies after intra-cytoplasmic injection of single spermatozoon into an oocyte. *Lancet*, 340, 17–19

# Reproductive medicine: basic concepts

# 2

*David A. Viniker*

## INTRODUCTION

The objective of this chapter is to briefly outline the fundamentals of reproductive medicine. Reproduction, with the perpetuation of the species, is the fundamental biological function. Basic physiological concepts are addressed and an overview of hormonal therapy is presented. Finally, the interface between patient and clinician is discussed.

When obstetrics and gynaecology became a speciality in its own right in the 1920s, it was essentially surgical. There was a noticeable change in philosophy with regard to training for the aspiring gynaecologist only 25–30 years ago. Until then, a general surgical training was considered advantageous if not essential. The advent of refined techniques, including hormone assay, ultrasound, embryology and hormone therapy have changed the face of the speciality so that the balance of therapy has shifted increasingly in a medical direction[1].

It is no longer feasible for the busy clinician, with a reproductive endocrinological interest, to personally undertake every aspect of care. The specialist nurse (Chapter 17) can be trained to undertake many tasks including day-to-day monitoring of agreed treatment protocols, postcoital tests, intrauterine inseminations and introduction of hormone implants. As the specialist nurse spends more time with the patient than the clinician, she is ideally placed to assist in patient counselling, particularly in relation to treatment protocols. Radiologists (Chapter 6), embryologists (Chapters 13 and 14) and trained counsellors (Chapter 16) each have an essential input. Clinicians should welcome the arrival of these skilled professionals into the team, ensuring that their patients reap the full rewards of modern investigation and treatment. Prescribing hormones is only part of therapy in reproductive medicine. Perhaps more than any other discipline, it involves patient involvement and choice.

## PHYSIOLOGICAL CONCEPTS

### Hormones

A hormone is a substance produced in a special tissue, usually within an endocrine gland, which is released into the bloodstream where it travels to distant responsive cells where the hormone exhibits characteristic effects. Hormones are extremely potent, for, although they are released in tiny amounts, their effects are profound. Oestradiol implants which are introduced under the skin, usually when the ovaries are no longer functional (Chapter 28), are smaller than an airgun pellet and most of the implant is the substance used to release the hormone. A typical oestradiol implant contains only one twentieth of a gram of oestradiol. This may be adequate for a year, to maintain generalized well-being, relieve menopausal symptoms, and significantly reduce the incidence and complications of the menopause including cardiac disease and osteoporosis. Hormones act by attaching to receptor sites on the cells of their target tissues (Figure 1) and this triggers a response.

### Neuroendocrinology

The fundamental concept of endocrinology is that endocrine tissues secrete hormones into the bloodstream which regulate the function of cells in selected target organs. The fundamental

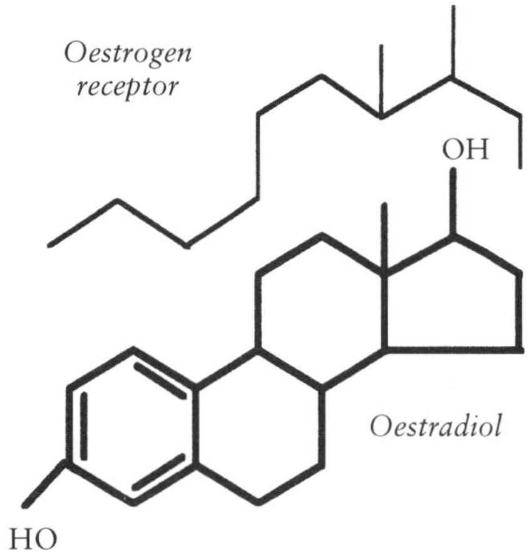


**Figure 1** Oestrogen receptor, schematic example

concept of neuroscience is that the nervous system functions by the discrete interactions of its individual components, the neurons or nerve cells. Neurons transmit information rapidly along their often considerable length and communicate with other target neurons, glandular cells or muscle cells by secreting chemical neurotransmitters.

In the early 1950s, the posterior pituitary was found to consist of the axons of hypothalamic neurons which released their hormones directly into the circulation. The nervous and endocrine systems were found to be even more closely interrelated with the recognition of a portal system carrying hormones secreted from the hypothalamus to the anterior pituitary. The chemical structures of neurotransmitters within the nervous system are remarkably similar to hormones regulating the activity of the endocrine system. Hormones secreted by the endocrine system feed back to the nervous system to complete the cycle. By the late 1950s it was recognized that the nervous system and endocrine system were so interdependent that they should be studied as one science, known as neuroendocrinology.

The response of the central nervous system to blood-borne steroid hormones allows for a co-ordinated feedback regulation to control hypothalamic physiotropic releasing and inhibiting factors. Methodology is rapidly evolving for the detection of steroid responsive elements (receptor sites) in the brain[2]. Isolation and purification of hormone receptors in peripheral tissues are now relatively refined[3]. Steroid binding to neurons is similar to that of other tissues. Initially, the steroid molecule binds with discrete soluble receptor proteins which are normally sited at the plasma membrane. After binding, the hormone receptor complex moves to the nucleus where regulation of cell function is modified[4].

The oestrogen receptor sites in the brain show remarkable similarity between species, with concentrations in the anterior hypothalamic and preoptic areas. The distribution of cerebral testosterone binding sites is similar, although at the cellular level there are differences.

## The menstrual cycle

As with any medical discipline, it is essential for the clinician supervising the treatment of patients with reproductive medical problems to have an understanding of the relevant physiology. From the menarche to the menopause, the endometrium is continually changing its histological structure under the influence of the sex steroids (oestrogens and progesterone) with menstruation marking just one of these cyclical changes. The menstrual cycle is interrupted by pregnancy when decidualization occurs. The menstrual cycle is controlled by hypothalamic, pituitary and ovarian hormones (Figure 2).

## Hypothalamus

The hypothalamus provides the link between the brain and the pituitary gland by producing releasing and inhibiting factors which control the pituitary's secretion of hormones into the peripheral circulation. In all, there are five releasing hormones including gonadotrophin releasing hormone (GnRH) which is a decapeptide. Thyrotrophin releasing hormone has only three peptides, whereas the largest, growth hormone releasing factor, has 44 peptides. Reproductive dysfunction can occur with functional abnormalities of any of these releasing factors

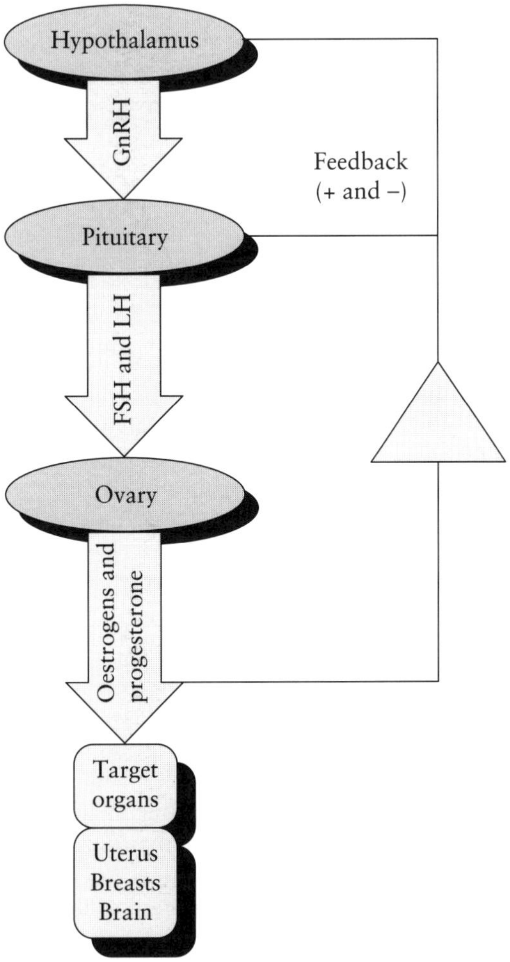


**Figure 2** The hypothalamic–pituitary–ovarian axis. GnRH = gonadotrophin releasing hormone; FSH = follicle stimulating hormone; LH = luteinizing hormone

which may be associated with syndromes including Cushing's and acromegaly.

## Pituitary

The anterior pituitary is responsible for producing the two gonadotrophic hormones, luteinizing hormone (LH) and follicle stimulating hormone (FSH). These have similar structures, with two glycosylated polypeptide (α and β) subunits. The α subunits of LH, FSH, thyroid stimulating hormone (TSH) and human chorionic gonadotrophin (hCG, which is produced by trophoblast cells during pregnancy) are identical[5]. Ovarian control of pituitary function is principally through a negative feedback by oestradiol but there is at least one additional non-steroidal regulator called inhibin.

The presence of prolactin, the hormone which promotes lactation, has been assumed for many years and was characterized early in many species. Human prolactin was not characterized until 1970 as it was overshadowed by human growth factor which has lactogenic activity and is present in greater quantity[6]. Bioassays, used to determine hormone concentrations by observing the response of target cells, have been largely superseded by radioimmunoassay (RIA). The concentrations of LH, FSH and prolactin are measured by specific radioimmunoassays using antisera raised against the purified hormones.

## Ovaries

The first primordial follicles, consisting of a primary oocyte together with pregranulosa cells, start to appear in the fetus at 16 weeks. It is believed that primordial follicle formation is concluded 6 months postpartum[7] (Figure 3). Factors determining the quantity of oocytes formed in the ovaries and their recruitment are unknown, although oocyte quality is believed to affect the rate of atresia[8]. An exact explanation for the emergence of a single dominant follicle from the pool of developing follicles has yet to be established[9].

There are three phases of follicular development[10]. During the preantral growth phase, primordial follicles mature to secondary follicles. In the tonic (periantral) growth phase, class 1 follicles mature to class 4 follicles and there is a 600-fold increase in the granulosa cell complement. The preantral and periantral growth phases take place during the three cycles before ovulation. It is in the late luteal phase of the third cycle that follicles reach class 5 and in 5-day steps they pass through classes 6 to 8, the exponential growth phase. It is during this phase that selection of a dominant follicle is achieved. Eighty-five days are taken for a class

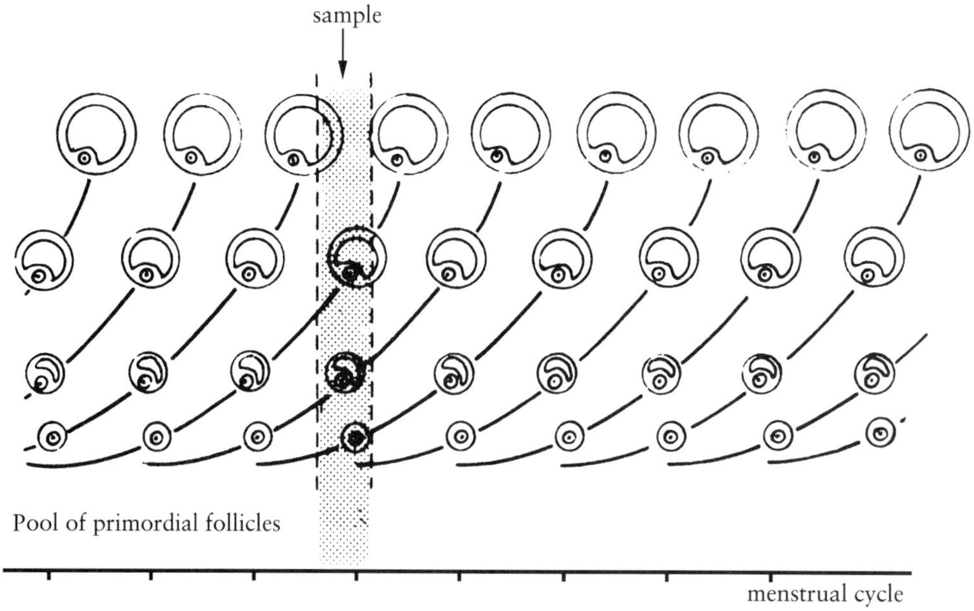


**Figure 3** Growth of ovarian follicles in a non-synchronous pattern. Reproduced from Gougeon, A. (1996). Dynamics of follicular growth in the human: a model from preliminary results. *Hum. Reprod.*, **1**, 81–7, by permission of Oxford University Press

1 follicle to become a mature follicle ready for ovulation (Figure 3).

Between ten and 30 primordial follicles (about 600 each month), which have been in a dormant state, become active each day. The vast majority of these follicles will die (atresia) at some stage of development. Only a small minority of follicles reach class 5 development at the critical time when there is a rise of FSH around the time of menstruation. A rise in FSH is associated with the reduced negative feedback of oestradiol in association with the demise of the corpus luteum in the preceding cycle. It seems unlikely that all primordial follicles are capable of full development. We know from routine *in vitro* fertilization (IVF) that on average only about ten follicles are recruited during several days of superovulation gonadotrophin therapy (see Chapter 10).

The two-cell theory is generally accepted as the rationale for follicular development. Luteinizing hormone acts on the theca cells which generate androgen production whilst FSH is responsible for growth of the follicle. Follicle-stimulating hormone receptors are only found on granulosa cells where the FSH is responsible for the aromatase enzyme that converts androgens to oestradiol (Figure 4). Luteinizing hormone receptors, which are not present in the early follicle, develop as the follicle enlarges and LH can then drive the granulosa cells further. As the follicle grows, oestradiol levels rise and this seems to trigger a surge of GnRH from the hypothalamus, which in turn produces the preovulatory surge of LH resulting in ovulation (Figure 5).

Our understanding of physiological principles develops in parallel with technology. The latest technological innovation in reproductive endocrinology has been the production of recombinant FSH (Chapter 29). Patients with hypogonadotrophic hypogonadism, when given recombinant FSH, produce follicles and mature ova capable of fertilization and pregnancy although oestradiol levels remain low. This means that oestradiol does not appear to have a direct action on the developing ovum[9]. Oestradiol is required in natural cycles, to inform the hypothalamus that there is a maturing follicle; this seems to promote the surge of

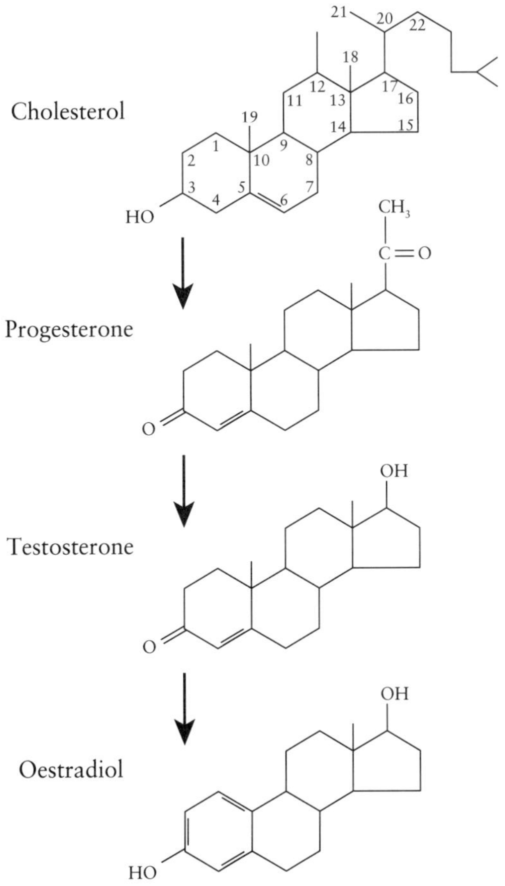


**Figure 4** Steroid structures, a simplified representation of the metabolic pathways

GnRH before ovulation. Oestradiol sensitizes the gonadotropes in the pituitary to GnRH in preparation for the GnRH increase. This facilitates a response to the preovulatory surge of LH essential for ovulation. Oestradiol is required to promote endometrial proliferation before ovulation and to encourage progesterone receptors in the late proliferative endometrium. Progesterone can act on the primed endometrium to allow implantation and create the environment required to nurture the early embryo.

When pregnancy has not occurred, the corpus luteum dies (luteolysis). Whereas in some species the mechanism for luteolysis is known (e.g. prolactin is responsible in the rat), the mechanism for luteolysis in the human remains to be determined[9]. Luteinizing hormone is essential in the maintenance of the corpus luteum up to the point of luteolysis. Pulses of GnRH, which in turn result in LH pulses, continue around the time of luteolysis but only hCG can prevent luteolysis.

By day 6 of the cycle, a dominant follicle is generally distinguishable. It has increased vascularization which results in preferential gonadotrophin support[11]. The dominant follicle produces rising levels of oestradiol which initially inhibits FSH production to levels that are insufficient to maintain other follicles. Studies in monkeys, who were given oestradiol antibodies, have demonstrated that negative feedback of oestradiol can be overridden. When FSH is not suppressed, more than one dominant follicle can be recruited[12]. In IVF programmes, gonadotrophin administration is employed to recruit several follicles. Inhibin, activin and follistatin are polypeptides produced by the ovary and are also thought to play a part in dominant follicle selection in natural cycles[13,14].

### Steroid hormones

Steroids are a subgroup of lipids, which share a structure that is characterized by four fused rings (perhydrocyclopentanophenanthrene, Figure 4). The rings are formed by polymerization of isoprene units which have five carbon atoms:

$$\begin{array}{c} \quad CH_3 \\ \quad | \\ H_2C = C - CH = CH_2 \end{array}$$

Cholesterol (chole, bile and stereos, solid) was the first of this group to be purified and gave us the group name 'steroids'. Details of the chemical pathways from cholesterol, through pregnenolone, progesterone, the androgens including androstenedione and testosterone, to the oestrogens have been presented by O'Malley and Stroit[15].

Sex hormone-binding globulin (SHBG) is a glycoprotein synthesized in the liver. The binding affinity of SHBG for testosterone is 30 000

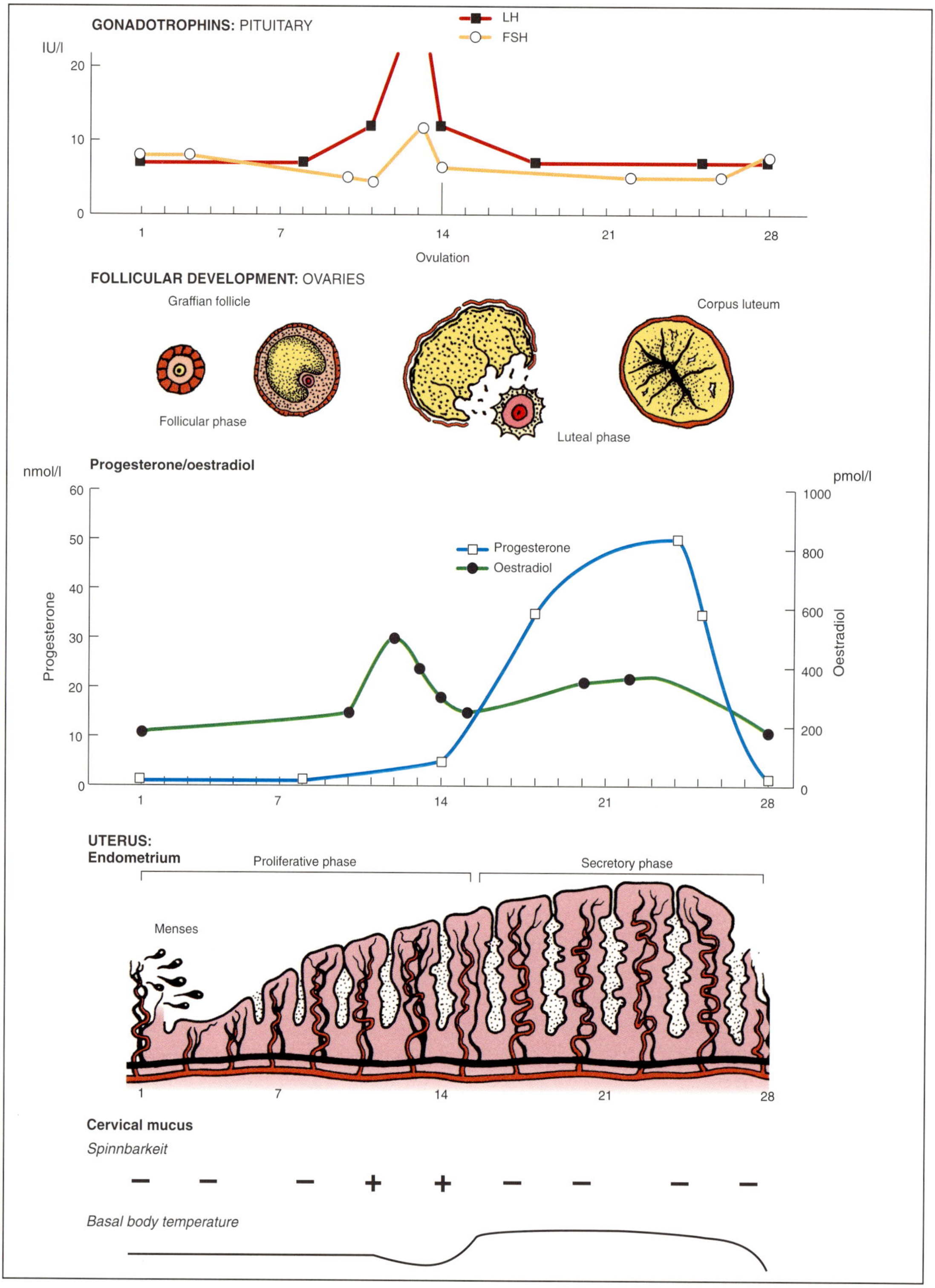


**Figure 5** Changes occurring during the menstrual cycle in the pituitary hormones, ovarian steroid levels and the uterus

times greater than albumin. The oestradiol affinity of SHBG is only about 30% when compared to testosterone. Women in their reproductive years have double the concentration of SHBG compared to men as oestrogens tend to encourage SHBG production whereas androgens are inhibitory. Women with hirsutism associated with hyperandrogenism have relatively low SHBG levels which result in increased levels of free androgens.

### Biorhythms and physiological clocks in reproductive medicine

A hypothalamic pacemaker, the suprachiasmatic nucleus[16], is mainly responsible for controlling a variety of biological rhythms influencing physiological activity. Releasing hormones are discharged episodically in pulses from the hypothalamus into the portal system, to the pituitary gland. External stimuli including darkness and light (circadian rhythm) and the sleep–wake cycles[17] may modulate releasing hormone pulse frequency. Sleep cycles are present in the fetus from about 30 weeks gestation[18]. Abnormalities of these biorhythms may be responsible for some types of reproductive dysfunction.

There remain many questions in reproductive physiology that are as yet unanswered. Perhaps the most intriguing of these questions relates to the timing of individual ovum maturation. It has been estimated that there are approximately 300 000 primordial follicles in a girl at the time of puberty. If these were to go into an active phase of maturation evenly throughout her reproductive years, there would be about 20 ova becoming active daily. The rate is probably higher in the earlier years and lower later on during planned conception cycles. Although the exact mechanism remains to be established, it would seem that, from a functional point of view, each primordial follicle behaves as if it were stamped with a date and perhaps even a time for it to start its maturation process – an egg timer hypothesis (Chapter 30).

There is some evidence that there is an oocyte maturation inhibitor, although its chemistry remains unknown[19]. Ovulation induction regimens are not triggering the follicular maturation process. They are providing a more sustained optimum hormonal balance so that those primordial follicles that have already commenced their intrinsic programmed maturation, and have reached class 5 around that time, are more likely to progress (recruitment). We know that if gonadotrophin therapy is given to a woman during her reproductive years in one month for the purposes of superovulation, a number of active follicles develop. If pregnancy does not ensue, then the treatment can be repeated a few weeks later and a different group of follicles develops. We can only deduce that this second group of primordial follicles was time-tabled to commence final maturation at this time and not before.

The working hypothesis that each primordial follicle is programmed to start maturation on a particular day may explain one or two other clinical entities. In the resistant ovary syndrome, it would seem likely that no primordial follicles are programmed to start maturation during the episode of amenorrhoea. As there are no active follicles, oestrogen levels are low and FSH is high. However, periods can resume and occasionally spontaneous pregnancy can occur[20] when an ovum starts to mature at its programmed time.

Many women presenting with apparently postmenopausal bleeding in their late forties or early fifties are often convinced that the bleed was typical of a period, with associated features such as 'premenstrual' mastalgia and tension. This could be explained if we accept that there was probably a primordial follicle scheduled to mature at this time; investigation of the bleeding must, nevertheless, be undertaken.

If primordial follicles are 'stamped' for a date to start maturation, are they also timed (Chapter 30)? Perhaps the essential hormonal balance required to ensure follicular maturation is limited to a narrow window of just a few hours? This would have implications for ovulation stimulation regimens.

A more detailed presentation of the endocrine changes controlling the menstrual cycle is outside the scope of this book. For the reader who would like to explore this subject in greater depth, the author would particularly recommend three texts (Yen and Jaffe[21]; Ferin, Jewelewicz and Warren[22]; Adashi, Rock and Rosenwaks[23]). The physiology of puberty is discussed in Chapter 3 and that of the menopause in Chapter 28.

## PHARMACOLOGY IN REPRODUCTIVE MEDICINE

### Introduction

Before considering drug therapy in reproductive medicine, an appreciation of the physiology of the hypothalamic–pituitary–ovarian axis, as previously briefly outlined, is essential. Biological mechanisms operate to maintain balance within cells, tissues, organs, individuals, species and beyond. Over the last three or four decades, there has been a remarkable explosion in the depth of knowledge about the physiological mechanisms in reproductive physiology. Pharmacologists have been able to develop drugs of incredible power, allowing the clinician to regularly prescribe treatments that were unimaginable even at the conclusion of the Second World War.

Cortisol, progesterone, testosterone (and other androgens) and oestradiol (and other oestrogens) are on a common metabolic pathway (Figure 4). Androgens and oestrogens are present in men and women although androgens predominate in the male whereas oestrogens predominate in the female. Abnormalities in the balance of hormones that may respond to reproductive hormone treatment include:

(1) Precocious or delayed puberty (Chapter 3);

(2) Amenorrhoea (Chapter 4);

(3) Hirsutism (Chapter 5);

(4) Anovulatory infertility (Chapters 7 and 8); and

(5) Premenstrual syndrome (Chapter 29).

Furthermore, we are able to prescribe hormonal therapy to prevent undesirable pregnancy (Chapter 22) and replace ovarian hormones beyond the menopause to alleviate symptoms and reduce long-term morbidity and mortality (Chapter 28).

The fundamental considerations of prescribing in reproductive medicine are presented in Figure 6. Hormonal therapy essentially uses drugs that are:

(1) Hormones found in nature and purified, e.g. human menopausal gonadotrophins, conjugated equine oestrogens and 'natural progesterone';

(2) Synthetic hormone replicas, e.g. recombinant FSH;

(3) Synthetic agents that are similar to natural hormones, e.g. dydrogesterone, medroxyprogesterone acetate and GnRH agonists; and

(4) Agents that activate receptors, as part of their structure resembles that of a natural hormone, e.g. clomiphene citrate.

Most drugs in general, and certainly hormones in particular, work by their action on receptor sites. Progesterone is a precursor of glucocorticoids and mineralocorticoids. There is great similarity in the molecular structure of the sex steroids, the mineralocorticoids and the glucocorticoids. Hormones, prescribed in

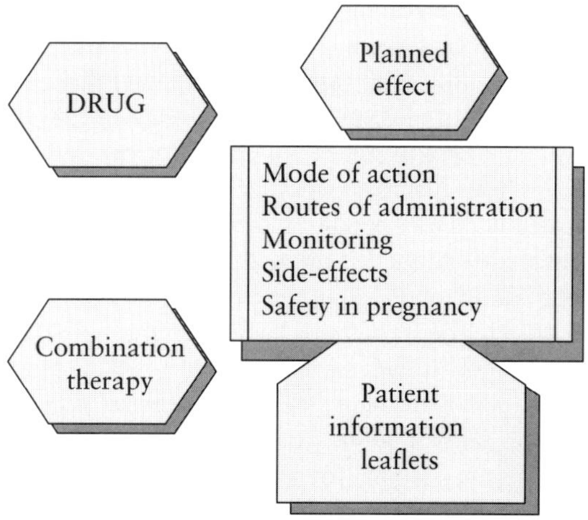


**Figure 6** Fundamentals of prescribing in reproductive medicine

anticipation of their action on one set of receptors, may also activate other receptors leading to side-effects. Thus progestogens, for example, and particularly norethisterone, may have androgenic side-effects and fluid retention may be a feature of several agents. Hormones acting on receptor sites may activate enzyme activity. FSH, for example, does not stimulate hormone production in the ovary but activates enzymes that allow conversion of androgens to oestradiol.

The action of one hormone treatment may be altered by others. A course of progestogen will not result in a withdrawal bleed in a patient with amenorrhoea and low oestrogen levels (hypogonadotrophic hypogonadism, Chapter 4, or hypergonadotrophic hypogonadism, see Chapter 28) but the same patient would have a positive result if primed with oestrogen.

A drug may act by blocking a receptor. Clomiphene, for example, is thought to act mainly by blocking the oestrogen feedback mechanism (Chapter 8). Gonadotrophin releasing hormone agonists may initially have a positive action (flare response) resulting in increased gonadotrophin output from the pituitary. Then they block the receptor sites resulting in suppression of gonadotrophin levels (down-regulation); this action is utilized in some infertility regimens and in particular in IVF (Chapter 10).

Some drugs have significant action on different receptor sites and these combined actions can be utilized therapeutically. Tibolone activates both oestrogen and progestogen receptor sites so that it has a place in oestrogen replacement therapy whilst protecting the endometrium (see Chapter 28); it may possibly have some beneficial androgenic action. Tamoxifen has anti-oestrogenic activity, which is of benefit in breast cancer therapy and also for infertility (see Chapter 8). It has oestrogenic effects too, so that it may relieve some menopausal symptoms but may also cause hyperplasia or even malignancy of the endometrium (see Chapter 28).

Frequently, combinations of hormones are prescribed, the most obvious examples being the combined oestrogen/progestogen oral contraceptive pills (Chapter 22) and hormone replacement therapy when the patient has not had hysterectomy (Chapter 28). The combination of GnRH down-regulation, gonadotrophin therapy, hCG and hormone support after embryo transfer (Chapter 17, Figure 1) is probably the most complex of regimens currently employed in reproductive medicine.

The pharmacological principles of drug action with particular reference to reproductive medicine have been described by James[24]. It is self-evident that when prescribing therapy for a woman during her reproductive years, great care should be taken to avoid drugs that could have an adverse effect in a possible pregnancy.

## Routes of administration

### *Oral administration*

Tablets and capsules administered orally are designed to break down, permitting absorption of the drug in the proximal third of the small bowel. There have been major pharmaceutical developments and refinements over the last 20 years. Blood from the small bowel enters the portal system and a major proportion of an orally administered drug may be metabolized by the liver on its 'first pass'. It is for this reason that other routes of administration may be chosen.

Gastric emptying varies between individuals and this may explain some differences in drug response. Absorption of hormones may be reduced by chronic bowel absorption problems or an acute gastrointestinal illness. This may lead to unwanted pregnancy in patients taking oral contraceptives, or irregular bleeding in women taking oral contraceptive pills or hormone replacement therapy.

### *Vaginal or rectal routes*

Rectal or vaginal progesterone is frequently prescribed for patients with premenstrual syndrome (PMS) and also in infertility treatment protocols. The majority of units performing IVF strongly believe in hormonal support after embryo transfer (Chapter 10) and progesterone administered rectally or vaginally is a common route of administration. There is evidence confirming efficacy of hormonal support of the luteal phase and early pregnancy in IVF[25]. Interestingly, there is little scientific evidence to suggest that such treatment is beneficial for patients with recurrent early pregnancy loss (Chapter 21).

Some drugs, notably bromocriptine and carbegoline may cause nausea, probably by direct action on the gastric and intestinal mucosa. The vagina may then prove to be a useful alternative route of administration (Chapter 4).

*Intramuscular and subcutaneous administration*
Lipid solubility is less of a problem with drugs administered by these routes and absorption is more predictable. Patients can be taught to self inject or, in infertility, the partner may feel more involved if he learns to give the injections. A depot preparation of medroxyprogesterone acetate provides a reliable method of contraception (Chapter 22).

Subcutaneous hormone implants of oestrogen and testosterone are frequently used in hormone replacement therapy (Chapter 28). GnRH analogues can also be given, usually once each month to suppress endogenous gonadotrophin and oestrogen production for endometriosis and also for patients with fibroids before surgery (Chapters 23, 24, 26 and Figure 7).

*Transdermal route*
The transdermal route is favoured by some patients having hormone replacement therapy. There are a variety of oestradiol patches and one is combined with a progestogen patch (Chapter 28). Progesterone and oestrogen gels are available in some countries.

*Nasal route*
Gonadotrophin-releasing hormone agonists, including buserelin and nafarelin, are frequently administered by nasal spray in the treatment of endometriosis (Chapter 23), preoperative preparation for fibroids (Chapters 24 and 25), preparation of the endometrium before endometrial ablation (Chapter 25) and in infertility regimens (Chapters 8 and 10).

*Intrauterine route*
The levonorgestrel intrauterine system (Mirena®, Pharmacia-Leiras) is a special intrauterine contraceptive device which releases the equivalent of two progesterone-only pills per week. It is currently licensed for contraception only (Chapter 22) but it has been shown to have a role in the management of dysfunctional uterine bleeding (Chapter 26).

In premenopausal women, it provides not only contraception but also protection with oestrogen replacement therapy (Chapter 28). It may prove to have a role in the management of premenstrual syndrome, allowing oestrogen therapy without cyclical progestogen administration (Chapter 27).

A variety of further applications have been or could be suggested. For example, whilst it is generally accepted that GnRH agonists or continuous progestogen therapy have a direct action on endometriotic tissue, it is also possible that, by reducing endometrial proliferation and therefore retrograde menstruation, there is a potential reduction of new endometriotic lesions. It may therefore be that the levonorgestrel intrauterine device might find a place in the management of endometriosis.

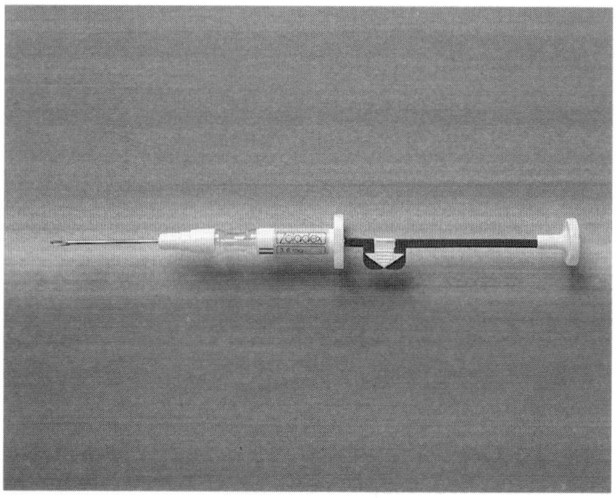

**Figure 7** Goserelin, a GnRH agonist, comes preloaded in a sterile syringe. After local anaesthesia, the plastic guard is removed and the implant is injected subcutaneously

### Oestrogens

Oestradiol is the predominant oestrogen produced by the ovary although oestrone also plays a significant role. The characteristic action of oestrogens is their relationship to sexual heat or oestrus in lower animals. In women, libido is more complex, with emotion having a more significant role than hormones. Androgens play a major part in male libido but are less important in females. Oestrogens are a major component in the development of secondary sexual characteristics including body shape and skin texture. They are instrumental in the development of the secondary sex organs: breasts, uterus and Fallopian tubes, vulva and vagina.

An interesting variation of hormone action is the effect of oestrogens which increase SHBG levels and therefore reduce the free androgen levels. This is of benefit to some women presenting with hirsutism.

### Progesterone and progestogens

Progesterone is produced by the corpus luteum and placenta and is essential in the maintenance of pregnancy. It has an action on the secondary sex organs but only if they are primed by oestrogens.

Progestogen therapy is employed in menstrual cycle regulation, i.e. amenorrhoea (Chapter 4), infertility (Chapter 8), contraception (Chapter 22), menorrhagia (Chapter 26), premenstrual syndrome (Chapter 27) and hormone replacement therapy (Chapter 28).

### Gonadotrophin releasing hormone analogues and gonadotrophins

Gonadotrophin releasing hormone is released by the hypothalamus and controls release of the gonadotrophic hormones FSH and LH. Analogues of GnRH may initially have a stimulatory or flare response which is followed by inhibitory action. This down-regulation is used in IVF protocols (Chapter 10) so that circulating gonadotrophins are exogenous and there is no physiological LH surge to cause unplanned ovulation. Suppression of gonadotrophins and therefore oestrogen is beneficial in preoperative preparation for fibroids (Chapters 24 and 25) and also in endometriosis (Chapter 23). Gonadotrophins are used in infertility regimens (Chapters 8 and 10).

### Anti-hormones

An anti-hormone prevents the action of a hormone on a receptor site. Anti-hormones have an increasing role in therapy. Clomiphene and tamoxifen are anti-oestrogens used in infertility and tamoxifen is widely used in breast cancer treatment. Cyproterone is an anti-androgen competing with androgens at the receptor sites. Spironolactone is an aldosterone antagonist that has anti-androgenic activity. Mifepristone is a synthetic steroid which is an anti-progesterone agent. It is licensed in the UK as an abortifactant up to 63 days gestation in combination with a prostaglandin analogue. Gonadotrophin releasing hormone analogues initially have a stimulatory action on the pituitary but then have an anti-GnRH effect and block gonadotrophin output. When administered in intermittent bolus by a pump, GnRH agonists are effective at inducing ovulation (Chapter 8). A new generation of GnRH antagonists, which have only anti-GnRH activity and no initial flare response, is under evaluation.

### Monitoring hormone levels

Monitoring the hormone response to therapy should be primarily clinical with serial hormone estimations being requested only if management is likely to be altered. For example, when patients report a good response to oestrogen replacement therapy, there is no advantage in checking oestradiol levels (Chapter 28). Testosterone estimations may be wise when administering androgens. In other situations, hormone concentrations are essential. High oestrogen levels during gonadotrophin therapy for IVF may indicate risk of ovarian hyperstimulation (Chapter 10). Mid-luteal phase progesterone estimations may indicate a need to adjust ovulation induction treatment (Chapter 8). Testosterone and SHBG levels provide a measure of response to treatment for hirsutism (Chapter 5).

A 33-year-old lady with a history of abdominal pain, endometriosis, irritable bowel syndrome and hirsutism was happy for a while with a combination of cyclical cyproterone acetate and oestradiol. She then reported a slight increase in the hirsutism and the laboratory reported a testosterone level of 12.2 nmol/l whereas it had been 0.6 nmol/lm (normal range 0.4–3.5 nmol/l). The laboratory had double checked the level and a second sample was reported at 11.0 nmol/l. Ultrasound of the pelvis and adrenal gland was unremarkable and her hormone profile was otherwise unremarkable. A further blood sample was sent to another laboratory which reported the testosterone at 0.7 nmol/l!

Hormone levels may be subject to diurnal variation and may also be dependent on their timing in relation to the next menstrual period. When laboratory results do not reflect the clinical picture, caution is required. In a study of four commercially available methods used to measure oestradiol samples, there was a significant variation of results[26]. The discrepancy was attributed to high SHBG levels and other metabolites.

Ultrasound examination of the pelvic organs provides a valuable method of measuring the response to hormone administration (Chapter 5). Follicular development and endometrial thickness measurements with ovulation induction agents is the most obvious example (Chapters 8 and 10).

## COMMUNICATIONS

### Physician–patient communication

Good physician–patient communication lies at the heart of clinical practice, although scientific appraisal of this essential aspect of the art of medicine appears to receive relatively little attention[27]. Historically, it was accepted that the physician, acting in the best interests of the ever appreciative patient, made all the decisions, which were accepted without question. Only the physician had the knowledge and the patient was shielded from worrying about decision making. Beneficence, however, is no longer acceptable. There has been an insidious change in the physician–patient relationship. Patients have increasingly and appropriately taken a more active role in decisions about their care[28] and perhaps the ideal situation is reached when the relationship becomes one of partnership.

The majority of patients, although not all, are keen to receive information[28]. Whilst there may be widespread belief amongst doctors that the information they regularly provide is easily understood and remembered, there is a wealth of literature to the contrary[29]. Patients may forget information given to them even within a short time of leaving the consulting room[30,31]. In the study by Joyce and colleagues[31], not one patient remembered everything and, on average, less than half of the total items were recalled.

Patients have difficulty in remembering information given to them for a variety of reasons. These include anxieties about the seriousness of their condition[30], concern about the investigations and treatment, and the incomprehensible terminology[32]. The more patients are told, the smaller the proportion they retain[30,33]. Statements, such as 'a further visit is required', are usually remembered, whereas statements about prognosis are more readily forgotten[30]. Patients aged greater than 56 years recall more than patients aged between 15 and 35 years[30]. Research has been conducted into patient recall of information but the value of the information that they remember and their comprehension of the retained information have not been evaluated[34].

Patient recall of information received during consultation increased from an average of 55% to 70% with provision of additional patient information including a brief booklet[35]. Information which helps patients to understand may reduce suffering, improve compliance with treatment, speed successful outcome and increase patient satisfaction[34]. A randomized controlled trial, following notification of abnormal cervical cytology, demonstrated higher patient acceptability, effectiveness and compliance amongst the group of patients receiving educational brochures compared to controls[36].

A variety of methods have been employed to improve patient recall of their consultation, including audiotape recording[29], videocassette[37] and information leaflets (pamphlets). During a personal review of the literature, the author found relatively few studies evaluating the benefits of patient educational methods in reproductive medicine in comparison to other medical disciplines. A comprehensive search of studies conducted from 1960 to 1992, comparing two or more patient teaching strategies and reaching strict inclusion criteria, was conducted by Theis and Johnson[38]. They found a total of 72 acceptable papers and these were analysed. There were 16 papers on cardiovascular conditions, eight on respiratory medicine and seven about diabetes mellitus. There were papers from fifteen other branches of medicine and one from midwifery, but there were no papers from reproductive medicine, gynaecology or obstetrics. Audiotapes proved to be the most effective method and computer assisted instruction came next. Pamphlets proved to be more effective than verbal teaching.

It is well recognized that some patients tend to manipulate clinical staff[39]. A few patients tend to demand a special relationship with their doctor who, to begin with, may accept the patient's view that the case is special and, furthermore, that it has probably been badly handled by previous doctors. At times, the behaviour of these patients may cause conflict among staff, some of whom react against her whilst others are on her side, at least initially. Loopholes are found in the practice organisation which are exploited, leading to confusion and anger[39]. Recognition of such behavioural disorder may assist the doctor to retain an objective professional approach despite provocation and perhaps avoid conflict. An extreme form of this manipulative behaviour, Main's syndrome, has been described by a psychiatrist[40]. An early emotional disturbance can often be found in these patients who are commonly female[40].

### *Physician–patient communication in reproductive medicine*

In reproductive medicine, there are complex issues to be addressed. It is relatively easy for a patient to understand that a joint is worn out or inflamed or that a heart valve is leaking. The interplay of the various hypothalamic, pituitary and ovarian hormones and their effect on the genital tract, fertility, general health and psyche is only superficially understood even by reproductive endocrinologists. Couples presenting with infertility may wish to comprehend ovulation, Fallopian tube function, male fertility tests, hormone results, modes of action of ovulation induction agents, prognosis, as well as receive pre-conception counselling.

There is a vast array of patient information leaflets in reproductive medicine. These are available, for example, from the RCOG Press (Royal College of Obstetricians and Gynaecologists), the American Society for Reproductive Medicine, The Human Fertilisation and Embryology Authority, The Family Planning Association, pharmaceutical companies, and many user groups. They are generally of a high standard and clearly receive time and care in their production. Preparing one's own patient information leaflets (Chapter 30) provides two advantages. First, they can be regularly updated to accommodate the alterations in practice as the subject advances and facilities develop locally. Second, there is inevitably a variation, at least in emphasis if not necessarily in content, between mass-produced leaflets and the way that doctors, as individuals, provide explanations to their patients. Kripalani[41] has provided helpful guidelines for designing patient information leaflets. Although patient information leaflets prepared in-house require time for initial production and subsequent updating, they are probably time-savers in the long-term.

Gynaecological problems are of a particularly sensitive and emotional nature. For example, following pregnancy loss or failed assisted conception treatment cycles, some degree of reactive depression is common. This depression is associated with reduced patient concentration and comprehension which, on occasion, may lead to patients inappropriately blaming clinical staff for their failure to achieve parenthood. Specialist counselling is often vital. Patients' expectations are increasing as a result of media coverage and political involvement such as 'The Patient's Charter' (grammatically suggesting that there is only one patient). Despite our best efforts, patient satisfaction is often less than the doctor expects, considering the care that the team have provided. Physicians have the responsibility to assist patients in the management of their clinical problems but this can only be accomplished with the cooperation of the patient; we cannot insist on patient conformity[42].

In busy hospital clinics, the doctor must take a clinical history and examine the patient, mentally summarize the clinical and investigation findings, organize future investigations, explain these to the patient and plan treatment together, ensure adequate medical records and communicate with other clinicians involved in the patient's care. About a quarter of consultation time is utilized giving information to the patient. It is incumbent on the physician to assist patient understanding of their clinical problem, and to encourage patient participation in treatment planning. Invariably there are a variety of treatment options and patients must be given ample opportunity for informed choice. Leaflets, given together with verbal information from the clinician, reinforce recall and increase satisfaction and compliance. When this is achieved, treatment efficacy is enhanced[43].

At times, the circumstances of a patient with reproductive endocrinological problems can be particularly complex. No leaflet, or combination of leaflets, can overcome this difficulty. Providing the patient with a copy of the detailed letter to the general practitioner may fill a potential information gap. For further clarification, it is our routine practice to provide a brief clinical summary at the beginning of all patient related letters. There can be no doubt that doctors have a responsibility for patient education, although a sensible balance is required between reality and utopia[44].

## Physician–physician communication

There is a perceptible trend in gynaecology away from an essentially surgical speciality towards greater reliance on medical therapy[1]. Subspecialization outside university hospitals, despite the reservations expressed by others[1], does not necessarily create immense organisational difficulties. Some of my colleagues concentrate on oncology, minimally invasive surgery, fetal– maternal medicine, undergraduate and postgraduate education and management. The author enjoys a busy general obstetric and gynaecology practice with subspecialty interests in reproductive medicine and the obstetric care of patients who initially presented with infertility.

In the United Kingdom, consultants should generally see patients with non-urgent problems at the request of their general practitioners and it is current government policy to enhance the role of primary healthcare. There is a tendency amongst general practitioners to increase their involvement, even with decisions about tertiary referrals[45]. The majority of general practitioners have speciality interests just as consultants have their subspecialty interests. Gynaecological problems are common and most can be successfully managed within the primary care sector, leaving the more persistent or complex to be referred for specialist advice. Those general practitioners who have particular interests in gynaecology and have been appropriately trained, should be encouraged to use their skills for the benefit of their patients[46]. Others, who have different speciality interests, should feel comfortable in referring their patients to the gynaecologist relatively early. Consultants would appreciate an indication at the time of referral as to the degree of involvement that general practitioner colleagues would wish to pursue once hospital diagnostic and surgical procedures have been performed and initial treatment planning accomplished[47].

## REFERENCES


1. Smith, S. K. (1996). Gynaecology – medical or surgical. *Br. Med. J.*, **312**, 592–3
2. Keefer, D. A. and Stumpf, W. E. (1975). Atlas of estrogen-concentrating cells in the central nervous system of the squirrel monkey. *J. Comp. Neurol.*, **160**, 419–41
3. Romano, G. J., Krust, A. and Pfaff, D. W. (1989). Expression and estrogen regulation of progesterone receptor mRNA in neurons of the mediobasal hypothalamus: an *in situ* hybridization study. *Mol. Endocrinol.*, **3**, 1295–300
4. Pfaff, D. W. and McEwen, B. S. (1983). Actions of estrogens and progestins on nerve cells. *Science*, **219**, 808–14
5. Parsons, T. F., Bloomfield, G. A. and Pierce, J. G. (1983). Purification of an alternate form of the alpha subunit of the glycoprotein hormones from bovine pituitaries and identification of its O-linked oligosaccharide. *J. Biol. Chem.*, **258**, 240–4
6. Catt, K. J. and Dufau, M. L. (1991). Gonadotropic hormones: biosynthesis, secretion, receptors, and actions. In Yen, S. S. C. and Jaffe, R. B. (eds.) *Reproductive Endocrinology, Physiology, Pathology and Clinical Management*, 3rd edn., pp. 105–55. (Philadelphia, London, Toronto, Montreal, Sydney and Tokyo: W.B. Saunders Company)
7. Adashi, E. Y. (1995). The ovarian follicular apparatus. In Adashi, E. Y., Rock, J. A. and Rosenwaks, Z. (eds.) *Reproductive Endocrinology, Surgery, and Technology*, pp. 17–40. (Philadelphia and New York: Lippincott-Raven)
8. Baird, D. T. (1990). Biology of the menopause. In Drife, J. O. and Studd, J. W. W. (eds.) *HRT and Osteoporosis*, pp. 3–10. (London: Springer-Verlag)
9. McNeilly, A. F. (1995). Control of ovarian function. Presented at the *Infertility Meeting*, July, Royal College of Obstetricians and Gynaecologists, London
10. Gougeon, A. (1985). Dynamics of follicular growth in the human: a model from preliminary results. *Hum. Reprod.*, **1**, 81–7
11. Zeleznik, A. J., Schuler, H. M. and Reichert, L. E. Jr (1981). Gonadotrophin-binding sites in the rhesus monkey ovary: role of the vasculature in the selective distribution of human chorionic gonadotrophin to the preovulatory follicle. *Endocrinology*, **109**, 356–62
12. Zeleznik, A. J., Hutchinson, J. S. and Schuler, H. M. (1987). Passive immunization with anti-oestradiol antibodies during the luteal phase of the menstrual cycle potentiates the perimenstrual rise in serum gonadotrophin concentration and stimulates follicular growth in the cynomolgus monkey (*Macaca fascicularis*). *J. Reprod. Fertil.*, **80**, 403–10
13. Schwall, R. H., Mason, A. J., Wilcox, J. N., Bassett, S. G. and Zeleznik, A. J. (1990). Localization of inhibin/activin subunit mRNAs within the primate ovary. *Mol. Endocrinol.*, **4**, 75–9
14. Halvorson, L. M. and DeCherney, A. H. (1996). Inhibin, activin, and follistatin in reproductive medicine. *Fertil. Steril.*, **65**, 459–69
15. O'Malley, B. W. and Stroit, C. A. (1991). Steroid hormones: metabolism and mechanism of action. In Yen, S. S. C. and Jaffe, R. B. (eds.) *Reproductive Endocrinology, Physiology, Pathology and Clinical Management,* 3rd edn., p. 156. (Philadelphia and London: W.B. Saunders) 3rd edn
16. Albers, H. E., Lydic, R., Gander, P. H. and Moore-Ede, M. C. (1984). Role of the suprachiasmatic nuclei in the circadian timing system of the squirrel monkey. I. The generation of rhythmicity. *Brain Res.*, **300**, 275–84
17. Moore-Ede, M. C., Czeisler, C. A. and Richardson, G. S. (1983). Circadian timekeeping in health and disease. Part 2. Clinical implications of circadian rhythmicity. *N. Engl. J. Med.*, **309**, 530–6
18. Viniker, D. A. (1983). Perinatal Cerebral Function Monitoring, *M.D. Thesis*, University of London
19. Adashi, E. Y. (1991). The ovarian life cycle. In Yen, S. S. C. and Jaffe, R. B. (eds.) *Reproductive Endocrinology, Physiology, Pathophysiology and Clinical Management*, pp. 181–237. (Philadelphia, London, Toronto, Montreal, Sydney and Tokyo: W.B. Saunders Company)
20. Gossain, V. V., Carella, M. J. and Rovner, D. R. (1993). Pregnancy in a patient with premature ovarian failure. *J. Med.*, **24**, 393–402
21. Yen, S. S. C. and Jaffe, R. B. (1991). *Reproductive Endocrinology, Physiology, Pathology and Clinical Management*, 3rd edn. (Philadelphia: W.B. Saunders)
22. Ferin, M., Jewelewicz, R. and Warren, M. (1993). *The Menstrual Cycle. Physiology,*

*Reproductive Disorders and Infertility*. (New York: Oxford University Press)
23. Adashi, E. Y., Rock, J. A. and Rosenwaks, Z. (1995). *Reproductive Endocrinology, Surgery, and Technology*. Volume 1, Part 1. (Philadelphia: Lippincott-Raven)
24. James, I. M. (1996). Pharmacological principles of drug action. In Ginsberg, J. (ed.) *Drug Therapy in Reproductive Medicine*. (London, Sydney and Auckland: Arnold)
25. Weckstein, L. N., Jacobson, A., Galen, D., Hampton, K., Ivani, K. and Andres, J. (1993). Improvement of pregnancy rates with oocyte donation in older recipients with the addition of progesterone vaginal suppositories. *Fertil. Steril.*, **60**, 573–5
26. Cook, N. J. and Read, G. F. (1995). Oestradiol measurement in women on oral hormone replacement therapy: the validity of commercial test kits. *Br. J. Med. Sci.*, **52**, 97–101
27. Charney, E. (1972). Patient-doctor communication. Implications for the clinician. *Pediatr. Clin. N. Am.*, **19**, 263–79
28. Deber, R. B. (1994). Physicians in health care management: 7. The patient-physician partnership: changing roles and the desire for information. *Can. Med. Assoc. J.*, **151**, 171–6
29. Butt, H. R. (1977). A method for better physician-patient communication. *Ann. Int. Med.*, **86**, 478–80
30. Ley, P. and Spelman, M. S. (1965). Communications in an out-patient setting. *Br. J. Soc. Clin. Psychol.*, **4**, 114–16
31. Joyce, C. B. R., Caple, G., Mason, M., Reynolds, E. and Mathews, J. A. (1969). Quantitative study of doctor-patient communication. *Q. J. Med.*, **38**, 183–94
32. Ley, P., Bradshaw, P. W., Eaves, D. and Walker, C. M. (1973). A method of increasing patients' recall of information presented by doctors. *Psychol. Med.*, **3**, 217–20
33. Ley, P. (1979). Memory for medical information. *Br. J. Soc. Clin. Psychol.*, **18**, 245–55
34. Tuckett, D. and Williams, A. (1984). Approaches to the measurement of explanation and information-giving in medical consultations: a review of empirical studies. *Soc. Sci. Med.*, **18**, 571–80
35. Ley, P., Whitworth, M. A., Skilbeck, C. E., Woodward, R., Pinsent, R. J. F. H., Pike, L. A., Clarkson, M. E. and Clark, P. B. (1976). Improving doctor-patient communication in general practice. *J. R. Coll. Gen. Pract.*, **26**, 720–4
36. Stewart, D. E., Buchegger, P. M., Lickrish, G. M. and Sierra, S. (1994). The effect of education brochures on follow-up compliance in women with abnormal Papanicolaou smears. *Obstet. Gynecol.*, **83**, 583–5
37. Pace, P. W. (1983). Videocassette use in diet instruction. *J. Am. Diet. Assoc.*, **83**, 166–9
38. Theis, S. L. and Johnson, J. H. (1995). Strategies for teaching patients: a meta-analysis. *Clin. Nurse Spec.*, **9**, 100–20
39. Working Party of The Royal College of General Practitioners (1972). *The Future General Practitioner*, pp. 160–5. (London: British Medical Journal)
40. Main, T. F. (1957). Ailment. *Br. J. Med. Psychol.*, **30**, 129–45
41. Kripalani, S. (1995). The write stuff. Simple guidelines can help you write and design effective patient education materials. *Tex. Med.*, **91**, 40–5
42. Hartmann, R. A. and Kochar, M. S. (1994). The provision of patient and family education. *Patient Educ. Counsel.*, **24**, 101–8
43. Gruninger, U. J. (1995). Patient education: an example of one-to-one communication. *J. Hum. Hypertens.*, **9**, 15–25
44. Ehlers, A. P. (1989). The physician's responsibility for patient education between utopia and reality. *Gynakologe*, **22**, 360–3
45. Bridger, S. and Cairns, S. R. (1996). Survey of general practitioners' views of consultants' non urgent referral of outpatients to other consultants. *Br. Med. J.*, **312**, 821–2
46. Seamark, C. J. and Seamark, D. A. (1996). Gynaecological problems should continue to be treated in primary care initially. *Br. Med. J.*, **312**, 1672–3
47. Viniker, D. A. (1996). GPs' participation in decisions about non-urgent tertiary referral is appropriate. *Br. Med. J.*, **313**, 112

# Puberty and its problems

# 3

*Charles G. D. Brook*

## INTRODUCTION

Puberty is the process by which reproductive capability is acquired.

## PHYSIOLOGY OF PUBERTY

The fetal hypothalamo–pituitary–gonadal axis becomes active at around 20 weeks of gestation. The secretion of testosterone from the fetal testis, which causes sexual differentiation in the male, is under the control of placental human chorionic gonadotrophin (hCG) stimulation before 20 weeks of gestation. Since congenital luteinizing hormone (LH) deficiency results in ambiguity of the genitalia, the integrity of the adult cascade of gonadotrophin-releasing hormone (GnRH) stimulating LH and follicle stimulating hormone (FSH), which stimulate gonadal activity, is important to the fetus. In mid-gestation, gonadotrophin levels are extremely high and decrease thereafter but gonadotrophin concentrations around the time of birth are at least as high as they become in puberty and only reach a nadir by 8 years of age[1].

During early childhood, occasional peaks of gonadotrophin are seen at night in both girls and boys. Towards the end of the first decade of life, nocturnal pulsatile gonadotrophin secretion becomes a regular event and this stimulates the gonadal secretion of testosterone and oestradiol. Because these levels rise during the night and early morning, there is no point in measuring sex steroid concentrations in boys and girls in early puberty.

As time passes, the amplitude of gonadotrophin pulsatility increases (Figure 1) and the consequently rising levels of sex steroids bring about the physical changes of puberty. In order to attain reproductive capability, and especially to sustain an LH surge for ovulation in the female, 24-h gonadotrophin pulsatility is required (Figure 1). The reason that some girls develop in puberty but have an anovulatory cycle is not infrequently due to the fact that they have failed to develop 24-h gonadotrophin pulsatility. Upsets of a physical or emotional kind, especially those involving starvation, will immediately inhibit gonadotrophin pulsatility and interfere with reproductive capability. The recovery from anorexia mirrors the gonadotrophin changes of puberty.

### Physical changes at puberty

*Boys*

The consequence of gonadotrophin secretion is an enlargement of the testicular volume from the prepubertal size of 2 ml to 4 ml. The testes enlarging under the influence of LH start to secrete testosterone and this causes enlargement of the penis, increased rugosity of the scrotum and the appearance of pubic hair (Figure 2). In a patient who has failure of development of the seminiferous tubules (e.g. after testicular irradiation for leukaemic deposits), Leydig cell hyperplasia will cause the testes to attain a volume of about 8 ml (the size of a walnut): the remainder of adult testicular volume (15–25 ml) comprises seminiferous tubular development.

During the early stages of pubertal development in boys, the gradual deceleration of growth rate which characterizes the late childhood growth curve continues, so that boys entering puberty late (see below) may become very small in relation to their peers before the

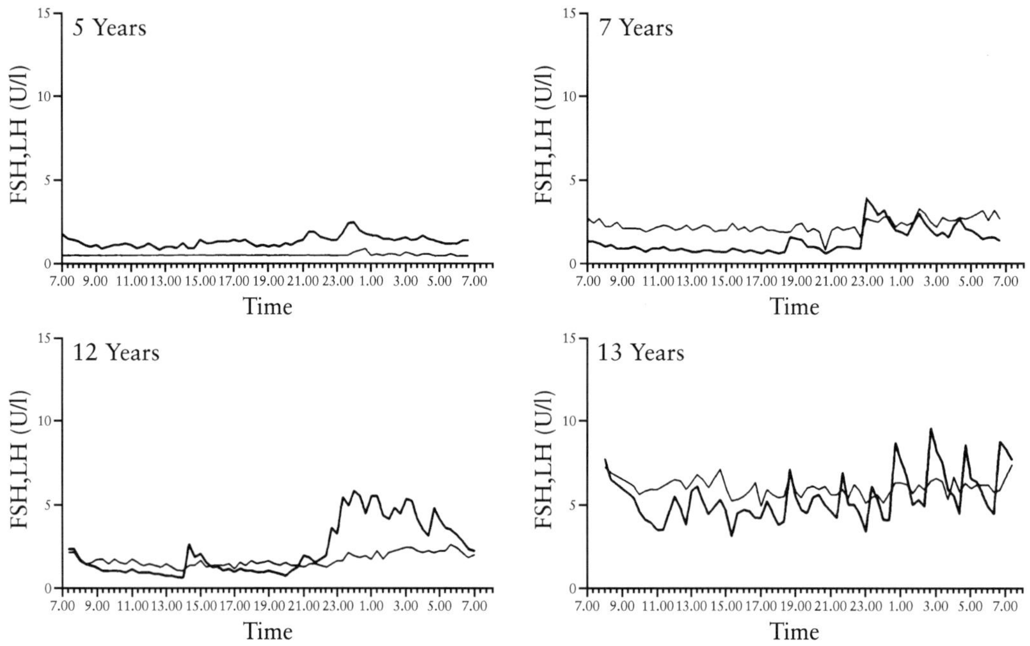


**Figure 1** Changing gonadotrophin pulsatility with age. Note nocturnal pulses at age 7, amplifying at age 12 and becoming 24-h at age 13. Follicle stimulating hormone (FSH), thinner trace; luteinizing hormone (LH), thicker trace

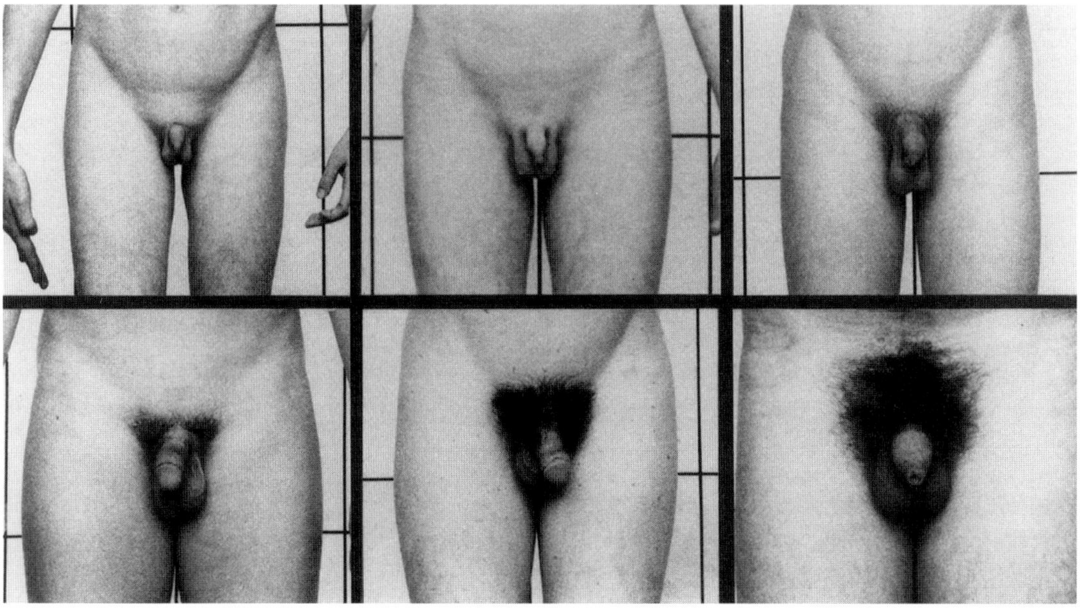

**Figure 2** Stages of genital and pubic hair 1–6 in boys

puberty growth spurt supervenes. The reason for this is that testosterone is not a very good stimulator of growth hormone secretion: it has to be aromatized in the hypothalamus to oestradiol. Consequently, the level of testosterone needs to be higher in a boy for the hypothalamo–pituitary axis to be exposed to the same concentration of oestradiol as occurs much earlier in puberty in the girl. As soon as there is sufficient oestradiol circulating in girls for breasts to develop, a growth spurt supervenes. In boys, by contrast, the onset of the growth spurt occurs approximately 18 months to 2 years later than the onset of the growth spurt in a girl, thus allowing the boy to attain a height about 10 cm taller than that of his female counterpart before a growth spurt starts.

Testosterone is a better anabolic hormone than oestradiol and the peak rate of the growth spurt in males is greater than that in females. Males stop growing sooner than girls after the peak height velocity of adolescence has been reached. The consequence of an increased height attained before the onset of the puberty growth spurt, plus the higher peak growth rate, less the reduction in time for growth after the peak height velocity has been attained results in the average boy being 12.6 cm or 5 inches taller than the average girl[2].

*Girls*

Rising levels of oestradiol in girls bring about changes in breast development (Figure 3) and an increase in growth rate secondary to an increase in growth hormone secretion.

It is much easier to follow what is happening in girls thanks to the availability of pelvic ultrasound. The prepubertal ovary is not quiescent and usually shows a few follicles (Figure 4a), but the prepubertal uterus is small and tubular with no endometrial echo (Figure 4d). As nocturnal pulsatile gonadotrophin secretion becomes regular, the ovary changes to a multicystic appearance (Figure 4b) and the uterus responds by becoming pear-shaped (Figure 4e). Twenty-four hour gonadotrophin secretion is associated with the normal adult female

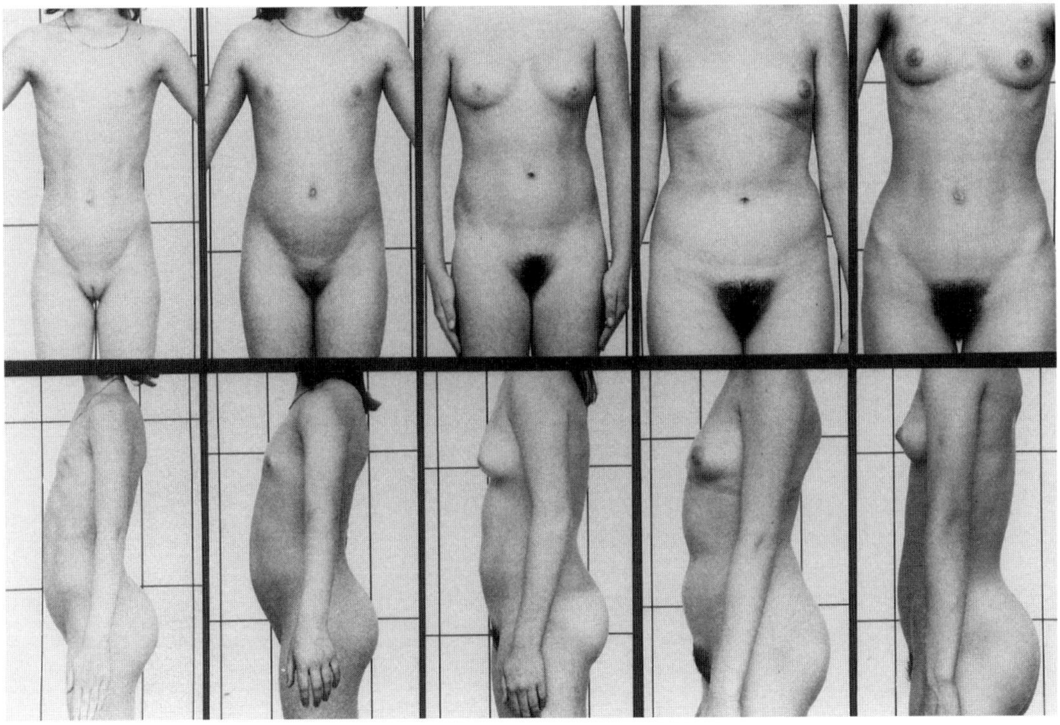

**Figure 3** Stages of breast and pubic hair 1–5 in girls

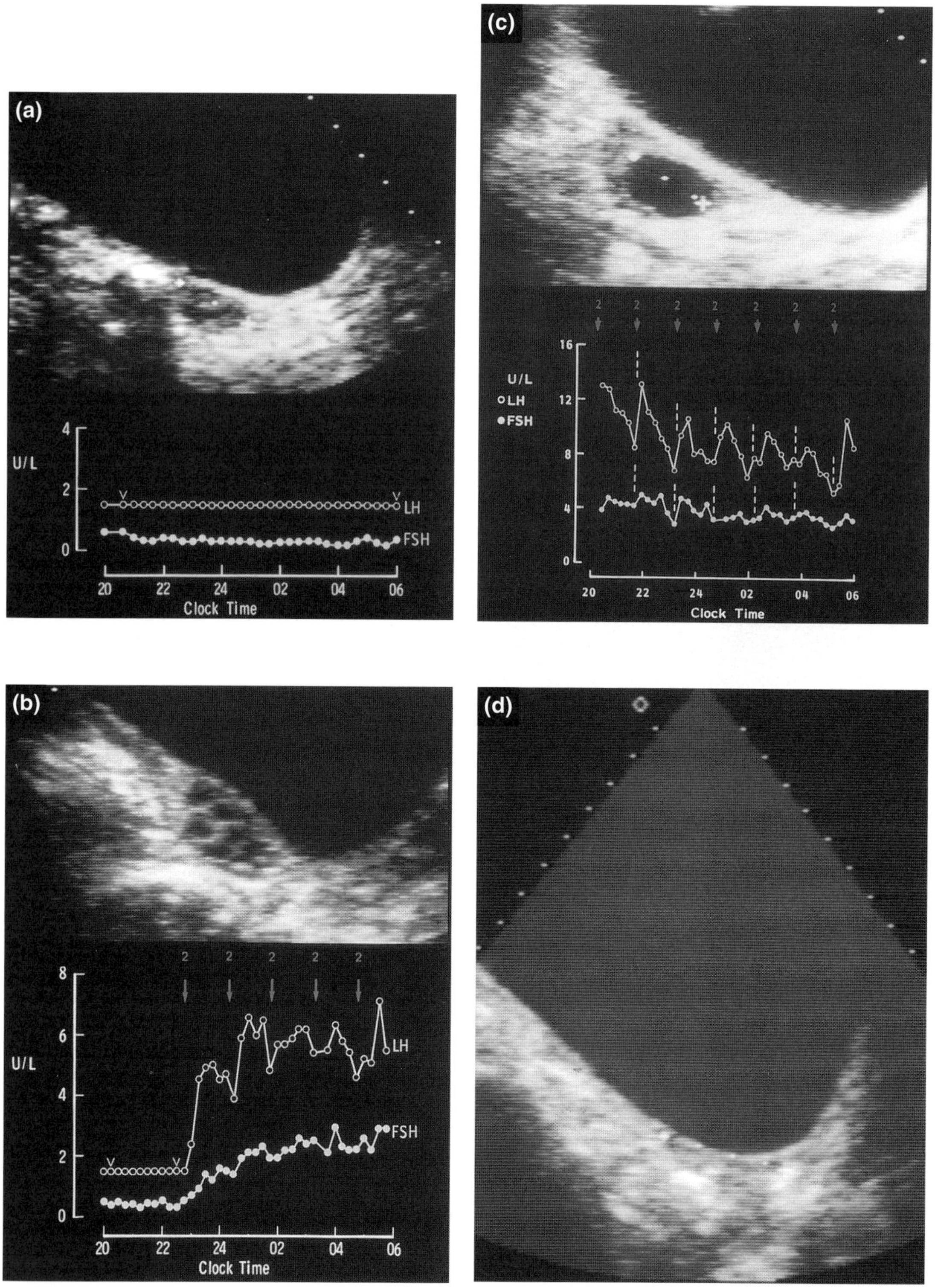
(a)
U/L
LH
FSH
20 22 24 02 04 06
Clock Time
(c)
U/L
LH
FSH
20 22 24 02 04 06
Clock Time
(b)
U/L
LH
FSH
20 22 24 02 04 06
Clock Time
(d)

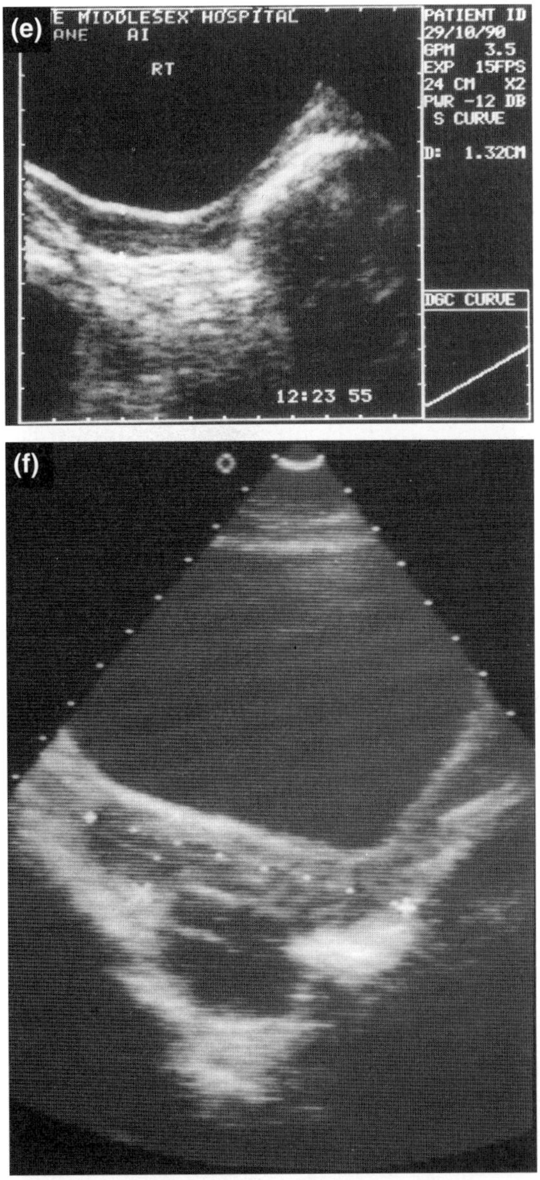


Figure 4 Pelvic ultrasound images of ovaries and uterus with gonadotrophin profiles in puberty. (i) Prepuberty: note no ovarian follicles (a), no gonadotrophin pulses and small uterus (d); (ii) mid-puberty: note multicystic ovaries (b), nocturnal luteinizing hormone (LH) and follicle-stimulating hormone (FSH) pulses and enlarging uterus (e); (iii) late puberty: note ovary with dominant follicle (c), 24-h gonadotrophin pulses and adult uterus with endometrial thickening (f) with the dominant follicle below it

appearance of ovaries with a dominant follicle and an adult uterus with an endometrial echo (Figures 4c, 4f)[3,4].

The growth of pubic hair in girls is due to the secretion of adrenal androgens. Adrenarche precedes gonadarche by about 3 years and pubic hair development in prepubertal children is a frequent occurrence. Because the differential diagnosis can be rather sinister (see below), the early development of pubic hair should be taken seriously but it is usually physiological. Nevertheless, oestrogens are clearly facilitative of pubic hair development in girls: patients with gonadal dysgenesis (e.g. Turner syndrome) may have scanty pubic hair at the age of about 15 years but, as soon as they are treated with oestrogens to induce puberty, pubic hair growth normalizes rapidly. There is clearly, therefore, a contribution of ovarian oestradiol secretion to pubic hair development but patients with Addison disease or adrenocorticotrophic hormone (ACTH) deficiency do not develop pubic hair, even if they go through puberty spontaneously or as a result of pubertal induction.

## Timing of onset of puberty

Fifty percent of girls show signs of breast development soon after their 11th birthday (Figure 5) and 97% of girls show signs of breast development by shortly after their 13th birthday. Serious consideration about pathology needs to be given to a girl who has no signs of breast development by her 14th birthday. Menarche comes late in the sequence of pubertal development, not until breast stage 4 and pubic hair stage 4 have been attained and the peak of the growth spurt of puberty has been passed. Fifty percent of girls have started menstruating by their 13th birthday and 97% have done so by their 15th birthday. The age of menarche ceased declining 30 years ago[5].

Fifty percent of boys show testicular enlargement by their 12th birthday and 97% have done so by their 14th birthday. As previously indicated, the peak height velocity of adolescence comes late in the sequence of pubertal development and not until genitalia stage 4 and

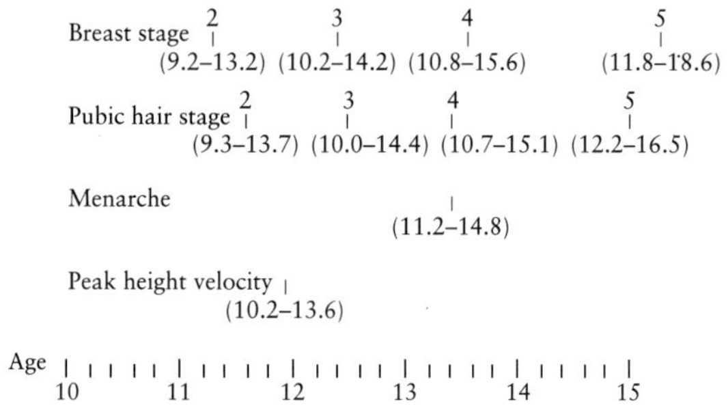


Figure 5 Timing of events in puberty in girls

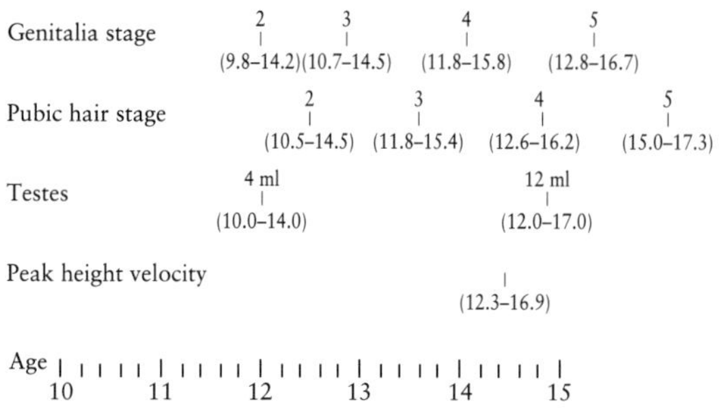


Figure 6 Timing of events in puberty in boys

testicular volumes of 10 ml have been attained. Fifty percent of boys have attained the peak height velocity of adolescence by their 14th birthday and 97% by their 16th birthday (Figure 6).

The onset of sperm production is usually in the 13th year with a range of 12–16 years. Thus sperm production precedes the peak of the adolescent growth spurt, is achieved at a testicular volume of less than 10 ml (6 ml testicular volumes in some boys) and occurs much earlier in the sequence of pubertal changes than the menarche in girls. Consequently, contrary to popular belief, a boy is actually capable of fathering a child before a girl of similar age is capable of conceiving one.

In females, gonadotrophins and oestradiol are produced throughout childhood. The amplitude of the hormonal levels and the duration of pulsatile secretion gradually increase through puberty and endometrial hyperplasia is the result of this stimulation. When the degree of hyperplasia is sufficient to break down when oestrogen support is withdrawn, menarche occurs. From the point of view of the endocrinologist, therefore, menarche is a relatively minor event. It remains, however, the only pubertal change in either sex which is readily identifiable as a single event in time and, for this reason, the various factors which influence menarche have attracted considerable attention, from which we may learn much about puberty.

In the1970s, it was widely believed that the occurrence of menarche was dependent upon the attainment of a 'critical' body weight. However, since the number of girls menstruating is distributed about the critical weight in a Gaussian fashion and as the weight of girls at menarche is also normally distributed, it is unlikely that menarche is initiated by the attainment of a particular body weight or, as has also been suggested, by the development of a specific relationship between the amounts of water and fat which contribute to body weight. Loss of weight or extreme devotion to exercise may delay puberty or influence reproductive ability in the human female, largely because of the effects that nutrition and exercise may have on the amplitude of pulsatile GnRH secretion.

Environmental influences on the timing of puberty are readily apparent. In many countries, there are clear differences among socioeconomic classes. Children of higher socioeconomic classes enter puberty earlier than their less advantaged peers. This may be a consquence of (probably infantile) better nutrition but the menarcheal difference between the social classes has largely disappeared in wealthy parts of the world so superabundant nutrition is not advantageous in this respect, even though obese children, certainly those obese from early infancy, have a tendency to be tall and to develop early in puberty.

The appearance of axillary hair does not bear a constant relationship to the development of breasts because adrenal androgen secretion is primarily responsible for axillary hair growth and oestrogens play little part. Axillary hair stage 2 (appearance of hair) occurs at a mean age in girls of 12.5 years and is adult in amount and distribution (stage 3) at a mean age of 13.9

years[6]. The apocrine glands of the axilla and vulva begin to function at about the same time as axillary and pubic hair appears but, in the case of the axilla, this may antedate the rest of pubertal development by some years.

In boys, axillary hair stages 2 and 3 are attained at mean ages of 14.3 and 15.6 years, each with a standard deviation of about 1 year[6]. The appearance of axillary hair is approximately coincident with peak height velocity of adolescence. Facial hair begins to appear at the corners of the upper lip at the age of about 15 years and spreads to the cheek at 16 years, but spread to the chin is rarely seen until growth of the genitalia is complete.

The breaking of the voice is a late event in male puberty. Fifty percent of boys' voices start to break at 15 years and are definitely broken about 1 year later[6].

## Changes in body proportions

During adolescence, the growth of nearly all parts of the skeleton is accelerated. The maximum rate of growth attained is similar in the legs and trunk but the total gain in sitting height during the adolescent growth spurt is greater than that in leg length because the spurt in sitting height lasts for a longer time. Most of the sex difference in adult height is due to different rates of growth of the trunk rather than of the legs. The mean gain in sitting height during puberty is 15.4 cm for boys and 13.5 cm for girls, compared to 12.1 and 11.5 cm for the increase in growth of the legs. The spurt in sitting height continues for about 6 months longer in boys than in girls[7]. The widths of the shoulders and the hips show growth spurts at the same time as the trunk.

Most facial measurements show accelerated growth and, in the face, the greatest increase is in the length of the mandible so that the jaw becomes considerably longer in relation to the front part of the face and projects more after puberty. This effect is increased in late puberty and early adult life when the growth of the chin is completed by further acquisition of bone at the mandibular symphysis. The forward projection of the maxilla is also increased by accelerated growth above the upper incisor teeth.

## Body composition

Most children put on fat from the age of about 8 years up to adolescence, but the rate of gain decreases when the adolescent growth spurt occurs. The rate of fat gain reaches its minimum at about the same time as the growth of the body as a whole attains its maximum rate: in boys, fat is actually lost during the adolescent spurt. In other words, the limbs become thinner in adolescent boys in contrast to those of girls which typically get fatter, although they do so more slowly during the adolescent spurt than before or after.

The thickness of muscle shows a maximum rate of increase in boys at about the same time as the peak height velocity of adolescence but the changes in subcutaneous fat are in the opposite direction.

These changes lead to differences in physical performance. In girls, there is continuous improvement throughout childhood but performance reaches a plateau at an average age of about 14 years. Motor performance in boys increases until at least 17 or 18 years of age and probably into the early 20s, that is after growth in size and development of the secondary sexual characteristics have been completed for some time. There is, therefore, a period which may last for several years when a boy looks 'grown up' but has not attained his adult strength. This fact may be responsible for the popular concept that boys 'outgrow their strength' at adolescence.

Muscular endurance, as well as strength, increases at puberty. This is due not only to the development of the skeleton and muscles but also to changes in the cardiovascular, respiratory and haemopoietic systems, presumably secondary to testosterone and erythropoietin secretion.

All of the changes in strength and physical performance take place in association with puberty, regardless of the age at which this occurs. Thus the boy who experiences puberty early becomes not only bigger than his peers but has other advantages in sport and physical activities of all kinds. These advantages may be lost when the boys who mature later undergo the corresponding changes and it is sometimes beneficial to warn early maturing boys and girls that their advantages may be only temporary, while late maturers may need to be reassured that they will eventually be comparable with their peers both in size and physical performance.

### Puberty and skeletal maturation

It is well known that the ossification of the skeleton provides an index of a child's progress in growth towards his or her final stature. The degree of ossification may be quantified by a number of techniques and the result is usually expressed as a 'bone age'. This can be used to predict final height within known probability limits which vary with age. The predictive value of bone age in relation to the events of puberty is much less clear than in the case of stature. It is true that children whose puberty is delayed usually have delayed bone ages but it is seldom possible to ascertain whether or not the subject had similarly delayed skeletal maturation during childhood. Children with precocious puberty have advanced bone ages but this is probably the direct result of their high level of circulating sex steroid hormones. There is little information about the skeletal maturation of such children before the development of precocious puberty.

There is no closer relationship between the onset of puberty in normal children and their chronological age than with their bone age. The bone age at which puberty begins in boys or girls varies just as much as their chronological ages and the bone age of a prepubertal child cannot give a useful prediction as to when puberty will begin[8]. A girl may begin to experience breast development when her skeletal age is anything between 8 and 14 years and this is true also of genital development in boys. Menarche, on the other hand, is associated more closely with bone age, probably because the oestradiol concentration affects both the uterus and skeletal maturity. Most girls menstruate when their bone ages are between 13 and 14 years and probably less than 20% are outside these limits. This information may be helpful in assessing girls whose breast and pubic hair development appears nearly complete but who complain of primary amenorrhoea.

## DISORDERS OF PUBERTY

### Early puberty

Signs of puberty appearing in girls before the age of 8 years and in boys before the age of 9 years should be regarded with suspicion, especially in boys. An audit of 213 children (197 girls and 16 boys) presenting to my department with sexual precocity showed that 91 girls and four boys had central precocious puberty, a female to male ratio of 23 : 1; a cause was identified in all the boys but only in six girls[9].

It is important to distinguish signs of puberty (sexual secondary characteristics) which are not part of the overall pattern of pubertal development from the early onset of puberty consonant in all modalities (Table 1).

*Sexual precocity in females*

Breast development is very common in the newborn female. This is usually the consequence of maternal oestrogen and it disappears within the first 3–6 months of birth. Sometimes, it persists or arises *de novo* during the first 2 or 3 years of postnatal life. In the absence of pubic hair and rapid growth, this condition is called *premature thelarche*. Pelvic ultrasound will reveal a small tubular uterus and an ovary with a single large follicle or microcyst (Figure 7c)[10]. We have shown this to be due to nocturnal gonadotrophin secretion when, contrary to the pattern in normal puberty, FSH concentrations exceed those of LH[11].

The characteristic of premature thelarche is that the breasts vary in size, as also does the size of the ovarian microcysts. Oestradiol concentrations are rarely above the limit of detection of a normally targeted oestradiol assay and measurements of gonadotrophin concentrations are not helpful. A GnRH

**Table 1** Causes of early sexual development

| |
|---|
| *Centrally mediated precocious puberty (consonant pubertal development)* |
| Idiopathic: exclusively female |
| Secondary: equal sex distribution |
| tumours |
| hydrocephalus |
| trauma |
| radiotherapy |
| sexual abuse |
| *Abnormal patterns of gonadotrophin secretion leading to isolated breast development* |
| Premature thelarche |
| Thelarche variant |
| Hypothyroidism |
| *Gonadotrophin independent precocious puberty* |
| Testotoxicosis |
| McCune–Albright syndrome |
| *Virilization* |
| Adrenarche |
| Congenital adrenal hyperplasia |
| Cushing disease |
| Adrenal tumours |
| *Others* |
| Gonadotrophin or sex steroid secreting tumours |
| Exogenous steroids |

stimulation test will reveal gonadotrophin secretion, with FSH concentrations exceeding those of LH. Because the oestradiol concentrations are very low, rates of growth in patients with premature thelarche are not increased and I have yet to see vaginal bleeding in association with the waxing and waning of ovarian follicular development.

This condition needs to be distinguished from the isolated breast development or testicular enlargement seen in patients with primary (usually acquired autoimmune) hypothyroidism. This condition is seen rarely before the age of 5 years, in contrast to premature thelarche which presents at a much younger age. Oestrogen secretion is the consequence of FSH drive of the gonads secondary to thyrotrophin releasing hormone (TRH) stimulation.

The characteristics of true *precocious puberty* are the development of breasts, pubic hair, a growth spurt and a considerable advance in bone age. Pelvic ultrasonography reveals a multifollicular ovarian appearance (Figure 7a) and a uterus of which the diameter of the fundus exceeds that of the cervix; there is considerable advance in bone age. This is consonant with puberty beginning at an abnormally early age.

Girls with this condition need a detailed history and a careful physical examination to rule

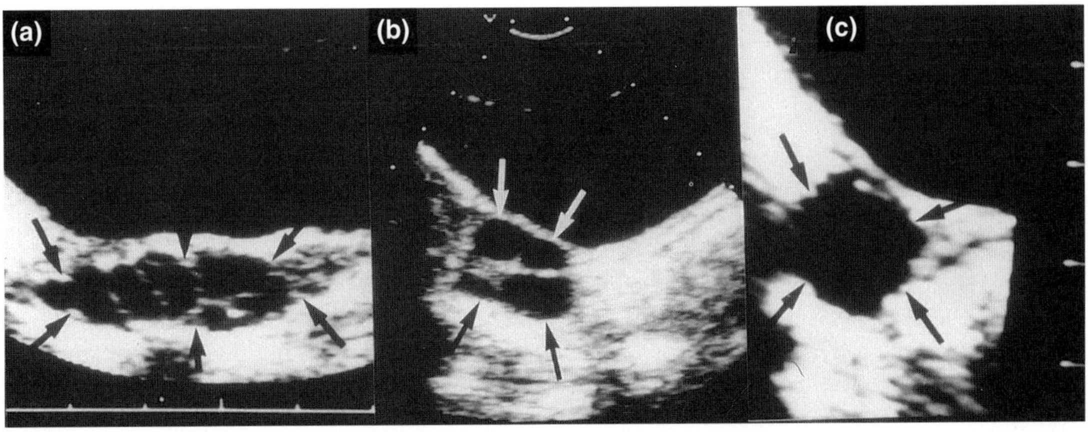


**Figure 7** Pelvic ultrasound appearances of (a) central gonadotrophin dependent precocious puberty: note the many 4–5-mm follicles; (b) thelarche variant: note five follicles only of up to 10-mm diameter; and (c) premature thelarche: note the single large 12-mm follicle

out an intracranial lesion as a cause of early pubertal development. There is argument about whether all girls with central precocious puberty require an imaging procedure of the central nervous system, preferably a magnetic resonance imaging (MRI) scan. The threshold for performing this investigation in a girl with early puberty should be low, but, as the author has never seen a girl presenting with precocious puberty due to a central lesion without some other pointer to the presence of that lesion (see audit quoted above), it is not his practice always to submit such patients to an imaging procedure.

In 1990 we recognized a condition which we called *thelarche variant*[12]. We think that this condition is identical to that described in Paris[13], of which the hallmarks are an increased growth rate, breast development without pubic hair, little change in uterine dimensions and a moderate advance in bone age. Profiles of gonadotrophin secretion show a pattern similar to that seen in premature thelarche with FSH secretion predominating over LH and an ovarian ultrasound image which is intermediate between that of premature thelarche and central precocious puberty (Figure 7b). Since the clinical evolution of this condition is entirely benign and since gonadotrophin suppression makes no difference to the outcome, the central nature of the FSH drive of ovarian development is in doubt. Since final height is not affected in premature thelarche and thelarche variant, these conditions need no treatment.

*Sexual precocity in boys*

Boys presenting with enlarging genitalia, pubic hair and increased growth need careful examination to determine testicular volume. This is because the majority of patients with such physical signs are manifesting adrenarche (and will have small testes), although some will have congenital adrenal hyperplasia diagnosed late. Such patients need adrenal investigation.

Where the testes are enlarged and consonant with the other signs of puberty, it is important to distinguish gonadotrophin dependent (central) precocious puberty from gonadotrophin independent precocious puberty. Basal measurements of LH and FSH may well reveal a clear difference, with undetectable concentrations in the latter condition, but a test of gonadotrophin secretion following an injection of GnRH will make the situation entirely clear. In precocious puberty, the gonadotrophin response will be exuberant, whereas it will be suppressed in gonadotrophin independent precocious puberty.

*Testoxicosis* is a form of hereditary precocious puberty where a mutation of the LH receptor gene causes a constant activation of the G protein even in the absence of ligand[14]. This condition may also be seen in association with other abnormalities, such as polyostotic fibrous dysplasia of bone and cutaneous pigmentation (McCune–Albright syndrome), which is much more common in girls. In this condition, there are activating mutations of the G protein in the affected cells[15] and such mutations may also occur in the pituitary gland, causing Cushing disease, in the thyroid gland, causing thyrotoxicosis, and in the adrenal gland, causing Cushing syndrome. Gonadotrophin independent precocious puberty gives way to gonadotrophin dependent puberty which usually commences at the normal age.

Since the author has neither seen nor heard of a boy with idiopathic central (gonadotrophin dependent) precocious puberty, all boys with consonant signs of puberty need detailed neuroimaging procedures. This does not necessarily mean that they require neurosurgical or other intervention (a hypothalamic hamartoma is perhaps best watched rather than operated) but a cause must always be found.

Primary hypothyroidism in boys causes testicular enlargement due to FSH secretion without other signs of puberty secondary to LH and testosterone secretion.

*Management of premature sexual development*

Premature thelarche and thelarche variant need no treatment. Indeed treatment is without effect and should be avoided.

Treatment of gonadotrophin independent precocious puberty should be avoided if possible. It does not influence long-term prognosis, which is benign, and is usually without effect. Since the only effective treatments interfere with steroid synthesis, drugs such as ketoconazole, an inhibitor of cytochrome P450 enzymes, have a generalized action in inhibiting steroid biosynthesis and thus there is a risk of inducing adrenal insufficiency and there is occasionally hepatic dysfunction. Testolactone, which inhibits the aromatization of testosterone to oestradiol and thereby abolishes the actions of testosterone, and spironolactone have both been used in the treatment of gonadotrophin independent precocious puberty but without much effect. Cyproterone acetate and medroxyprogesterone have side-effects, and the reports of hepatic carcinoma in patients treated with large doses of the former agent cause particular concern. My view is that gonadotrophin independent precocious puberty should be tolerated, not treated.

Central precocious puberty can be treated with gonadotrophin releasing hormone analogues, usually given (at the time of writing) as long-acting depot preparations by monthly injection to abolish gonadotrophin pulsatility. This is highly effective in stopping pubertal development but it makes no difference to final height achieved, even though height predictions may initially improve. Precocious puberty in girls is associated with the development of polycystic ovaries and the exhibition of gonadotrophin releasing hormone analogues increases this incidence, which is made still worse if growth hormone is used[16]. The physician has, therefore, to be very clear what is the object of treating central precocious puberty.

There are problems in three areas: premature sexual development itself, especially menstruation; psychological disturbance, especially masturbation in boys; impaired growth prognosis. The first and second may demand treatment but the third is not influenced by it. I am increasingly persuaded that discretion may be the better part of valour and learning to cope with the symptoms and psychological disadvantages of precocious puberty may be preferable to chemotherapeutic manoeuvres.

**Late puberty**

Ninety-seven percent of girls have developed signs of puberty by 13.2 years and 97% of boys by 14.2 years. Most of those who have not developed signs of puberty by these ages have delayed activation of the hypothalamo–pituitary–gonadal axis and will develop signs of puberty eventually. The majority of these cases are idiopathic and boys presenting with so-called constitutional delay of puberty outnumber girls by at least 20 to 1. This is probably because the male pituitary is relatively insensitive to GnRH stimulation[17] (which may be why precocious puberty is more common in

**Table 2** Causes of pubertal delay and pubertal failure

| |
|---|
| *Causes of pubertal delay* |
| Constitutional delay |
| Chronic disease |
|   asthma |
|   gastrointestinal problems |
|   renal failure |
| Undernutrition |
| Physical exercise (excessive) |
| Anorexia nervosa |
| *Hypothalamic and pituitary causes of pubertal failure – low gonadotrophins* |
| Congenital defects |
|   Kallman syndrome |
|   congenital adrenal hypoplasia |
|   septo-optic dysplasia |
|   developmental defects of the pituitary |
|   hypogonadotrophic hypogonadism (often presents as bilateral undescended testes) |
| Brain tumours: direct effects or following radiotherapy or surgery |
| Haemochromatosis/iron overload |
| *Gonadal causes of pubertal failure – elevated gonadotrophins* |
| Radiotherapy or chemotherapy |
| Females |
|   Turner syndrome |
|   premature menopause |
| Males |
|   anorchia |
|   bilateral orchidectomy |
|   orchitis |

girls) and it is certainly more difficult to suppress the gonadotrophin secretion of girls with precocious puberty than it is of boys.

Any chronic disease may delay puberty, for example inflammatory bowel disease, asthma, cystic fibrosis and renal disease. The combination of high levels of exercise and low weight seen in athletes and ballet dancers is a cause of significant delay in puberty.

Since it is difficult, if not impossible, to distinguish hypogonadotrophic hypogonadism from constitutional delay of puberty, it is often better to treat a patient with significantly delayed puberty and then to revisit the diagnosis later. It is obviously important to exclude organic disease and it is wise to measure the prolactin concentration to exclude the presence of a prolactinoma. It is, however, also important to distinguish gonadal failure as a cause of delayed puberty, especially in girls. Measurement of basal levels of gonadotrophins will achieve this separation and the causes of delayed puberty are shown in Table 2.

A plan for the investigation of delayed puberty is shown in Figure 8. Some individuals have signs of puberty at presentation and require no more than a measurement of height, assessment of pubertal stage and bone age with follow-up to make sure that puberty progresses. Children with no signs of puberty should have measurement of height, assessment of pubertal stage and bone age, measurements of gonadotrophin and prolactin concentrations

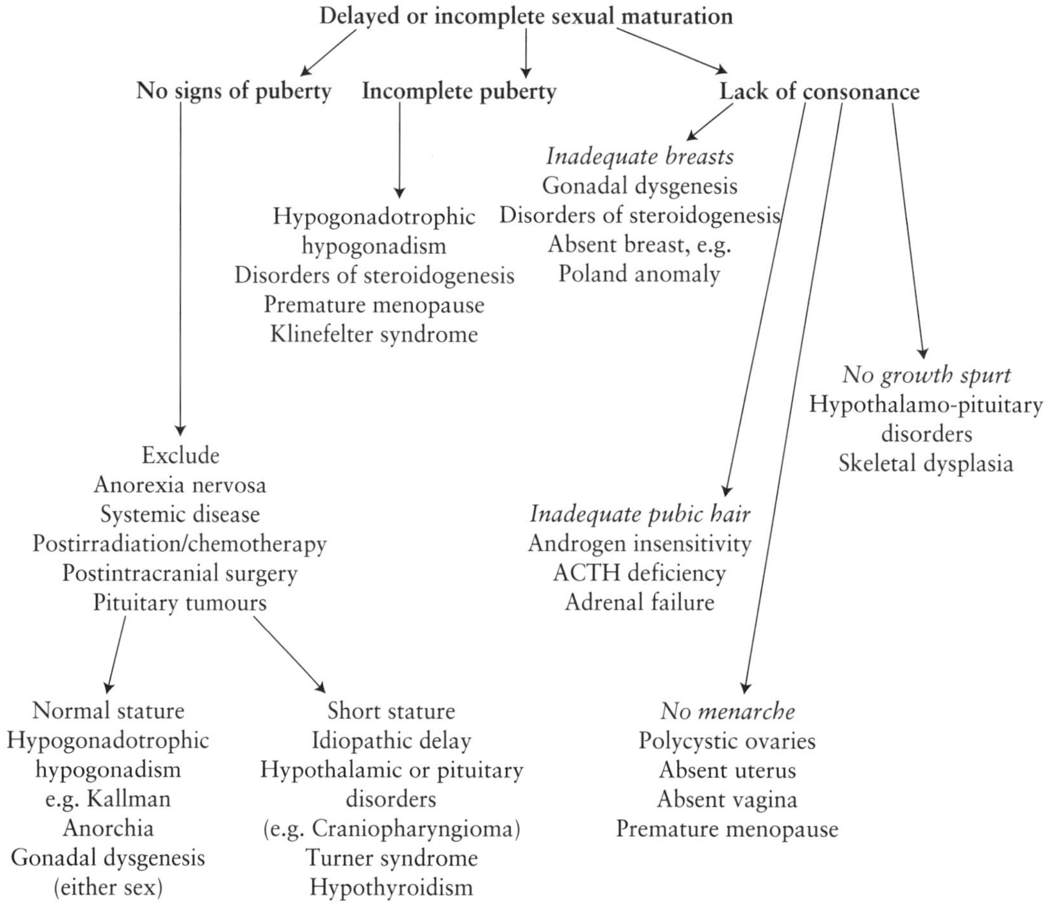


**Figure 8** Algorithm for the investigation of delayed puberty. ACTH = adrenocorticotrophic hormone

(to exclude a prolactinoma) and a test of thyroid function.

Basal concentrations of gonadotrophins will be expected to be low in children of pubertal age and are measured to exclude gonadal failure. There is no advantage in measuring the response of gonadotrophin to GnRH stimulation, since children with hypogonadotrophic hypogonadism may respond and children with constitutional delay of puberty may not do so. A 24-h profile of gonadotrophin secretion does not help the differential diagnosis. Since steroid levels are low for much of the day in early puberty, there is little point in measuring basal concentrations.

In girls, a pelvic ultrasound examination may help by showing signs of ovarian activity or a change in the shape of the uterus. Many girls with Turner syndrome do not have a typical phenotypic appearance and chromosomes should be checked if there is suspicion; for example, if the girl is unusually short when compared to her parents or if gonadotrophin concentrations are unexpectedly raised.

In children growing slowly in late prepuberty, there may be a temptation to undertake investigation of growth hormone secretion. This should be resisted because basal and stimulated levels are low at this time. If it is necessary to predict whether they will rise as spontaneous puberty is entered, a test of growth hormone secretion can be carried out after a dose of sex steroids has been administered or else a therapeutic trial of low-dose sex steroid treatment can be initiated to see if growth is induced.

### *Treatment of pubertal delay and pubertal failure*

The psychological problems associated with pubertal delay mean that treatment can be of benefit. In girls, a small dose of oestrogen given orally or transdermally often stimulates the hypothalamo–pituitary–ovarian axis and growth and breast development can be precipitated with very small doses of sex steroid (2–5 μg ethinyloestradiol orally) and no further intervention is needed after a short period. If pubertal development becomes arrested, a schedule of treatment is shown in Table 3.

Because the growth spurt in puberty in boys happens late, there is not only a problem with late puberty but also with late growth. As well as using testosterone to induce puberty (Table 3), it is possible to advance the onset of the growth spurt by using anabolic steroids. These precipitate a growth spurt which becomes sustained[18]. We have used pulsatile administration of GnRH to induce puberty in both boys and girls[17] but do not favour this for routine practice. Boys with anorchia may wish to have silicone implants to improve cosmetic appearance.

Growth hormone should not be used to treat the short stature of delayed puberty. Not only

**Table 3** Scheme for induction of puberty. These schema are designed to be introduced in the prepubertal patient aged 10+ years. They may be entered beyond the first dose in patients with arrested puberty but should not be accelerated on grounds of age alone

*Boys*

Testosterone esters (e.g. Sustanon)
- 50 mg i.m. every 6 weeks for 6 months
- 50 mg i.m. every 4 weeks for 6 months
- 100 mg i.m. every 4 weeks for 6 months
- 100 mg i.m. every 3 weeks for 6 months
- 250 mg i.m. every 4 weeks for 6 months

then as dictated by clinical state and measurements of trough concentrations of testosterone, luteinizing hormone and follicle stimulating hormone

*Girls*

Ethinyloestradiol
- 2 μg daily for 6 months
- 5 μg daily for 6 months
- 10 μg daily for 6 months
- 15 μg daily for 6 months*
- 20 μg daily for 6 months**
- 30 μg daily *sine die***

*A progestogen (e.g. levonorgestrel 30 μg daily for 1 week in 4) should be introduced at this stage or earlier if breakthrough bleeding supervenes; **these doses can be given in combination with a progestogen in an oral contraceptive pill but some infertile girls prefer to take two separate medications does it accelerate pubertal development[19] but it is also less effective in promoting final height as compared with small doses of anabolic steroids[18]. It should be reserved for patients with true insufficiency of growth hormone secretion developing at puberty.

Individuals with hypergonadotrophic hypogonadism should be treated with sex steroids to induce puberty at the normal time. The pubertal growth spurt induced by oestrogen in girls with Turner syndrome is less than in normal girls because of the skeletal dysplasia which is associated with the syndrome (and is no better when the puberty is spontaneous). There may be a place for the pharmacological action of growth hormone in this situation.

A child who arrests growth in puberty requires investigation to exclude a brain tumour. Some of these individuals have a hypothalamic defect which means that they can produce GnRH sufficient to start puberty but not to complete it[20]. The onset of severe illness, such as inflammatory bowel disease, can halt pubertal development, as can the development of anorexia nervosa.

Gynaecomastia is extremely common in puberty but, in some boys, especially in those in whom testicular testosterone secretion is inadequate, such as undiagnosed Klinefelter syndrome, the problem may be severe and cause great embarrassment. Mastectomy can cure the problem but if inadequate testosterone secretion is expected and hypergonadotrophic hypogonadism is likely to occur, gynaecomastia can be prevented by adequate testosterone treatment.

*Polycystic ovaries*

The endocrine and reproductive consequences of polycystic ovaries were described as the polycystic ovarian (Stein Leventhal) syndrome before the introduction of ultrasound. The introduction of this technique has demonstrated that 22–25% of adult women have ovaries with a polycystic appearance (Figure 9)[21]. While some women have symptoms referable to their polycystic ovaries, ranging from mild hirsutism and menstrual irregularity to classical polycystic ovarian syndrome (obesity, insulin resistance, excessive androgen secretion, amenorrhoea, hirsutism and acanthosis nigricans), many do not.

In children, the prevalence of polycystic ovary appearance at ultrasound rises from about 6% at 6 years of age to 22–25% at the end of puberty[3]. Many such affected children never have symptoms referable to their polycystic ovaries, but a few girls do develop the classic polycystic ovarian syndrome by the end of puberty and need to be treated in a way identical to that of adults. Polycystic ovaries are the most common cause of delayed menarche in girls who are otherwise well developed in puberty and some girls develop a pattern of irregular menses similar to that seen in some adult women with the condition.

There is no way to predict which child with polycystic ovaries will become symptomatic. Adolescents with polycystic ovaries on ultrasound should be encouraged to avoid becoming obese in order to avoid menstrual irregularities, insulin resistance and excessive androgen secretion. As long as a girl is well oestrogenized, has a normal bone mineral density and is happy, there is no need to induce cycle control just because of amenorrhoea secondary to polycystic ovaries.

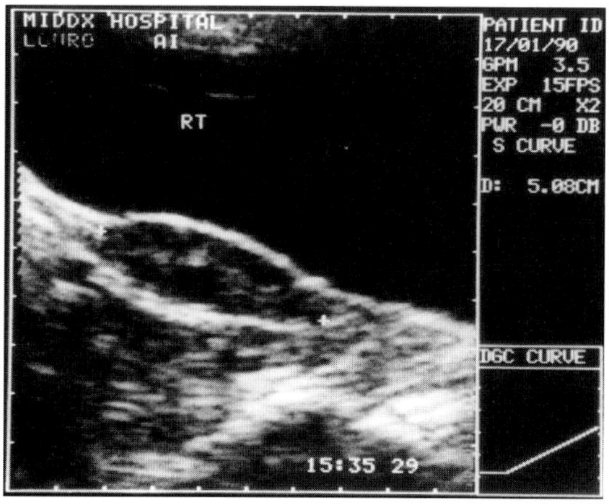


**Figure 9** Pelvic ultrasound appearance of polycystic ovary

## REFERENCES

1. Bridges, N. A., Matthews, D. R., Hindmarsh, P. C. and Brook, C. G. D. (1994). Changes in gonadotrophin secretion during childhood and puberty. *J. Endocrinol.*, **141**, 169–76
2. Gasser, T., Kohler, W., Muller, H. G., Largo, R., Molinari, L. and Prader, A. (1985). Human height growth: correlational and multivariate structure of velocity and acceleration. *Ann. Hum. Biol.*, **12**, 501–15
3. Bridges, N. A., Cooke, A., Healy, M. J. R., Hindmarsh, P. C. and Brook, C. G. D. (1993). Standards for ovarian volume in childhood and puberty. *Fertil. Steril.*, **60**, 456–60
4. Bridges, N. A. (1995). The endocrine and physical events of puberty. *D. M. Thesis*, University of Southampton
5. Dann, T. C. (1996). Trend towards earlier menarche stopped thirty years ago. *Br. Med. J.*, **312**, 1419
6. Billewicz, W. Z., Fellowes, M. and Thompson, A. M. (1981). Pubertal changes in boys and girls in Newcastle-upon-Tyne. *Ann. Hum. Biol.*, **8**, 211–19
7. Tanner, J. M., Whitehouse, R. H. and Takaishi, M. (1966). Standards from birth to maturity for height weight height velocity and weight velocity: British children 1965. *Arch. Dis. Child.*, **41**, 454–71 and 613–35
8. Marshall, W. A. (1974). Interrelationships of skeletal maturation, sexual development and somatic growth in man. *Ann. Hum. Biol.*, **1**, 29–40
9. Bridges, N. A., Christopher, J. A., Hindmarsh, P. C. and Brook, C. G. D. (1994). Sexual precocity: sex incidence and aetiology. *Arch. Dis. Child.*, **70**, 116–18
10. Freedman, S. M., Kreitzer, B. M., Elkowitz, S. S., Soberman, N. and Leonidas, J. C. (1993). Ovarian microcysts in girls with isolated premature thelarche. *J. Pediatr.*, **122**, 246–9
11. Stanhope, R., Abdulwahid, N. A., Adams, J. and Brook, C. G. D. (1986). Studies of gonadotrophin pulsatility in pelvic ultrasound examinations distinguish between isolated premature thelarche in central precocious puberty. *Eur. J. Pediatr.*, **145**, 190–4
12. Stanhope, R. and Brook, C. G. D. (1990). Thelarche variant: a new syndrome of precocious sexual development? *Acta Endocrinol.*, **123**, 480–6
13. Fontoura, M., Brauner, R., Prevot, C. and Rappaport, R. (1989). Precocious puberty in girls: early diagnosis of a slowly progressing variant. *Arch. Dis. Child.*, **64**, 1170–6
14. Shenker, A., Laue, L., Kosugi, S., Merendino, J. J., Minegishi, T. and Cutler, G. B. (1993). A constitutively activating mutation of the luteinising hormone receptor in familial male precocious puberty. *Nature (London)*, **365**, 652–4
15. Weinstein, L. S., Shenka, A., Gejman, P. V., Mareno, M. J., Friedman, E. and Spiegel, A. M. (1991). Activating mutations of the stimulatory G protein in the McCune-Albright syndrome. *N. Engl. J. Med.*, **325**, 1688–95
16. Bridges, N. A., Cooke, A., Healy, M. J. R., Hindmarsh, P. C. and Brook, C. G. D. (1995). Ovaries in sexual precocity. *Clin. Endocrinol.*, **42**, 135–40
17. Stanhope, R., Brook, C. G. D., Pringle, P. J., Adams, J. and Jacobs, H. S. (1987). Induction of puberty by pulsatile GnRH. *Lancet*, **2**, 552–5
18. Buyukgebiz, A., Hindmarsh, P. C. and Brook, C. G. D. (1990). Treatment of constitutional delay of growth and puberty with oxandrolone compared with growth hormone. *Arch. Dis. Child.*, **65**, 448–52
19. Darendeliler, F., Hindmarsh, P. C., Preece, M. A., Cox, L. and Brook, C. G. D. (1990). Growth hormone increases the rate of pubertal maturation. *Acta Endocrinol.*, **122**, 414–16
20. Barkan, A. L., Reame, N. E., Kelch, R. P. and Marshall, J. C. (1985). Idiopathic hypogonadotrophic hypogonadism in men: dependence of the hormone responses to GnRH on the magnitude of the endogenous GnRH secretory defect. *J. Clin. Endocrinol. Metab.*, **61**, 1118–25
21. Polson, D. W., Adams, J., Wadsworth, J. and Franks, S. (1988). Polycystic ovaries: a common finding in normal women. *Lancet*, **1**, 870–2

# Amenorrhoea and anovulation 4

*Adam H. Balen*

## INTRODUCTION

Amenorrhoea is the absence of menstruation, either temporarily or permanently. It may occur as a normal physiological condition, before puberty or during pregnancy, lactation or the menopause, or as a feature of a systemic or gynaecological disorder. In this chapter, we outline a classification of amenorrhoea (Table 1) and the management of the different causes, with particular reference to its occurrence during the reproductive years.

## PRIMARY AMENORRHOEA

Failure to menstruate by the age of 16 in the presence of normal secondary sexual development, or 14 in the absence of secondary sexual characteristics, warrants investigation[1]. This distinction helps to differentiate reproductive tract anomalies from gonadal quiescence and gonadal failure. Primary amenorrhoea may be a result of congenital abnormalities in the development of ovaries, genital tract or external genitalia or a disturbance of the normal endocrinological events of puberty. However, most of the causes of secondary amenorrhoea can also cause primary amenorrhoea, if they occur before the menarche. Delayed puberty is often constitutional, but it is important to exclude primary ovarian failure or hypothalamic/pituitary dysfunction[2]. Overall it is estimated that endocrine disorders account for approximately 40% of the causes of primary amenorrhoea, the remaining 60% having developmental abnormalities[3] (Table 2).

**Table 1** Classification of amenorrhoea

| | |
|---|---|
| Hypothalamic | functional<br>weight-related, exercise-related<br>tumours<br>hypogonadotrophic hypogonadism (Kallman's syndrome) |
| Pituitary | tumours (non-functional)<br>hyperprolactinomas<br>hypopituitarism |
| Ovarian | polycystic ovary syndrome<br>ovarian failure |
| Uterine | Asherman's syndrome<br>congenital anomalies |
| General | chemo/radiotherapy<br>debilitating illness |

## SECONDARY AMENORRHOEA

Cessation of menstruation for 6 consecutive months in a woman who has previously had regular periods is the usual criterion for investigation. However, more recently 3 or 4 months

**Table 2** The aetiology of primary amenorrhoea in 90 consecutive patients attending the Endocrine Clinic at the Middlesex Hospital

| *Cause* | % |
|---|---|
| Premature (primary) ovarian failure | 36 |
| Hypogonadotrophic hypogonadism | 34 |
| Polycystic ovary syndrome | 17 |
| Hypopituitarism | 4 |
| Hyperprolactinaemia | 3 |
| Weight-related amenorrhoea | 2 |
| Congenital abnormalities | 4 |

of amenorrhoea has been considered pathological[4,5]. Women with secondary amenorrhoea must have a patent lower genital tract, an endometrium that is responsive to ovarian hormone stimulation and ovaries that have responded to pituitary gonadotrophins (Table 3).

## HISTORY, EXAMINATION AND INVESTIGATION OF AMENORRHOEA

A thorough history and a careful examination of stature and body form, secondary sexual development and external genitalia should always be carried out before further investigations are instigated. A history of secondary amenorrhoea may be misleading, as the 'periods' may have been the result of exogenous hormone administration. In most cases, however, a history of secondary amenorrhoea excludes congenital abnormalities. A family history of fertility problems, autoimmune disorders or premature menopause may also give clues to the aetiology.

A bimanual examination is inappropriate in a young woman who has never been sexually active, and examination of the external genitalia of an adolescent should be undertaken in the presence of a patient's mother. Furthermore, it may be more appropriate to defer this from the first consultation in order to assure sensitivity in future management. A transabdominal ultrasound examination of the pelvis is an excellent non-invasive method of obtaining valuable information in these patients. However, examination under anaesthetic is sometimes indicated, particularly in cases of intersex.

**Table 3** The aetiology of secondary amenorrhoea in 570 patients attending the Endocrine Clinic at the Middlesex Hospital

| *Cause* | % |
|---|---|
| Polycystic ovary syndrome | 36.9 |
| Premature ovarian failure | 23.6 |
| Hyperprolactinaemia | 16.9 |
| Weight-related amenorrhoea | 9.8 |
| Hypogonadotrophic hypogonadism | 5.9 |
| Hypopituitarism | 4.4 |
| Exercise-related amenorrhoea | 2.5 |

When it has been established that the internal and external genitalia are normally developed, it is important to exclude pregnancy in women of any age. Measurements of height and weight should be taken in order to calculate a patient's body mass index (BMI). The normal range is 20–25 kg/m$^2$, and a value above or below this range may suggest a diagnosis of weight-related amenorrhoea (which is a term usually applied to underweight women).

A baseline assessment in all patients should include measurement of serum prolactin and gonadotrophin concentrations and an assessment of thyroid function. Prolactin levels may be elevated in response to a number of conditions, including stress, a recent breast examination, or even having a blood test. However, such elevation is moderate and transient. A more permanent, but still moderate, elevation (> 700 IU) can be associated with hypothyroidism and is also a common finding in women with polycystic ovary syndrome (PCOS), in which prolactin levels up to 2000 IU/l have been reported[6]. PCOS may also result in amenorrhoea, which can therefore create diagnostic difficulties, and hence difficulties with appropriate management, for those women with hyperprolactinaemia and polycystic ovaries. Amenorrhoea in women with PCOS is secondary to acyclical ovarian activity and continuous oestrogen production. A positive response to a progestogen challenge test[7], which induces a withdrawal bleed, will distinguish patients with PCOS-related hyperprolactinaemia from those with polycystic ovaries and unrelated hyperprolactinaemia, because the latter causes oestrogen deficiency and therefore failure to respond to the progestogen challenge.

A serum prolactin concentration of > 1500 IU/l warrants further investigation. Computerized tomography or magnetic resonance imaging of the pituitary fossa may be used to exclude a hypothalamic tumour, a non-functioning pituitary tumour compressing the hypothalamus or a prolactinoma. Serum prolactin concentrations of > 5000 IU/l are usually associated with a macroprolactinoma, which by definition is > 1 cm in diameter.

The patient's oestrogen status may be assessed clinically by examination of the lower genital tract, or by means of a progestogen challenge[8]. Serum measurements of oestradiol are unhelpful, as they vary considerably, even in a patient with amenorrhoea. If the patient is well oestrogenized, the endometrium will be shed on withdrawal of the progestogen.

Serum gonadotrophin measurements help to distinguish between cases of hypothalamic or pituitary failure and gonadal failure. Elevated gonadotrophin concentrations indicate a failure of negative feedback as a result of primary ovarian failure. A serum follicle stimulating hormone (FSH) concentration of > 15 IU/l that is not associated with a preovulatory surge suggests impending ovarian failure. FSH levels of > 40 IU/l are suggestive of irreversible ovarian failure. The exact values vary according to individual assays, and so local reference levels should be checked[9].

An elevated luteinizing hormone (LH) concentration, when associated with a raised FSH concentration, is indicative of ovarian failure. However, if LH is elevated alone (and is not attributable to the preovulatory LH surge), this suggests PCOS. This may be confirmed by a pelvic ultrasound scan[10]. Rarely, an elevated LH level in a phenotypic female may be due to testicular feminization (androgen resistance syndrome).

Failure at the level of the hypothalamus or pituitary is reflected by abnormally low levels of serum gonadotrophin concentrations, and gives rise to hypogonadotrophic hypogonadism. Kallman's syndrome is the clinical finding of hyposmia and/or colour blindness associated with hypogonadotrophic hypogonadism. It is difficult to distinguish between hypothalamic and pituitary aetiology, as both respond to stimulation with gonadotrophin releasing hormone (GnRH). A skull X-ray should be performed, and computerized tomography (CT) or magnetic resonance imaging (MRI), if indicated.

Karyotyping of women with primary amenorrhoea, or those under 30 with gonadotrophin levels compatible with premature ovarian failure, should be performed, as some chromosomal abnormalities (e.g. Turner's syndrome) may be associated with premature ovarian failure. An autoantibody screen should also be undertaken in women with a premature menopause (under the age of 40 years).

A history of a recent endometrial curettage or endometritis in a patient with normal genitalia and normal endocrinology, but with absent or only a small withdrawal bleed following a progestogen challenge, is suggestive of Asherman's syndrome. Hysteroscopy will confirm the diagnosis.

Measurement of bone mineral density is indicated in amenorrhoeic women who are oestrogen deficient. Measurements of density are made at the lumbar spine and femoral neck. The vertebral bone is more sensitive to oestrogen deficiency and vertebral fractures tend to occur in a younger age group (50–60 years) than fractures at the femoral neck (70+ years). However, it should be noted that crush fractures can spuriously increase the measured bone mineral density. An X-ray of the dorsolumbar spine is therefore often complementary, particularly in patients who have lost height.

Amenorrhoea may also have long-term metabolic and physical consequences. In women with PCOS and prolonged amenorrhoea, there is a risk of endometrial hyperplasia and adenocarcinoma. If, on resumption of menstruation, there is a history of persistent intermenstrual bleeding, or, on ultrasound examination, there is a postmenstrual endometrial thickness of > 10 mm, then an endometrial biopsy is indicated.

Serum cholesterol measurements are important because of the association of an increased risk of heart disease in women with premature ovarian failure. Women with PCOS[11], although not oestrogen deficient, may have a subnormal high-density lipoprotein (HDL) : total cholesterol ratio. This is a consequence of the hypersecretion of insulin that occurs in many women with PCOS, and may increase the lifetime risk of heart disease.

## PRIMARY AMENORRHOEA DUE TO DEVELOPMENTAL ABNORMALITIES

### Turner's syndrome

Turner's syndrome is the commonest cause of gonadal dysgenesis. In its most severe form the XO genotype is associated with the classical Turner's features, including short stature, webbing of the neck, cubitus valgus, widely spaced nipples, cardiac and renal abnormalities and often autoimmune hypothyroidism[12]. Spontaneous menstruation may occur (particularly when there is mosaicism), but premature ovarian failure usually ensues. It is important to determine the karyotype, because the presence of a Y chromosome in an individual with gonadal dysgenesis necessitates removal of gonadal tissue because of an increased risk of malignancy[13]. Serum gonadotrophin concentrations are elevated compared with levels in adolescents of the same age and may approach the menopausal range.

Management includes low-dose oestrogen therapy to promote breast development without further disturbing linear growth[14]. Treatment with growth hormone has also benefited some individuals[15]. Cyclical oestrogen plus progestogen may be used as maintenance therapy. A regular withdrawal bleed is essential in order to prevent endometrial hyperplasia. Spontaneous conception has been reported in patients with Turner's syndrome, but is rare. However, the possibility of assisted conception and oocyte donation[16] should be discussed at an early age.

### Müllerian duct abnormalities

In the absence of a Y chromosome, testis and testosterone, the Wolffian ducts regress after the 6th week of embryonic life[17]. The Müllerian ducts then develop into the uterus and Fallopian tubes, and fuse caudally with the urogenital sinus to form the vagina. Abnormalities in the process of fusion may be either medial or vertical and result in primary amenorrhoea[18]; complete or partial Müllerian agenesis may also occur. Renal developmental abnormalities are commonly seen in association with abnormalities of the genital tract, so assessment by intravenous urography is advisable before corrective surgery is attempted[19].

Women with Müllerian agenesis (Mayer–Rokitansky–Kuster–Hauser syndrome) have a 46,XX genotype and a normal female phenotype, with spontaneous development of secondary sexual characteristics, as ovarian tissue is present and functions normally. The external genitalia have a normal appearance, but the vagina is short and blind-ending, such that either surgery or gradual dilatation is necessary to achieve a capacity appropriate for normal sexual function. Hormone treatment is not required, as ovarian oestrogen output is normal. Indeed, ovulation occurs and oocyte retrieval could theoretically be performed in order to achieve a 'biological' pregnancy through the services of a surrogate mother.

Girls who are phenotypically normal but have absent pubic and axillary hair in the presence of normal breast development have androgen insensitivity (testicular feminization syndrome). In this condition, the karyotype is 46,XY and, whilst testes are present, there is an insensitivity to secreted androgens because of abnormalities in the androgen receptors. After puberty gonadal tissue should be removed to prevent malignant transformation, which occurs in about 5% of cases[20]. Exogenous oestrogen should then be prescribed; cyclical treatment is not required, because the uterus is absent. The syndrome may be diagnosed in infancy if a testis is found in either the labia or an inguinal hernia, in which case both testes should be removed at this time, because of the potential risk of malignancy. Some cases, however, only present at puberty with primary amenorrhoea, and removal of abdominal testes should then be performed.

Careful psychological assessment and counselling is obligatory to allow an understanding of the gonadal dysfunction and necessity for hormone treatment. It may be helpful to describe the gonads as ovaries that have been incompletely formed and which are therefore prone to develop cancer if they are not removed. Surgery may be necessary to enable sexual function. Patients with these problems should be referred to centres where there are specialists experienced in these conditions, where a comprehensive team approach can be provided[21].

There are several uncommon intersex disorders that result in primary amenorrhoea and, although their management must be individualized, it will often broadly follow the above outline. Examples are male pseudohermaphroditism caused by 5α-reductase deficiency, and female pseudohermaphroditism, caused by congenital adrenal hyperplasia. In contrast to the testicular feminization syndrome, in these conditions there is deficient or absent breast development, yet normal or increased pubic and axillary hair[22].

Amenorrhoea, secondary to an imperforate hymen or transverse vaginal septum, presents classically with cyclical abdominal pain and swelling. Surgical correction is usually straightforward, although damage may have already occurred to the Fallopian tubes as a result of retrograde menstrual flow. When there is a transverse septum it has been found to be high in 46% of patients, in the middle of the vagina in 40% and low in the remaining 14%. It is the patients in the last two groups who have higher pregnancy rates after surgery[23].

## HYPOTHALAMIC CAUSES OF PRIMARY AMENORRHOEA

Kallman's syndrome is an autosomal dominant condition that causes isolated deficiency of GnRH secretion and is associated with hyposmia and colour blindness. Pubertal development does not occur spontaneously and should be induced with low-dose oestrogen therapy followed by a cyclical oestrogen/progesterone preparation[2]. If the patient is particularly anxious about future fertility, a non-therapeutic trial of exogenous pulsatile GnRH administration, via a miniature portable infusion pump[24], confirms pituitary responsiveness. However, induction of ovulation can be achieved, bypassing the pituitary, by direct administration of either human menopausal gonadotrophin (hMG) (Humegon, Organon, UK) or with recombinant FSH (Puregon, Organon, UK). However, hMG is a more suitable choice for these patients, as it also contains LH, which is necessary to stimulate oestrogen biosynthesis[25].

## SECONDARY AMENORRHOEA

### Genital tract abnormalities

Asherman's syndrome is a condition in which intrauterine adhesions prevent normal growth of the endometrium[26]. This may be the result of a too vigorous endometrial curettage, or may follow endometritis. Typically amenorrhoea is not absolute, and it may be possible to induce a withdrawal bleed. Diagnosis and treatment by adhesiolysis is carried out hysteroscopically. Following surgery, a 3-month course of cyclical progesterone/oestrogen should be given. Some clinicians insert a Foley catheter into the uterine cavity for 7–10 days postoperatively[1], or an intrauterine contraceptive device for 2–3 months[27], in order to prevent recurrence of adhesions.

Cervical stenosis is an occasional cause of secondary amenorrhoea. It was relatively common following a traditional cone biopsy for the treatment of cervical intraepithelial neoplasia. However, modern procedures, such as laser or loop diathermy, have fewer postoperative cervical complications[28]. Treatment for cervical stenosis consists of careful cervical dilatation.

### Systemic disorders causing secondary amenorrhoea

Chronic disease may result in menstrual disorders as a consequence of the general disease state, weight loss or the effect of the disease process on the hypothalamic–pituitary axis. Furthermore, a chronic disease that leads to immobility, such as chronic obstructive airways disease, may increase the risk of amenorrhoea-associated osteoporosis.

In addition, certain diseases affect gonadal function directly. Women with chronic renal failure have a discordantly elevated LH[29], possibly as a consequence of impaired clearance[30]. Prolactin is also elevated in these women, due to failure of normal dopamine inhibition.

Diabetes mellitus may result in functional hypothalamic–pituitary amenorrhoea[31]. Liver disease affects the level of circulating sex hormone binding globulin, and thus free hormone levels, thereby disrupting the normal feedback mechanisms. Metabolism of various hormones, including testosterone, is also liver dependent; both menstruation and fertility return after liver transplantation[32].

Endocrine disorders such as thyrotoxicosis and Cushing's syndrome are commonly associated with gonadal dysfunction[33]. Autoimmune endocrinopathies may be associated with premature ovarian failure, because of ovarian antibodies.

Management of these patients should concentrate on the underlying systemic problem and on preventing complications of oestrogen deficiency. If fertility is required, it is desirable to achieve maximal health and, where possible, to discontinue the use of teratogenic drugs.

### Weight-related amenorrhoea

Weight can have profound effects on gonadotrophin regulation and release. Weight disorders are common. In one study up to 35% of women attending a London endocrine clinic had secondary amenorrhoea associated with weight loss[22]. The normal BMI is 20–25 kg/m$^2$. A regular menstrual cycle will not occur if the BMI is less than 19 kg/m$^2$. Fat appears to be critical to a normally functioning hypothalamic–pituitary–gonadal axis. It is estimated that at least 22% of body weight should be fat in order to maintain ovulatory cycles[34]. This level enables the extra-ovarian aromatization of androgens to oestrogens, and maintains appropriate feedback control of the hypothalamic–pituitary–ovarian axis[35]. Therefore, girls who are significantly underweight prior to puberty may have primary amenorrhoea, whilst those who are significantly underweight after puberty will have secondary amenorrhoea.

The clinical presentation depends upon the severity of the nutritional insult and its age of onset. To cause amenorrhoea, the loss must be 10–15% of the women's normal weight for height. Weight loss may be due to a number of causes, including self-induced abstinence, starvation, illness and exercise. However, whatever the precipitating cause, the net result is impairment of gonadotrophin secretion[36]. In severe weight loss, oestrogen may be catabolized to the anti-oestrogen 2-hydroxy-oestrone, rather than to the usual oestradiol, which may further suppress gonadotrophin secretion. This pathway is enhanced by cigarette smoking. Weight-related gonadotrophin deficiency is more pronounced with LH than with FSH[37]. This and the reduction in pulsatility of gonadotrophin secretion may result in a 'multicystic' pattern in the ovary. This appearance is typical of normal puberty and is seen when there are several cysts (about 5–10 mm in diameter) together with a stroma of normal density.

Studies have documented the prevalence of weight-related amenorrhoea to be between 9.8% and 35%[14,22,38–40]. Anorexia nervosa is at the extreme end of a spectrum of eating disorders and is invariably accompanied by menstrual disturbance; indeed, it may account for between 15 and 35% of patients with amenorrhoea. Women with anorexia nervosa should be managed in collaboration with a psychiatrist, and it is essential to encourage weight gain as the main therapy.

An artificial cycle may be induced with the combined oral contraceptive. However, this may corroborate the denial of weight loss as being the underlying problem. Similarly, although it is possible to induce ovulation with GnRH[41] or exogenous gonadotrophins[42], treatment of infertility in the significantly underweight patient is associated with a significant increase in intrauterine growth retardation and neonatal problems[42,43]. Furthermore, since three-quarters of the cell divisions that occur during pregnancy do so during the first trimester, it is essential that nutritional status is optimized before conception. Low birth weight is also now being related to an increased risk of cardiovascular disease, obstructive lung disease and schizophrenia in adult life[44].

Weight-related amenorrhoea may also have profound long-term effects on bone mineral density[45]. Oestrogen deficiency, reduced calcium and protein intake, reduced levels of vitamin D[46] and elevated cortisol levels[47] can all contribute to osteoporosis. The age of onset of anorexia nervosa is also important, as prolonged amenorrhoea before the normal age at which peak bone mass is obtained (approximately 25 years) increases the likelihood of severe osteoporosis.

World-wide, involuntary starvation is the commonest cause of reduced reproductive ability, resulting in delayed pubertal growth and menarche in adolescents[48] and infertility in adults. Acute malnutrition, as seen in famine conditions and during and after the Second World War, has profound effects on fertility and fecundity[35]. Ovulatory function usually returns quickly on restoration of adequate nutrition. The chronic malnutrition common in developing countries has less profound effects on fertility, but is associated with small and premature babies.

### Psychological stress

Studies have failed to demonstrate a link between stressful life events and amenorrhoea of longer than 2 months[40]. However, stress may lead to physical debility such as weight loss, which may then cause menstrual disturbance.

### Exercise-related amenorrhoea

Menstrual disturbance is common in athletes undergoing intensive training. Between 10 and 20% have oligomenorrhoea or amenorrhoea, compared with 5% in the general population[49]. Amenorrhoea is more common in athletes of under 30 years and is particularly common in women involved in endurance events (such as long-distance running). Up to 50% of competitive runners training 80 miles (approximately 130 km) per week may be amenorrhoeic[50].

The main aetiological factors are weight and percentage body fat content, but other factors have also been postulated. Physiological changes are consistent with those associated with starvation and chronic illness. In order to conserve energy, there may be a fall in thyroid-stimulating hormone (TSH), a reduction in tri-iodothyronine (T3) and an elevation of the inactive reverse-T3[51]. Exercise also leads to a fall in levels of circulating insulin and insulin-like growth factor-1 (IGF-1), and therefore decreases their stimulation of the pituitary and ovary. Prolactin and circulating androgen levels show no consistent changes with exercise.

Ballet dancers provide an interesting, and much studied, subgroup of sportswomen, because their training begins at an early age. They have been found to have a significant delay in menarche (15.4 compared to 12.5 years) and a retardation in pubertal development that parallels the intensity of their training[52]. Menstrual irregularities are common and up to 44% have secondary amenorrhoea[53]. In a survey of 75 dancers 61% were found to have stress fractures and 24% had scoliosis; the risk of these pathological features was increased if menarche was delayed or if there were prolonged periods of amenorrhoea[53]. These findings may be explained by delayed pubertal maturation, resulting in attainment of a greater than expected height and a predisposition to scoliosis, as oestrogen is required for epiphyseal closure.

Exercise-induced amenorrhoea has the potential to cause severe long-term morbidity, particularly with regard to osteoporosis. Studies on young ballet dancers have shown that the amount of exercise undertaken by these dancers does not compensate for these osteoporotic changes[53]. Oestrogen is also important in the formation of collagen, and soft tissue injuries are also common in dancers[54].

Whereas moderate exercise has been found to reduce the incidence of postmenopausal osteoporosis[55], young athletes may be placing themselves at risk at an age when the attainment of peak bone mass is important for long-term skeletal strength. Appropriate advice should be given, particularly regarding diet, and the use of a cyclical oestrogen/progestogen preparation should be considered.

### Hypothalamic causes of secondary amenorrhoea

Hypothalamic causes of amenorrhoea may be either primary or secondary. Primary hypothalamic lesions include craniopharyngiomas, germinomas, gliomas and dermoid cysts. These hypothalamic lesions either disrupt the normal pathway of prolactin inhibitory factor (dopamine), thus causing hyperprolactinaemia, or compress and/or destroy hypothalamic and pituitary tissue. Treatment is usually surgical, with additional radiotherapy if required. Hormone replacement therapy is required to mimic ovarian function and, if the pituitary gland is damaged either by the lesion or by the treatment, replacement thyroid and adrenal hormones are required.

Secondary hypogonadotrophic hypogonadism may result from systemic conditions including sarcoidosis and tuberculosis, as well as following head injury or cranial irradiation. Sheehan's syndrome, the result of profound and prolonged hypotension on the sensitive pituitary gland, enlarged by pregnancy, may also be a cause of hypogonadotrophic hypogonadism in someone with a history of a major obstetric haemorrhage[56]. It is essential to assess pituitary function fully in all these patients and then instigate the appropriate replacement therapy. Ovulation may be induced with hMG or pulsatile subcutaneous GnRH.

### Pituitary causes of secondary amenorrhoea

Hyperprolactinaemia is the commonest pituitary cause of amenorrhoea. This may be physiological as during lactation, iatrogenic or pathological. A non-functioning tumour in the region of the hypothalamus or pituitary, which disrupts the inhibitory influence of dopamine on prolactin secretion, and pituitary adenomas, will both cause hyperprolactinomas. Other known causes are certain drugs, particularly prothiazines and metoclopramide that act as dopamine antagonists.

In women with amenorrhoea associated with hyperprolactinaemia the main symptoms are usually those of oestrogen deficiency[57]. In contrast, when hyperprolactinaemia is associated with PCOS, the syndrome is characterized by adequate oestrogenization, polycystic ovaries on ultrasound scan and a withdrawal bleed in response to a progestogen challenge test. Galactorrhoea may be found in up to a third of hyperprolactinaemic patients, although its appearance is neither correlated with prolactin levels nor with the presence of a tumour[58]. Approximately 5% of patients present with visual field defects[59].

Prolactin-secreting microadenomas are usually associated with a moderately elevated prolactin level (1500–4000 mU/l) and are unlikely to show up on a lateral skull X-ray. Macroadenomas, however, are associated with a prolactin level of > 5000 IU/l, and are by definition > 1 cm in diameter. On lateral skull X-ray the typical appearance is of an asymmetrically enlarged pituitary fossa, with a double contour to its floor and erosion of the clinoid processes. CT and MRI scans now allow detailed examination of the extent of the tumour and any suprasellar extension.

The management of hyperprolactinaemia is by the use of a dopamine antagonist, usually bromocriptine. Other longer-acting preparations are available to patients who develop unacceptable side affects such as nausea, vomiting, headache and postural hypotension[60]. If the hyperprolactinaemia is drug induced, the relevant preparation should be changed. Surgery is reserved for those patients with pituitary tumours who are unresponsive to drug treatment or who are unable to tolerate it. Transsphenoidal adenectomy is also required if there is suprasellar extension of the tumour that has not regressed during treatment with bromocriptine.

Women with a microadenoma who wish to conceive can stop bromocriptine treatment when pregnancy is diagnosed, without further monitoring, as tumour expansion is unlikely. However, macroadenomas have a 25% chance of expanding during pregnancy if bromocriptine treatment has not been instigated. In cases with suprasellar expansion, follow-up CT or MRI scanning should be performed after three months of treatment to ensure tumour regression, before it is safe to embark on pregnancy. Only if there is continuing suprasellar expansion is it necessary to continue with bromocriptine during pregnancy, and it is these patients alone who also require expert assessment of their visual fields during pregnancy.

Most patients with hyperprolactinaemia need treatment in order to correct amenorrhoea and oestrogen deficiency, improve libido and achieve tumour shrinkage. If the patient taking bromocriptine requires contraception, it is safe to prescribe a combined contraceptive preparation containing up to 30–35 μg of ethinyloestradiol. If the serum prolactin level is found to be elevated and the patient has a regular cycle, no treatment is necessary, unless the cycle is anovulatory and fertility is desired. Amenorrhoea is the 'bioassay' of prolactin excess and should be corrected for its sequelae, rather than for the serum level of prolactin. Since the finding of osteoporosis in association with hyperprolactinaemia, there has been a debate as to whether the hyperprolactinaemia itself has a direct effect on bone[61]. Current thinking is that it is the degree of oestrogen deficiency rather than prolactin excess that is important; decalcification is reversible to an extent that is dependent on the preceding duration of amenorrhoea[62]. Hyperprolactinaemic women with regular cycles have a normal bone mineral content.

**Ovarian causes of amenorrhoea**

*Premature ovarian failure*

Ovarian failure, by definition, is the cessation of periods accompanied by raised gonadotrophin levels prior to the age of 40 years. It may occur at any age. The exact incidence of this condition is unknown, as many cases go unrecognized, but estimates vary at 1–5% of the female population. Studies of amenorrhoeic women report the incidence of premature ovarian failure to be 10–36%[63].

Chromosomal abnormalities are common in women with primary amenorrhoea. Hague and colleagues[64] found chromosomal abnormalities in 70% of patients with primary amenorrhoea and in 2–5% of women with secondary amenorrhoea due to premature ovarian failure. Ovarian failure occurring before puberty is usually due to a chromosomal abnormality, or a childhood malignancy that required chemotherapy or radiotherapy. Adolescents who lose ovarian function soon after menarche are often found to have a Turner's mosaic (46,XX/45,X) or an X-chromosome trisomy (47,XXX).

Overall, the most common cause of premature ovarian failure is autoimmune disease, with infection, previous surgery, chemo- and radiotherapy also contributing to the aetiology of premature ovarian failure. Ovarian autoantibodies can be measured and have been found in up to 69% of cases of premature ovarian failure. However, the assay is expensive and not readily available in most units. It is therefore important to consider other autoimmune disorders, and screen for autoantibodies to the thyroid gland, gastric mucosa parietal cells and adrenal gland, if there is any clinical indication[65].

Prior to the absolute cessation of periods of true premature ovarian failure, some women experience an intermittent return to menses, interspersed between variable periods of amenorrhoea. Gonadotrophin levels usually remain moderately elevated during these spontaneous cycles, with plasma FSH levels of 15–20 IU/l[66]. This occult ovarian failure, or resistant ovary syndrome, is associated with the presence of primordial follicles on ovarian biopsy, and pregnancies are sometimes achieved, although the ovaries are usually resistant to exogenous gonadotrophins as they are to endogenous hormones. It is probable that reports of pregnancy in women with premature ovarian failure represent cases of fluctuating ovarian function rather than successes of treatment.

It is possible, however, to achieve pregnancy by oocyte donation, as part of *in vitro* fertilization treatment[67]. Experimental work in animals has succeeded in transplanting primordial follicles into irradiated ovaries, with subsequent ovulation and normal pregnancy. This is obviously still a remote prospect in humans, even if it were considered to be ethically acceptable[68].

The diagnosis and consequences of premature ovarian failure require careful counselling of the patient. It may be particularly difficult for a young woman to accept the need to take oestrogen preparations that are clearly labelled as being intended for older postmenopausal women, whilst at the same time having to come to terms with the inability to conceive naturally. The short- and long-term consequences of ovarian failure and oestrogen deficiency are similar to those occurring in the 5th and 6th decades. However, the duration of the problem is much longer and therefore hormone replacement therapy is advisable to reduce the consequences of oestrogen deficiency in the long-term.

Younger women with premature loss of ovarian function have an increased risk of osteoporosis. A recent study[69] of 200 amenorrhoeic women between the ages of 16 and 40 demonstrated a mean reduction in bone mineral density of 15% as compared with a control group and after correction for body weight, smoking and exercise. The degree of bone loss was correlated with the duration of the amenorrhoea and the severity of the oestrogen deficiency, rather than the underlying diagnosis, and was worse in patients with primary amenorrhoea compared with those with secondary amenorrhoea. A return to normal oestrogen status may improve bone mass, but bone mineral density is unlikely to improve more than 5–10% and it probably does not return to its normal value. However, it is not certain if the radiological improvement seen will actually reduce the risk of fracture, as remineralization is not equivalent to the restrengthening of bone. Early diagnosis and early correction of oestrogen status is therefore important.

Underproduction of progesterone may also be important in the pathogenesis of osteoporosis. Progesterone promotes bone formation and accelerates remodelling, whereas oestrogen acts to prevent bone resorption and decrease remodelling through receptors on the osteoblasts. Therefore, an intact ovulatory unit is optimal for normal bone formation.

Women with premature ovarian failure have an increased risk of cardiovascular disease. Oestrogens (HRT) have been shown to have beneficial effects on cardiovascular status in women. They increase the levels of cardioprotective HDL but also total triglyceride levels, whilst decreasing total cholesterol and low density lipoprotein (LDL) levels. The overall effect is of cardiovascular protection.

Women with hypo-oestrogenic amenorrhoea require hormone replacement. A cyclical oestrogen/progestogen preparation is required for patients with a uterus, in order to prevent endometrial hyperplasia, which is a high-risk consequence of prolonged unopposed oestrogen therapy. The hormone replacement preparations prescribed for menopausal women are also preferred for young women. The reason for this is that even modern low-dose combined oral contraception preparations contain at least twice the amount of oestrogen that is recommended for hormone replacement therapy, in order to achieve a contraceptive suppressive effect on the hypothalamic–pituitary axis. Hormone replacement therapy also contains 'natural' oestrogens rather than the synthetic ethinyloestradiol that is found in most combined oral contraceptives[70].

It should be noted that there is mounting evidence to suggest a slight increase in the risk of developing breast cancer with longer durations of hormone replacement therapy[71,72]. However, it is difficult to extrapolate these large studies to small numbers of younger women who constitute a separate population with different risk factors. On balance the beneficial effects of hormone replacement in reducing osteoporosis and cardiovascular mortality are thought to outweigh the risk of breast cancer, particularly in women with premature ovarian failure[73]. It is sensible to perform annual breast examination, especially for nulliparous women, those who have not breast fed their children and certainly those with a family history of breast cancer. Mammography in normal young women, with active glandular breasts may be difficult to interpret, and so the role of mammography as a screening procedure in young women taking hormone replacement therapy is uncertain.

While hormone replacement therapy is likely to be advantageous to the future well-being of a woman with premature ovarian failure, it is also important to advise on general measures to minimize the detrimental effects of amenorrhoea that may have occurred prior to recognition of the problem. It is therefore important to advise against cigarette smoking, and advocate a balanced diet, exercise and maintenance of a normal BMI.

In order to protect against osteoporosis a daily dose of 2 mg oral oestradiol, 0.625 mg oral conjugated equine oestrogens or 50 µg transdermal oestradiol is required. If the patient is found to have significant osteoporosis (bone mineral density < 50% of normal) after 3 years of hormone replacement therapy, the adjuvant use of cyclical bisphosphonate and calcium therapy may enhance the rate of increase of bone mineral content.

### Iatrogenic causes of amenorrhoea

There are many iatrogenic causes of amenorrhoea, which may be either temporary or permanent. These include radiation to the abdomen/pelvis or chemotherapy for malignant conditions. Both these treatments may result in permanent gonadal damage; the amount of damage is directly related to the age of the patient, the cumulative dose and the patient's prior menstrual status.

Gynaecological procedures such as oophorectomy, hysterectomy and endometrial resection inevitably result in amenorrhoea. Hormone replacement should be prescribed for these patients where appropriate.

Hormone therapy itself can be used deliberately to disrupt the menstrual cycle. However, iatrogenic causes of ovarian quiescence have the same consequences of oestrogen deficiency due to any other aetiology. Therefore, the use of GnRH analogues in the treatment of oestrogen-dependent conditions (e.g. precocious puberty, endometriosis, uterine fibroids) results in a significant decrease in bone mineral density in as little as 6 months, although the demineralization is reversible with the cessation of therapy, especially for the treatment of benign conditions in young women who are in the process of achieving their peak bone mass. The concurrent use of an androgenic progestogen may protect against bone loss.

## REFERENCES

1. Doody, K. M. and Carr, B. R. (1990). Amenorrhea. In Chihal, H. J. and London, S. N. (eds.) *Menstrual Cycle Disorders, Obstet. Gynecol. Clin. N. Am.*, pp. 361–87. (Philadelphia: WB Saunders)
2. Brook, C. G. D. (1985). Management of delayed puberty. *Br. Med. J.*, **290**, 657–8
3. Ross, G. T. and Vandewiele, R. (1985). The ovary. In Wilson, J. D. and Foster, D. (eds.) *Textbook of Endocrinology*, pp. 279–350. (Philadelphia: WB Saunders)
4. Pettersson, F., Fries, H. and Nillius, S. J. (1973). Epidemiology of secondary amenorrhea. *Am. J. Obstet. Gynecol.*, **117**, 80–6
5. Jacobs, H. S., Hull, M. G. R., Murray, M. A. F. and Franks, S. (1975). Therapy-orientated diagnosis of secondary amenorrhoea. *Horm. Res.*, **6**, 268–87
6. Conway, G. S., Honour, J. W. and Jacobs, H. S. (1989). Heterogeneity of polycystic ovary syndrome: clinical, endocrine and ultrasound features in 556 cases. *Clin. Endocrinol.*, **30**, 459–70
7. Lunenfeld, B. and Insler, V. (1974). Classification of amenorrhoea states and their treatment by ovulation induction. *Clin. Endocrinol.*, **3**, 223–37
8. Hull, M. G. R., Knuth, U. A., Murray, M. A. F. and Jacobs, H. S. (1979). The practical value of the progestogen challenge test, serum oestradiol estimation or clinical examination in assessment of the oestrogen state and response to clomiphene in amenorrhoea. *Br. J. Obstet. Gynaecol.*, **86**, 799–805
9. Seth, J., Hanning, I., Jacobs, H. S. and Jeffcoate, S. L. (1989). Measuring serum gonadotrophins: a cautionary note. *Lancet*, **1**, 671
10. Adams, J., Polson, D. W. and Franks, S. (1986). Prevalence of polycystic ovaries in women with anovulation and idiopathic hirsutism. *Br. Med. J.*, **293**, 355–9
11. Conway, G. S. (1990). Insulin resistance and the polycystic ovary syndrome. *Contemp. Rev. Obstet. Gynaecol.*, **2**, 34–9
12. Turner, H. H. (1938). A syndrome of infantilism, congenital webbed neck, and cubitus valgus. *Endocrinology*, **23**, 566

13. Hall, J. G., Sybert, V. P. and Williamson, R. A. (1982). Turner's syndrome. *West. J. Med.*, **137**, 32
14. Ducharme, J. R. (1985). Puberty: physiology and pathophysiology in girls. In Studd, J. (ed.) *Progress in Obstetrics and Gynaecology*, Vol. 5, pp. 195–221. (Edinburgh: Churchill Livingstone)
15. Hindmarsh, P. C., Bridges, N. A. and Brook, C. G. D. (1991). Wider indications for treatment with biosynthetic human growth hormone in children. *Clin. Endocrinol.*, **34**, 417–28
16. Lutjen, P., Trounson, A., Leeton, J., Findlay, J., Wood, C. and Renou, P. (1984). The establishment and maintenance of pregnancy using *in vitro* fertilization and embryo donation in a patient with primary ovarian failure. *Nature (London)*, **307**, 174–5
17. Ulfelder, H. and Robboy, S. J. (1976). The embryonic development of the human vagina. *Am. J. Obstet. Gynecol.*, **126**, 769
18. Rock, J. A. (1986). Anomalous development of the vagina. *Semin. Reprod. Endocrinol.*, **4**, 1
19. Fore, S. R., Hammond, C. B., Parker, R. T. *et al.* (1975). Urologic and genital anomalies in patients with congenital absence of the vagina. *Obstet. Gynecol.*, **46**, 410–16
20. Manuel, M., Katayama, K. P. and Jones, H. W. (1976). The age of occurrence of gonadal tumors in intersex patients with a Y chromosome. *Am. J. Obstet. Gynecol.*, **124**, 293
21. Goodall, J. (1991). Helping a child to understand her own testicular feminisation/Y chromosome. *Lancet*, **337**, 33–5
22. Franks, S. (1987). Primary and secondary amenorrhoea. *Br. Med. J.*, **294**, 815–19
23. Rock, J. A., Zacur, H. A., Dlugi, A. M., Jones, H. W. and TeLinde, R. W. (1982). Pregnancy success following surgical correction of imperforate hymen and complete transverse vaginal septum. *Obstet. Gynecol.*, **59**, 448–51
24. Mason, W. P., Adams, J., Morris, D. V., Tucker, M., Price, J., Voulgaris, Z., Van der Spuy, Z. M., Sutherland, I., Chambers, G. R., White, S., Wheeler, M. J. and Jacobs, H. S. (1984). The induction of ovulation with pulsatile luteinising hormone-releasing hormone. *Br. Med. J.*, **288**, 181–5
25. Shoham, Z., Balen, A. H., Patel, A. and Jacobs, H. S. (1991). Results of ovulation induction using human menopausal gonadotropins or purified follicle-stimulating hormone in hypogonadotrophic hypogonadism patients. *Fertil. Steril.*, **56**, 1048–53
26. Asherman, J. G. (1950). Traumatic intrauterine adhesions. *J. Obstet. Gynaecol. Br. Empire*, **57**, 892–6
27. Jewelewicz, R. and van de Wiele, R. L. (1980). Clinical course and outcome of pregnancy in 25 patients with pituitary microadenomas. *Am. J. Obstet. Gynecol.*, **136**, 339–43
28. Baggish, M. S. (1980). High power density carbon dioxide laser therapy for early cervical neoplasia. *Am. J. Obstet. Gynaecol.*, **136**, 117–25
29. Steinkampf, M. P. (1990). Systemic illness and menstrual dysfunction. In Chihal, H. J. and London, S. N. (eds.) *Menstrual Cycle Disorders, Obstet. Gynecol. Clin. N. Am.*, pp. 311–19. (Philadelphia: W B Saunders)
30. de Kretser, D. M., Atkins, R. C. and Paulsen, C. A. (1973). Role of the kidney in the metabolism of luteinising hormone. *J. Endocrinol.*, **58**, 425
31. Djursing, H. (1987). Hypothalamic–pituitary–gonadal function in insulin treated diabetic women with and without amenorrhoea. *Dan. Med. Bull.*, **34**, 139
32. Cundy, T. F., O'Grady, J. G. and Williams, R. (1990). Recovery of menstruation and pregnancy after liver transplantation. *Gut*, **31**, 337–8
33. Kaufman, F. R., Kogut, M. D., Donnell, G. N., Goebelsmann, U., March, C. and Koch, R. (1981). Hypergonadotrophic hypogonadism in female patients with galactosemia. *N. Engl. J. Med.*, **304**, 994–8
34. Frisch, R. E. (1976). Fatness of girls from menarche to age 18 years, with a nomogram. *Hum. Biol.*, **48**, 353–9
35. Van der Spuy, Z. M. (1985). Nutrition and reproduction. In Jacobs, H. S. (ed.) *Reproductive Endocrinology, Clinics in Obstetrics and Gynaecology*, Vol. 12, pp. 579–604. (London: WB Saunders)
36. Fishman, J. and Bradlow, H. L. (1976). Effect of malnutrition on the metabolism of sex hormones in man. *Clin. Pharmacol. Ther.*, **22**, 721–8
37. Warren, M. P. and Vande Wiele, R. L. (1973). Clinical and metabolic features of anorexia nervosa. *Am. J. Obstet. Gynecol.*, **117**, 435–49
38. Tan, S. L. and Jacobs, H. S. (1991). Causes of primary amenorrhoea. In Tan, S. L. and Jacobs,

H. S. (eds.) *Infertility: Your Questions Answered*, p. 62. (Singapore: McGraw-Hill)
39. Reindollar, R. H., Novak, M., Tho, S. P. T. and McDonough, P. G. (1986). Adult-onset amenorrhea: a study of 262 patients. *Am. J. Obstet. Gynecol.*, **155**, 531–43
40. Bachmann, G. A. and Kemmann, E. (1982). Prevalence of oligomenorrhea and amenorrhea in a college population. *Am. J. Obstet. Gynecol.*, **144**, 98–102
41. Nillius, S. J. and Wide, L. (1977). The pituitary responsiveness to acute and chronic administration of gonadotropin-releasing hormone in acute and recovery stages of anorexia nervosa. In Vigersky, R. A. (ed.) *Anorexia Nervosa*, pp. 225–41. (New York: Raven Press)
42. Van der Spuy, Z. M., Steer, P. J., McCusker, M., Steele, S. J. and Jacobs, H. S. (1988). Outcome of pregnancy in underweight women after spontaneous and induced ovulation. *Br. Med. J.*, **296**, 962–5
43. Treasure, J. L. and Russell, G. F. M. (1988). Intrauterine growth and neonatal weight gain in babies of women with anorexia nervosa. *Br. Med. J.*, **296**, 1038
44. Barker, D. J. P. (1990). The fetal and infant origins of adult disease. *Br. Med. J.*, **301**, 111
45. Szmukler, G. I., Brown, S. W., Parsons, V. and Darby, A. (1985). Premature loss of bone in chronic anorexia nervosa. *Br. Med. J.*, **290**, 26–7
46. Fonseca, V., Houlder, S., Thomas, M., D'Souza, V., Wakeling, A. and Dandoma, P. (1985). Osteopenia in women with anorexia nervosa. *N. Engl. J. Med.*, **313**, 326–7
47. Biller, B. M. K., Saxe, V., Herzog, D. B., Rosenthal, D. I., Holzman, S. and Klibanski, A. (1989). Mechanisms of osteoporosis in adult and adolescent women with anorexia nervosa. *J. Clin. Endocrinol. Metab.*, **68**, 548–53
48. Kulin, H. E., Bwibo, N., Mutie, D. and Santner, S. J. (1982). The effect of chronic childhood malnutrition on pubertal growth and development. *Am. J. Clin. Nutrition*, **36**, 527–36
49. Schwartz, B., Cumming, D. C., Riordan, E., Selye, M., Yen, S. S. C. and Rebar, R. W. (1981). Exercise-associated amenorrhoea: a distinct entity? *Am. J. Obstet. Gynecol.*, **141**, 662–70
50. Cumming, D. C. and Rebar, R. W. (1983). Exercise and reproductive function in women. *Am. J. Indust. Med.*, **4**, 113–25
51. Suda, A. K., Pittman, C. S., Shimuzu, T. and Chambers, J. B. (1978). The production and metabolism of 3,3′,5′-triiodothyronine in normal and fasting subjects. *J. Clin. Endocrinol. Metab.*, **47**, 1311–19
52. Warren, M. P. (1980). The effects of exercise on pubertal progression and reproductive function in girls. *J. Clin. Endocrinol. Metab.*, **51**, 1150–7
53. Warren, M. P., Brooks-Gunn, J., Hamilton, L. H., Warren, L F. and Hamilton, W. G. (1986). Scoliosis and fractures in young ballet dancers. *N. Engl. J. Med.*, **314**, 1348–53
54. Bowling, A. (1989). Injuries to dancers: prevalence, treatment and perception of causes. *Br. Med. J.*, **298**, 731–4
55. Aloia, J. F., Cohn, S. H., Ostuni, J. A., Cane, R. and Ellis, K. (1978). Prevention of involutional bone loss by exercise. *Ann. Intern. Med.*, **89**, 356–8
56. Sheehan, H. L. (1939). Simmond's disease due to post-partum necrosis of the anterior pituitary. *Q. J. Med.*, **8**, 277
57. Jacobs, H. S. (1981). Management of prolactin-secreting pituitary tumours. In Studd, J. (ed.) *Progress in Obstetrics and Gynaecology*, Vol. 1, pp. 263–76. (Edinburgh: Churchill Livingstone)
58. Jacobs, H. S., Franks, S., Murray, M. A. F., Hull, M. G. R., Steele, S. J. and Nabarro, J. D. N. (1976). Clinical and endocrinological features of hyperprolactinaemic amenorrhoea. *Clin. Endocrinol.*, **5**, 439–54
59. Nabarro, J. D. N. and Franks, S. (1978). Prolactin and amenorrhoea. In Jacobs, H. S. (ed.) *Advances in Gynaecological Endocrinology. Proceedings of 6th Study Group of Royal College of Obstetricians and Gynaecologists*, pp. 248–61. (London: Royal College of Obstetricians and Gynaecologists)
60. Shoham, Z., Homburg, R. and Jacobs, H. S. (1991). CV 205-502 – effectiveness, tolerability and safety over 24 month study. *Fertil. Steril.*, **55**, 501–6
61. Schlecte, J. A., Sherman, B. and Martin, R. (1983). Bone density in amenorrheic women with and without hyperprolactinaemia. *J. Clin. Endocrinol. Metab.*, **56**, 1120–3
62. Klibanski, A., Biller, B. M. K., Rosenthal, D. I., Schoenfeld, D. A. and Saxe, V. (1988). Effects of prolactin and estrogen deficiency in amenorrheic bone loss. *J. Clin. Endocrinol. Metab.*, **67**, 124–30
63. Cust, M. P. (1991). The treatment of early ovarian failure. *Curr. Obstet. Gynaecol.*, **1**, 15–20

64. Hague, W. M., Tan, S. L., Adams, J. and Jacobs, H. S. (1987). Hypergonadotrophic amenorrhoea – etiology and outcome in 93 young women. *Int. J. Gynaecol. Obstet.*, **25**, 121–5
65. Mignot, M. H., Drexhage, H. A., Kleingeld, M., Van de Plassche-Boers, E. M., Rao, B. R. and Schoemaker, J. (1989). Premature ovarian failure. II: Considerations of cellular immunity defects. *Eur. J. Obstet. Gynaecol. Reprod. Biol.*, **30**, 67–82
66. Cameron, I. T., O'Shea, F. C., Rolland, J. M., Hughes, E. G., de Kretser, D. M. and Healy, D. L. (1988). Occult ovarian failure: a syndrome of infertility, regular menses and elevated follicle-stimulating hormone concentrations. *J. Clin. Endocrinol. Metab.*, **67**, 1190–4
67. Lutjen, P., Trounson, A., Leeton, J., Findlay, J., Wood, C. and Renou, P. (1984). The establishment and maintenance of pregnancy using *in vitro* fertilization and embryo donation in a patient with primary ovarian failure. *Nature (London)*, **307**, 174–5
68. Gosden, R. G. (1990). Restitution of fertility in sterilized mice by transferring primordial ovarian follicles. *Hum. Reprod.*, *5*, 499–504
69. Prior, J. C. (1990). Progesterone as a bone-trophic hormone. *Endocr. Rev.*, **1**, 386–98
70. Hunt, K. and Vessey, M. (1991). The risks and benefits of hormone replacement therapy: an updated review. *Curr. Obstet. Gynaecol.*, **1**, 21–7
71. Bergkvist, L., Adami, H.-O., Persson, I., Hoover, R. and Schairer, C. (1989). The risk of breast cancer after estrogen and estrogen–progestin replacement. *N. Engl. J. Med.*, **321**, 293–7
72. Hunt, K., Vessey, M., McPherson, K. and Colememan, M. (1987). Long-term surveillance of mortality and cancer incidence in women receiving hormone replacement therapy. *Br. J. Obstet. Gynaecol.*, **94**, 620–35
73. Hunt, K., Vessey, M. and McPherson, K. (1990). Mortality in a cohort of long-term users of hormone replacement therapy: an updated analysis. *Br. J. Obstet. Gynaecol.*, **97**, 1080–6

# Polycystic ovary syndrome and hirsutism

# 5

*Deborah J. Harrington and Adam H. Balen*

## AETIOLOGY AND PATHOPHYSIOLOGY

The polycystic ovary syndrome (PCOS) is one of the most common endocrine disorders, although its aetiology remains unknown. This heterogeneous disorder may present, at one end of the spectrum, with the single finding of polycystic ovarian morphology as detected by pelvic ultrasound. At the other end of the spectrum, symptoms such as obesity, hyperandrogenic manifestations, menstrual cycle disturbance and infertility may occur either singly or in combination (Table 1). Metabolic disturbances (elevated serum concentrations of luteinizing hormone (LH), testosterone, insulin and prolactin) are common and may have profound implications on the long-term health of women with PCOS. The polycystic ovary syndrome is a familial condition, possibly autosomal dominant, with premature balding being the male phenotype[1]. It appears to have its origins during adolescence and is thought to be associated with increased weight gain during puberty[2]. However, the polycystic ovary gene (or genes) has not yet been identified and the effect of environmental influences such as weight changes and circulating hormone concentrations, and the age at which these occur, is unknown.

High-resolution ultrasound scanning has made an accurate estimate of the prevalence of polycystic ovaries possible. Several studies have estimated the prevalence of polycystic ovaries in 'normal adult' women and have found rates of approximately 20%[3–7] but it is not known at what age they first appear. Detecting polycystic ovaries in girls relies upon transabdominal scanning, which in a study by Fox and colleagues[8] failed to detect 30% of polycystic ovaries compared to 100% detection rate with a transvaginal scan. Bridges and associates[9] performed 428 ovarian scans in girls aged

**Table 1** The spectrum of clinical manifestations of the heterogeneous polycystic ovary syndrome

| *Symptoms* | *% patients affected* | *Associated endocrine manifestations* | *Possible late sequelae* |
|---|---|---|---|
| Obesity | 38 | ↑ androgens (testosterone and androstenedione) | diabetes mellitus (11%) |
| Menstrual disturbance | 66 | | cardiovascular disease |
| Hyperandrogenism | 48 | ↑ luteinizing hormone | hyperinsulinaemia |
| Infertility | 73 of anovulatory infertility | ↑ LH : FSH ratio | low LDL |
| | | ↑ free oestradiol | endometrial carcinoma |
| | | ↑ fasting insulin | hypertension |
| Asymptomatic | 20 | ↑ prolactin | |
| | | ↓ sex hormone binding globulin | |

↑ = increase in serum concentration; ↓ = decrease in serum concentration; LH = luteinizing hormone; FSH = follicle stimulating hormone; LDL = low density lipids between 3 and 18 years and found polycystic ovaries in 101 girls (24% of the total). The rate of detection of polycystic ovaries was 6% in 6-year-old girls, rising to 18% in those aged 10 years and 26% in those aged 15 years. The implication of this study is that polycystic ovaries are present before puberty and are more easy to detect in older girls as the ovaries increase in size.

Prior to puberty, there appear to be two periods of increased ovarian growth. The first is at adrenarche, in response to increased concentrations of circulating androgens, and the second, just before and during puberty, due to rising gonadotrophin levels, the actions of growth hormone, and insulin-like growth factor-1 (IGF-1) and insulin on the ovary.

Sampaolo and co-workers[10] reported a study of 49 obese girls at different stages of puberty, comparing their pelvic ultrasound features and endocrine profiles with 35 age- and pubertal stage-matched controls. They found that obesity was associated with a significant increase in uterine and ovarian volume. They also found that obese postmenarchal girls with polycystic ovaries had larger uterine and ovarian volumes than obese postmenarchal girls with normal ovaries. Sampaolo concludes that obesity leads to hyperinsulinism, which causes both hyperandrogenaemia and raised IGF-1 levels, which augment the ovarian response to gonadotrophins. This implies that obesity may be important in the pathogenesis of polycystic ovaries, but further study is required to evaluate this. It is known that obesity is not a prerequisite for the polycystic ovary syndrome. Indeed, in a series of 1741 women with polycystic ovaries in a study by Balen and colleagues[11], only 38.4% of patients were overweight (body mass index (BMI) > 25 kg/m$^2$).

Many women with polycystic ovaries detected by ultrasound do not have overt symptoms of PCOS, although symptoms may develop later, after a gain in weight, for example. Ovarian morphology using the criteria described by Adams and associates[12] (ten or more cysts, 2–8 mm in diameter, arranged around an echo-dense stroma) appears to be the most sensitive diagnostic marker for polycystic ovaries. The classical features of oligo/amenorrhoea, obesity, and/or clinical symptoms of hyperandrogenism in addition to the ultrasound features of the polycystic ovary are diagnostic of the polycystic ovary syndrome. Polycystic ovaries may be associated with several endocrinopathies. Studies comparing women with polycystic ovaries to normal controls have shown elevated concentrations of LH, LH : FSH (follicle stimulating hormone) ratio, fasting insulin, testosterone and androstenedione and reduced concentration of sex hormone-binding globulin (SHBG). However, the classical hormone changes are not seen in all patients. Indeed, Fox and colleagues[8] found that isolated measurements of serum concentrations of androgens, oestradiol, gonadotrophins and the LH : FSH ratio confirmed the finding in only 75% of women with ultrasound-confirmed polycystic ovaries and oligo/amenorrhoea. Single hormone measurements may be unreliable as serum hormone concentrations vary with time. For example, sampling LH every 20 min over a 6-h period gives a variability of 38% in the follicular phase and 92% in the luteal phase of normal women.

## HETEROGENEITY OF POLYCYSTIC OVARY SYNDROME

The findings of a large series of 1741 women with polycystic ovaries detected by ultrasound scan, attending the Middlesex Hospital Endocrine Unit, are summarized in Table 2[11]. The frequency distributions of serum concentrations of FSH, LH, testosterone and prolactin and the body mass index, ovarian volume, uterine cross-sectional area and endometrial thickness were determined and correlated with the symptoms and signs of PCOS. Thirty-eight per cent of the women were overweight (BMI > 25 kg/m$^2$). Obesity was significantly associated with an increased risk of hirsutism, menstrual cycle disturbance and an elevated serum testosterone concentration. Obesity was also associated with an increased rate of infertility and menstrual cycle disturbance (Figure 1). A rising serum concentration of testosterone was associated with an increased risk of

**Table 2** Characteristics of 1741 women with ultrasound-detected polycystic ovaries

| *Characteristic* | *Normal range* | *Mean* | *5–95th centiles* |
|---|---|---|---|
| Age (years) | | 31.5 | 14–50 |
| Ovarian volume ($cm^3$) | | 11.7 | 4.6–22.3 |
| Uterine cross-sectional area ($cm^2$) | | 27.5 | 15.2–46.3 |
| Endometrium (mm) | | 7.5 | 4.0–13.0 |
| Body mass index ($kg/m^2$) | 19–25 | 25.4 | 19.0–38.6 |
| Follicle stimulating hormone (IU/l) | 1–10 | 4.5 | 1.4–7.5 |
| Luteinizing hormone | 1–10 | 10.9 | 2.0–27.0 |
| Testosterone (nmol/l) | 0.5–2.5 | 2.6 | 1.1–4.8 |
| Prolactin (mU/l) | < 350 | 342 | 87–917 |

hirsutism, infertility and cycle disturbance. Twenty-six per cent of patients with primary infertility and 14% of patients with secondary infertility had a BMI of more than 30 $kg/m^2$. The rates of infertility and menstrual cycle disturbance also increased with increasing serum LH concentrations greater than 10 IU/l. The serum LH concentration of those with primary infertility was significantly higher than that of women with secondary infertility (i.e. those with at least one previous pregnancy) and both were higher than the LH concentration of those with proven fertility (Figure 2). The ovarian volume was significantly correlated with the serum concentrations of testosterone and LH and the BMI, which also correlated with uterine cross-sectional area. Ovarian morphology appears to be the most sensitive marker of PCOS, compared to the classical endocrine features of raised serum LH and testosterone, which were found in only 39.8% and 28.9% of patients, respectively, in the Middlesex Hospital study.

## HYPERSECRETION OF LUTEINIZING HORMONE

Hypersecretion of LH occurs in approximately 40% of women who have polycystic ovaries. The risk of infertility and miscarriage is raised in these patients. Several hypotheses have been suggested to explain this over-secretion of LH. These include increased pulse frequency of gonadotrophin releasing hormone (GnRH), increased pituitary sensitivity to GnRH, hyperinsulinaemic stimulation of the pituitary gland and disturbance of the ovarian steroid–pituitary feedback mechanism. However, none of these fully explain hypersecretion of LH. Since the isolation and characterization of inhibin and activin, it has become apparent that there are several non-steroidal gonadal signals that influence gonadotrophin secretion and help control reproductive function. Inhibin exerts negative feedback on pituitary gonadotrophin production, particularly affecting FSH secretion. More recently, several groups have suggested that a non-steroidal peptide named gonadotrophin surge inhibiting or attenuating factor (GnSIF/GnSAF) acts via a feedback pathway on the pituitary and preferentially affects LH secretion. The precise mechanism of action of the GnSAF will not be known until the hormone is isolated. However, one theory is that it may act by returning the LH responsiveness of the pituitary gland back to the unprimed state following each pulse of GnRH. Thus LH levels are kept low during follicular phase preceding the surge. However, increased stimulation by GnRH overcomes this suppressive action, allowing the pituitary to become ‘primed’ by the GnRH and therefore permitting the LH surge. Evidence to support this hypothesis has come from women with hypogonadotrophic hypogonadism (HH), who also have polycystic ovaries detected by pelvic ultrasound. When these women were treated with pulsatile GnRH

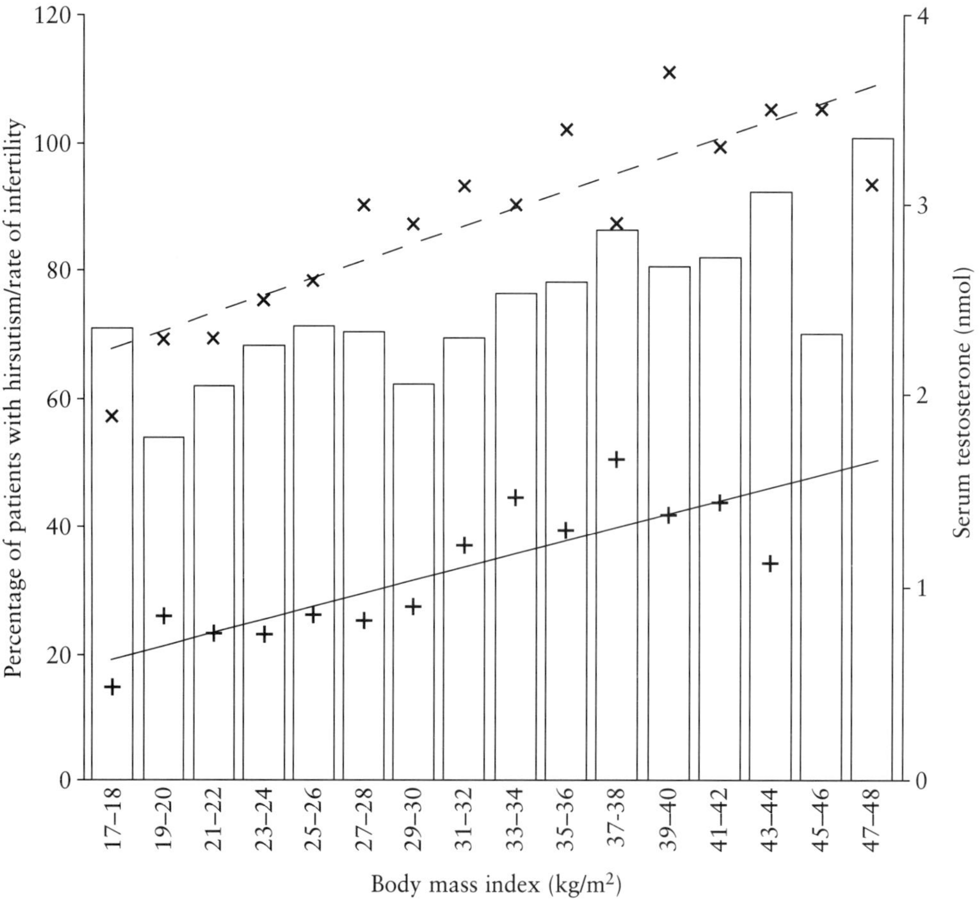


**Figure 1** Relationship of body mass index to the rate of hirsutism (shown in columns) and serum testosterone concentration (×). The rate of infertility is also indicated (+)

to induce ovulation, they had significantly higher serum LH concentrations than women with HH and normal ovaries[13]. This suggests that the cause of hypersecretion of LH involves a perturbation of ovarian–pituitary feedback.

## MANAGEMENT OF THE POLYCYSTIC OVARY SYNDROME

The clinical management of a woman with PCOS should be focused on her individual problems. An increasing BMI has been found to be correlated with an increased rate of hirsutism, cycle disturbance and infertility. Obese women (BMI > 30 kg/m$^2$) should therefore be encouraged to lose weight. Weight loss improves the endocrine profile[14], the likelihood of ovulation and a healthy pregnancy. A recent study by Clark and associates[15] looked at the effect of a weight loss programme on women with at least a 2-year history of anovulatory infertility, clomiphene resistance and a BMI > 30 kg/m$^2$. Weight loss had a significant effect on endocrine function, ovulation and subsequent pregnancy. Twelve of the 13 subjects resumed ovulation, 11 becoming pregnant (five spontaneously). Fasting insulin and serum testosterone concentrations were both shown to decrease.

Women with PCOS have a greater frequency of both hyperinsulinaemia and insulin resistance. Obese women with PCOS hypersecrete

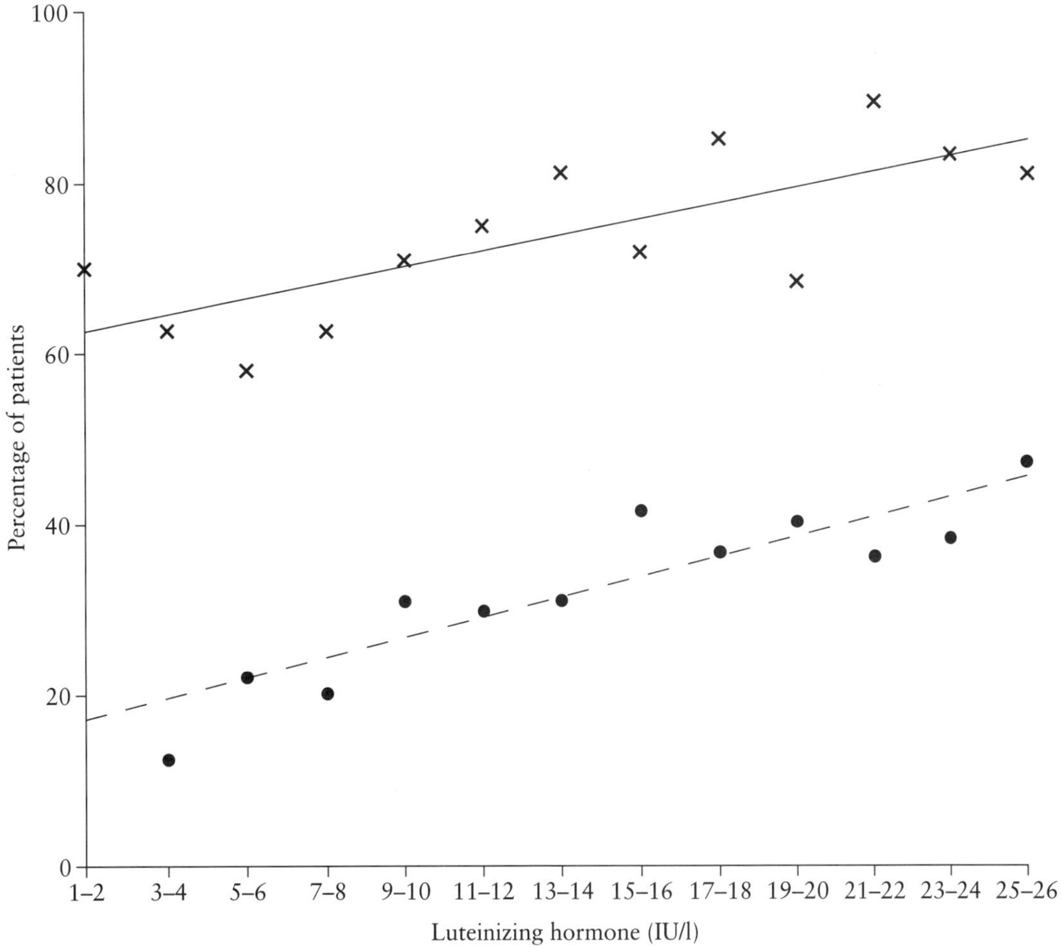


**Figure 2** Relationship between serum concentration of luteinizing hormone and rates of infertility (●) and cycle disturbance (×)

insulin which stimulates ovarian secretion of androgens. The prevalence of diabetes in obese women with PCOS is 11%[16] and so an assessment for possible impaired glucose tolerance is important in these women.

## HYPERANDROGENISM AND HIRSUTISM

Serum concentrations of testosterone may be elevated in women with PCOS. The bioavailability of testosterone is affected by the serum concentration of SHBG. High levels of insulin lower the production of SHBG and so increase the free fraction of androgen. However, a testosterone concentration greater than 5 nmol/l should be investigated to exclude androgen secreting tumours of the ovary or adrenal gland, Cushing's syndrome and late-onset congenital adrenal hyperplasia. Elevated serum androgen concentrations stimulate peripheral androgen receptors, resulting in an increase in 5$\alpha$-reductase activity, directly increasing the conversion of testosterone to the more potent metabolite, dihydrotestosterone. Symptoms of hyperandrogenism include hirsutism, which can be a distressing condition. Hirsutism is characterized by terminal hair growth in a male pattern of distribution, including chin, upper lip, chest, upper and lower back, upper and lower abdomen, upper arm, thigh and buttocks. A standardized scoring system, such as the modified Ferriman and Gallwey score, should be used to evaluate the degree of hirsutism before and during treatments. Treatment options include cosmetic and medical therapies. Medical regimens stop further progression of hirsutism and decrease the rate of hair growth. However, drug therapies may take 6–9 months or longer before any benefit is perceived and so physical treatments including electrolysis, waxing and bleaching may be helpful whilst waiting for medical treatments to work. Symptoms of hyperandrogenism can be treated by a combination of an oestrogen (such as ethinyloestradiol, or a combined contraceptive pill) and the anti-androgen cyproterone acetate (50–100 mg). Oestrogens lower circulating androgens by a combination of a slight inhibition of gonadotrophin secretion and gonadotrophin-sensitive ovarian steroid production and by an increase in hepatic production of SHBG, resulting in lower free testosterone. The cyproterone is taken for the first 10 days of a cycle (the 'reversed sequential' method) and the oestrogen for the first 21 days. After a gap of exactly 7 days, during which menstruation usually occurs, the regimen is repeated. As an alternative, the preparation Dianette® (Schering Health, Sussex, UK) contains ethinyloestradiol in combination with cyproterone, although at a lower dose (2 mg). Cyproterone acetate acts as a competitive inhibitor at the androgen receptor. Serum levels of LH, FSH, oestradiol, androstenedione, total and free testosterone are lowered, whilst SHBG increases. However, there is an increase in triglycerides, apolipoprotein A1, A2 and B. Cyproterone acetate can cause liver damage and liver function should be checked periodically.

Other anti-androgens such as spironolactone, ketoconazole and flutamide have been tried, but are not widely used in the UK due to their adverse side-effects. Vidal-Puig and coworkers[17] treated 26 women with hirsutism, acne and oligomenorrhoea with low dose ketoconazole for 9 months. Ketoconazole is a known inhibitor of P450 steroidogenic enzymes. All patients showed a significant decrease in hirsutism and circulating total testosterone, dehydroepiandrosterone sulphate (DHEAS) and LH. However, the side-effects of dyspepsia, dysfunctional uterine bleeding, alopecia and raised transaminase levels resulted in 30% being withdrawn from the trial. Spironolactone, an androgen inhibitor and diuretic, acts as an inhibitor of 5α-reductase activity. However, it is not widely used due to side-effects including menorrhagia, dizziness and mild hypotension. Flutamide, a non-steroidal pure anti-androgen is used in the USA as an adjuvant treatment for prostate cancer. In a prospective study of 11 patients with PCOS and 25 patients with idiopathic hirsutism, both groups showed a 60% decrease in Ferriman Gallwey score and a decrease in total and free testosterone levels. However, both fatal and non-fatal hepatotoxicity have been described with flutamide and so this treatment is rarely used in the UK. Indeed, in a randomized controlled trial of patients with moderate to severe hirsutism treated with flutamide for 9 months, 0.36% of patients had a hepatic reaction. It is also essential to take contraceptive precautions whilst using anti-androgens.

Hyperandrogenism may also have long-term consequences, including an increased risk of cardiovascular disease, android obesity, elevated blood pressure, insulin resistance, atherogenic lipid profiles and an increased risk of developing diabetes.

## MENSTRUAL IRREGULARITY

If menstrual irregularity (amenorrhoea or oligomenorrhoea) is a problem, the easiest approach is the use of a low dose combined oral contraceptive preparation. This will result in an artificial cycle and regular shedding of the endometrium. An alternative is a progestogen (such as medroxyprogesterone acetate or dydrogesterone) for 12 days every 1–3 months to induce a withdrawal bleed. It is also important once again to encourage weight loss. Women with PCOS are thought to be at increased risk of cardiovascular disease, and so a modern 'lipid friendly' combined contraceptive pill should be used.

In women with anovulatory cycles, the action of oestradiol on the endometrium is unopposed because of the lack of cyclical progestone secretion. This may result in episodes of irregular uterine bleeding, and in the long term endometrial hyperplasia and even endometrial cancer. An ultrasound assessment of endometrial thickness provides a bioassay for oestradiol production by the ovaries and conversion of androgens in the peripheral fat. If the endometrium is thicker than 15 mm a withdrawal bleed should be induced and if the endometrium fails to shed then endometrial sampling is required to exclude endometrial hyperplasia or malignancy. The only young women (< 35 years) to develop endometrial carcinoma, which has a mean age of occurrence of 61 years in the UK, are those with anovulation secondary to PCOS or oestrogen-secreting tumours.

## INFERTILITY

Hypersecretion of LH is particularly associated with menstrual disturbances and infertility[11,18,19]. Indeed, it is this endocrine feature that appears to result in reduced conception rates and increased rates of miscarriage in both natural and assisted conception. Whilst it has been suggested that the finding of a persistently elevated early to mid-follicular phase LH concentration in a woman who is trying to conceive indicates the need to suppress LH levels by pituitary desensitization with a gonadotrophin releasing hormone agonist, prospective randomized studies have not shown this approach to be of proven benefit. Before commencing ovulation induction, it is always important to investigate the couple thoroughly by checking for other endocrine abnormalities, Fallopian tube patency and semen analysis.

Ovulation can be induced with the anti-oestrogens, clomiphene citrate (50–100 mg) or tamoxifen (20–40 mg), on days 2–6 of a natural or artifically induced bleed. Whilst clomiphene is successful in inducing ovulation in over 80% of women, pregnancy only occurs in 30–40%. A daily dose of more than 100 mg rarely confers any benefit and can cause thickening of the cervical mucus, which can impede passage of sperm through the cervix. A post-coital test, or assessment of cervical mucus, is therefore advisable once treatment has started. Clomiphene can cause an exaggerated release of LH and therefore a mid-follicular phase LH concentration should be measured. A starting dose of 50 mg of clomiphene is given for 3 months, but may be increased up to 100 mg if needed. Once an ovulatory dose has been reached, the cumulative conception rate continues to increase for up to ten to 12 cycles. However, clomiphene is only licensed for 6 months' use in the UK because of the suggested increased risk of ovarian cancer with prolonged use[20], and so we would advise careful counselling of patients if clomiphene citrate therapy is continued beyond 6 months.

The therapeutic options for patients with anovulatory infertility who are resistant to anti-oestrogens are either parenteral gonadotrophin therapy or laparoscopic ovarian diathermy. Balen and co-workers[21] recently published the cumulative conception and live birth rates in 103 women with PCOS who did not ovulate with anti-oestrogen therapy and who were then treated with gonadotrophin therapy. Whilst the cumulative conception and live birth rates after 6 months were 62% and 54%, respectively, and after 12 months 73% and 62%, respectively (Figure 3), the rate of multiple pregnancy was 19% and there were three cases of moderate to severe ovarian hyperstimulation syndrome[21]. Because the polycystic ovary is very sensitive to stimulation by exogenous hormones, it is very important to start with very low doses of gonadotrophins and follicular development must be carefully monitored by ultrasound scans. The advent of transvaginal ultrasonography has enabled the multiple pregnancy rate to be reduced to approximately 7% because of its higher resolution and clearer view of the developing follicles. Close monitoring should enable treatment to be suspended if three or more mature follicles develop, as the risk of multiple pregnancy obviously increases.

Women with the polycystic ovary syndrome are also at increased risk of developing the

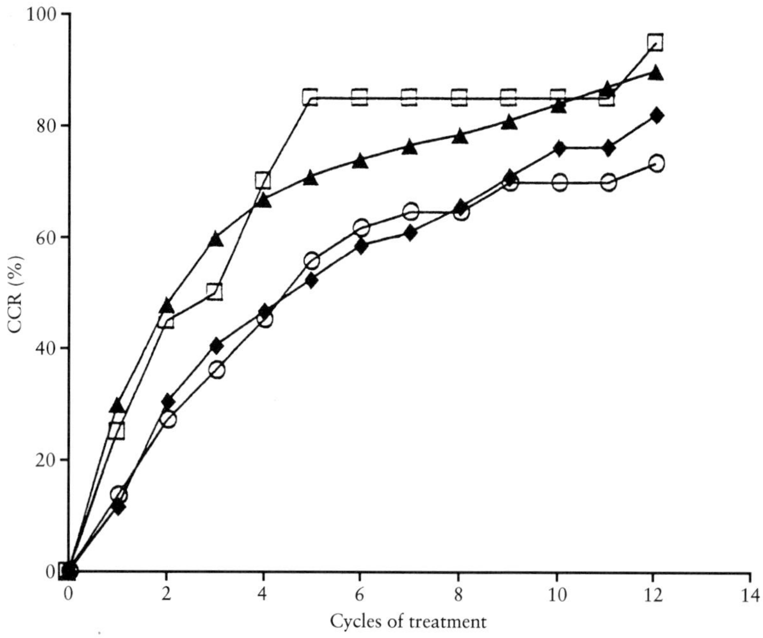


**Figure 3** Cumulative conception rates (CCR) after one course of ovulation induction treatment for patients with polycystic ovary syndrome (O; *n* = 103), hypogonadotrophic hypogonadism (✦; *n* = 77) and weight-related amenorrhoea (□; *n* = 20) compared with the CCR of a normal population (▲). Data from references 21 and 27. Reproduced with permission from Balen *et al.* (1994). *Human Reproduction,* 9, 1563–70[21]

ovarian hyperstimulation syndrome (OHSS). This occurs if too many follicles (> 10 mm) are stimulated and results in abdominal distension, discomfort, nausea, vomiting and sometimes difficulty in breathing[22]. The mechanism for OHSS is thought to be secondary to activation of the ovarian renin–angiotensin pathway and excessive secretion of vascular epidermal growth factor (VEGF). The ascites, pleural and pericardial effusions exacerbate this serious condition and the resultant haemoconcentration can lead to thromboembolism. The situation worsens if a pregnancy has resulted from the treatment as human chorionic gonadotrophin (hCG) from the placenta further stimulates the ovaries. Hospitalization is sometimes necessary in order for intravenous fluids and heparin to be given to prevent dehydration and thromboembolism. Although severe OHSS is rare, it is potentially fatal and should be avoidable with appropriate monitoring of gonadotrophin therapy.

Ovarian diathermy is free of the risks of multiple pregnancy and ovarian hyperstimulation and does not require intensive ultrasound monitoring. Laparoscopic ovarian diathermy (LOD) has taken the place of wedge resection of the ovaries (which resulted in extensive periovarian and tubal adhesions), and it appears to be as effective as routine gonadotrophin therapy in the treatment of clomiphene-insensitive PCOS[23]. Only minimal damage to the ovary is required to stimulate ovulation[24]. In a study by Balen and associates[25], ten patients who had been unresponsive to treatment with clomiphene citrate underwent ovarian diathermy. Six patients received bilateral LOD and four had unilateral LOD. Five patients ovulated spontaneously within 6 weeks of LOD. The remaining five subsequently ovulated in response to clomiphene or gonadotrophin therapy. Three of the four patients who received unilateral diathermy ovulated spontaneously, all from the contralateral ovary in the first cycle and then alternatively from each ovary. There were no significant differences in the baseline hormones of the responders and those of the non-responders. However, there was a significant fall of the serum LH concentration post-treatment in the responders. Rossmanith and co-workers[26] found an attenuation of GnRH-stimulated LH secretion after laparoscopic ovarian diathermy. This result again suggests that it is an abnormality in the ovary that is responsible for the hypersecretion of LH.

The mechanism of ovulation induction by LOD is uncertain, but it appears that minimal damage to an unresponsive ovary either restores an ovulatory cycle or increases the sensitivity of the ovary to exogenous stimulation. The finding of an attenuated response of LH secretion to stimulation with GnRH[26] suggests an effect on ovarian pituitary feedback and pituitary sensitivity to GnRH. One hypothesis is that the response of the ovary to injury results in the local release of growth factors that stimulate follicular growth and the production of GnSAF/GnSIF which leads to a fall in serum LH concentrations.

## CONCLUSIONS

Polycystic ovary syndrome is the most common endocrine abnormality affecting women. It is also the most common cause of anovulatory infertility. Modern ultrasound techniques using clear diagnostic criteria have allowed the prevalence of the disorder to be estimated. The aetiology of polycystic ovary syndrome is unknown, but a genetic defect inherited in an autosomal dominant pattern, and affecting the regulation of enzymes responsible for ovarian androgen production, has been suggested.

The management and treatment of polycystic ovary syndrome should be tailored to the individual. Women who are overweight should be encouraged to lose weight and can be expected to experience an improvement in the symptoms of menstrual disturbance, infertility and hyperandrogenism. Attainment of normal weight may decrease the long-term risk of cardiovascular disease and non-insulin dependent diabetes mellitus. If the serum concentration of luteinizing hormone is elevated, there is a strong association with infertility and treatment strategies include pituitary desensitization and laparoscopic ovarian diathermy. The long-term sequelae, particularly with regard to lipid metabolism, diabetes and the effects of unopposed oestrogens, on the endometrium need careful appraisal and counselling as soon as the diagnosis is made, and possibly long-term follow-up.

## REFERENCES


1. Carey, A. H., Chan, K. L., Short, D., White, D., Williamson, R. and Franks, S. (1993). Evidence for a single gene defect causing polycystic ovaries and male pattern baldness. *Clin. Endocrinol.*, **38**, 653–8
2. Balen, A. H. and Dunger, D. (1995). Pubertal maturation of the internal genitalia. *Ultrasound Obstet. Gynecol.*, **6**, 164–5
3. Polson, D. W., Wadsworth, J., Adams, J. and Franks, S. (1988). Polycystic ovaries: a common finding in normal women. *Lancet*, **2**, 870–2
4. Tayob, Y., Robinson, G., Adams, J., Nye, M., Whitelaw, N., Shaw, R. W., Jacobs, H. S. and Guillebaud, J. (1990). Ultrasound appearance of the ovaries during the pill-free interval. *Br. J. Fam. Plann.*, **16**, 94–6
5. Gadir, A. A., Khatim, M. S., Mowafi, R. S., Alnaser, H. M. I., Muharib, N. S. and Shaw, R. W. (1992). Implications of ultrasonically detected polycystic ovaries. Correlations with basal hormone profiles. *Hum. Reprod.*, **7**, 453–7
6. Clayton, R. N., Ogden, V., Hodgekinson, J., Worsick, L., Rodin, D. A., Dyer, S. and Meade, T. W. (1992). How common are polycystic ovaries in normal women and what is their significance for the fertility of the population? *Clin. Endocrinol.*, **37**, 127–34
7. Farquhar, C. M., Birdsall, M., Manning, P. and Mitchell, J. M. (1994). Transabdominal versus transvaginal ultrasound in the diagnosis of polycystic ovaries on ultrasound scanning in a population of randomly selected women. *Ultrasound Obstet. Gynecol.*, **4**, 54–9
8. Fox, R., Corrigan, E., Thomas, P. A. and Hull, M. G. R. (1991). The diagnosis of polycystic ovaries in women with oligo-amenorrhoea:

predictive power of endocrine tests. *Clin. Endocrinol.*, **34**, 127–31
9. Bridges, N. A., Cooke, A., Healy, M. J. R., Hindmarsh, P. C. and Brook, C. G. D. (1993). Standards for ovarian volume in childhood and puberty. *Fertil. Steril.*, **60**, 456–60
10. Sampaolo, P., Livien, C., Montanari, L., Paganelli, A., Salesi, A. and Lorini, R. (1994). Precocious signs of polycystic ovaries in obese girls. *Ultrasound Obstet. Gynecol.*, **4**, 1–6
11. Balen, A. H., Conway, G. S., Kaltsas, G., Techatraisak, K., Manning, P. J., West, C. and Jacobs, H. S. (1995). Polycystic ovary syndrome: the spectrum of the disorder in 1741 patients. *Hum. Reprod.*, **10**, 2705–12
12. Adams, J., Franks, S., Polson, D. W., Mason, H. D., Abdulwahid, N., Tucker, M., Morris, D. V., Price, J. and Jacobs, H. S. (1985). Multifollicular ovaries: clinical and endocrine features and response to pulsatile gonadotrophin releasing hormone. *Lancet*, **2**, 1375–8
13. Schachter, M., Balen, A. H., Patel, A. and Jacobs, H. S. (1996). Hypogonadotrophic patients with ultrasonographically detected polycystic ovaries have aberrant gonadotrophin secretion when treated with pulsatile GnRH – a new insight to the pathophysiology of polycystic ovary syndrome. *Fertil. Steril.*, in press
14. Kiddy, D. S., Hamilton-Fairly, D., Seppala, M., Koistman, R., James, V. H. T., Reed, M. J. and Franks, S. (1989). Diet induced changes in sex hormone binding globulin and free testosterone in women with normal or polycystic ovaries: correlation with serum insulin-like growth factor 1. *Clin. Endocrinol.*, **31**, 757–63
15. Clark, A. M., Ledger, W., Galletly, C., Tomlinson, L., Blaney, F., Wang, X. and Norman, R. J. (1995). Weight loss results in significant improvement in pregnancy and ovulation rates in anovulatory obese women. *Hum. Reprod.*, **10**, 2705–12
16. Conway, G. S., Agrawal, R., Betteridge, D. J. and Jacobs, H. S. (1992). Risk factors for coronary artery disease in lean and obese women with the polycystic ovary syndrome. *Clin. Endocrinol.*, **37**, 119–25
17. Vidal-Puig, A. J., Munos-Torres, M., Jodere-Gimeno, E., Garcia-Calvente, C. J., Lardelli, P., Ruiz-Regena, M. E. and Escobar-Jimenez, F. (1994). Ketoconazole therapy: hormonal and clinical effects in non-tumoral hyperandrogenism. *Eur. J. Endocrinol.*, **130**, 333–8
18. Regan, L., Owen, E. J. and Jacobs, H. S. (1990). Hypersecretion of LH, infertility and miscarriage. *Lancet*, **336**, 1141–4
19. Balen, A. H., Tan, S. L. and Jacobs, H. S. (1993). Hypersecretion of luteinising hormone – a significant cause of infertility and miscarriage. *Br. J. Obstet. Gynaecol.*, **100**, 1082–9
20. Rossing, M. A., Daling, J. R., Weiss, N. S., Moore, D. E. and Self, S. G. (1994). Ovarian tumours in a cohort of infertile women. *N. Engl. J. Med.*, **331**, 771–6
21. Balen, A. H., Braat, D. D. M., West, C., Patel, A. and Jacobs, H. S. (1994). Cumulative conception and live birth rates after the treatment of anovulatory infertility. *Hum. Reprod.*, **9**, 1563–70
22. Brinsden, P. R., Wada, I., Tan, S. L., Balen, A. H. and Jacobs, H. S. (1995). Diagnosis, prevention and management of the ovarian hyperstimulation syndrome. *Br. J. Obstet. Gynaecol.*, **102**, 767–72
23. Gadir, A. A., Khatim, M. S., Mowafi, R. S., Alnaser, H. M., Alzaid, H. G. and Shaw, R. W. (1990). Ovarian electrocautery versus hMG and pure FSH therapy in the treatment of patients with PCOS. *Clin. Endocrinol.*, **33**, 585–92
24. Armar, N. A., McGarrigle, H. H. G., Honour, J. W., Holownia, P., Jacobs, H. S. and Lachelin, G. C. L. (1990). Laparoscopic ovarian diathermy in the management of anovulatory infertility in women with polycystic ovaries: endocrine changes and clinical outcome. *Fertil. Steril.*, **53**, 45–9
25. Balen, A. H. and Jacobs, H. S. (1994). A prospective study comparing unilateral and bilateral laparoscopic ovarian diathermy in women with the polycystic ovary syndrome. *Fertil. Steril.*, **62**, 921–5
26. Rossmanith, W. G., Keckstein, J., Spatzier, K. and Lauritzen, C. (1991). The impact of ovarian laser surgery on the gonadotrophin secretion in women with PCOS. *Clin. Endocrinol.*, **34**, 223–30
27. Tietze, C. (1968). Fertility after discontinuation of oral and intrauterine contraception. *Int. J. Fertil.*, **13**, 385–9

# The role of ultrasound in reproductive medicine

# 6

*Pat Thurley*

## INTRODUCTION

Ultrasound is used as the main imaging technique throughout the management of the infertile couple. It has a role to play in the initial assessment of any abnormalities within the female pelvis.

Since the first workers, Hansmann and Hackloer in 1976[1], demonstrated that it was possible to visualize ovarian follicles and monitor their growth, ultrasound has been used extensively to assess follicular development. Ultrasound is used as a visible guide for oocyte recovery and other interventional procedures. Finally, ultrasound can be used to assess early gestation and any complications such as ectopic pregnancy at a very early stage.

## INSTRUMENTATION

Successful imaging of the female pelvis depends on two factors, the quality of the imaging and the experience of the ultrasound operator. It is important to have a machine that gives high-quality transvaginal ultrasound images. A transabdominal probe to assess the large fibroid uterus and high ovary out of reach of the transvaginal probe is also essential. The transabdominal probe gives a global observation which is helpful in orientating the transvaginal scan.

The transvaginal probe uses a higher frequency (5.0–7.5 MHz) which improves resolution of the image of the uterus and adnexae (Figure 1). The frequency of the probe is related to the depth of penetration. The axial resolution increases from 0.67 mm for a 3.5 MHz transducer to 0.32 mm for a 7.5 MHz transducer. On the other hand, a 7.5 MHz transducer has a depth of view of only 7.0 cm whereas the 5 MHz has one of 14.0 cm. Most transducers are of a single frequency but some manufacturers offer a dual or multiple frequency transducer. For the novice, a 5 MHz probe with a wide field of view (scanning angle) is probably the best because it allows easier orientation.

The foot plate of the probe is usually situated at the end of the probe, sometimes slightly angulated and, in some mechanical sector probes, it can be rotated. There are advantages[2] with all of these probes. The rotating mechanical sector is easy to use but has the disadvantage of a poorer near-field image. Most of the probes will have a needle guide for biopsy and aspiration (Figure 2). Transvaginal ultrasound needle guidance is commonly used for harvesting oocytes for assisted reproduction in the *in vitro* fertilization (IVF) procedure[3].

Colour flow imaging and duplex Doppler technology are now widely available. The equipment tends to be more expensive and there are many pitfalls for the inexperienced. At its simplest, colour flow will differentiate dilated Fallopian tubes from prominent veins. More complex duplex Doppler may be used to characterize the waveform pattern of the uterine and ovarian vessels, so providing interesting information in the management of infertility. However, at present, many of these applications are in the process of being evaluated.

Most patients accept transvaginal scanning. Some prefer it to having an uncomfortably full bladder as required for transabdominal scans. Some urine in the bladder can be helpful in positioning the uterus for transvaginal scanning. It is important to make sure that the condom which covers the transvaginal probe and

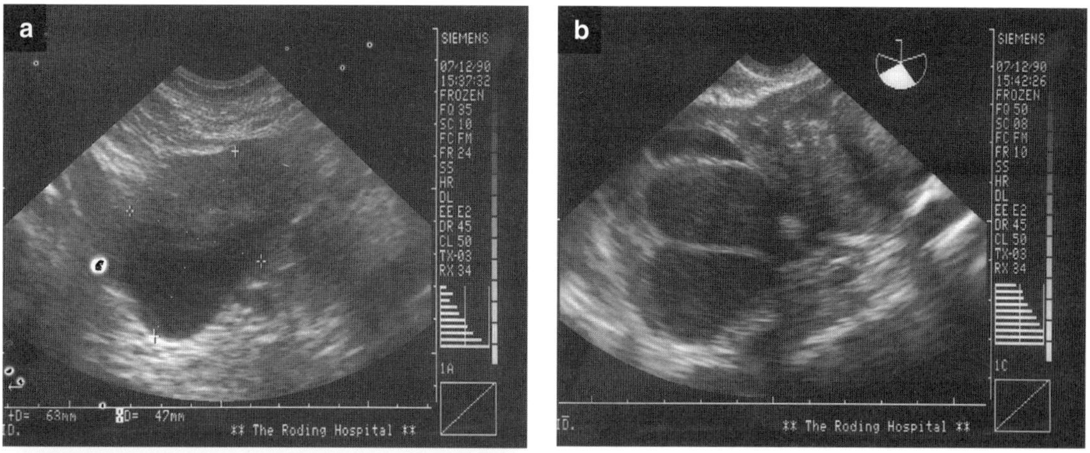


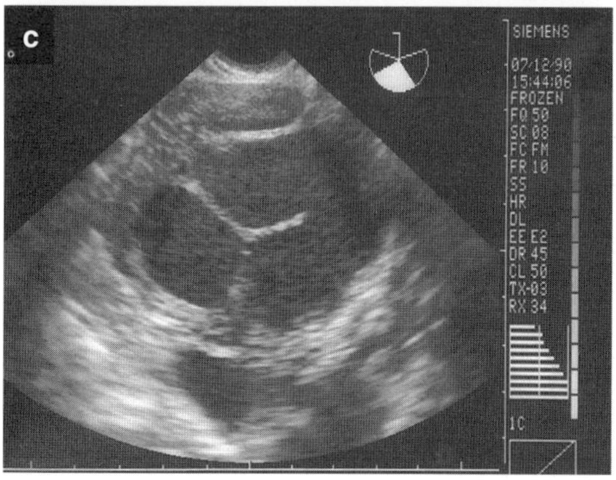


**Figure 1** Comparison of transabdominal and transvaginal scanning in an adnexal mass. (a) Transabdominal scan shows a vague transonic mass; (b) and (c) transvaginal scans show this to be a dilated tube with probable pus within it

the lubricating gel are not spermicidal when scanning infertile patients!

## THE INITIAL ASSESSMENT OF THE FEMALE PELVIS

### The uterus

Uterine pathology accounts for only a small percentage of cases of infertility. It is the ultrasonographer's role to describe the pathology e.g. fibroids, and the clinician's role to assess their importance as a contributory factor in the couple's infertility.

Müllerian duct abnormalities (MDA) which result from non-development or varying degrees of non-fusion of the Müllerian ducts are a small but important cause of infertility and pregnancy loss. Transvaginal and transabdominal ultrasound will visualize the endometrial cavity and uterine outline, thus differentiating unicornuate, bicornuate and septate uteri (Figure 3). Transvaginal ultrasound combined with hysterosalpingography have resulted in diagnostic rates as high as 90% in differentiating septate from bicornuate uteri[4]. This is important as the surgical management is different in these two conditions. However, the most consistently accurate imaging technique for evaluating Müllerian duct abnormalities is MRI[5]. With bicornuate uteri, the endometrial cavities are more divergent (> 105° angle) than with the septate uteri (< 75° angle). However, there is overlap and the external contour differentiates the two, as the bicornuate uterus has a heart-shaped external configuration. It is most important to evaluate the renal tract in these patients.

Endometrial adhesions or synechiae and endometrial polyps are usually best imaged with hysterosalpingography. Recently, with the introduction of sonohysterography using saline[6] (or a specially manufactured echogenic contrast media) transvaginal ultrasound can be employed to assess the endometrial cavity (Figure 4). Saline is introduced into the endometrial cavity during transvaginal ultrasound scanning. It allows the differentiation of intracavitary endometrial and submucosal

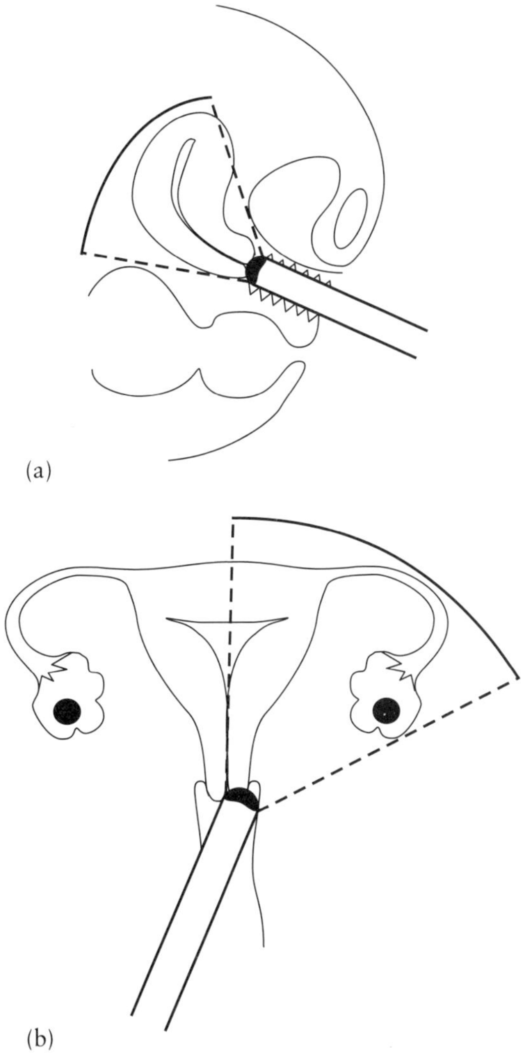


**Figure 2** Positioning of the probe in transvaginal scanning. (a) Longitudinal view of the anteverted uterus; (b) probe rotated through 90° and positioned in the lateral fornix to visualize the adnexae

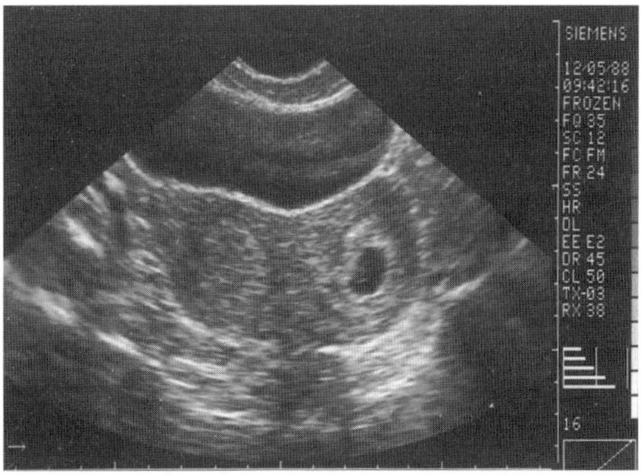


**Figure 3** Bicornuate uterus with an early gestational sac and yolk sac in one endometrial cavity

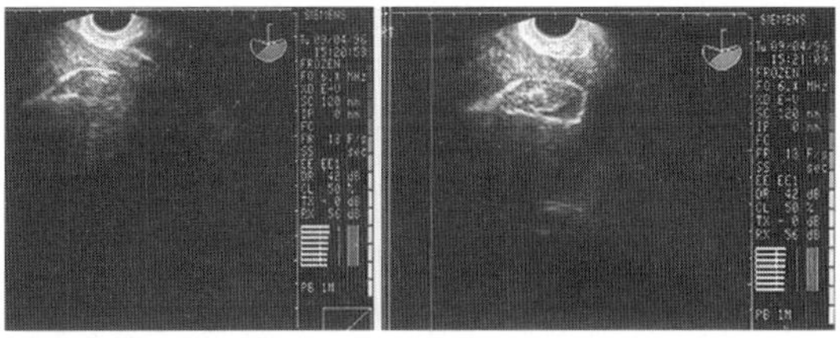

**Figure 4** Echogenic contrast within the endometrial cavity outlining a polypoid submucosal fibroid

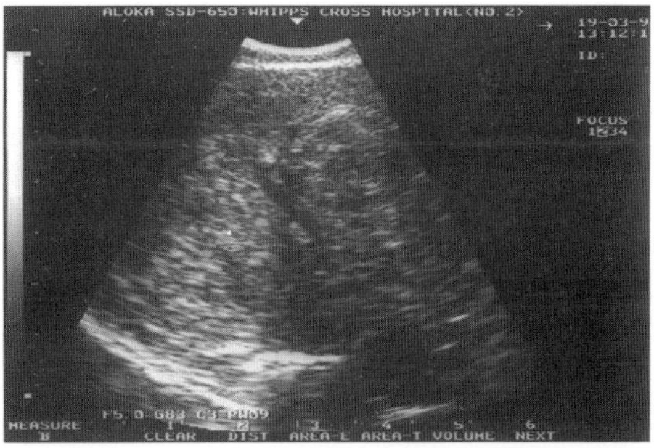


**Figure 5** Fluid seen in the endometrial cavity emphasizing the position of the submucosal fibroid

abnormalities without the use of ionizing radiation (Figures 5 and 6).

Leiomyomata can play a role in infertility and will increase pregnancy wastage. They may occlude the tubal ostia, distort the endometrial cavity and interfere with the blood flow. The accuracy of ultrasound in detecting fibroids is 65–93%[7]. The fibroids may appear hypoechoic, isoechoic or hyperechoic on ultrasound. Calcified fibroids cause acoustic shadowing and may prevent good visualization of the endometrial cavity (Figure 7). Small isoechoic fibroids may be difficult to see. Scanning in the second half of the cycle when the endometrium is thickest will improve visualization of the endometrial cavity and its relationship to the fibroids[8].

If surgery is being considered, hysteroscopy combined with transvaginal ultrasound is useful for submucosal fibroids. Magnetic

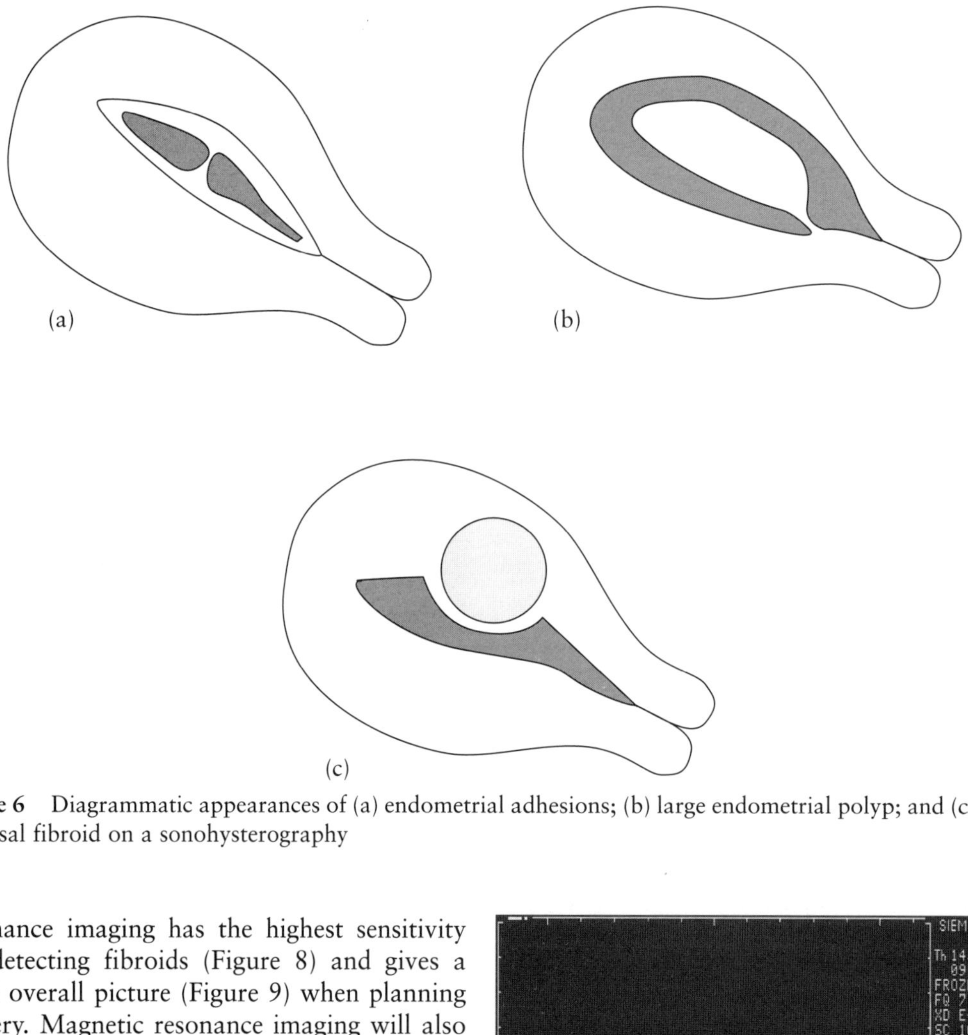


**Figure 6** Diagrammatic appearances of (a) endometrial adhesions; (b) large endometrial polyp; and (c) submucosal fibroid on a sonohysterography

resonance imaging has the highest sensitivity for detecting fibroids (Figure 8) and gives a good overall picture (Figure 9) when planning surgery. Magnetic resonance imaging will also differentiate leiomyomas from adenomyosis, unlike other imaging techniques.

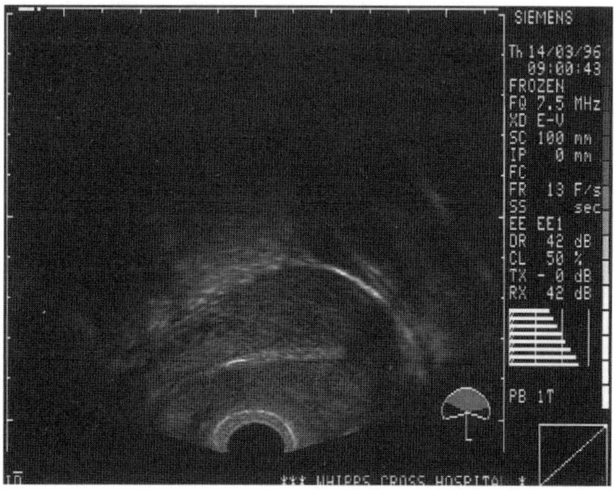


**Figure 7** Small hyperechoic fibroid of the fundus of the uterus demonstrating acoustic shadowing

## The Fallopian tubes

Tubal disease is found to play a role in 30–50%[9] of female infertility. In view of this and the concern over long-term effects of infertility drugs, it is advisable to assess tubal patency early in the initial assessment.

Hysterosalpingography and laparoscopy and dye insufflation (lap and dye) have been the traditional methods of assessing tubal patency (Figure 10), with lap and dye perhaps being the gold standard, as hysterosalpingography has a false-positive rate of 6–20%, probably due to cornual spasm, and a false-negative rate of 8–24%, possibly due to difficulty in assessing peritubal adhesions. However, hysterosalpingo-

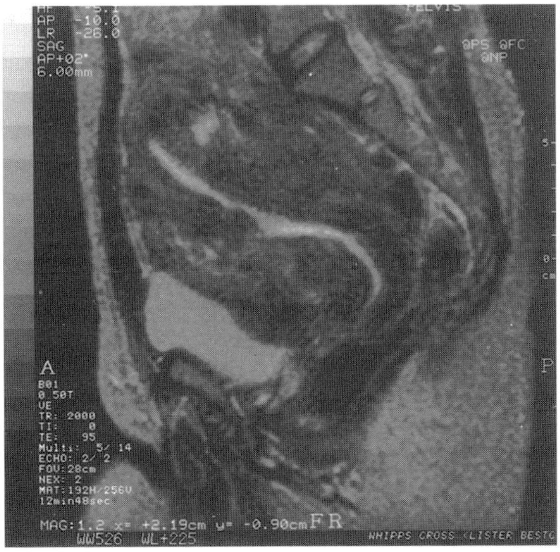

**Figure 8** A sagittal magnetic resonance imaging scan through a large fibroid uterus. The fibroids are of low signal (black) and are seen well in relation to the high-signal endometrium

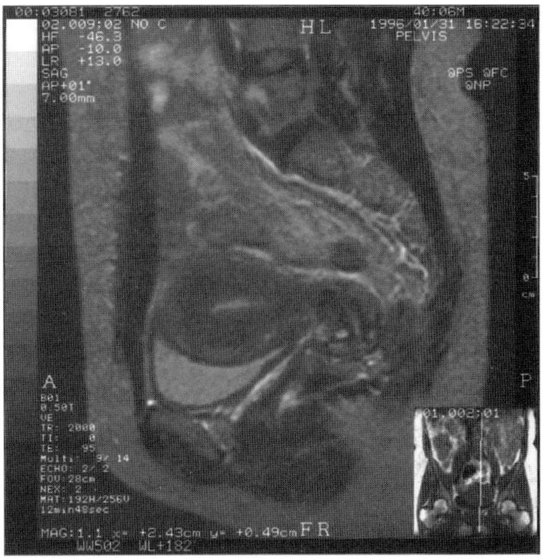

**Figure 9** Diffuse adenomyosis of the myometrium demonstrated with magnetic resonance imaging. Notice the low signal, which has spread beyond the junctional zone between the high signal endometrium and the grey myometrium

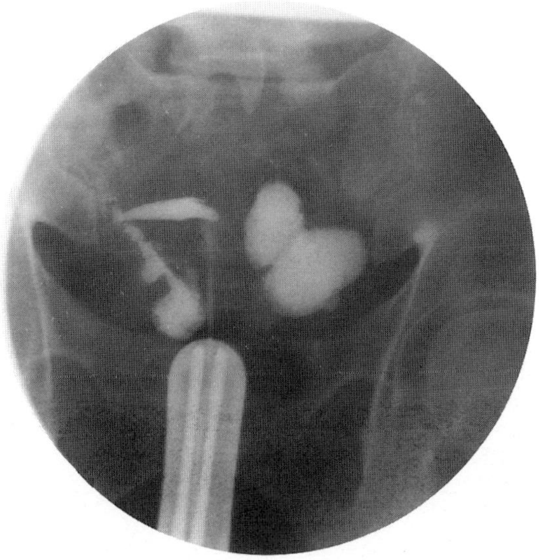

**Figure 10** Hysterosalpingography showing bilateral hydrosalpinges

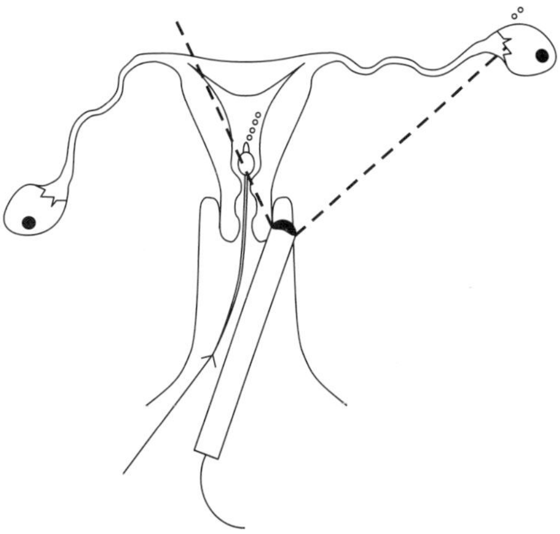

**Figure 11** Hysterosalpingo-contrast sonography (HyCoSy): the catheter balloon is within the endometrial cavity. The transvaginal probe is positioned to visualize the contrast flow down the proximal tube

graphy is better at assessing the tubal mucosa in conditions such as salpingitis isthmica nodosa, where many small diverticuli are visualized.

Recently, an echogenic contrast medium has been developed for transvaginal ultrasound assessment of the tube. It involves passing a small catheter into the uterine cavity and slowly injecting the contrast while scanning the cornu of the uterus and Fallopian tubes (Figure 11)[10]. Flow down the tubes can be easily seen and denotes tubal patency. Data from a recent cross-over multicentre trial show that hysterosalpingo-contrast sonography (HyCoSy) (Figure 12) demonstrates a sensitivity of 86% and a positive predictive value of 90% compared with X-ray hysterosalpingography[11,12].

The future role of HyCoSy seems to lie in the hands of gynaecologists and sonographers who perform transvaginal ultrasound at their initial assessment clinics. In this situation, the addition of the HyCoSy technique would be quite simple and, if tubal patency was demonstrated, the patient could proceed immediately to medical treatment. If the results are inconclusive, the patient could then proceed to X-ray hysterosalpingography or lap and dye according to local practice.

Hysterosalpingo-contrast sonography requires considerable competence in transvaginal scanning and there is a concern that flow into a large hydrosalpinx may give normal flow in the proximal tubes.

Transvaginal ultrasound will demonstrate a hydrosalpinx following fimbrial adhesions due to infection. A dilated Fallopian tube is characteristically tubular or fusiform. Recognition of an inner mucosal layer reliably differentiates a dilated tube from other pelvic cysts. Sometimes the dilated Fallopian tube will demonstrate small polypoid nodules projecting into the lumen (cog-wheel sign)[13,14]. With chronic pelvic inflammation, adhesions will form and transvaginal ultrasound may demonstrate lack of movement between the uterus and ovaries.

## The ovary

On transvaginal scanning, the ovaries usually lie between the uterus and the pelvic side wall and are closely related to the internal iliac vessels. They may, however, lie in the pouch of Douglas or higher in the pelvis. Sometimes, manual compression of the abdomen may be necessary to bring the ovary into view with transvaginal ultrasound. The small follicles of the ovary enable it to be easily identified.

On the initial assessment scan, various ovarian pathologies may be visualized. Simple functional cysts are commonly seen and reflect the fact that the ovary is a very dynamic organ. Most functional cysts measure less than 5.0 cm in diameter and usually resolve within one or two menstrual cycles. The follicular cyst is a smooth-walled unilocular cyst with no internal echoes and a well-defined margin. A corpus luteal cyst may have evidence of internal haemorrhage and the wall is usually thickened and irregular. It may have a net of internal echoes (Figure 13) or a polypoid appearance. In fact, the corpus luteal cyst is a great mimic of other disease processes, ranging from ectopic pregnancy to neoplasia.

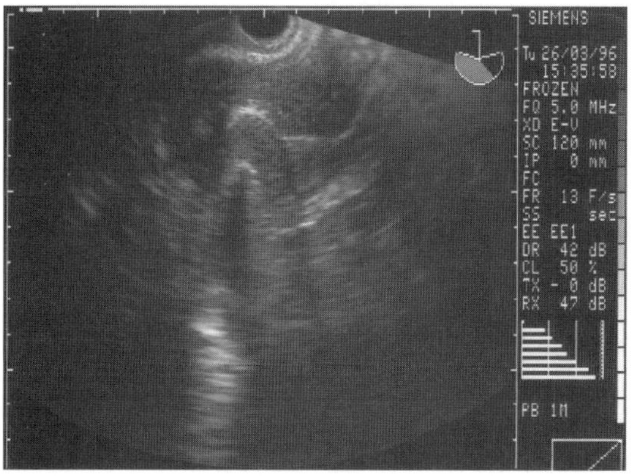


**Figure 12** Hysterosalpingo-contrast sonography (HyCoSy): echogenic (white) contrast can be seen in the endometrial cavity and going down the left tube

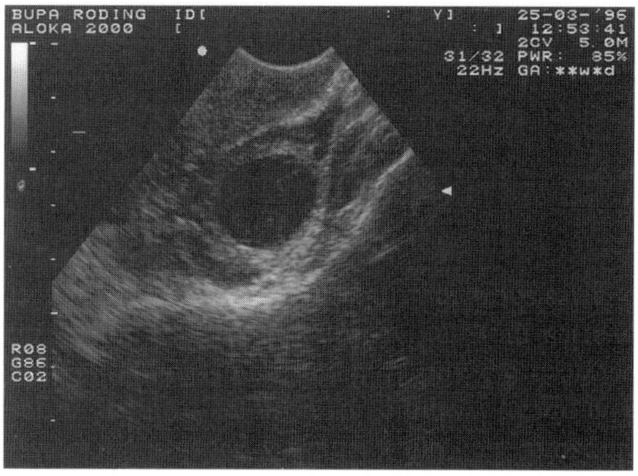


**Figure 13** Corpus luteum showing a net of internal echoes compatible with haemorrhage

It is essential to relate the ultrasound findings to the clinical situation and, if necessary, repeat the scan in 6 weeks' time when the luteal cyst will have regressed. It appears that these simple cysts do not significantly affect the overall folliculogenesis during ovarian stimulation in an IVF programme[15].

Endometriosis commonly involves the ovary and the posterior leaf of the broad ligament. If chocolate cysts have developed, they may be visualized as cystic structures containing uniform or homogeneous internal echoes. They may be very thin-walled or be seen within thick walls, representing adhesions (Figure 14). Endometriosis of the bladder may also be seen easily on ultrasound, usually as a polypoid, ill-defined mass projecting into the bladder. Adhesions, caused by endometriosis, may be suggested on ultrasound (Figure 15) by an unusual position of the ovary and immobility of the ovary on transvaginal ultrasound.

Laparoscopy provides an accurate means of diagnosing small deposits of endometriosis which will not be visualized by ultrasound. Recently magnetic resonance imaging has been shown to be very good at imaging endometriosis, especially in a pelvis with many adhesions when laparoscopy may be less useful[16]. Ultrasound has a role in assessing the response of endometriosis to hormonal treatment.

Transvaginal ultrasound is very important in diagnosing polycystic ovaries as the hormonal levels of luteinizing hormone (LH) may lie within the normal range in a significant percentage of patients with polycystic ovaries (Chapter 4). The ultrasonographer must also be careful not to over-diagnose polycystic ovary syndrome (PCOS) in patients with normal ovulation. There has been much discussion over the years as to which are the best ultrasound criteria used to diagnose polycystic ovaries. On average, the ovarian volume is greater in polycystic ovaries. The volume of the ovary may be measured using a simplified formula for an ellipsoid, i.e. $0.5 \times$ length $\times$ width $\times$ thickness. The mean volume in normal women varies between 6.5 and 10.0 $cm^3$ and some polycystic ovaries may fall within this range. Polycystic ovaries show multiple small (2–8 mm diameter;

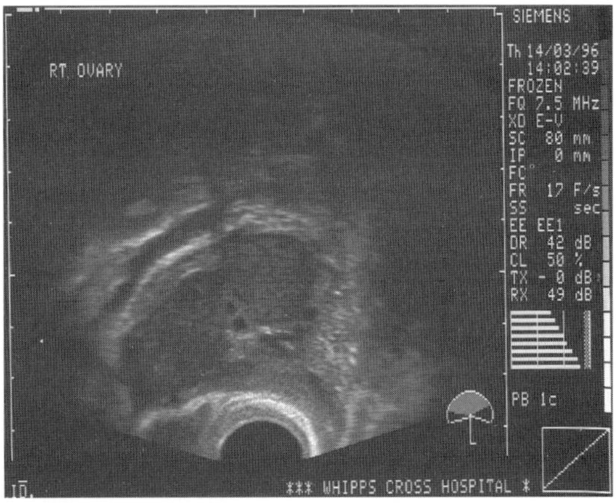


**Figure 14** Typical endometriomas of the ovary with homogeneous low level echoes

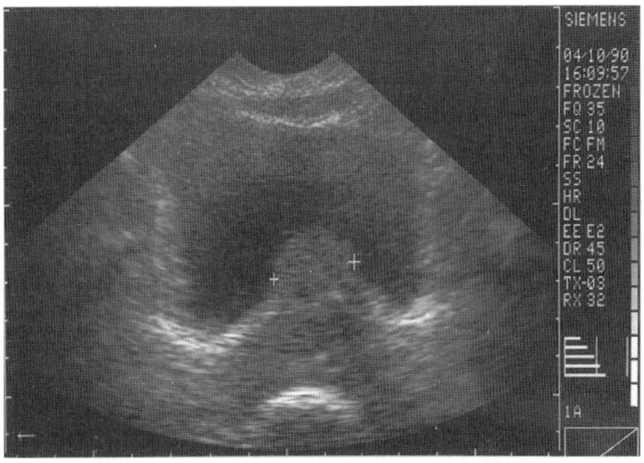


**Figure 15** Transverse scan of the bladder showing endometriosis involving the posterior bladder wall

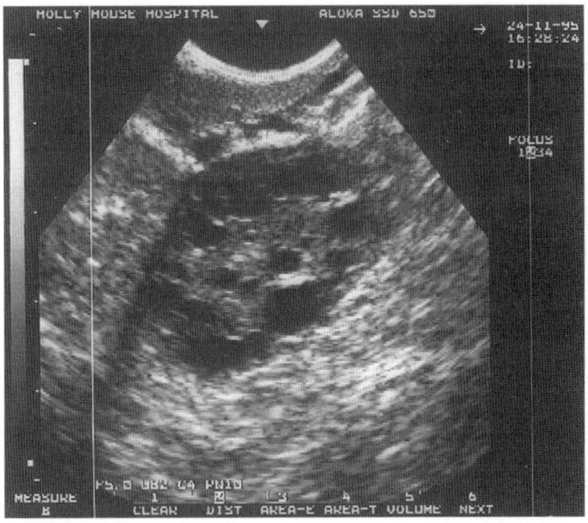


**Figure 16** Typical appearance of a polycystic ovary with many small, less than 1.0 cm follicles on transvaginal scan

Figure 16) cysts usually lying peripherally but they may also be distributed throughout the stroma. The stroma may be of increased echogenicity[17] (probably reflecting the direct action of both luteinizing hormone (LH) and insulin). The combination of ovarian volume and follicular size appears to be the most sensitive method of discriminating polycystic ovaries from normal ovaries[18].

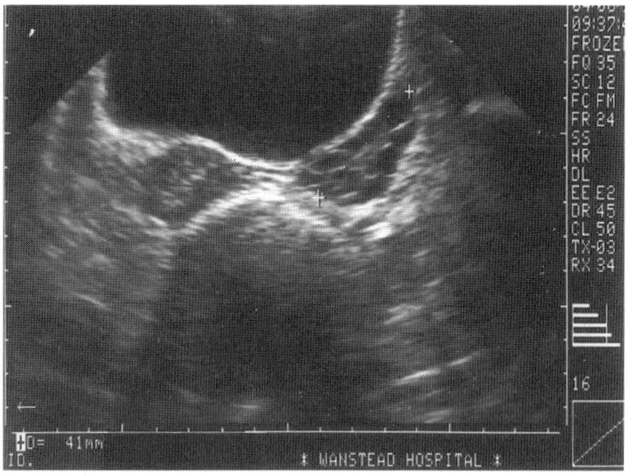


Figure 17 Transabdominal scan of a polycystic ovary. Note the echogenic stroma and the lack of detail compared with Figure 16

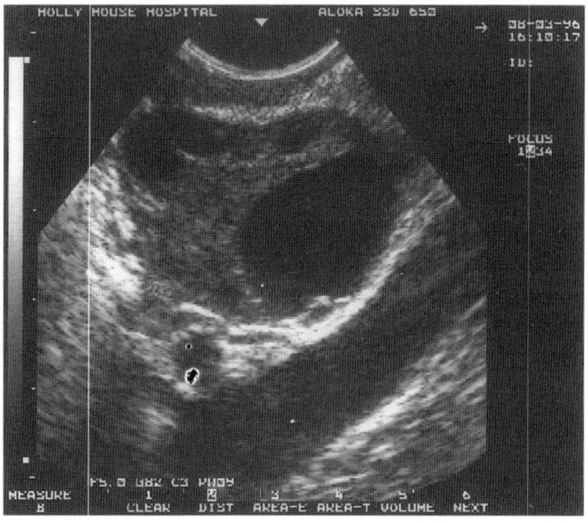


Figure 18 Transvaginal ultrasound of a normal ovary with a developing follicle on day 13 of the cycle. Note the relationship of the ovary to the internal iliac vessel

The ovarian shape in polycystic ovaries is variable; it may be round but it is often long and thin. The endometrium tends to be of a thickness greater than 5.0 mm and of a homogeneous nature (Figure 17), which may be the result of increased estrogen levels[19]. Diagnosis of PCOS in infertility is important as it predisposes to ovarian hyperstimulation syndrome during infertility treatment.

However, most initial scans of the pelvis in the infertile patient are normal. It is sensible to perform the initial scan on days 11–13 so that any developing follicles can be visualized and thus avoid a further scan to assess follicular development.

## ULTRASOUND OF THE NORMAL OVARIAN CYCLE

The transvaginal scan can visualize follicles as small as 2.0 mm. Growth of the follicles parallels the hormonal changes of the normal menstrual cycle. Thus by day 5–7, several follicles will be recognized as small cysts of diameter 2–4 mm. Serial scans will show the emergence of the dominant follicle, which will grow approximately 1.4–2.2 mm per day with slightly greater growth of 2–3 mm per day just before ovulation (Figure 18). At the time of ovulation, the follicle diameter will range from 16 to 35 mm with most lying between 18 and 24 mm[20,21]. Measurement of the diameter of the mature follicle may be difficult if it is ovoid; in this case, an average of the diameter in three planes may be used.

The ovulatory phase occurs with the onset of the LH surge, the development of the cumulus oophorus and the separation of the granulosa cell layer from the thecal cells. The cumulus oophorus is only 1.0 mm in diameter and, although some authors report detection of this 1–2 days before ovulation and of seeing a 'double contour' to the follicle just before ovulation[23], other authors using transvaginal scanning have failed to confirm this[22]. These signs are not consistent enough to time ovulation reliably so the follicular diameter is used to assess maturation in infertility treatment; most centres use 1.8 cm as the size at which ovulation is initiated by hCG administration.

After ovulation, there is collapse of the follicle wall, development of internal echoes and formation of the corpus luteum. As mentioned earlier, this has a variable appearance and size from a thick-walled cyst to a more complex mass with internal haemorrhage. No relationship has been shown between the corpus luteum size and progesterone levels in the luteal phase. Duplex Doppler shows a high diastolic flow in the ovary containing the corpus luteum, which may be helpful in identifying the corpus luteum (Figure 19).

In anovulatory cycles, there is poor follicular development and the follicle rarely reaches 14 mm in diameter and then collapses prematurely.

Occasionally, the dominant follicle fails to rupture and continues to grow in the luteal phase of the cycle, the so-called luteinizing unruptured follicle. It appears to change in structure and secrete progesterone in normal quantities and thus is difficult to diagnose. There is some uncertainty of the incidence of luteinized unruptured follicle syndrome[23,24].

## ULTRASOUND IN INDUCED OVULATORY CYCLES

The role of ultrasound in induced cycles is to establish that the ovary is responding to stimulation, to ensure that the dominant follicle reaches a minimum size and to ascertain the number of preovulatory follicles to avoid multiple pregnancies and over-stimulation. Post-ovulation scanning will show that ovulation has occurred and help with the diagnosis of ovarian hyperstimulation.

In general, infertility treatment is time-consuming for the patient and the number of scans to track the follicles should be kept to a minimum. It is helpful if the sonographer is part of the infertility team and follows the patient throughout the treatment, as this will usually give more consistent measurements. In induced cycles using clomiphene citrate or other antiestrogen, a scan should be performed on day 8. This scan should demonstrate developing follicles of 8–10 mm diameter. With clomiphene-induced ovulation, follicular development may be different from natural cycles, with each follicle growing at an individual rate. If the day 8 scan does not show any follicular development, the dose of clomiphene may be increased. The plasma estradiol levels may not give good correlation with follicular size in induced cycles, as three small follicles may give the same level as one large follicle, thus emphasizing the value of ultrasound in assessing follicular growth. Following the initial day 8 scan on a clomiphene cycle, it is only necessary to scan again in 3–4 days to ascertain the growth of a dominant follicle.

If gonadotrophins are being used to stimulate the ovary (usually after the failure of clomiphene), repeat scans every 2–4 days will assess the follicular growth and, when one follicle reaches 1.8 cm diameter, human chorionic gonadotrophin (hCG) should be given to

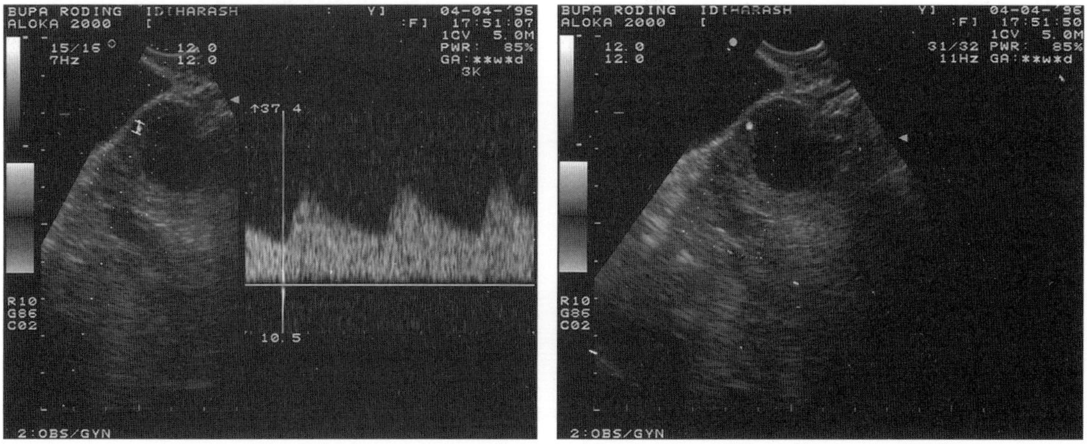


**Figure 19** Typical corpus luteum with intraovarian Doppler trace showing high diastolic flow

induce ovulation, which should occur 36 h later. If multiple follicular development is seen, i.e. three follicles greater than 16 mm or six follicles greater than 14 mm, hCG should not be given because of the risk of multiple pregnancy and ovarian hyperstimulation syndrome[24].

The protocol for ultrasound scanning will vary between units. For example, some units will only perform a day 12 scan if clomiphene is being given. It is also important to tailor the programme to the individual patient's needs.

Usually an assessment of the endometrium is made just before the administration of hCG; the thickness, appearance and perhaps the blood flow to the endometrium are measured to assess if it is ready for implantation.

## SUPEROVULATION AND *IN VITRO* FERTILIZATION

In IVF, the aim is to produce a reasonable number of eggs for fertilization and thus increase the number of embryos available for fresh embryo transfer and cryopreservation. This is achieved by stimulating the ovary to produce a reasonable number of follicles.

Many centres now give a gonadotrophin releasing hormone (GnRH) agonist to suppress the normal pituitary and ovary before stimulating the ovaries with gonadotrophin. This makes monitoring of the follicular development much easier as there is no LH surge and ovulation can be controlled.

Ultrasound can be used, together with estradiol levels, to ascertain suppression of the ovaries. On ultrasound examination there should only be tiny follicles in the ovaries and a thin endometrium (less than 4.0 mm).

Human menopausal gonadotrophin (hMG), together with a GnRH agonist, are then given to stimulate follicular development. Ultrasound examination may be performed daily after day 8 of stimulation or less often if the ovaries have been down-regulated. More frequent ultrasound assessments are necessary in gonadotrophin-alone cycles to monitor the ovaries once the dominant follicle is formed. Stimulation is continued until there are three follicles of 1.8 cm diameter. At each scan, the number and size of the follicles are documented and it is important to measure the follicular diameters in at least two places as they tend to be compressed by each other.

The estradiol level is measured before hCG administration and, if it is too high, the cycle may be aborted to avoid ovarian hyperstimulation syndrome, especially in polycystic ovary syndrome (see Chapter 4).

There is a window of 2–3 days within which to give hCG if GnRH agonists have been given. The eggs are collected 36 h after hCG administration, usually by transvaginal ultrasound guidance.

### Ultrasound in the detection of complications of infertility treatment: ovarian hyperstimulation syndrome

This occurs more commonly in patients with polycystic ovary syndrome and in superovulatory induction. It occurs when hyperstimulation of the ovaries is associated with an abnormality of fluid balance, leading to accumulation of fluid in the extracellular space and electrolyte disturbances. Ultrasound can be used to assess the size of the ovaries and categorize the severity of the disease[25]. Mild cases show ovarian enlargement up to 5.0 cm, moderate cases show larger ovaries up to 10 cm, and severe cases show ovaries greater than 10 cm with ascites and pleural effusions and haemoconcentration. The enlarged ovaries are full of many cysts, separated by thick septae (Figure 20), as the result of massive follicular luteinization, and therefore only follows hCG administration. It is made worse with successful pregnancy and endogenous hCG production.

Sometimes these patients will present in casualty with a distended, acute abdomen. Ultrasound of the ovaries will quickly confirm the diagnosis and prevent unnecessary surgery. It is a severe condition that may be fatal and therefore it is important to withhold hCG if oestrogen levels are too high, i.e. if on scan there are more than 20 follicles greater than 12.0 mm diameter present or the serum estradiol levels are greater than 10 000 pmol/l. Then

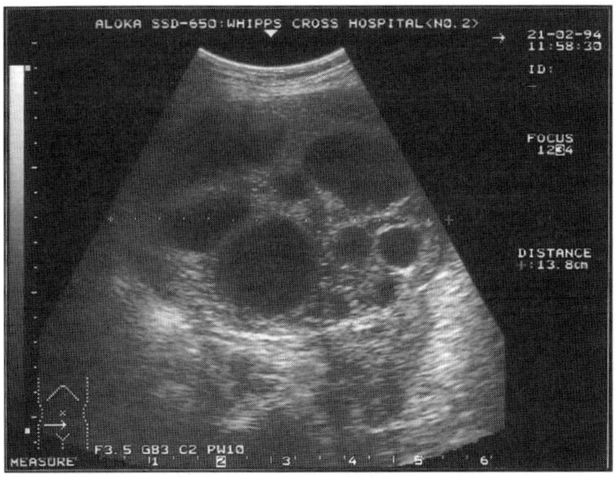


**Figure 20** The enlarged multicystic ovary of moderate ovarian hyperstimulation syndrome

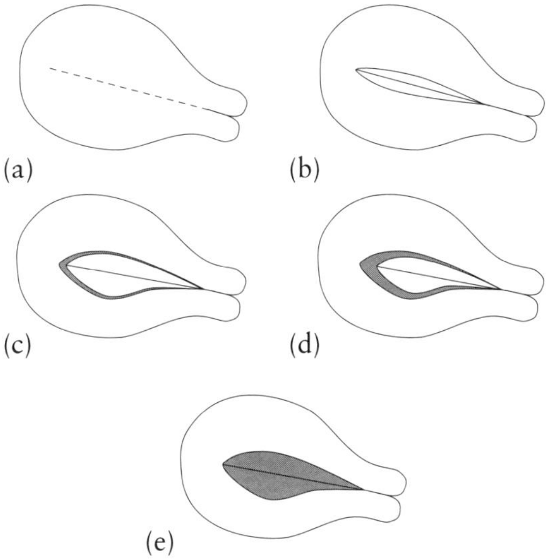


**Figure 21** Simple outlines of endometrial appearances during the menstrual cycle: (a) menstrual phase; (b) proliferative phase, isoechoic with myometrium; (c) preovulatory phase, increasing echogenicity and thickness; (d) periovulatory phase, three layer appearance; and (e) secretory phase, thick and echogenic

treatment should either be abandoned before the administration of hCG injection or the embryos should be cryopreserved to be used in another cycle.

## Oocyte retrieval

The majority of centres now use a transvaginal probe with an appropriate needle guide attached alongside the probe[26] so that the needle can be directed into each follicle in turn under direct visual guidance. The ultrasound probe needs to be placed in the lateral fornix as near to the ovary as possible. A high-frequency 5.0–7.5 MHz probe is advisable for high-resolution imaging. The success rate is comparable to that achieved using the laparoscopic technique. Transvaginal ultrasound has an advantage in patients with adhesions which may prevent access to the ovary laparoscopically. Rarely, the ovary is inaccessible transvaginally and a transuterine or transabdominal approach may be required. Transvaginal ultrasound may also be used to guide the necessary canalization of the Fallopian tube via the uterus for gamete or zygote intrafallopian transfer techniques.

## The endometrium in assisted conception

The endometrium changes thickness and appearance during the menstrual cycle both in spontaneous and induced cycles (Figure 21)[27]. In the menstrual phase, the endometrium appears as a thin, broken echogenic surface. In the proliferative phase, it thickens, measuring 3–5 mm, and becomes isoechoic with the myometrium. As ovulation approaches, the endometrium becomes more echogenic, perhaps due to secretions within the tortuous glands. In the periovulatory period, there is usually a hypoechoic area within the inner endometrium, giving a multilayered appearance to the endometrium rather like a hamburger (Figure 22). During the secretory phase, the endometrium reaches its greatest thickness and echogenicity. Drugs used in assisted conception may alter the development of the endometrium[28].

It is tempting to try to relate thickness or texture of the endometrium on ultrasound to the success or failure of pregnancy but numerous studies have failed to show a statistical association. One study showed that a multilayered appearance to the endometrium seemed to make a statistically significant difference in the pregnancy rate[28]. Other workers have

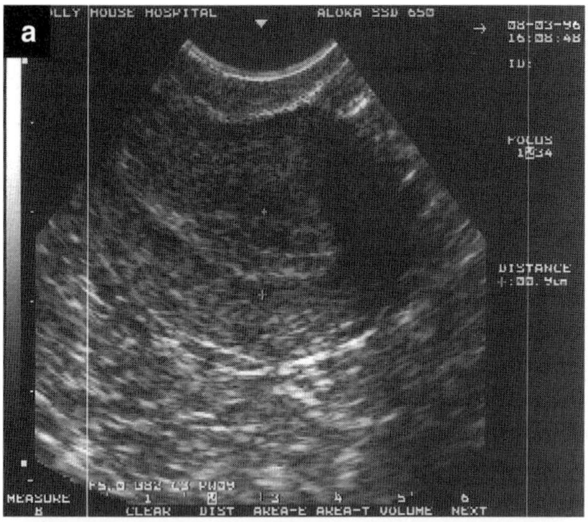


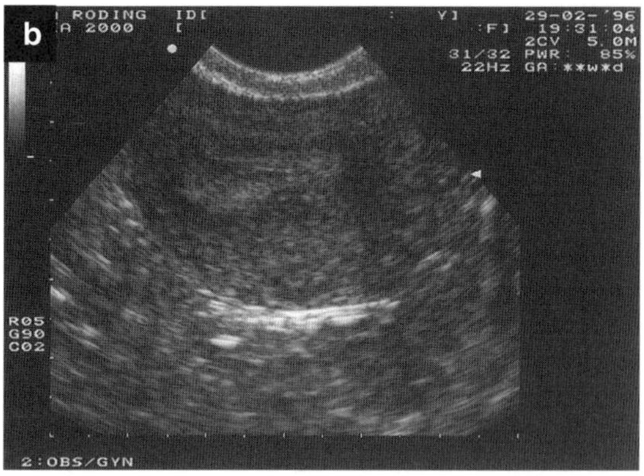


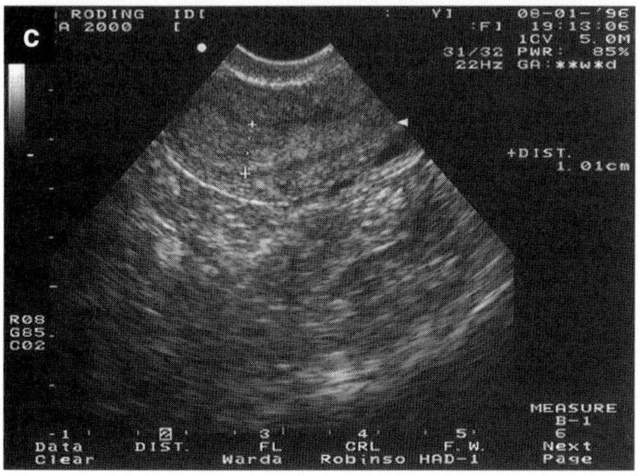


**Figure 22** The appearance of the endometrium in different phases of the endometrial cycle: (a) typical three layer appearance of the endometrium on day 13 with 9.0 mm thickness; (b) more echogenic secretory endometrium on day 16; and (c) more homogeneously echogenic endometrium in secretory phase of cycle

found that the uniformly echogenic endometrium was the least successful. In IVF treatment cycles, it is important to know whether the endometrium will be receptive and implantation will occur. If the endometrium is unreceptive, it may be advantageous to freeze the embryos and implant them in a frozen embryo transfer cycle at a later stage. Conversely, if the endometrium is receptive, it might be advisable to implant only two embryos to prevent triplet pregnancy.

Transvaginal scanning with colour flow imaging of the uterine arteries shows changes in the blood flow during the menstrual cycle[29]. These studies have shown that the chances of implantation are low if the pulsatility index (PI) is over 3[30].

Colour Doppler transvaginal ultrasound allows easier identification of the uterine arteries which may be difficult to see on just the B-scan image. Once identified, it is then impossible to place the pulsed Doppler gate on the vessel and obtain a trace of the flow velocity waveforms during systole and diastole. The pulsatility index is given by (peak systolic – peak diastolic shift frequency)/mean shift frequency, and is a useful way of expressing the blood flow impedance distal to the point of sampling. Most colour Doppler machines will calculate this once the cursors have outlined the flow velocity waveforms.

A low value for the PI (when there is good diastolic flow) indicates decreased impedance to blood flow in the distal uterine and endometrial vessels (Figure 23).

There are, however, many pitfalls for the unwary in using colour Doppler. It is important to achieve a low angle between the ultrasound beam and the direction of blood flow to obtain an accurate trace (from the Doppler formula, velocity = frequency shift × cos B, where B is the angle between the line of the ultrasound beam and the direction of the flow).

Technical errors are easily caused by improper setting of the colour flow parameters such as colour velocity scale, colour sensitivity and colour wall filter, especially in the low-flow setting used in transvaginal gynaecology

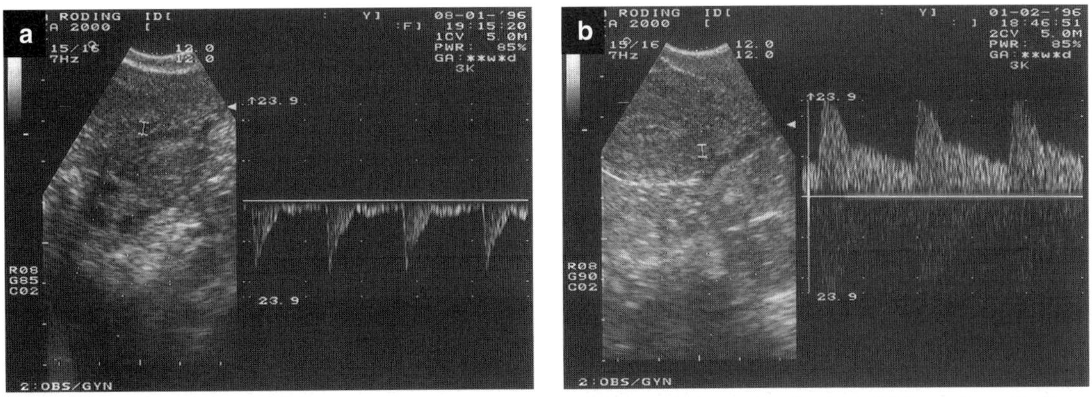

**Figure 23** Doppler flow changes in the uterine arteries during the menstrual cycle: (a) low diastolic flow and prominent notch seen early in menstrual cycle; and (b) high diastolic flow in the mid-cycle (notice three-layered endometrium)

scanning. For those interested, the author recommends a recent review article on this subject[31].

A recent paper[32] investigated the vascular penetration of the endometrium in mid-cycle using colour Doppler transvaginal ultrasound. It was found that absent subendometrial and interendometrial vascularization on the day of hCG administration appears to be a useful predictor of failure of implantation in IVF treatment cycles, irrespective of the morphological appearance of the endometrium.

The morphological appearance of the endometrium is subjective and will differ with transabdominal and transvaginal scanning. Thus a more objective and reproducible test for the likely failure of implantation is to be welcomed. One suggestion is a uterine biophysical profile, scoring all the parameters which can be measured with ultrasound that are likely to influence implantation[33].

## Assessment of early pregnancy in assisted conception

There is considerable anxiety for all concerned while waiting to discover whether or not there has been successful implantation. Transvaginal Doppler of the ovarian arteries and measurement of the resistance index (RI) of the Doppler wave form to the corpus luteum showed a significant difference in RI in those women who became pregnant. No patient with an RI of greater than 0.5 became pregnant after IVF or gamete intrafallopian transfer (GIFT). These measurements were taken 3 and 10 days after implantation[34].

Pregnancies resulting from IVF procedures have a higher rate of early obstetric complications than do spontaneous pregnancies. There is a higher incidence of ectopic implantation, reportedly occurring in 5–11% of cases[35]. This may be due to damaged Fallopian tubes, the site of implantation and the migration of the embryo. The frequency of heterotopic pregnancy is increased, occurring in as many as 2.9% of all IVF pregnancies[36]. In these cases, the presence of a normal intrauterine pregnancy should not prevent an ultrasound search for an ectopic pregnancy. There is also a higher rate of miscarriage, though this may only affect one fetus of a multiple pregnancy[37]. Miscarriage rates following IVF are increased in women with polycystic ovary syndrome and reduced by pituitary desensitization with buserelin. Serial measurement of the β-hCG levels will give a good indication of whether there is a viable intrauterine pregnancy, ectopic pregnancy or failed pregnancy. However, with multiple pregnancies, it is more difficult to assess and transvaginal ultrasound at 28 days and 42 days after implantation will be performed in most centres. It is also very encouraging for the patient if a viable pregnancy can be visualized.

## THE NORMAL ULTRASOUND FEATURES OF EARLY PREGNANCY

With the advent of transvaginal scanning it became possible clearly to see and measure the gestational sac and early embryo.

### Gestational sac

The first reliable sign of pregnancy is the visualization of the gestational sac, which is seen as a ring-like structure with an echogenic rim around it (Figure 24). With good transvaginal equipment, this can be seen as early as 4 weeks and 1 or 2 days' menstrual age[38]. It is usually located in the upper part of the endometrium, usually in an eccentric position. It is round, up to a size of 1.0 cm diameter and a healthy sac grows approximately 1.0 mm per day[39]. The level of β-hCG at which an intrauterine pregnancy can be detected by ultrasound should be ≥ 1000 IU/l (First International Reference Preparation). Repeat β-hCG levels can be helpful as a guide to the ultrasonographer searching for an ectopic pregnancy, when the levels will show a slower rise than normal. An ectopic pregnancy can be associated with some fluid in the endometrial cavity, the so-called decidual cast. However, the gestational sac is seen actually within the endometrium and has a definite echogenic outline on transvaginal ultrasound. Colour Doppler appearances may also be helpful in differentiating the tiny gestational sac from a pseudosac.

### Yolk sac

At the beginning of the 5th week, the yolk sac becomes visible within the gestational sac, in fact within the chorionic cavity (Figure 25)[40]. The yolk sac is a circular, well-defined echo-free area, usually near one wall of the gestational sac. It is approximately 3–4 mm in diameter within a gestational sac of 8–10 mm diameter. On scanning, only the walls of the yolk sac at right angles to the beam may be seen but, on movement of the probe, its circular nature becomes apparent. The yolk sac grows slowly until it reaches a maximum diameter of 6.0 mm at 10 weeks.

As the amniotic cavity develops and fills the chorionic sac, the yolk sac gradually moves away from the embryo to lie between the amniotic and chorionic membranes (Figure 26).

Absence of a yolk sac in early pregnancy obviously indicates a poor outcome. Some workers have used measurements of the yolk sac size very early in gestation as a useful marker of pregnancy outcome[41]. Seeing the yolk sac in a possible small ectopic gestational sac is very helpful in detecting early ectopic pregnancies.

### Embryo

The embryo is first seen as a straight echogenic line adjacent to the yolk sac at approximately 40 days' gestation[42]. Sometimes the embryonic heart pulsations are seen more clearly than the embryo!

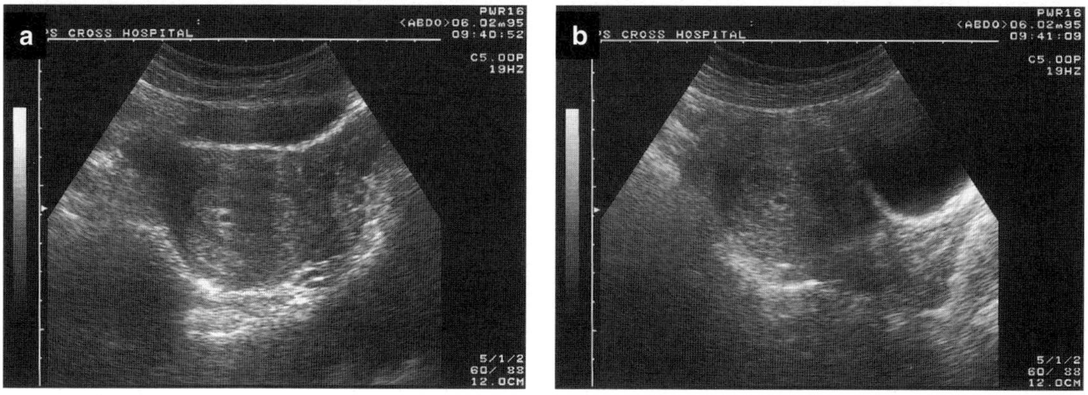


**Figure 24** An early 4–5-week gestational sac seen lying within the thickened endometrium

When the embryo reaches a crown–rump length of 5.0 mm, it should be consistently seen as separate from the yolk sac, with a pulsating cardiac echo. This corresponds to a gestational age of 6 weeks and 4 days and a gestational sac diameter of 15–20 mm.

A blighted ovum is a failed pregnancy when the embryo has failed to develop, although the gestational sac is present. With transvaginal ultrasound, a gestational sac of 18 mm without a visible embryo is unequivocal evidence of a failed anembryonic pregnancy.

In order to prevent mistakes in assessing pregnancy viability by ultrasound in early pregnancy, the Royal Colleges of Radiologists and Obstetricians and Gynaecologists have proposed the following guidelines[43]: 'All ultrasound scans should be transvaginal if any doubt exists. The following features should be noted:

(1) If a gestational sac has a mean diameter of greater than 20 mm with no evidence of an embryo or yolk sac, this is highly suggestive of a blighted ovum.

(2) If the embryo has a crown–rump length greater than 6.0 mm with no evidence of heart pulsations, this is highly suggestive of a missed abortion.

(3) When the mean gestational sac diameter is less than 20 mm or the crown–rump length is less than 6.0 mm, a repeat examination should be performed 1 week later to assess growth.

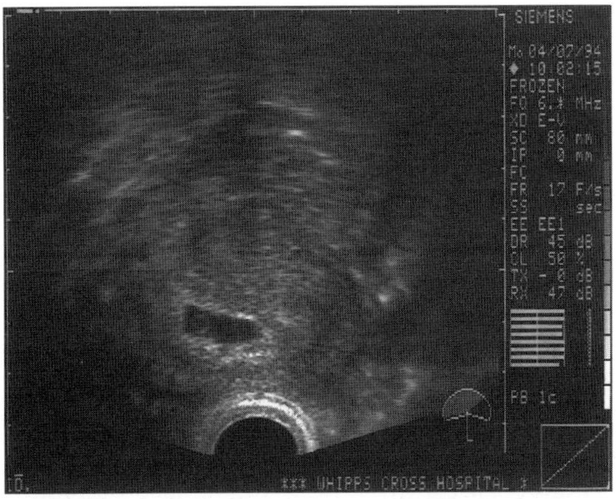


**Figure 25** An early 5–6-week gestational sac showing a normal yolk sac

There is a higher miscarriage rate with assisted conception techniques. If in doubt about the viability, it seems sensible to wait and see. However, in the situation of a suspected early ectopic pregnancy, there is a greater degree of clinical urgency.

### Ectopic pregnancy

In natural pregnancy, the appearance of a normal intrauterine pregnancy usually rules out an associated ectopic pregnancy as this will only occur in 1 in 30 000 pregnancies. However, following IVF and GIFT, the incidence of heterotopic pregnancy has been reported to be as high as 1 in 100 pregnancies[45].

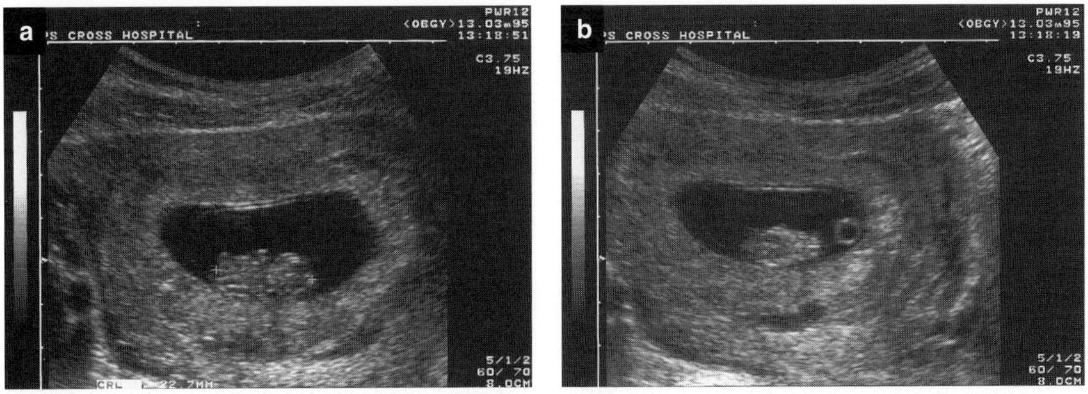


**Figure 26** 8–9-week pregnancy showing (a) measurement of the crown–rump length and (b) the yolk sac lying between the amniotic and chorionic membranes

Transvaginal ultrasound has a reported accuracy of greater than 90%[46] and should routinely be used in the search for an ectopic pregnancy. The detection rates for ectopics vary with authors and some find associated colour Doppler studies helpful in increasing the detection rate but there are pitfalls for the inexperienced[31]. When a viable embryo is seen in an extrauterine sac adjacent to an ovary containing a corpus luteum, the diagnosis is not difficult (Figure 27).

In assessing the possibility of an ectopic pregnancy, it is helpful to know the quantitative measurements of serum β-hCG in the maternal blood. These values will tend to be lower than those of a normal intrauterine pregnancy.

The uterine appearances in ectopic pregnancy are variable but may be helpful[47]. Usually the uterus is empty and a decidual reaction may be present (if the patient has not bled). An endometrial fluid collection or pseudogestational sac is found in 10–20% of cases and should be differentiated from an intrauterine gestational sac. Adnexal findings vary from a viable ectopic embryo to an adnexal mass with the appearance of a gestational sac, to a complex adnexal mass which represents haemorrhage. Levels of β-hCG may be low in the latter cases.

During transvaginal scanning it is helpful to look for free fluid in the peritoneum and assess its echogenicity. Free blood in the peritoneum will have internal echoes (Figure 28). This may be the only sonographic finding of an ectopic.

A haemorrhagic corpus luteum may be mistaken for a haemorrhagic ectopic pregnancy; in fact it often is! The corpus luteum usually lies within the ovary and usually contains more echoes. It is helpful to recognize the corpus luteum during the search for an ectopic as the ectopic is often on the same side as the corpus luteum. Unfortunately, the colour Doppler ring of colour in the wall of the corpus luteum is similar to that seen around the gestational sac. Unusual sites of ectopic pregnancies include the cervix and uterine cornu. The cornual pregnancy is difficult to diagnose. However, it must be considered if the myometrial covering is eccentric and the main endometrial cavity appears separate from it. It is important to make the diagnosis because of the associated mortality. With early diagnosis of asymptomatic ectopics, especially in heterotopic pregnancies, there is the opportunity for expectant management or non-surgical intervention, usually under ultrasound guidance[48].

## SCREENING FOR FETAL ABNORMALITIES

It is appropriate to mention screening for chromosomal abnormalities in relation to assisted conception. The successful pregnancy is especially precious, often occurring in the older age

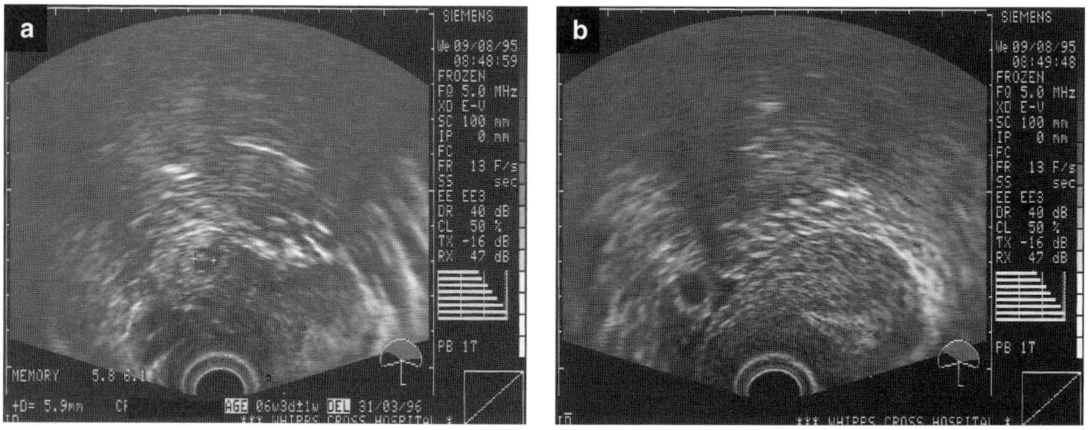


**Figure 27** Six-week ectopic pregnancy showing 6.0-mm embryo on one wall of the yolk sac. (a) Ectopic pregnancy; (b) empty endometrial cavity

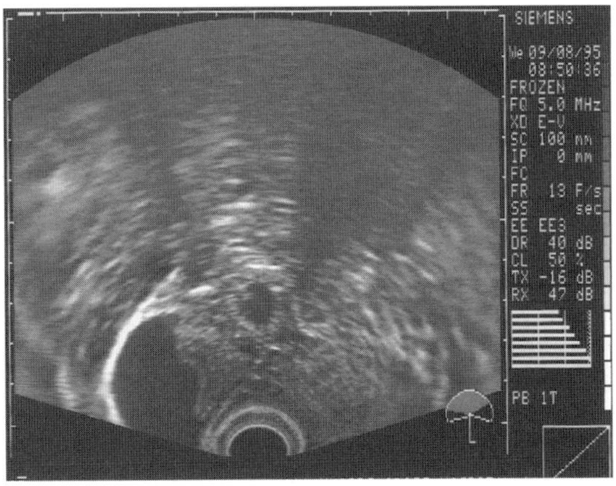


**Figure 28** An ectopic pregnancy with blood in the peritoneal cavity

group and involving multiple pregnancies. Multiple gestation makes serum testing for chromosomal abnormalities difficult and invasive tests are to be avoided if possible.

Ultrasound examination in the first trimester of pregnancy is an alternative (or complement) to serum testing for fetal chromosomal abnormalities. Increased fetal nuchal translucency thickness at 10–14 weeks of gestation is a common phenotypic expression of trisomies 21, 18 and 13, Turner's syndrome and triploidy. This method can potentially identify more than 80% of affected fetuses for a false-positive rate of less than 5%[49].

Nuchal translucency is defined as an anechoic area in between the skin and the soft tissue overlying the cervical spine. It can be measured using transabdominal ultrasound in most cases and scanning at around 11 weeks' gestation. The measurement is made by obtaining a sagittal section of the fetus as for the measurement of the fetal crown–rump length. The maximum thickness of the subcutaneous translucency between the skin and the soft tissue overlying the cervical spine is measured. It is important to see the amniotic membrane separate from the skin and this is achieved by waiting for movement of the fetus away from the amniotic membrane (Figure 29). The nuchal fold is regarded as abnormal if it measures more than 2.5 mm (Figure 30). Higher cut-off values may be taken but these will lead to a

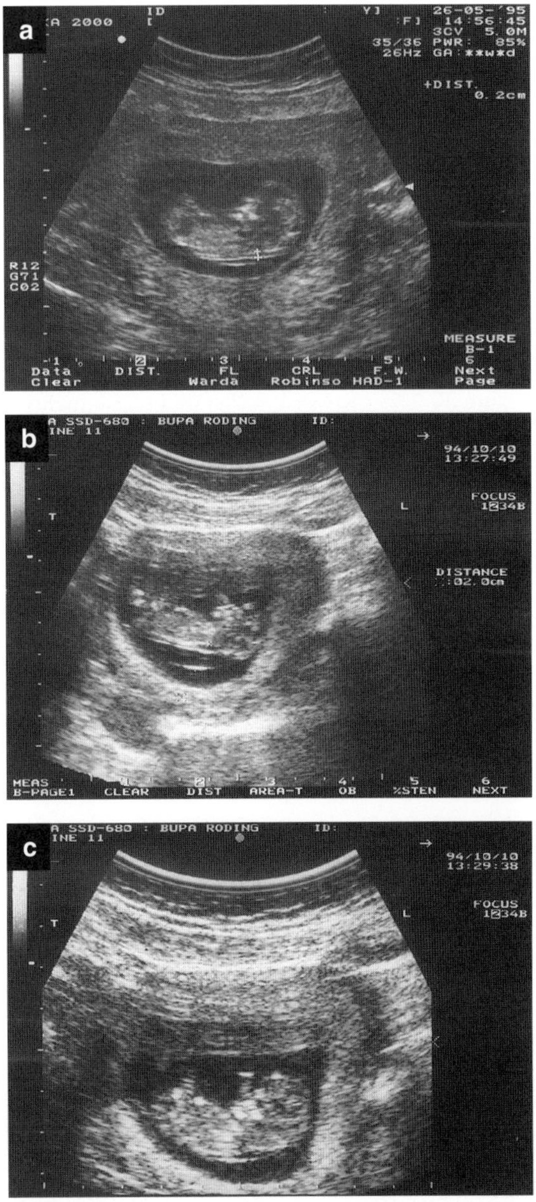


**Figure 29** (a) Nuchal fold measurement; (b) nuchal fold seen well separated from amniotic membrane on fetal movement; (c) fetus lying on amniotic membrane

lower pick-up rate of chromosomal abnormalities. This is only a screening test and further invasive definitive tests will be needed before diagnosis. This test is especially useful in multiple pregnancies where maternal serum screening is not accurate. The nuchal increased

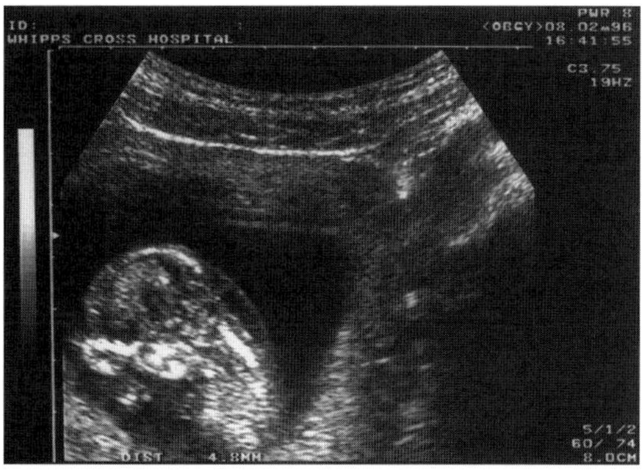


**Figure 30** An increased nuchal fold of 6.0 mm in a case of trisomy 18

translucency also acts as a marker if the parents are considering selective termination after chromosome analysis. There is less risk of miscarriage from selective fetocide before 16 weeks.

Although complications of pregnancy in *in vitro* assisted conception cycles are higher, the rate of fetal abnormality does not appear to be increased.

## CONCLUSION

Ultrasound is *the* imaging tool of reproductive medicine. The ultrasonographer should be an integral part of the reproductive medicine team and the ultrasound findings should always be correlated with the clinical and biochemical results. New developments such as power colour Doppler (which gives vascular colour without reliance on the angle of the ultrasound beam) will improve and increase the use of ultrasound. Ultrasound will also be increasingly used for direct minimal invasive procedures in this field.

## REFERENCES


1. Hackloer, B. J., Fleming, R., Robinson, H. P., Adam, A. H. and Coutts, J. R. T. (1979). Correlation of ultrasonic and endocrinologic assessment of human follicular development. *Am. J. Obstet. Gynecol.*, **135**, 122–8
2. Price, R. R. and Fleischer, A. C. (1991). Sonographic instrumentation. In Fleischer, A. C., Romero, R., Manning, F. A., Jeanty, P. and James, A. E. Jr (eds.) *The Principles and Practice of Ultrasonography in Obstetrics and Gynaecology*, 4th edn., pp. 25–38. (Norwalk, Cambridge: Appleton and Lange)
3. Cohen, J., Debache, C., Pen, J. P., Junra, A. M. and Cohen-Bacrie, P. (1986). Transvaginal sonographically controlled ovarian puncture of oocyte retrieval for *in vitro* fertilization. *J. In Vitro Fertil. Embryo Transfer*, **3**, 309–13
4. Reuter, R. L., Daly, D. C. and Cohen, S. M. (1989). Septate versus bicornuate uteri: errors in imaging diagnosis. *Radiology*, **172**, 749–52
5. Woodward, P. J., Wagner, B. J. and Farley, T. E. (1993). MR imaging in the evaluation of female infertility. *Radiographics*, **13**, 293–310
6. Cullinan, J. A., Fleischer, A. C., Kepple, D. M. and Arnold, A. L. (1995). Sonohysterography: a technique for endometrial evaluation. *Radiographics*, **15**, 501–14
7. Gutmann, J. N. (1992). Imaging in the evaluation of female infertility. *J. Reprod. Med.*, **37**, 54–61
8. Dudiak, C. M., Turner, D. A. and Patel, S. K. (1988). Uterine leiomyomas in the infertile patient. *Radiology*, **167**, 627–30
9. Krysiewicy, S. (1992). Infertility in women: diagnostic evaluation with hysterosalpingography and other imaging techniques. *Am. J. Roentgenol.*, **159**, 253–61
10. Campbell, S., Bourne, T. H., Tan, S. L. and Collins, W. P. (1994). Hysterosalpingo-contrast sonography and its future role in investigation of infertility in Europe. *Ultrasound Obstet. Gynecol.*, **4**, 245–53
11. Ayida, G., Kennedy, S., Barlow, D. and Chamberlain, P. (1996). A comparison of patient tolerance of HyCoSy and X-ray H.S.G. for outpatient investigation of infertile women. *Ultrasound Obstet. Gynecol.*, **7**, 201–4
12. Volpi, E., Zuccaro, G., Patriari, A., Rustichelli, S. and Sismondi, P. (1996). Transvaginal sonographic tubal patency testing using air and saline solution as contrast media in a routine infertility clinic setting. *Ultrasound Obstet. Gynecol.*, **7**, 43–8
13. Tessler, F. N., Persella, R. R., Fleischer, A. C. and Grant, E. G. (1989). Endovaginal sonographic disorders of dilated Fallopian tubes. *Am. J. Roentgenol.*, **153**, 523–5

14. Timor-Tritsch, I. E., Rottem, S. and Lewit, N. (1991). The Fallopian tubes. In Timor-Tritsch, I. E. and Rottem, S. (eds.). *Transvaginal Sonography*, 2nd edn. (New York: Elsevier)
15. Rizk, B., Tan, S., Kingsland, C., Steer, C., Mason, B. and Campbell, S. (1990). Ovarian cyst aspiration and outcome of *in vitro* fertilization. *Fertil. Steril.*, **54**, 661–5
16. Kaori Togashi, K., Nishimura, I., Kimura, I. and Tsuda, Y. (1991). Endometrial cysts: diagnosis with M. R. imaging. *Radiology*, **180**, 73–8
17. Pache, T., Hop, W., Wladimiroff, J., Schipper, J. and Fauser, B. (1991). Transvaginal sonography and abnormal ovarian appearance in menstrual cycle disturbances. *Ultrasound Med. Biol.*, **17**, 589–93
18. Pache, T. D., Wladimiroff, J. W., Hop, W. C. J. and Fauser, B. C. J. M. (1992). How to discriminate between normal and polycystic ovaries. Transvaginal U/S study. *Radiology*, **183**, 421–3
19. Beires, J., Montenegro, N. and Pignatelli, D. (1994). Polycystic ovarian syndrome and the current contribution of ultrasound. In Kurjak, A. (ed.) *Ultrasound and the Ovary*, pp. 179–87. (Carnforth, UK: Parthenon)
20. Hamilton, C. J. C. M., Evers, J. L. H., Tan, F. E. S. and Hoogland, H. J. (1987). The reliability of ovulation prediction by a simple sonographic follicle measurement. *Hum. Reprod.*, **2**, 103–7
21. Smith, D. H., Picker, R. H., Sinosich, M. and Saunders, D. M. (1980). Assessment of ovulation by ultrasound and oestradiol levels during spontaneous and induced cycles. *Fertil. Steril.*, **33**, 387–90
22. Zandt-Stastny, D., Thorsen, M. K. and Middleton, W. D. (1989). Inability of sonography to detect imminent ovulation. *Am. J. Roentgenol.*, **152**, 91–5
23. Ritchie, W. G. M. (1986). Sonographic evaluation of normal and induced ovulation. *Radiology*, **161**, 1–10
24. Balen, F. G., Balen, A. H. and Tan, S.-L. (1994). The ovary and assisted reproduction. In Kurjak, A. (ed.) *Ultrasound and the Ovary*, pp. 83–98. (Carnforth, UK: Parthenon)
25. Rankin, R. N. and Hutton, L. C. (1981). Ultrasound in ovarian hyperstimulation syndrome. *J. Clin. Ultrasound*, **9**, 473–6
26. Levy, S., Leeton, J. and Renou, P. (1987). Transvaginal recovery of oocytes for *in vitro* fertilization using vaginal ultrasound. *J. In Vitro Fertil. Embryo Transfer*, **4**, 51–5
27. Tickman, D., Arger, P. and Turek, R. (1986). Sonographic assessment of the endometrium in patients undergoing *in vitro* fertilization. *J. Ultrasound Med.*, **5**, 197
28. Fleischer, A. C., Herbert, C. and Hill, G. (1991). Transvaginal sonography of the endometrium during induced cycles. *J. Ultrasound Med.*, **10**, 93
29. Steer, C. V., Campbell, S., Pampiglione, J. S., Kingsland, C. R., Mason, B. A. and Collins, W. P. (1990). Transvaginal colour flow imaging of the uterine arteries during the ovarian and menstrual cycles. *Hum. Reprod.*, **5**, 391–5
30. Steer, C. V., Campbell, S. and Tan, S. L. (1992). Transvaginal colour Doppler: a new technique for use after *in vitro* fertilization to identify optimum uterine conditions before embryo transfer. *Fertil. Steril.*, **57**, 372–6
31. Pellerito, J. S., Tioiano, R. N., Quedeus-Case, C. and Taylor, K. J. W. (1995). Common pitfalls of endovaginal color Doppler flow imaging. *Radiographics*, **15**, 37–47
32. Zaidi, J., Campbell, S., Pittrof, R. and Tam, S. L. (1995). Endometrial thickness, morphology, vascular penetration and velocimetry in predicting implantation in an *in vitro* fertilization programme. *Ultrasound Obstet. Gynecol.*, **6**, 191–8
33. Applebaum, M. (1995). The uterine biophysical profile (Letter to the Editor). *Ultrasound Obstet. Gynecol.*, **5**, 67–8
34. Baker, R. J., McSweeney, M. B., Gill, R. W., Porter, R. N., Picker, R. H., Warren, P. S., Kossof, G. and Saunders, D. M. (1988). Transvaginal pulsed Doppler ultrasound assessment of blood flow to the corpus luteum in IVF patients following embryo transfer. *Br. J. Obstet. Gynaecol.*, **95**, 1226–30
35. Kurjak, A. (1989). *Ultrasound and Infertility*. (Boca Raton, FL: CRC Press)
36. Molloy, D., Deambrosis, W. and Keeping, D. (1990). Multiple-sited (heterotopic) pregnancy after *in vitro* fertilization. *Fertil. Steril.*, **53**, 1068
37. Wax, M. R., Frates, M., Benson, C. B., Yeh, J. and Doubilet, P. M. (1992). First trimester findings in pregnancies after *in vitro* fertilization. *J. Ultrasound Med.*, **11**, 321–5
38. Takeuchi, H. (1992). Transvaginal ultrasound in the first trimester of pregnancy. *Early Hum. Dev.*, **29**, 381–4

39. Rossavik, I. K., Torjusen, G. O. and Gibbons, W. E. (1988). Conceptual age and ultrasound measurements of gestational sac and crown–rump length in *in vitro* fertilization pregnancies. *Fertil. Steril.*, **49**, 1012–15
40. Jauniaux, E., Jurkovic, D. and Henriet, Y. (1991). Development of the secondary human yolk sac: correlation of sonographic and anatomical features. *Hum. Reprod.*, **6**, 1160–3
41. Stampone, C., Nicotra, M., Muttinelli, C. and Cosmi, E. V. (1996). Transvaginal sonography of the yolk sac in normal and abnormal pregnancy. *J. Clin. Ultrasound*, **24**, 3–9
42. Gruboeck, K., Zosmer, N. and Jurkovic, D. (1996). Ultrasound features of early pregnancy development. In Jurkovic, D. and Jauniaux, E. (eds.) In *Ultrasound and Early Pregnancy*, pp. 41–53. (Carnforth, UK: Parthenon)
43. Standing Joint Committee on Obstetric Ultrasound of the two Colleges (1995). *Guidance on Ultrasound Procedures in Early Pregnancy*
44. Balen, A. H., Tan, S. L., MacDougall, J. and Jacobs, H. S. (1993). Miscarriage rates following *in vitro* fertilization are increased in women with polycystic ovaries and reduced by pituitary desensitization with buserelin. *Hum. Reprod.*, **8**, 959–64
45. Molloy, D., Hynes, J., Deanbrosis, W., Harrison, K., Keeping, D. and Hennessey, J. (1990). Multiple-sites (heterotopic) pregnancy after *in vitro* fertilization and gamete intrafallopian transfer. *Fertil. Steril.*, **53**, 1068–71
46. Remysen, A. (1988). Vaginal sonography in ectopic pregnancy. *J. Ultrasound Med.*, **7**, 381–7
47. Nyberg, D. A. (1992). Ectopic pregnancy. In Patterson, A. S. (ed.) *Transvaginal Ultrasound*, pp. 105–32. (St. Louis: Mosby)
48. Hacker, E. and Jurkovic, D. (1996). Ultrasound in the diagnosis and non-surgical management of ectopic pregnancy. In Jurkovic, D. and Jauniaux, E. (eds.) *Ultrasound in Early Pregnancy*, pp. 65–80. (Carnforth, UK: Parthenon)
49. Pandya, P. P., Johnson, S., Malligianis, P. and Nicolaides, K. H. (1996). First trimester foetal nuchal translucency and screening for chromosomal abnormalities. In Jurkovic, D. and Jauniaux, E. (eds.) *Ultrasound and Early Pregnancy*, pp. 81–94. (Carnforth, UK: Parthenon)

# Investigations for infertility management

# 7

*David A. Viniker*

## INTRODUCTION

The objectives in requesting investigations for couples with infertility are initially to identify factors that may be contributing to delay in achieving a successful pregnancy and subsequently to monitor the response to treatment that has been instituted.

Infertility is usually defined as involuntary failure to conceive after 1 year of unprotected sexual intercourse. In its wider sense, infertility refers to couples who are having difficulty producing a baby and would therefore include pregnancy problems such as recurrent abortion. Between 80 and 90% of couples will have achieved a pregnancy within the first year and about 95% by 2 years[1]. It has been estimated that one couple in six will have been concerned about their fertility and about 10% of couples are currently experiencing fertility difficulties[2]. In Denmark, a study of 3743 randomly selected women aged 15–44 reported that 26.2% of those planning a family had experienced fertility delays[3].

Primary infertility usually refers to patients with no previous history of a successful pregnancy, although some would limit primary infertility to no previous pregnancy. It might also be appropriate to consider whether the infertility is primary or secondary for each partner as well as for the current partnership.

In western society, falling perinatal and infant mortality rates have tended to reduce the desire to produce large families. Healthy offspring rather than quantity is the requisite. Effective family planning methods, such as the combined oral contraceptive pill, allow modern couples the facility to delay child bearing until socially convenient. In France, the average age of first pregnancy is 28 years compared to 24 years in 1970 and there has been a doubling in the proportion of women giving birth after 30 years of age since 1972[4].

Fertility declines with advancing female age[5]. The prevalence of infertility is increased to 25% in women in their late thirties. From the age of 40 onwards, fertility declines even more rapidly[6]. There is also evidence of declining fertility with age of the male partner[4,7]. Cigarette smoking has an adverse effect on female fertility[8] and smoking in pregnancy reduces the future fertility of the unborn child[9]. There is a five-fold increase in infertility for patients with a history of ectopic pregnancy[10].

There was a 25% increase in the number of couples requesting fertility services in the USA from 1982 to 1988[11]. The prevalence of infertility remained unaltered over a 10-year period but the proportion seeking medical assistance increased significantly[2]. Furthermore, there has probably been an increase in the number of visits to the fertility clinics per couple in association with the increasing number of available treatments. The media, including magazines, newspapers, radio and television, serve to inform the public of the advances in medical technology, and reproductive medicine is a popular topic. Only 30 years ago the treatment of infertility was relatively primitive. We have now reached a situation where even in the presence of azoospermia, it may be possible to aspirate a few non-motile sperm and fertilization can be achieved by intracytoplasmic sperm injection (Chapter 14).

The three most common causes of infertility are ovulatory dysfunction, Fallopian tube problems and male factor infertility (Chapter 11).

## OVULATORY DYSFUNCTION

### Pathophysiology

Failure of ovulation is the cause of infertility in about 21% of couples referred to an infertility clinic[12]. The commonest cause of anovulation is polycystic ovary syndrome. We now know that polycystic ovaries are common, occurring in one woman in five (Chapter 5). Anovulatory infertility is suggested by amenorrhoea, oligomenorrhoea or irregular menstruation. Occasionally, despite apparently normal menstrual cycles, there may prove to be evidence of ovulatory problems detectable on ultrasound or serum progesterone levels. With the exception of premature menopause, a successful outcome can be expected in 96% of patients with infertility and amenorrhoea and in 78% when there is oligomenorrhoea[12].

The majority of patients with amenorrhoea have previously experienced menstruation (secondary amenorrhoea). The physiology of ovulation is discussed in Chapter 2. Primary amenorrhoea has usually been investigated before the patient presents with infertility. The investigation and management of primary amenorrhoea is discussed in Chapter 4. In the years leading up to the menopause, follicle stimulating hormone (FSH) levels tend to rise[13,14]. Primary ovarian failure is indicated by repeatedly elevated FSH levels (> 30 IU/l = hypergonadotrophic hypogonadism). This initial rise in FSH level is related to decreased levels of inhibin but normal oestradiol levels.

A 30-year-old woman presented to us for consideration of *in vitro* fertilization (IVF) with a regular spontaneous 28-day cycle for several months after discontinuation of hormone replacement therapy (HRT) for premature menopause. Her gonadotrophins proved to be in the menopausal range and her previous gynaecologist confirmed that 4 years earlier she had presented with irregular periods and her FSH had been repeatedly greater than 50 IU/l. Buckler and colleagues[13] identified a group of infertile women with regular menstruation and persistently elevated FSH with presumed incipient ovarian failure. Suppression of gonadotrophins by combined oestrogen–progesterone preparations may result in subsequent apparent ovulation, although unfortunately conception would be exceptional. It would seem that diminished inhibin secretion results in elevation of the FSH in association with incipient ovarian failure. Elevated FSH levels on day 3 above 15 IU/l are associated with poor success rates in IVF[15] and at levels greater than 25 IU/l pregnancy is unlikely to occur. When the FSH is elevated, it is prudent to repeat the investigation. Careful and cautious counselling is required as even an isolated high reading may suggest the possibility of a premature menopause in a young woman. These women may subsequently resent delay if expedited investigation and treatment have not been pursued. In a series of 67 women aged under 35 years who had an FSH of greater than 20 IU/l, 17 subsequently ovulated spontaneously and six conceived; ovulation induction therapy (including clomiphene citrate, gonadotrophins and bromocriptine) was of no value in these patients whilst the FSH remained elevated[16].

In hypogonadotrophic hypogonadism, the FSH and LH are low (< 5 IU/l). Women with hypogonadotrophic hypogonadism have deficient gonadotrophin releasing hormone (GnRH) pulsatile secretion, usually in association with low weight and/or stress. As oestrogen levels are low there is little endometrial activity and when challenged with a progestogen (e.g. medroxyprogesterone acetate 10 mg) daily for 5 days, there is no withdrawal bleed. The majority of these patients with a negative progestogen challenge do not ovulate with oral ovulation stimulation; gonadotrophin therapy is usually required to achieve a pregnancy.

Hypersecretion of LH is associated with poor conception rates and increased risk of miscarriage. In 1985, fertilization of oocytes was noted to be reduced in association with raised basal LH levels during the follicular phase[17,18]. In a prospective study[19], 193 women who were planning to conceive were recruited. These women had regular spontaneous menstrual cycles and had no significant medical or gynaecological pathology. Blood samples in the early follicular phase were assayed for LH. Luteinizing hormone levels of less than 10 IU/l were recorded in 147 women; 88% of these women conceived and 12% of these miscarried. Luteinizing hormone levels greater than 10 IU/l were present in 46 women and in this group only 67% conceived; 65% of these miscarried.

Gonadotrophin-releasing hormone analogues administered during early pregnancy reduce LH levels but do not improve the pregnancy outcomes of patients with hypersecretion of LH[20]. Clifford and co-workers[21] have recently reported the results from their controlled trial of women with habitual abortion. They found that prepregnancy suppression of high LH hormone concentrations with a GnRH analogue did not improve the outcome of pregnancy. In all, 46 out of 56 patients with high LH, who did not receive GnRH analogues, conceived and 76% of these had a live birth. They concluded that hypersecretion of LH does not seem to be causally related to early pregnancy loss.

Galactorrhoea (inappropriate lactation) is a symptom of hyperprolactinaemia. Ovulatory disorders may be a manifestation of hyperprolactinaemia. Hyperprolactinaemia may be associated with medication, including antidepressants, cimetidene and methyldopa. Prolactin levels may be slightly elevated in patients with polycystic ovary syndrome and hypothyroidism. Higher levels may be found with pituitary adenomas and radiological examination of the pituitary fossa is indicated in these cases. Routine prolactin measurement in women with normal menstrual cycles is probably of no value[22].

### Assessment of ovulation

Many women experience a change in their mucus just before ovulation, the mucus becoming more watery. Mid-cycle pain is often associated with ovulation but can be severe and occasionally be the cause of apareunia during the fertile phase.

The basal temperature chart provides a simple and inexpensive indication of ovulation. The temperature can be taken orally with a regular thermometer that should be easy to read. The clinic nurse can teach patients how to use this instrument; the temperature should be taken before the day's activity begins. Sexual intercourse should be recorded on the chart and this may show that timing of intercourse may be inappropriate. Typically, the temperature falls and then rises by 0.5°C around the time of ovulation. The temperature remains elevated throughout the luteal phase and is a marker of progesterone activity. The rise of the temperature in association with ovulation is apparent only retrospectively and couples should appreciate that it is not a useful predictor of imminent ovulation[23]. A sustained elevation of the temperature in association with failure to menstruate is usually diagnostic for pregnancy. With experienced observers and agreed criteria, meaningful interpretation of basal temperature charts is enhanced[24].

Home testing for the LH surge, which uses monoclonal technology, provides a valuable method for determining the timing of ovulation, and potentially reduces the stress and costs of fertility programmes[25]. These home tests can be even more reliable than laboratory serum analyses[26] and can be easily and accurately read by patients[27]. The LH predictor test is a better predictor of the next menstrual period than basal temperature charting[28]. Perhaps surprisingly, these tests in one study did not improve timing of postcoital tests compared with cycle averaging or reviewing basal temperature charts[29].

In a series of untreated conceptual cycles, the mid-luteal progesterone was in excess of 28 nmol/l[30] and 30 nmol/l is generally accepted as evidence of ovulation. Pregnancy has been reported in cycles with a mid-luteal phase progesterone level of 12 nmol/l[31]. Progesterone is released in a pulsatile fashion[32] and there may be some advantage in assaying more than one sample before diagnosing anovulation[33]. There is a suggestion that slightly higher levels of midluteal phase progesterone should occur in patients receiving clomiphene or tamoxifen if pregnancy is to occur[30,31].

Ultrasound is playing an increasingly important part in the investigation and treatment of infertility. An initial single ultrasound evaluation of the pelvis provides a useful assessment of the pelvic anatomy. If this scan is scheduled for the 12th day of the menstrual cycle there should be a dominant follicle of at least 12 mm in a 28-day cycle and the endometrium should be well developed with adequate oestrogenic activity. It would seem possible that ultrasonic evaluation of tubal patency might also be undertaken at this time. Pelvic ultrasound may demonstrate uterine pathology including fibroids and congenital anomaly. Ovarian cysts and endometriomas should be evident. Polycystic ovaries have a characteristic picture (Chapter 6). Serial scans, usually on alternate days through the second half of the follicular phase, should demonstrate normal follicular development in the diameter of a dominant follicle at a rate of about 1 mm daily. Normal ovulation has a characteristic ultrasound appearance. There is a variation in the temporal relationship between urine LH surge and timing of ovulation, as seen ultrasonically, varying from 1 to 2 days[34].

### Luteal phase deficiency

Until the advent of progesterone assay and ultrasound, endometrial biopsy, to evaluate secretory changes, was regarded as the best investigation to evaluate ovulation. If there is a lag of greater than 2 days between the maturation of secretory changes of the endometrium compared to the day of the cycle then a state of luteal phase deficiency is diagnosed. Luteal phase defect can be found occasionally in 30% of normal women and an association with infertility should only be assumed if it is found in two cycles. Decreased progesterone production by the corpus luteum is assumed to be responsible but this may follow inadequate FSH levels in the follicular phase, abnormal LH secretion or abnormal response of the endometrium. Decreased inhibin levels in the early and mid-follicular phases might indicate a defect of the preovulatory follicle, possibly secondary to defects in gonadotrophin secretion[33].

The inadequate luteal phase is a loose term without consistent definition. A shortened luteal phase, borderline progesterone estimations, and reduced secretory changes on histological assessment of the endometrium have all been cited as diagnostic features.

The length of the luteal phase was assessed in a series of 92 healthy volunteer women and 95 women with unexplained infertility. All 187 women had regular ovulatory menstrual cycles. There was a short luteal phase in 9% of the infertile group and 8% of the control group, suggesting no clinical significance related to a shortened luteal phase[35]. The rate of rise of the postovulatory basal body temperature chart does not differentiate between normal and luteal phase deficiency cycles[36]. Successful conception can occur with a luteal phase of just 10 days. Adequate endometrial biopsies can be obtained for diagnosis of luteal phase defect with a Pipelle endometrial suction curette[37] (see Figure 1 in Chapter 26).

A rapid urinary LH monoclonal test has been shown to be the best method to predict the next menstrual period and to time the optimum day for endometrial assessment[28]. It has been recommended that the endometrial biopsies should be taken 2 days before the next period and a monoclonal human chorionic gonadotrophin (hCG) test be performed to exclude pregnancy before sampling[38]. There is considerable variation in histological dating of secretory endometrium particularly in the late luteal phase even by the same pathologist repeating examinations on the same specimens. Furthermore, there is variation of maturation of the endometrium between cycles within the same subject[39].

The significance of this condition and the relevance and success of treatment is contentious. Some studies suggest that luteal phase deficiency is not more common in infertile women[40]. It may be that only more severe degrees of luteal phase deficiency are of practical importance, with delays of 5 or more days on endometrial biopsy[41].

A recent detailed histological dating study of the endometrium with serum progesterone measurements found endometrial abnormality in 43% of infertile women compared to 9% in a group of fertile women[42]. There was no concomitant defect of the corpus luteum suggesting a primary endometrial problem. Luteal phase defects may be associated with an increased risk of spontaneous abortion and ectopic pregnacy[43].

### Luteinized unruptured follicle syndrome

Luteinized unruptured follicle syndrome was initially described from laparoscopic observations when there was apparent endocrine evidence of ovulation but no sign of a corpus haemorrhagicum[44]. Abdulla and colleagues[31] reported a mean progesterone level of 66.2 nmol/l in a group of women having luteinized unruptured follicle cycles. Negative LH tests at the time of expected LH surge often correlate with luteinized unruptured follicles[45]. Ultrasound scanning has shown that, with normal follicular development and with normal mid-luteal progesterone, failure of follicular rupture is unusual[46]. Even with daily ultrasound examination, the typical collapse of the follicle can be missed[47]. The luteinized unruptured follicle syndrome is not generally recognized as a significant and recurring cause of infertility[48] and routine ultrasound screening for this condition is not indicated. We suspect that this syndrome represents evidence of ovulatory dysfunction which requires ovulation induction to overcome the problem.

## ENDOMETRIOSIS

Endometriosis may be defined as histological evidence of endometrial glands and stroma outside the uterine cavity. That severe endometriosis with structural damage to the tubes and ovaries is a cause of infertility has never been questioned. Endometriosis might be suggested by a history of pelvic pain, dysmenorrhoea, dyspareunia and menorrhagia and on clinical examination there may be pelvic masses or tenderness. The significance of milder forms of endometriosis as a cause of infertility, however, has been the subject of debate. There is an increased prostanoid content and macrophage activity in the peritoneal fluid associated with endometriosis and this may alter sperm function and tubal motility. There is also evidence of disturbed immune mechanisms. Endometriosis might be the consequence, rather than the cause, of a multitude of abnormalities found in infertility patients[49].

Endometriosis has been reported to be more common in infertile women, ranging from 20 to 40%[50], although estimating the incidence of endometriosis in the general population must be subject to inaccuracy as the diagnosis would require an invasive procedure. Higher pregnancy rates have been reported in a small donor insemination programme in women without endometriosis compared to those found to have endometriosis[51]. Assessment of the severity of endometriosis using the revised American Fertility Society classification allows a degree of comparison, although a study of the laparoscopic videotapes of 20 patients with endometriosis showed considerable variation of scoring between observers and also by the same observer on re-evaluation of the same patient[52].

In women with primary infertility, mild endometriosis is more common when there are male factor problems, suggesting that, in these women, infertility predisposes to endometriosis rather than endometriosis being a cause for the infertility[53]. Bancroft and co-workers[54] compared pituitary–ovarian function in 22 women with minor degrees of endometriosis but otherwise unexplained infertility and a control group of ten healthy and fertile women. Abnormalities including low concentration of progesterone during the luteal phase and luteinized unruptured follicles were found in 82% of the index group; the endometriosis was not considered to be the cause of the endocrine disturbances.

Mild endometriosis is extremely common; with scrutiny and appreciation of the various forms of lesions, it can probably be found at least intermittently in the majority of women, so that it should no longer be considered as a pathological state[55]. In 1955, Buxton and Southam[56] observed, from a series of 1607 infertile couples, that uncomplicated endometriosis could not be incriminated statistically as an infertility factor and that the treatment of endometriosis to alleviate infertility would be of no benefit. Forty years later, this prediction seems to find support. As treatment of mild endometriosis apparently confers no improvement in pregnancy rates (Chapters 8 and 23), there would appear to be no obvious advantage in performing laparoscopy to make a diagnosis of mild endometriosis or to otherwise exclude it as a 'cause' of infertility.

## THE TUBAL FACTOR AND TUBAL FUNCTION TESTS

### Physiology and pathology

The Fallopian tubes have three functions. It is in the Fallopian tubes that ova are fertilized by ascending spermatozoa. Cilial action actively transports the ova to the uterine cavity. During their passage along the tubes, ova are nourished by secretions within the tube.

Approximately 14% of infertility is attributable to the 'tubal factor'[12]. Ascending infection to the Fallopian tubes following pregnancy or through sexual transmission accounts for the majority of patients with Fallopian tube problems. *Chlamydia trachomatis* infection is increasingly recognized as a significant pathogen[57,58] in tubal factor infertility. *Chlamydia trachomatis* antibody has a high correlation with tubal factor infertility and may become a part of baseline infertility investigation[59]. There is a five-fold increase of tubal factor infertility following ruptured appendix but simple appendectomy uncomplicated by rupture is not associated with fertility difficulty[60]. Tuberculosis of the Fallopian tubes is still occasionally found, although it was more prevalent 50 years ago[61].

### The development of tubal patency: tests and their possible therapeutic effects

Tubal function tests, generally employed, provide evidence of patency only. Rubin[62] published the earliest work on the subject by demonstrating that, if the tubes are patent, oxygen introduced through the cervix would pass into the peritoneal cavity. Cron[63] used carbon dioxide instead of oxygen as it is more readily absorbed, resulting in less discomfort. He introduced the concept that investigation of tubal patency might be therapeutic. In some patients with long histories of infertility, patency was only confirmed after initial difficulty; some of these patients conceived soon after the test. Rubin[64], in 1932, drew attention to isthmotubal spasm and he also considered that tubal insufflation was therapeutic as well as diagnostic. Green-Armytage[65] observed that the site of tubal occlusion could be demonstrated by hysterosalpingography and he believed that this technique was even more therapeutic than insufflation. In his classical lecture on 'Facts and fantasy in the study of female infertility', Stallworthy[66] accepted that conceptions following tubal function tests were facts but he believed that claims that these investigations were therapeutic were fantasy.

For some years, investigations were undertaken to establish the best 'therapeutic' agent for hysterosalpingography. However, Buxton and Southam[56] observed more pregnancies in the control group than in a group who had insufflation and Sharman[61] found no significant difference in conception rates between hysterosalpingography and non-hysterosalpingography groups. However, the case for a therapeutic role of hysterosalpingography, particularly with oil-soluble contrast media, continues to find scientific support[67].

The arrival of fibre-optic light technology, and the first reports of the laparoscope in the English literature, opened up the world of direct visualization of the pelvic organs. When combined with methylene blue dye insufflation, a new technique for assessing tubal patency became available[68]. Often hysterosalpingography and laparoscopy provide differing evidence on tubal patency. Asfari and Thompson[69] suggested that if conception does not occur within 6 months of hysterosalpingography when patency has been demonstrated, laparoscopy is indicated.

Laparoscopy and hysterosalpingography can provide evidence of tubal patency. Current routine techniques for the evaluation of the 'tubal factor' are basically patency tests; they do not assess other functions such as the ability of the fimbria to pick up oocytes.

There have been some attempts to evaluate other aspects of tubal function. Decker and Decker[70] deposited sterile suspensions of starch over the fimbria at laparotomy or culdoscopy. Twenty-four hours later they examined the cervical mucus on a slide by staining with iodine. Patients known to have healthy patent tubes all had positive starch tests. The test was negative in patients with known tubal occlusion. Four women with chronic tubal disease but evidence of patency from other tests had negative starch tests. Dapena[71] injected 3 ml of Vaseline droplets into the peritoneal cavity. The cervical mucus was subsequently examined microscopically. The Vaseline droplets had a similar diameter to ova. Pecoud and Lowy[72] injected indigo carmin into the peritoneal cavity in a series of 150 patients, who were also subjected to tubal insufflation, hysterosalpingography and laparoscopy or laparotomy. They found that the indigo carmin test was more reliable than hysterosalpingography. More recently, radionuclide migration has been advocated for the detection of diseased but patent tubes[73,74].

### Hysterosalpingography or laparoscopy and dye insufflation?

In a study of 104 infertile couples[75], the woman was submitted to both hysterosalpingography and laparoscopy with dye insufflation. There was an overall agreement between the two techniques in 62.5% of cases. It was concluded that whenever the hysterosalpingogram demonstrated tubal patency with free flow of dye, laparoscopic hydrotubation may be unnecessary. A meta-analysis of hysterosalpingography has suggested that evaluation of peritubal adhesions is not reliable[76]. To ensure differentiation between organic obstruction and spasm at the cornua, agents such as orciprenaline can be employed[77].

At one time, laparoscopy with dye insufflation was scheduled premenstrually so that a simultaneous endometrial biopsy obtained by curettage could be examined for secretory changes. Hysteroscopy provides direct visual assessment of the endometrial cavity. Some lesions, such as submucous fibroids and congenital septae, may be treated under direct hysteroscopic view. Hysteroscopy and endometrial curettage may be undertaken at the time of laparoscopy and dye insufflation although we do not believe that these investigations are indicated as part of the routine investigation of infertility.

Several experts have come to the conclusion that in the absence of clinical indicators of significant pelvic pathology and a normal hysterosalpingogram there is little to be gained by submitting infertile women to laparoscopy[78,79].

Endoscopy allows direct visualization of the tubal mucosa and correlations have been made between the morphology of the mucosa and the chance of subsequent pregnancy. A 3 mm endoscope can be introduced at laparoscopy into the fimbrial end of the tube[80]. Menashe and colleagues[81] have described transuterine insertion of a fibre optic device which allows assessment of all sections of the tubes.

Laparoscopy is an invasive technique carrying a degree of risk even in the hands of experts. The chance of laparotomy being required after a diagnostic procedure is 1.67 per thousand[82]. The major complication rate in a recently published series of 2324 laparoscopies was 0.22%; there were five major and 15 minor complications[83].

With careful clinical evaluation there would appear to be no advantage for routine laparoscopy and dye insufflation[84].

### Hysterosalpingo-contrast-sonography

In 1984, Richman and associates[85] described ultrasound assessment of the Fallopian tubes using ultrasound to demonstrate free fluid in the pelvis after introducing fluid through the cervix; there was good correlation with hysterosalpingography in a series of 35 infertile women. Others have also confirmed the value of transvaginal hysterosalpingo-contrast-sonography (Hy-Co-Sy)[86–88] with the suggestion that this technique could be used as an office screening procedure. The combination of air and saline has been shown to be an effective and cheap contrast medium in a series of 31 women[89]. Thirty-one infertile women were examined by transvaginal salpingosonography and the results compared to laparoscopy with dye insufflation. The ultrasound technique proved to be safe and comfortable for the patients and results were compatible in 85%. It is not yet clear whether the new contrast medium (Echovist, Schering) will prove better than saline and air[90] although it is apparent that the Echovist proves to enhance visualisation of the tubes. Colour Doppler ultrasonography may possibly enhance clarity.

Many studies try to compare the sensitivity and specificity of tubal patency tests, often accepting laparoscopy and dye as the 'gold standard' as this allows the gynaecologist direct visualization of the pelvic organs. It is apparent that air, carbon dioxide, X-ray contrast media, dye, saline and Echovist can pass along healthy Fallopian tubes. Ultimately the success of confirming patency will depend on the seal at the cervix and perhaps tubal spasm which can be overcome by agents such as amyl nitrate or Buscopan. From a theoretical point of view, there should be no advantage in confirming spill of the medium purely as a result of the visualization technique, whether this be by the laparoscope, radiology or ultrasound.

## UTERINE FACTORS

Uterine factors that could be associated with infertility relate to the endometrium and myometrium; the cervix is considered separately.

Uterine fibroids distorting the uterine cavity and congenital abnormality could be related to infertility. Ultrasound, hysterosalpingography and hysteroscopy allow assessment. Potentially, magnetic resonance imaging may prove to be of value in the investigation of infertility; unexpected pathology, particularly of the uterus, can be identified[91].

Arguably the most significant cause of infertility is implantation failure. From a practical point of view, the next area for significant development in the treatment of infertility lies in our understanding of embryo implantation. Only 12% of embryos transferred during IVF result in a live birth, although implantation is probably around 25% in natural conception[92]. Endometrial function can be assessed by ultrasound, histology and endometrial protein concentrations in endometrial washings.

A successful outcome of assisted fertility treatment is reduced to about 30% in women over 40 years of age[93]. The reduction in fertility with age could be related to oocytes or to uterine factors. In a donor oocyte IVF programme, the take-home-baby rate was initially reduced in recipients aged more than 40. Increasing the progesterone support for the women over 40 provided equivalent outcome success to younger recipients[93]. Batista and co-workers[94] studied the endometria of women aged 20–30 or 40–50 in association with hormone profiles and they found that it is follicular recruitment rather than luteal function or endometrial maturation that contributes to declining fertility with age. The incidence of early pregnancy loss doubles from the age of 20 to 40 years[95] and evidence from IVF with egg donation suggests that increased miscarriage problems in older women may be partly attributable to the uterus[96]. A recent study in Bologna, Italy, compared implantation and pregnancy rates in an oocyte donation programme with women of different ages sharing oocytes from the same donor; clinical pregnancy rates and ongoing pregnancy rates were twice as high in recipients less than 40 years old compared to older recipients[97].

An endometrial thickness of less than 8 mm tends to be associated with proliferative endometrium and greater than 9 mm with secretory endometrium but ultrasound does not accurately correlate with histological dating[98]. In a series of 59 women the endometrial thickness was assessed prior to embryo transfer. The mean endometrial thickness was 10.24 mm in conception cycles and there were only two pregnancies when the endometrium was less than 7.5 mm[99]. Further research is required to improve our understanding in this critical area of fertility investigation but successful treatment for implantation problems remains elusive[100].

## THE CERVICAL FACTOR AND THE POSTCOITAL TEST

The cervical mucus may be hostile during ovulation and the cervical factor has been considered to be responsible for up to 10% of couples presenting with infertility[101]. To investigate the cervical factor, a postcoital test is scheduled around the expected time of the LH surge which occurs about 36 h before ovulation. Cervical mucus is aspirated about 4–12 h after coitus and examined under the microscope; the couple have an opportunity to see the result for themselves. The spinnbarkheit (stretchability) of the mucus is noted.

Although the World Health Organization (WHO) recommend a cut-off level of 20 motile sperm per high power field, the range accepted by various European infertility centres ranges from one to 50[102]. Different clinics recommend wide variation in the time intervals between sexual intercourse and the postcoital test: some recommend a maximum interval of 2.5 h whilst others advocate a minimum of 9 h. The WHO recommended a time interval of 9–24 h[102]. Similar results are obtained whether the mucus be sampled high or low from the cervical canal[103].

Opinion varies on the value of this relatively simple investigation. Some authorities consider the postcoital test to be an essential early investigation of the infertile couple[104] whilst others find it to have little validity[105]. If the test is normal, it suggests that coital technique is satisfactory, ovulation is occurring, the male fertility test will be normal and the mucus is not hostile to sperm at this time. Some would advocate that if the postcoital test is normal, the only other essential factor to be investigated is the Fallopian tube. Whilst a positive test is reassuring, a negative test is more difficult to evaluate. On several occasions we have seen a negative test in a conception cycle. Oei and associates[106] undertook a systematic review of the literature relating to the postcoital test results and pregnancy. They concluded that to avoid over-treatment of the poorly defined condition known as ‘cervical factor infertility’, one motile spermatozoon per high-power field is probably the best cut-off point.

Another argument against the postcoital test is that the most common form of treatment, whether the test is positive or not, is intrauterine insemination. We believe that the majority of our patients find it reassuring to know that a cause for otherwise unexplained infertility has been determined. There are occasions when the postcoital test finds no sperm in the cervical mucus when there has been no history of coital problems. The test may be of greater value in units who use treatments specifically for the cervical factor such as preovulatory oestrogen or precoital sodium bicarbonate douching (Chapter 8).

A yellowish mucus may indicate chlamydia infection and appropriate cultures should be taken. If the sperm are moving but not progressing through the mucus there may be an antibody problem. An autoimmune cause is responsible for some cases of cervical factor infertility[107]. As the result of a postcoital test depends on a number of factors, it has been considered to be more useful as a prognostic indicator of pregnancy rather than a specific investigation of infertility. It has been shown that sperm antibodies in the circulation have no influence on fertility[108]. *In vitro* cross testing, utilizing donor mucus and sperm can indicate the origin of an abnormal postcoital test. A drop of the partner’s sperm and donor sperm are placed in contact with the patient’s mucus and also with donor mucus[109]. Penetration of the mucus is evaluated microscopically. These tests are less popular now that we have advanced treatments of assisted conception readily available.

Cervicitis and retroversion of the uterus cannot be implicated as causative factors in infertility[56].

## UNEXPLAINED INFERTILITY

Unexplained infertility is an arbitrary diagnosis derived by exclusion according to the protocols of the investigating department. We regard infertility as unexplained if there is a normal semen analysis, reasonable follicular development (> 12 mm) on the 12th day of the menstrual cycle and a mid-luteal progesterone level of at least 30 nmol/l, a normal hysterosalpingogram and a positive postcoital test.

Harrison[110] identified a factor considered to account for reduced fertility in all 316 patients achieving a pregnancy whilst attending the infertility clinic at The Chelsea Hospital for Women in the years 1976–7; 11% of these patients had more than one identifiable factor. The range in the reported incidence of unexplained infertility varies from 0 to 31% with an average of 17%[111]. This variation can be explained mainly by the different diagnostic criteria employed. The only confirmation of successful ovulation is pregnancy; all other tests are only suggestive of ovulation rather than diagnostic. Apparently normal semen analysis does not prove normal sperm function (Chapter 11). Current tubal function tests are essentially just tubal patency tests. Ultimately, only during *in vitro* investigation do we learn whether the spermatozoa and oocytes are capable of fertilization. Some authors include mild endometriosis as a cause of infertility. *In vitro* fertilization has also taught us that only 12% of pre-embryos will successfully implant. Recurrent failure of implantation in some women suggests that the endometrium may be a factor in infertility.

Immunological differences between the endometrium of women with unexplained infertility compared to fertile women has led to the suggestion that there may be an immunological factor in some cases of unexplained infertility[112]. Antiphospholipid antibodies, notably lupus anticoagulant and anticardiolipin, are more prevalent in women with unexplained infertility[113]. Low-dose aspirin administered as soon as pregnancy is confirmed significantly improves pregnancy continuation in patients with recurrent abortion and evidence of antiphospholipid syndrome (Chapter 21). We are not aware of any proven therapy for antiphospholipid syndrome increasing conception rates. It may be that we should consider investigating prolonged unexplained infertility with antiphospholipid studies and also chromosome analysis.

It may be frustrating for an infertile couple concluding their initial set of infertility investigations to learn that no explanation for their problem has been detected. Frequently, there is an interaction of female and male factors[114]. We try to place a more positive spirit on the situation for eventual success is more likely, even with low-tech treatment, than when infertility is attributable to male factor or tubal factor problems. The average spontaneous pregnancy rate with unexplained infertility over 3 years is 60%[115].

## PLANNING INVESTIGATION AND TREATMENT

It is essential that investigation and treatment should be planned and orderly. There should be no restriction to early patient access for advice. General practitioners are often well placed to offer early counselling. Guidelines for general practitioner management and referral of couples with infertility has been demonstrated to improve care, which is further enhanced by the introduction of infertility management protocols[116]. Basic advice on the fertile phase of the menstrual cycle may be all that is required. Some general practitioners may be able to enquire about possible difficulties with intercourse; sadly, we occasionally find evidence of coital problems on postcoital tests sometimes years after a couple first report fertility problems. Coital failure may account for 6% of infertility[12]. It would be inappropriate to delay infertility investigations if there is an abnormal menstrual cycle, a history suggesting possible tubal pathology or coital difficulties.

At Whipps Cross Hospital, my team has followed a protocol for initial investigation which was adopted and recommended by the North East Thames Region[117]. Figure 1 shows a flow

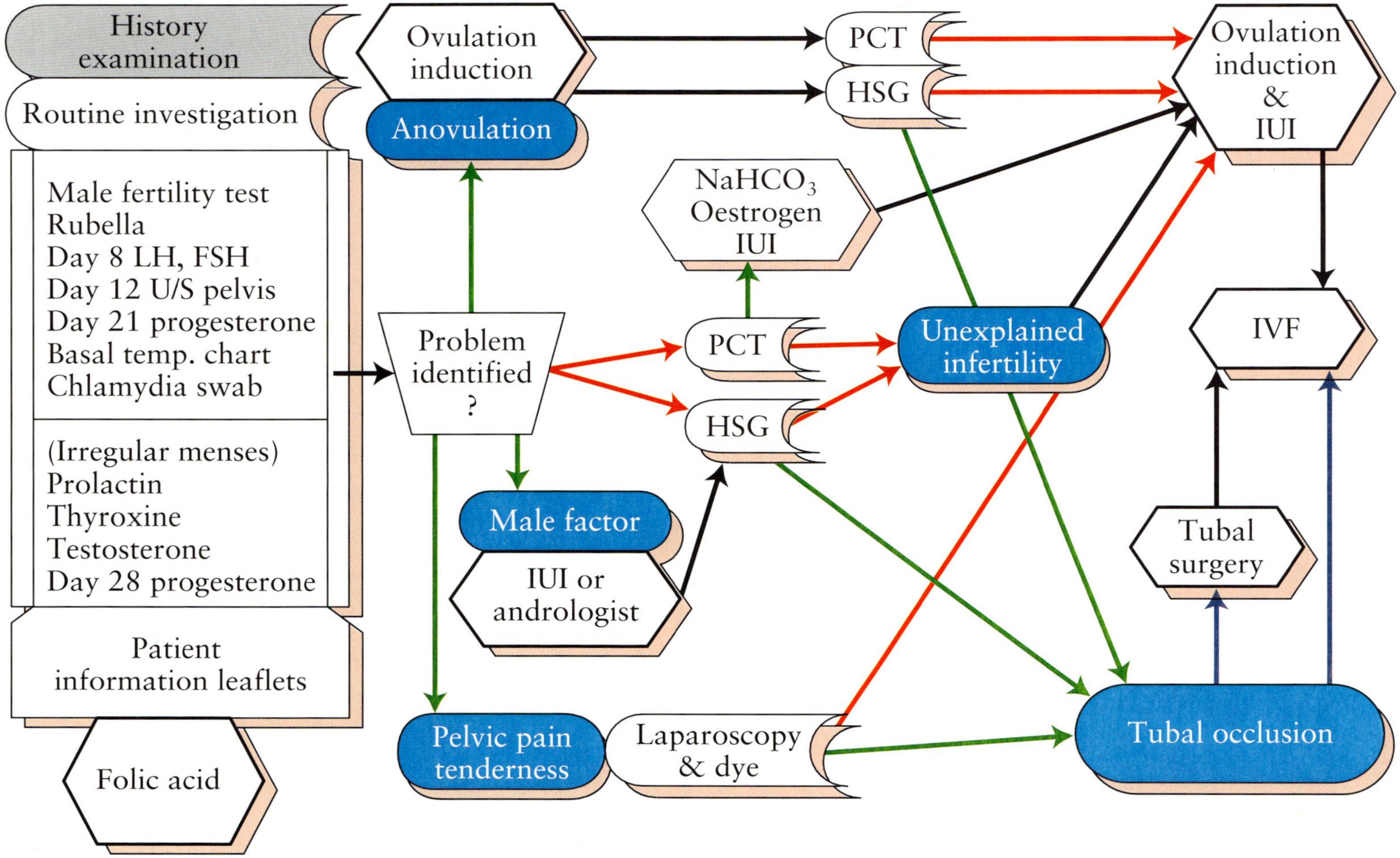


**Figure 1** Flow chart for the investigation and treatment of infertility. PCT, postcoital test; HSG, hysterosalpingogram; IUI, intrauterine insemination; IVF, *in vitro* fertilization; U/S, ultrasound. Green arrows represent 'yes' or a positive result, red arrows 'no' or a negative result, blue arrows options, and black arrows indicate the next step, with no choice

chart for the investigation and treatment of infertility. We encourage our general practitioner colleagues to commence investigations before referral. These investigations include a full blood count and rubella immunity screen, serum FSH and LH on the 8th day of the cycle, ultrasound examination of the pelvis on the 12th day and progesterone on day 21 of the menstrual cycle. A semen sample from the male partner is analysed. All referral letters from the general practitioners are reviewed personally and outstanding baseline investigations arranged before the initial consultation. If the menstrual cycle is irregular we also request prolactin, thyroxin, testosterone and day 28 progesterone estimations.

At the first hospital consultation, a full history is recorded in an orderly fashion with the assistance of a proforma, and the female partner is examined. Weight, height and blood pressure are recorded by the clinic nurse and a urine sample is analysed for protein and sugar. A general and pelvic examination is performed by a gynaecologist. A cervical smear is sent for cytological examination if indicated and a cervical swab sent for chlamydia.

Following the examination, we sit with the couple and review the salient points of the history, examination and initial investigation findings. It is essential to view the investigation of the infertile couple not only with the goal of conception but also with a wider outlook including future pregnancy and delivery. We explain that there are three major causes of infertility, viz. male factor, ovulatory dysfunction and problems with the Fallopian tubes.

The fertility team should ensure that patients are kept informed of investigation and treatment protocols and that they have some prognosis for the likelihood of success. To ensure that the couple has adequate information, we provide regularly updated patient information leaflets relating to the investigation and treatments of infertility, polycystic ovaries if applicable and also antenatal screening. These are produced in-house on word processor (Chapter 30). They have the advantage of being consistent with explanations offered during consultation and they can be readily updated. At each consultation the couple has an opportunity to have their questions answered.

If there is evidence of ovulatory problems, ovulation induction is commenced. If there is a history of significant pelvic pain, dyspareunia or tenderness on pelvic examination, laparoscopy with dye insufflation, hysteroscopy and endometrial curettage is scheduled. A poor male fertility test is an indication for an andrological evaluation or early introduction to our artificial insemination of partner's sperm programme. We encourage the use of basal temperature charts, not only as a guide to ovulation but also to chart the timing of investigations such as progesterone levels and postcoital tests and to determine whether intercourse is being appropriately timed.

When initial assessment indicates no obvious factors to account for the infertility, a hysterosalpingogram and postcoital test are scheduled. We emphasize that infertility can be unexplained in about a quarter of couples attending but there are still treatments that can enhance the chances of conception. Hysterosalpingography and a postcoital test are performed if conception has not occurred within 3 months of ovulation induction or artificial insemination. A mild analgesic is recommended, before the hysterosalpingogram, such as paracetamol about an hour before the appointment. Hysterosalpingography should be performed within a few days of a period finishing. We are considering assessing tubal patency by ultrasound at the time of the day 12 ultrasound examination. The majority of our patients do not require laparoscopy. We do not investigate for luteal phase deficiency or luteinized unruptured follicles as we consider these to be essentially evidence of ovulation dysfunction which should be subject to treatment with ovulation induction. We do not see a place for sperm antibody screening.

Pregnant women should always be given adequate counselling about current antenatal screening tests and their implications. For couples who have experienced fertility difficulties, the dilemma of opting into antenatal screening tests is particularly complicated as they might ultimately result in the discontinuation of a pregnancy that has been difficult to achieve and perhaps irreplaceable. The commonest group would be women in their late thirties or forties who may wish to be screened antenatally for Down's syndrome. Other examples would be communities at risk of thalassaemia or Tay Sacks disease. Infertility consultations provide an opportunity for preconception counselling. We believe that infertility couples should have an early opportunity to consider their options with regard to antenatal screening in anticipation of pregnancy.

The central theme of biology is reproduction, and for those unfortunate couples who have difficulties achieving parenthood there may be frustration, anxiety and depression. Perhaps surprisingly, little evidence of increasing psychopathology developed between assessment at the time of the initial visit to an infertility clinic and a second assessment about 8 months later[118]. There is no evidence that the psychological disturbance resulting from infertility reduces fertility potential. The importance of counselling for infertile couples is discussed in Chapter 16.

Infertility is associated with an increased incidence of early pregnancy loss[2,119] and ectopic pregnancy[120]. A recent prospective observational study of 200 couples planning to conceive found the maximum efficiency of human reproduction to be 30% conception rate per cycle; with sensitive early hCG testing it was shown that pregnancy wastage accounts for 31% of pregnancies[121]. Forty-one per cent of pregnancy losses were detected by hCG alone without apparent missed periods.

All complications in pregnancy following fertility difficulties are understandably prone to increased anxieties for the patient, who requires particularly skilful, sympathetic and experienced counselling by clinicians and often specialist counsellors.

## REFERENCES


1. Cooke, I. D., Salaiman, R. A., Lenton, E. A. and Parsons, R. J. (1981). Fertility and infertility statistics: their importance and application. *Clin. Obstet. Gynaecol.*, **8**, 531–48
2. Templeton, A., Fraser, C. and Thompson, B. (1991). Infertility – epidemiology and referral practice. *Hum. Reprod.*, **6**, 1391–4
3. Schmidt, L., Munster, K. and Helm, P. (1995). Infertility and the seeking of infertility treatment in a representative population. *Br. J. Obstet. Gynaecol.*, **102**, 978–84
4. Lansac, J. (1995). Delayed parenting: is delayed childbearing a good thing? (1995). *Hum. Reprod.*, **10**, 1033–6
5. Schwartz, D. and Mayaux, J. M. (1982). Female fecundity as a function of age: results of artificial insemination in 2193 nulliparous women with azoospermic husbands. *N. Engl. J. Med.*, **306**, 404–6
6. Soules, M. R. (1988). Prevention of infertility. *Fertil. Steril.*, **49**, 582–4
7. Mathieu, C., Ecochard, R., Bied, V., Lornage, J. and Czyba, J. C. (1995). Cumulative conception rate following intrauterine artificial insemination with husband's spermatozoa: influence of husband's age. *Hum. Reprod.*, **10**, 1090–7
8. Baird, D. D. and Wilcox, A. J. (1985). Cigarette smoking associated with delayed conception. *J. Am. Med. Assoc.*, **253**, 2979–83
9. Weinberg, C. R., Wilcox, A. J. and Baird, D. D. (1989). Reduced fecundability in women with prenatal exposure to cigarette smoking. *Am. J. Epidemiol.*, **129**, 1072–8
10. Thonneau, P., Quesnot, S., Ducot, B., Marchand, S., Fignon, A., Lansac, J. and Spira, A. (1992). Risk factors for female and male infertility: results of a case-control study. *Hum. Reprod.*, **7**, 55–8
11. Mosher, W. D. and Pratt, W. F. (1993). The demography of infertility in the United States. In Asch, R. H. and Studd, J. W. W. (eds.) *Annual Progress in Reproductive Medicine*, pp. 37–43. (Carnforth, UK: Parthenon Publishing)
12. Hull, M. G. R., Glazener, C. M., Kelly, N. J., Conway, D. I., Foster, P. A., Hinton, R. A., Coulson, C., Lambert, P. A., Watt, E. M. and Desai, K. M. (1985). Population study of causes, treatment and outcome of infertility. *Br. Med. J.*, **91**, 1693–7
13. Buckler, H. M., Evans, C. A., Mamtora, H., Burger, H. G. and Anderson, D. C. (1991). Gonadotrophin, steroid and inhibin levels in women with incipient ovarian failure during anovulatory and ovulatory rebound cycles. *J. Clin. Endocrinol. Metab.*, **72**, 116–24

14. MacNaughton, J., Banah, M., McCloud, P., Hee, J. and Burger, H. (1992). Age related changes in follicle stimulating hormone, luteinizing hormone, oestradiol and immunoreactive inhibin in women of reproductive age. *Clin. Endocrinol.*, **36**, 339–45
15. Toner, J. P., Philput, C. B., Jones, G. S. and Muasher, S. J. (1991). Basal follicle-stimulating hormone level is a better predictor of *in vitro* fertilization performance than age. *Fertil. Steril.*, **55**, 784–91
16. O'Herlihy, C., Pepperell, R. J. and Evans, J. H. (1980). The significance of FSH elevation in young women with disorders of ovulation. *Br. Med. J.*, **281**, 1447–50
17. Stanger, J. D. and Yovich, J. L. (1985). Reduced *in-vitro* fertilization of human oocytes from patients with raised basal luteinizing hormone levels during the follicular phase. *Br. J. Obstet. Gynaecol.*, **92**, 385–93
18. Homberg, R., Armar, N. A., Eshel, A., Adams, J. and Jacobs, H. S. (1988). Influence of serum luteinising hormone concentrations of ovulation, conception, and early pregnancy loss in polycystic ovary syndrome. *Lancet*, **297**, 1024–6
19. Regan, L., Owen, E. J. and Jacobs, H. S. (1990). Hypersecretion of luteinising hormone, infertility, and miscarriage. *Lancet*, **336**, 1141–4
20. Abu-Heija, A. T., Fleming, R., Yates, R. S. W. and Coutts, J. R. T. (1995). Pregnancy outcome following exposure to gonadotrophin-releasing hormone analogue during early pregnancy: comparisons in patients with normal or elevated luteinizing hormone. *Hum. Reprod.*, **10**, 3317–19
21. Clifford, K., Rai, R., Watson, H., Franks, S. and Regan, L. (1996). Does suppressing luteinising hormone secretion reduce the miscarriage rate? Results of a randomised controlled trial. *Br. Med. J.*, **312**, 1508–11
22. Glazener, C. M., Kelly, N. J. and Hull, M. G. (1987). Prolactin measurement in the investigation of infertility in women with a normal menstrual cycle. *Br. J. Obstet. Gynaecol.*, **94**, 535–8
23. Lenton, E. A., Weston, G. A. and Cooke, I. D. (1977). Problems in using body temperature recordings in an infertility clinic. *Br. Med. J.*, **1**, 803–5
24. Ayres-de-Campos, D., Silva-Carvalho, J. L., Oliveira, C., Martins-da-Silva, I., Silva-Carvalho, J. and Pereira-Leite, L. (1995). Interobserver agreement in analysis of basal body temperature graphs from infertile women. *Hum. Reprod.*, **10**, 2010–16
25. Leader, L. R., Russell, T., Clifford, K. and Stenning, B. (1991). The clinical value of Clearplan home ovulation detection kits in infertility practice. *Aust. NZ J. Obstet. Gynaecol.*, **31**, 142–4
26. Schmutzler, R. K., Diedrich, K. and Krebs, D. (1995). Value of the Clearplan Ovulation Test in sterility treatment. *Geburtshilfe. Frauenheilkd.*, **55**, 266–9
27. Rudy, E. B. and Estok, P. (1992). Professional and lay interrator reliability of urinary luteinizing hormone surges measured by OvuQuick test. *J. Obstet. Gynecol. Neonatal Nurs.*, **21**, 407–11
28. Martinez, A. R., Voorhorst, F. J. and Schoemaker, J. (1992). Reliability of urinary LH testing for planning of endometrial biopsies. *Eur. J. Obstet. Gynecol. Reprod. Biol.*, **43**, 137–42
29. Corsan, G. H., Blotner, M. B., Bohrer, M. K., Shelden, R. and Kemmann, E. (1993). The utility of a home urinary LH immunoassay in timing the postcoital test. *Obstet. Gynecol.*, **81**, 736–8
30. Hull, M. G., Savage, P. E., Bromham, D. R., Ismail, A. A. A. and Morris, A. F. (1982). The value of single serum progesterone measurement in the midluteal phase as a criterion of a potentially fertile cycle ('ovulation') derived from treated and untreated conception cycles. *Fertil. Steril.*, **37**, 355–60
31. Abdulla, U., Diver, M. J., Hipkin, L. J. and Davis, J. C. (1983). Plasma progesterone levels as an index of ovulation. *Br. J. Obstet. Gynaecol.*, **90**, 543–8
32. Fujimoto, V. Y., Clifton, D. K., Cohen, N. L. and Soules, M. R. (1990). Variability of serum prolactin and progesterone levels in normal women: the relevance of single hormone measurements in the clinical setting. *Obstet. Gynecol.*, **76**, 71–8
33. Soules, M. R., McLachlan, R. I., Ek, M., Dahl, K. D., Cohen, N. L. and Bremner, W. J. (1989). Luteal phase deficiency: characterization of reproductive hormones over the menstrual cycle. *J. Clin. Endocrinol. Metab.*, **69**, 804–12
34. Pearlstone, A. C. and Surrey, E. S. (1994). The temporal relation between the urine LH surge

and sonographic evidence of ovulation: determinants and clinical significance. *Obstet. Gynecol.*, **83**, 184–8
35. Smith, S. K., Lenton, E. A., Landgren, B. M. and Cooke, I. D. (1984). The short luteal phase and infertility. *Br. J. Obstet. Gynaecol.*, **91**, 1020–2
36. Downs, K. A. and Gibson, M. (1983). Basal body temperature graph and the luteal phase defect. *Fertil. Steril.*, **40**, 466–8
37. Hills, G. A., Herbert, C. M., Parker, R. A. and Wentz, A. C. (1989). Comparison of late luteal phase endometrial biopsies using the Novak curette or Pipelle endometrial suction curette. *Obstet. Gynecol.*, **73**, 443–5
38. Herbert, C. M., Hill, G. A., Maxson, W. S., Wentz, A. C. and Osteen, K. G. (1990). Use of a sensitive urine pregnancy test before endometrial biopsies taken in the late luteal phase. *Fertil. Steril.*, **53**, 162–4
39. Li, T. C., Dockery, P., Rogers, A. W. and Cooke, I. D. (1989). How precise is histologic dating of endometrium using the standard dating criteria? *Fertil. Steril.*, **51**, 759–63
40. Wentz, A. C., Kossoy, L. R. and Parker, R. A. (1990). The impact of luteal phase inadequacy in an infertile population. *Am. J. Obstet. Gynecol.*, **162**, 937–43
41. Downs, K. A. and Gibson, M. (1983). Clomiphene citrate therapy for luteal phase defect. *Fertil. Steril.*, **39**, 34–8
42. Batista, M. C., Cartledge, T. P., Zellmer, A. W., Merino, M. J., Nieman, L. K., Loriaux, D. L. and Merriam, G. R. (1996). A prospective controlled study of luteal and endometrial abnormalities in an infertile population. *Fertil. Steril.*, **65**, 495–502
43. Guillaume, A. J., Benjamin, F., Sicuranza, B., Deutsch, S. and Spitzer, M. (1995). Luteal phase defects and ectopic pregnancy. *Fertil. Steril.*, **63**, 30–3
44. Marik, J. and Hulka, J. (1978). Luteinized unruptured follicle syndrome: a subtle cause of infertility. *Fertil. Steril.*, **29**, 270–4
45. Martinez, A. R., Bernardus, R. E., Kucharska, D. and Schoemaker, J. (1991). Urinary luteinizing hormone testing and prediction of ovulation in spontaneous, clomiphene citrate and human menopausal gonadotrophin-stimulated cycles. *Acta Endocrinol. (Copenh.)*, **124**, 357–63
46. Coutts, J. R. T., Adam, A. H. and Fleming, R. (1982). The deficient luteal phase may represent an anovulatory cycle. *Clin. Endocrinol.*, **17**, 389–94
47. Speroff, L., Glass, R. H. and Kase, N. G. (1994). *Clinical Gynecologic Endocrinology and Infertility*, p. 832. (Baltimore: Williams and Wilkins)
48. Glazener, C. M., Kelly, N. J. and Hull, M. G. (1988). Luteal deficiency not a persistent cause of infertility. *Hum. Reprod.*, **3**, 213–17
49. Bancroft, K., Vaughan-Williams, C. A. and Elstein, M. (1989). Minimal-mild endometriosis and infertility. *Br. J. Obstet. Gynaecol.*, **96**, 445–60
50. Mahmood, T. A. and Templeton, A. (1990). The impact of treatment on the natural history of endometriosis. *Hum. Reprod.*, **5**, 965–70
51. Jansen, R. P. S. (1986). Minimal endometriosis and reduced fecundability: prospective evidence from an artificial insemination by donor program. *Fertil. Steril.*, **46**, 141–3
52. Hornstein, M. D., Gleason, R. E., Orav, J., Haas, S. T., Friedman, A. J., Rein, M. S., Hill, J. A. and Barbieri, R. L. (1993). The reproducibility of the revised American Fertility Society classification of endometriosis. *Fertil. Steril.*, **59**, 1015–21
53. Mahmood, T. A. and Templeton, A. (1989). The relationship between endometriosis and semen analysis: a review of 490 consecutive laparoscopies. *Hum. Reprod.*, **4**, 782–5
54. Bancroft, K., Vaughan-Williams, C. A. and Elstein, M. (1992). Pituitary-ovarian function in women with minimal or mild endometriosis and otherwise unexplained infertility. *Clin. Endocrinol. (Oxf.)*, **36**, 177–81
55. Koninckx, P. R. (1994). Is mild endometriosis a condition occuring intermittently in all women? *Hum. Reprod.*, **9**, 2202–5
56. Buxton, L. and Southam, A. (1955). A critical survey of present methods of diagnosis and therapy in human infertility. *Am. J. Obstet. Gynecol.*, **70**, 741–52
57. Shepard, M. K. and Jones, R. B. (1989). Recovery of *Chlamydia trachomatis* from endometrial and Fallopian tube biopsies in women with infertility of tubal origin. *Fertil. Steril.*, **52**, 232–8
58. Patton, D. L., Askienazy-Elbhar, M., Henry-Suchet, J., Campbell, L. A., Cappuccio, A., Tannous, W., Wang, S. P. and Kuo, C. C. (1994). Detection of *Chlamydia trachomatis* in Fallopian tube tissue in women with

postinfectious tubal infertility. *Am. J. Obstet. Gynecol.*, **171**, 95–101
59. Dabekausen, Y. A., Evers, J. L., Land, J. A. and Stals, F. S. (1994). *Chlamydia trachomatis* antibody testing is more accurate than hysterosalpingography in predicting tubal factor infertility. *Fertil. Steril.*, **61**, 833–7
60. Mueller, B. A., Daling, J. R., Moore, D. E., Weiss, N. S., Spadoni, L. R., Stadel, B. V. and Soules, M. R. (1986). Appendectomy and the risk of tubal infertility. *N. Engl. J. Med.*, **315**, 1506–8
61. Sharman, A. (1944). Some recent studies and investigations in sterility. *J. Obstet. Gynaecol. Br. Emp.*, **51**, 85–111
62. Rubin, I. C. (1920). Nonoperative determination of patency of Fallopian tubes in sterility. *J. Am. Med. Assoc.*, **74**, 1017
63. Cron, R. S. (1922). Carbon dioxide gas inflation as a means of determining the causes of sterility in women. *J. Am. Med. Assoc.*, **79**, 713–7
64. Rubin, I. C. (1932). Twelve years' experience with uterotubal insufflation; diagnostic and therapeutic. *Am. J. Obstet. Gynecol.*, **23**, 561–73
65. Green-Armytage, V. B. (1943). The lessons and virtues of salpingography. *J. Obstet. Gynaecol.*, **30**, 23–6
66. Stallworthy, J. (1948). Facts and fantasy in the study of female infertility. *J. Obstet. Gynaecol.*, **55**, 171–80
67. Watson, A., Vandekerckhove, P., Lilford, R., Vail, A., Brosens, I. and Hughes, E. (1994). A meta-analysis of the therapeutic role of oil soluble contrast media at hysterosalpingography: a surprising result? *Fertil. Steril.*, **61**, 470–7
68. Steptoe, P. C. (1967). *Laparoscopy in Gynaecology*. (Edinburgh: Livingstone)
69. Afsari, A. and Thompson, R. J. (1972). Current tests for tubal patency. Their study and comparison. *Med. Henry Ford Hosp. J.*, **20**, 125
70. Decker, A. and Decker, W. H. (1954). A tubal function test. *Obstet. Gynecol.*, **4**, 35–8
71. Dapena, J. E. (1974). Retrograde test for the study of Fallopian tubes. In *Abstracts of the 8th World Congress of Fertility and Sterility*, Buenos Aires, Argentina, November, abstr. 315
72. Pecoud, E. and Lowy, G. (1974). Investigation of tubal patency by the indigo carmin method. In *Abstracts of the 8th World Congress of Fertility and Sterility*, Buenos Aires, Argentina, November, abstr. 339
73. Gurgan, T., Kisnisci, H. A., Yarali, H., Develioglu, O., Zeyneloglu, H., Aksu, T. and Caner, B. (1991). Evaluation of the functional status of the Fallopian tubes in unexplained infertility with radionuclide hysterosalpingography. *Gynecol. Obstet. Invest.*, **32**, 224–6
74. McQueen, D., McKillop, J. H., Gray, H. W., Bessent, R. G. and Black, W. P. (1991). Investigation of tubal infertility by radionuclide migration. *Hum. Reprod.*, **6**, 529–32
75. Adelusi, B., Al-Nuaim, L., Makanjoula, D., Khashoggi, T., Chowdhury, N. and Kangave, D. (1995). Accuracy of hysterosalpingography and laparoscopic hydrotubation in diagnosis of tubal patency. *Fertil. Steril.*, **63**, 1016–20
76. Swart, P., Mol, B. W. J., van der Veen, F., van Beurden, M., Redekop, W. K. and Bossuyt, P. M. M. (1995). The accuracy of hysterosalpingography in the diagnosis of tubal pathology: a meta-analysis. *Fertil. Steril.*, **64**, 486–91
77. Sher, G. and Barnard, P. G. (1976). The alleviation of uterocornual spasm of the Fallopian tubes during hysterosalpingography by intravenous administration of orciprenaline. *S. Afr. Med. J.*, **50**, 1164–5
78. Abdalla, H. I. (1992). Active management of infertility. *Br. J. Hosp. Med.*, **48**, 28–33
79. Guzick, D. S. (1995). Do infertility tests discriminate between fertile and infertile populations? *Hum. Reprod.*, **10**, 2008–9
80. Brosens, I., Boeckx, W., Delattin, P., Puttemans, P. and Vasquez, G. (1987). Salpingoscopy: a new pre-operative diagnostic tool in tubal infertility. *Br. J. Obstet. Gynaecol.*, **94**, 768–73
81. Menashe, Y., Rosen, D. J., Surrey, E. and Kerin, J. F. (1993). Falloposcopy – a new method for evaluation and treatment of infertility due to tubal factors. *Harefuah*, **124**, 8–12
82. Chapron, C., Querleu, D., Mage, G., Madelnat, P., Dubuisson, J. B., Audebert, A., Erny, R. and Bruhat, M. A. (1992). Complications of gynecologic laparoscopy. Multicentric study of 7604 laparoscopies. *J. Gynecol. Obstet. Biol. Reprod. (Paris)*, **21**, 207–13
83. Bateman, B. G., Kolp, L. A. and Hoeger, K. (1996). Complications of laparoscopy – operative and diagnostic. *Fertil. Steril.*, **66**, 30–5
84. Daly, D. C. and Hager, M. (1994). Does a normal outpatient evaluation eliminate the need for diagnostic laparoscopy? In *American Society for Reproductive Medicine: Abstracts for the Scientific Oral and Poster Sessions*, November, p. S40

85. Richman, T. S., Viscomi, G. N., deCherney, A., Polan, M. L. and Alcebo, L. O. (1984). Fallopian tubal patency assessed by ultrasound following fluid injection. *Radiology*, **152**, 507–10
86. Deichert, U., Schleif, R., van de Sandt, M. and Juhnke, I. (1989). Transvaginal hysterosalpingo-contrast-sonography (Hy-Co-Sy) compared with conventional tubal diagnostics. *Hum. Reprod.*, **4**, 418–24
87. Mitri, F. F., Andronikou, A. D., Perpinyal, S., Hofmeyr, G. J. and Sonnendecker, E. W. W. (1991). A clinical comparison of sonographic hydrotubation and hysterosalpingography. *Br. J. Obstet. Gynaecol.*, **98**, 1031–6
88. Allahbadia, G. N. (1992). Fallopian tubes and ultrasonography: the Sion experience. *Fertil. Steril.*, **58**, 901–7
89. Heikkinen, H., Tekay, A., Volpi, E., Martikainen, H. and Jouppila, P. (1995). Transvaginal salpingosonography for the assessment of tubal patency in infertile women: methodological and clinical experiences. *Fertil. Steril.*, **64**, 293–8
90. Venezia, R. and Zangara, C. (1991). Echohysterosalpingography: new diagnostic possibilities with S HU 450 Echovist. *Acta Europ. Fertilitatis*, **22**, 279–82
91. de Souza, N. M., Brosens, J. J., Schwieso, J. E., Paraschos, T. and Winston, R. M. (1995). The potential value of magnetic resonance imaging in infertility. *Clin. Radiol.*, **50**, 75–9
92. Shushan, A., Eisenberg, V. H. and Schenker, J. G. (1995). Subfertility in the era of assisted reproduction: changes and consequences. *Fertil. Steril.*, **64**, 459–69
93. Meldrum, D. R. (1993). Female reproductive aging – ovarian and uterine factors. *Fertil. Steril.*, **59**, 1–5
94. Batista, M. C., Cartledge, T. P., Zellmer, A. W., Merino, M. J., Axiotis, C., Bremner, W. J. and Nieman, L. K. (1995). Effects of aging on menstrual cycle hormones and endometrial maturation. *Fertil. Steril.*, **64**, 492–9
95. Wilcox, A. J., Weinberg, C. R., O'Connor, J. F., Baird, D. D., Schlatterer, J. P., Canfield, R. F., Armstrong, E. G. and Nisulaa, B. C. (1988). Incidence of early loss of pregnancy. *N. Engl. J. Med.*, **319**, 189–94
96. Cano, F., Simon, C., Remohi, J. and Pellicer, A. (1995). Effect of aging on the female reproductive system: evidence for a role of uterine senescence in the decline in female fecundity. *Fertil. Steril.*, **64**, 584–9
97. Borini, A., Bianchi, L., Violini, F., Maccolini, A., Cattoli, M. and Flamigni, C. (1996). Oocyte donation program: pregnancy and implantation rates in women of different ages sharing oocytes from single donor. *Fertil. Steril.*, **65**, 94–7
98. Li, T. C., Nuttall, L., Klentzeris, L. and Cooke, I. D. (1992). How well does ultrasonographic measurement of endometrial thickness predict the results of histological dating? *Hum. Reprod.*, **7**, 1–5
99. Abdalla, H. I., Brooks, A. A., Johnson, M. R., Kirkland, A., Thomas, A. and Studd, J. W. W. (1994). Endometrial thickness: a predictor of implantation in ovum recipients? *Hum. Reprod.*, **9**, 363–5
100. Li, T. C. and Cooke, I. D. (1992). Uterine factors in infertility. *Curr. Opin. Obstet. Gynecol.*, **4**, 212–19
101. Margalloth, E. J., Sauter, E., Bronson, R. A., Rosenfeld, D. J., Scholl, G. M. and Cooper, G. W. (1988). Intrauterine insemination as treatment for antisperm antibodies in the female. *Fertil. Steril.*, **50**, 441–6
102. Oei, S. G., Kierse, M. J. N. C., Bloemenkamp, K. W. M. and Helmerhorst, F. M. (1995). European postcoital tests: opinions and practice. *Br. J. Obstet. Gynaecol.*, **102**, 621–4
103. Drake, T. S., Tredway, D. R. and Buchanan, G. C. (1979). A reassessment of the fractional postcoital test. *Am. J. Obstet. Gynecol.*, **133**, 382–5
104. Hull, M. G., Savage, P. E. and Bromham, D. R. (1982). Prognostic value of the postcoital test: prospective study based on time-specific conception rates. *Br. J. Obstet. Gynaecol.*, **89**, 299–305
105. Collins, J. A., So, Y., Wilson, E. H., Wrixon, W. and Casper, R. F. (1984). The postcoital test as a predictor of pregnancy among 355 infertile couples. *Fertil. Steril.*, **41**, 703–8
106. Oei, S. G., Helmerhorst, F. M. and Keirse, M. J. N. C. (1975). When is the post-coital test normal? A critical appraisal. *Hum. Reprod.*, **10**, 1711–14
107. Bronson, R. A. and Cooper, G. W. (1987). Effects of sperm-reactive monoclonal antibodies on the cervical mucus penetrating ability of human spermatazoa. *Am. J. Reprod. Immunol. Microbiol.*, **14**, 59–61

108. Eggert-Kruse, W., Christmann, M., Gerhard, I., Pohl, S., Klinga, K. and Runnebaum, B. (1989). Circulating antisperm antibodies and fertility prognosis: a prospective study. *Hum. Reprod.*, **4**, 513–20
109. Eggert-Kruse, W., Gerhard, I., Tilgen, W. and Runnebaum, B. (1989). Clinical significance of crossed *in vitro* sperm-cervical mucus penetration test in infertility investigation. *Fertil. Steril.*, **52**, 1032–40
110. Harrison, R. F. (1980). Pregnancy successes in the infertile couple. *Int. J. Fertil.*, **25**, 81–7
111. Taylor, P. J. and Collins, J. A. (1992). *Unexplained Infertility*, p. 5. (Oxford, New York and Tokyo: Oxford University Press)
112. Klentzeris, L. D., Bulmer, J. N., Warren, M. A., Morrison, L., Li, T. C. and Cooke, I. D. (1994). Lymphoid tissue in the endometrium of women with unexplained infertility: morphometric and immunohistochemical aspects. *Hum. Reprod.*, **9**, 646–52
113. Taylor, P. V., Campbell, J. M. and Scott, J. S. (1989). Presence of autoantibodies in women with unexplained infertility. *Am. J. Obstet. Gynecol.*, **161**, 377–9
114. Dunphy, B. C., Li, T. C., Macleod, I. C., Barratt, C. L., Lenton, E. A. and Cooke, I. D. (1990). The interaction of parameters of male and female infertility in couples with previously unexplained infertility. *Fertil. Steril.*, **54**, 824–7
115. Lobo, R. A. (1993). Unexplained infertility. *J. Reprod. Med.*, **38**, 241–9
116. Emslie, C., Grimshaw, J. and Templeton, A. (1993). Do clinical guidelines improve general practice management and referral of infertile couples. *Br. Med. J.*, **306**, 1728–31
117. Working Group (1993). *Fertility Services Guidance For Purchasers*. North East Thames Regional Health Authority
118. Connolly, K. J., Edelman, R. J., Cooke, I. D. and Robson, J. (1992). The impact of infertility on psychological functioning. *J. Psychosom. Res.*, **36**, 459–68
119. Jansen, R. P. (1982). Spontaneous abortion incidence in the treatment of infertility. *Am. J. Obstet. Gynecol.*, **143**, 451–73
120. Tuomivaara, L. and Ronnberg, L. (1991). Ectopic pregnancy and infertility following treatment of infertile couples: a follow-up of 929 cases. *Eur. J. Obstet. Gynecol. Reprod. Biol.*, **42**, 33–8
121. Zinaman, M. J., Clegg, E. D., Brown, C. C., O'Connor, J. and Selevan, S. G. (1996). Estimates of human fertility and pregnancy loss. *Fertil. Steril.*, **65**, 503–9

# Infertility treatment 8

*David A. Viniker*

## INTRODUCTION

The objective of treatment for couples with infertility is to achieve a successful pregnancy quickly and safely with the minimum intervention required, always recognizing the sensitivity of our patients and their need for information and input into decision making.

## INDUCTION OF OVULATION

With the exception of primary ovarian failure, ovulatory disorders can usually be successfully treated, and this treatment depends on the underlying cause of the problem. When weight loss is responsible for secondary amenorrhoea, weight gain alone may prove to be successful[1,2].

### Orally active agents

*Clomiphene citrate*

Clomiphene citrate, although not a steroid, has a biochemical configuration similar to that of estrogens. It modifies hypothalamic and pituitary activity by binding to estrogen receptors and also by inhibiting receptor replenishment. The hypothalamus assumes a falsely low reading of estrogen levels and gonadotrophin releasing hormone (GnRH) activity, and consequently follicle stimulating hormone (FSH) and luteinizing hormone (LH) output from the pituitary are increased.

Clomiphene therapy is traditionally started with 50 mg daily for 5 days. We generally commence anovulatory normoprolactinaemic patients on the 2nd day of the cycle, although there is probably no clinical advantage arising from the exact start day. In a series of 414 treatment cycles, there was no significant difference in terms of ovulation, pregnancy rates or outcome when clomiphene was begun on the 2nd, 3rd, 4th or 5th day of the cycle[3]. There is no accurate way of predicting the likely chance of ovulation occurring from a hormone profile[4]. Ovarian hyperstimulation can occur with clomiphene, although this is less common and not as severe as with gonadotrophin therapy. Increasing the dose of clomiphene increases the risk of hyperstimulation occurring. Twins occur in 5% of clomiphene-induced pregnancies but higher order pregnancies are unusual. I learnt recently that the wife of a schoolfriend of mine, who was treated in another clinic 20 years ago, delivered quintuplets following clomiphene 100 mg daily for 5 days; reassuringly, all five are healthy. Other side-effects of clomiphene therapy include hot flushes and headaches but these are not usually severe enough to discontinue treatment.

The majority of pregnancies will occur in the first few cycles. For early treatment of cycles, it has been suggested that simple monitoring with basal temperature alone is as good as urinary LH monitoring and ultrasound[5]. If there is no success with 50 mg, then the dose can slowly be increased in 50 mg increments up to 200 mg daily for 5 days[6].

Although attention has been drawn to the antiestrogenic activity of clomiphene, there may be no substance in the suggestion that the cervical mucus is adversely affected[7]. In contrast, Roumen and colleagues[8] found problems with the cervical mucus in some patients treated with clomiphene. Estrogen supplementation has been advocated in the preovulatory phase[9], although the benefits have been debated[10]. There would appear to be no increased risk of congenital abnormality in pregnancy after clomiphene ovulation induction[7,11]. Early pregnancy loss and ectopic pregnancy rates are not significantly increased in association with clomiphene-induced ovulation[12].

An analysis of 3837 women investigated for infertility in Seattle between 1974 and 1985 was reported in 1994[13]. There were 11 invasive or borderline malignant tumours against an expected number of 4.4. Nine of the women developing ovarian malignancy had taken clomiphene and five of these nine had taken the drug for 12 months or more. The relative risk for the women taking clomiphene for 12 months or more was 11.1; treatment with clomiphene for less than a year was not associated with increased risk. Subsequent to the Seattle report, The Committee on Safety of Medicines in the United Kingdom, whilst accepting that further studies are indicated to investigate the possible association between clomiphene and ovarian cancer, has stated that 'We recommend that clomiphene should not normally be used for more than six cycles'[14]. If it is clinically felt to be in the patient's interests to continue with clomiphene, it would certainly be wise to ensure that the patient is aware of current concerns relating to ovarian cancer and that she gives her fully informed consent.

Ovulation rates can be in the region of 90% but pregnancy rates do not exceed 60%. When there is evidence of follicular development with clomiphene but ovulation or pregnancy does not occur, human chorionic gonadotrophin (hCG) administration can increase the chance of conception. The hCG should be given when the leading follicle reaches approximately 18 mm diameter as visualized by ultrasound[15]. GnRH agonist can be used instead of hCG, resulting in a short flare response of endogenous LH and FSH release, but in a comparative study, pregnancy rates and early pregnancy losses were not significantly different[16].

*Tamoxifen*

Tamoxifen is an antiestrogen and it is generally considered to increase fertility rates in a similar way to clomiphene. Interestingly, it does not increase follicular phase FSH and LH levels, although there is an increase in estradiol levels and luteal phase progesterone[17,18]. It has, therefore, been postulated that tamoxifen improves folliculogenesis by direct action on the ovary rather than through the hypothalamic-pituitary axis.

Early studies indicated similar success rates between tamoxifen and clomiphene[19]. In one series of 66 anovulatory patients, both drugs achieved pregnancy rates of 80% within 9 months but there were fewer early pregnancy losses with clomiphene[20]. When clomiphene fails to achieve ovulation or pregnancy, tamoxifen may prove to be effective[21]. Roumen and colleagues[8] found better cervical mucus with tamoxifen than clomiphene but Elstein and Fawcett[22] found similar effects on the cervical mucus with the two agents. They suggested that their effect seemed to be related to end-organ sensitivity rather than to a specific agent.

Gulekli and associates[23] have recommended tamoxifen for patients with polycystic ovary syndrome who prove to be resistant to clomiphene before treatment with surgery or gonadotrophins. Tan and Jacobs[24] consider tamoxifen to be their first choice rather than clomiphene for patients with hypersecretion of LH. In one small trial, a combination of tamoxifen and clomiphene was shown to be more effective at inducing ovulation than clomiphene alone and there were also more pregnancies with no multiple pregnancies[25].

When used for short periods, tamoxifen does not appear to be associated with any increased risk of either ovarian or endometrial malignancy[26].

*Hyperprolactinaemia: bromocriptine*

Hyperprolactinaemia is associated with suppression of the pulsatile GnRH release, with associated reduction of gonadotrophin levels. In mild hyperprolactinaemia, there may be an inadequate luteal phase whereas in severe cases there may be amenorrhoea. Since 1976, bromocriptine, a dopamine agonist which inhibits prolactin secretion by the pituitary, has been the drug of choice.

Ovulation rates of 90% and pregnancy rates of 75% have been reported with bromocriptine in patients with microprolactinomas or idiopathic hyperprolactinaemia[27]. Whereas bromocriptine does not enhance pregnancy rates in unexplained infertility[28], pregnancy rates are increased in patients with galactorrhoea but normal prolactin levels[29]. Bromocriptine may also reduce LH secretion in patients with polycystic ovary syndrome who do not respond to clomiphene alone[30]. There would not appear to be any adverse effects on pregnancy outcome following cessation of bromocriptine or if bromocriptine is continued throughout pregnancy[31].

The standard dose of bromocriptine is 2.5 mg twice daily, although much higher doses are sometimes required to achieve normal prolactin levels. Side-effects frequently occur and include headache, nausea and diarrhoea. These problems can be reduced by prescribing a gradually escalating regime starting with half a tablet at night and increasing at 4-day intervals. Occasionally, the vaginal route of administration proves to be better tolerated. Although there is no evidence of teratogenicity, it is generally recommended that bromocriptine be withdrawn as soon as pregnancy is achieved. Recently, there have been some new agents that may prove to be better tolerated than bromocriptine: cabergoline may become the drug of choice[32], although it is currently relatively expensive.

*Gonadotrophins*

Successful induction of ovulation and subsequent pregnancy using gonadotrophins derived from cadaveric pituitaries was first described by Gemzell and co-workers in 1958[33], but supplies were extremely limited. Gonadotrophins have become commercially available using extraction techniques on urine from menopausal women (hMG) who have high levels of gonadotrophins. The most recent advance in gonadotrophin production involves recombinant DNA technology. The DNA code for FSH has been defined and can be incorporated with a larger circular piece of DNA. This recombinant DNA is inserted into mammalian cells which then produce the FSH. Recombinant human FSH has become available[34].

The objective of gonadotrophin therapy is to produce mature follicles which can be released by injection of hCG. The specific complications of gonadotrophin therapy are multiple pregnancy and ovarian hyperstimulation syndrome (Chapter 5). In one series of 143 pregnancies in 110 women receiving hMG, the multiple pregnancy rate was 26.8%[35]. It is wise to ensure that the couple have adequate counselling before commencing treatment. Protocols for hMG in superovulation/*in vitro* fertilization (IVF) are discussed in Chapter 10.

The increase in ovulation rate with gonadotrophin therapy may be related to rescue of early follicles that would have undergone atresia and small follicles continuing to mature. There is evidence of low-molecular weight molecules in the follicular fluid of maturing follicles that are presumed to be produced by the dominant follicle which alters receptor responsiveness of other follicles. Exogenous gonadotrophins must interfere with this balance[36].

For 'low-tech' treatment, the objective is to stimulate maturation, preferably of one follicle but with a maximum of three follicles. Patients who fail to ovulate or conceive with clomiphene or tamoxifen are candidates for gonadotrophin therapy. Tubal patency, normal prolactin levels and satisfactory semen analysis are essential prerequisites. Patients with hypergonadotrophic hypogonadism (menopausal gonadotrophin levels) do not respond to gonadotrophin therapy. Ovarian hyperstimulation syndrome is more commonly associated with polycystic ovary syndrome and, accordingly for these women, the quantity of gonadotrophin administered should be reduced.

There have been a variety of regimens for the administration of gonadotrophins. The *fixed regimen* involves a predetermined dose administered in a single intramuscular injection on 3 alternate days, e.g. days 1, 3 and 5 of the menstrual cycle followed by hCG, given 3 days later if the estrogen response is in the accepted range[37–39]. In a study of 77 women having 322 treatment cycles, Ellis and Williamson[39] reported 43 pregnancies (48%) with a 31.6%

multiple pregnancy rate. There was a 5% incidence of ovarian hyperstimulation and 0.62% severe hyperstimulation rate.

In the *variable regimen*, gonadotrophins tended to be administered daily, the dose being adjusted according to plasma or urinary estradiol values. Human chorionic gonadotrophin was given 24–48 h after the optimum estradiol level had been reached[40,41]. There is some evidence that individualized regimens are associated with improved pregnancy rates and reduced hyperstimulation when compared to fixed regimens[41]. A step-down dose regimen has been described with an initial dose of 1.5–2.5 ampoules of FSH, reducing by 0.5 ampoules/day with ultrasound monitoring. Pregnancy rates of 17% per cycle, multiple pregnancy rates of 8% and only 1.7% mild ovarian hyperstimulation suggest that further investigation should be considered[42].

In the early days of gonadotrophin therapy, the only investigation for monitoring ovarian response was by estrogen assay of urine or blood after establishing normal ranges. Ultrasound tracking of follicular development, initially transabdominally and, more recently, by the transvaginal route, has provided a valuable addition for the monitoring of gonadotrophin therapy (Chapter 6). The dangers of hyperstimulation can be reduced by monitoring estrogen concentration and follicular tracking by ultrasound[43]. Some units continue to monitor estrogen levels in addition to ultrasound, but it has been shown that ultrasound alone can be used safely and efficiently[44].

The development of follicles in normal and induced ovulation as visualized by ultrasound has been described[45]. In spontaneous cycles, follicular development can be seen around the 5th day and the dominant follicle becomes apparent by about day 9. The maximum preovulatory follicular diameter can vary from 14 to 28 mm, although pregnancy is unlikely to occur at less than 17 mm. Ultrasound has demonstrated that there is a rapid enlargement of the dominant follicle before ovulation. Ovulatory pain or 'Mittelschmerz' is related to this enlargement of the follicle and precedes ovulation. Transvaginal ultrasound is preferred by patients to transabdominal ultrasound[46]. The maximum follicular development in hMG cycles tends to be less than with spontaneous or clomiphene-induced cycles (15–18 mm); when hCG is administered, ovulation occurs 36 h later.

A combination of clomiphene and low dose gonadotrophin therapy has been shown to increase pregnancy rates in ovulation disorders and unexplained infertility, with a relatively low incidence of ovarian hyperstimulation[47]. Minimal stimulation with a combination of clomiphene 100 mg daily for 5 days followed by a single dose of hMG 150 IU proved to be as successful as hMG alone in a group of non-IVF patients requiring controlled ovarian stimulation[48]. Two ampoules of hMG were used in the combination regimen compared to an average of 17 ampoules in the hMG-only protocol. There was no significant difference in the pregnancy rates (14.8% vs. 16.2%). Economic considerations would suggest an advantage for the combination therapy but controlled studies would be required to confirm this.

As with clomiphene, there is concern that gonadotrophin therapy may be associated with an increased risk of ovarian cancer. In a study of 2197 ovarian cancer patients and 8893 controls in 12 US case-controlled studies in the years 1956–1986, Whittemore and colleagues[49] found an increased risk in nulliparous women that appeared to be due to infertility and an increased risk that might be due to the use of fertility drugs; the risk of ovarian malignancy decreases with increasing parity. The validity of Whittemore's research has been questioned[50], although further studies continue to support the view that there is an increased incidence of ovarian carcinoma following gonadotrophin therapy[51]. There has been an almost exponential increase over the last 20 years in the use of ovulation induction agents; clomiphene has increased 11-fold and hMG 30-fold[52]. In an extensive review of the literature, Tarlatzis and co-workers[53] concluded that the evidence does not support a direct causal relationship between ovarian stimulation and ovarian cancer. Bristow and Karlan[54] have undertaken a literature search to identify all case reports and all epidemiological studies of data relevant to infertility, infertility treatment and risk of ovarian cancer. They found four case–control studies, three retrospective cohort studies and a meta-analysis of three additional case–control studies. They concluded that infertility alone is an independent risk factor for the development of ovarian cancer. Nulliparous women who have not responded to infertility therapy are particularly at risk and this is irrespective of the use of fertility agents. There is a tendency to increasing exposure of young women to these agents; careful analysis of data as they unfold is essential. It would be prudent to advocate close clinical surveillance of women with infertility problems, before, during and after treatment for infertility

Incorporation of estrogen add-back therapy for induction of ovulation has been proposed by Goldstein and colleagues[55] in down-regulation regimens used with ovulation stimulation, as less gonadotrophin therapy is required. This was advocated for cost–benefit considerations and the authors also indicated that this might be of importance from the point of view of cancer risk. Further research is urgently required to determine if this association can be confirmed. The problem may prove difficult to resolve as one could not envisage a controlled trial with only one group receiving ovulation induction whilst the other relinquishes fertility treatment. We already have strong advice to withhold clomiphene after six cycles. We would need to know if the relationship is specific to individual agents or to ovulation induction in general. This has major implications for infertility management. For example, if the effect proves to be cumulative, then, theoretically, gonadotrophin therapy or IFV, carrying greater success rates per cycle, would be indicated earlier. Should the relationship prove to be directly related to the strength of ovulation stimulation, then gonadotrophin therapy would need to be minimized.

Endometrial thickness on the day of hCG administration, as measured by ultrasound, correlates with the likelihood of pregnancy. Success is most likely if the endometrial thickness is greater than 6 mm[56,57]. Clomiphene is associated with reduced endometrial thickness[44,58]; this can probably be improved by estrogen administration.

### Luteinized unruptured follicles and luteal phase deficiency

Patients with frequent episodes of luteinized unruptured follicles may respond to injections of 5000 units of hCG at the time of the natural LH surge[59]. Dehydrogesterone or progesterone vaginal pessaries have proved to be equally successful, both being significantly better at improving the endometrial defect than in a control group, in a group of 44 infertile patients with luteal phase deficiency[60]. In a subsequent study with clomiphene citrate, hCG and dehydrogesterone compared to clomiphene and hCG alone, it was found that the progestational agent was of little therapeutic value[61]. Clomiphene citrate may be effective for luteinized unruptured follicles, particularly if histological dating of endometrium is delayed by at least 5 days[62].

From a study of 14 patients with luteal phase deficiency, it has been demonstrated that down-regulation with GnRH analogue and subsequent hormone replacement therapy (HRT) provides a normal endometrium, whereas progesterone supplements administered by injection were not as successful[63]. Dydrogesterone supports a secretory endometrium for a limited time even in the absence of endogenous progesterone[64].

According to the two-cell theory of folliculogenesis, androgen production in the thecal cell compartment is a function of LH action, and granulosa cell aromatization of the androgens is a function of FSH. It is assumed that the combined action of both FSH and LH is required for follicular maturation. Although it is apparent that both FSH and LH are required for follicular development, the optimal ratio of these two agents has yet to be determined. The arrival of highly purified FSH has allowed comparative investigation of the effect of pure FSH compared to combined FSH and LH[65]. In severe hypogonadotrophic hypogonadism, pharmacological doses of FSH with small amounts of LH are able to stimulate ovarian follicular maturation. From a theoretical point of view, pure FSH might have advantages over hMG, which is a mixture of FSH and LH: this would particularly apply to patients with polycystic ovary syndrome who tend to have elevated LH levels. FSH therapy results in lower LH levels than hMG levels pharmacodynamically but clinical benefit has not yet been conclusively demonstrated[66,67]. A new set of gonadotrophins with different ratios of FSH and LH and also recombinant preparations will be available soon; these are the subject of a number of current trials to determine their relative therapeutic value.

*Gonadotrophin releasing hormone*

Premature luteinization associated with an LH surge may account for some failures to conceive with gonadotrophin therapy; this is particularly common in patients with polycystic ovary syndrome[68]. Suppression of spontaneous gonadotrophin release and mid-cycle surge can be achieved with long-acting GnRH agonists (down-regulation), allowing controlled exogenous gonadotrophin stimulation. In the first report of this combination, seven out of eight patients, who had failed to conceive with prolonged antiestrogen therapy, conceived quickly[69].

Gonadotrophin releasing hormone analogues have been in clinical use for more than a decade. Their initial effect is to cause an increase in gonadotrophin production, or 'flare-response', before gonadotrophin production is reduced (down-regulation). A new set of drugs, the GnRH antagonists, which have no flare response, are currently under investigation[70].

*Pulsatile gonadotrophin releasing hormone*

Clomiphene, tamoxifen, bromocriptine, hMG and hCG provide excellent results, whether used individually or in combinations, for the majority of women with ovulatory dysfunction. Some women have unacceptable side-effects or fail to respond adequately; pulsatile GnRH therapy has provided an additional option[71].

Pituitary secretion of gonadotrophins is dependent physiologically on pulsatile release of GnRH by the hypothalamus. Homberg and colleagues[72] reviewed 100 pregnancies achieved by administration of 15 μg of GnRH subcutaneously every 90 min with a miniaturized pump and monitored the response with ultrasound. There were seven multiple pregnancies and 28 early pregnancy losses. They concluded that this treatment was safe, simple and effective with little need for monitoring. There was no danger of hyperstimulation. Pulse frequencies for release of the GnRH set at 90- or 120-min intervals have been shown more reliably to induce follicular development than settings at 60- or 180-min intervals[73].

Effective follicular maturation and ovulation have been achieved with pulsatile hMG administration[74,75], with FSH[75,76] and with combinations of sequential FSH and pulsatile GnRH[77].

Women with regular menses, but persistently raised FSH levels, are probably in a state of incipient ovarian failure. Suppression of gonadotrophin production with an estrogen–progesterone preparation can lead to evidence of ovulation on withdrawal of the suppression, although unfortunately pregnancy would be unusual[78].

Laparoscopic ovarian electrocautery may prove to be more effective than medical treatment for patients with polycystic ovary syndrome who are resistant to clomiphene. This treatment is associated with reduction of LH concentrations and a return to a normal menstrual cycle in 41% of patients and a reduction in gonadotrophin requirements should additional therapy be needed[79]. Further studies on pregnancy rates and early pregnancy losses are indicated to establish the future role of ovarian electrocautery.

## ENDOMETRIOSIS

Prospective randomized trials comparing danazol[80], gestrinone[81], medroxyprogesterone acetate[82] and GnRH analogues[83] with controls in the treatment of mild endometriosis have shown no advantage in terms of pregnancy rates. There is no evidence that surgery, including minimally invasive techniques, confers any better results than medical treatment[84]. Whitelaw and associates[85] evaluated laser surgery in a group of 17 women with infertility of at least 1 year. Patients in the laser group had adhesiolysis and all visible endometriotic implants vaporized. Within 1 year of treatment, there were no pregnancies in the group submitted to laser, while two patients in the expectantly managed group conceived!

When there is severe endometriosis, pregnancy rates of 50% have been achieved following restoration of normal anatomy at laparotomy[86], and similar success rates may be possible with minimally invasive surgery[87].

## TUBAL SURGERY

The chance of pregnancy occurring after tubal surgery depends on the severity of the pathology[88,89]. Careful preoperative assessment, including semen analysis and often laparoscopy and hysterosalpingography, is required[88]. The commonest site of tubal damage is the distal end, with birth rates after surgery of about 25%[90]. About a quarter of subsequent pregnancies are ectopic. Surgery for proximal tubal occlusion is more successful, with live birth rates of 50% and ectopic rates of 10%[91,92]. Just over a half of intrauterine pregnancies following salpingostomy may occur more than 1 year after surgery[93]. Reversal of sterilization, with removal of clips and re-anastomosis, carries a relatively high pregnancy rate of up to 80%[94].

Microsurgical tubal surgery involves the use of magnification as well as the adoption of a set of techniques including special instruments, minimal handling of the Fallopian tubes and fine non-reactive suture material. There have been no controlled trials conclusively to prove an advantage over macrosurgical techniques, but several surgical teams have reported improved success rates after adopting microsurgery[95,96]. It is technically possible to transplant the Fallopian tube and large numbers of these organs would undoubtedly be donated by women undergoing sterilization or hysterectomy[97]. Research interest in this area seems to have diminished following the arrival of IVF.

In an early trial of hydrotubation with hydrocortisone and, in some cases, antibiotics, there appeared to be enhanced success rates[98]. A randomized, controlled trial, however, found no benefit with hydrotubation[99]. Similarly, the intraperitoneal instillation of Dextran 70 (Pharmacia AB, Sweden) appears to have no greater effect on reducing adhesion formation than saline[100].

*In vitro* fertilization provides an alternative to tubal surgery (Chapter 10). For mild tubal disease and previous sterilization, tubal surgery is generally the treatment of first choice. With severe tubal pathology, IVF carries a much better success rate. For intermediate pathology, the optimal method in terms of success is less certain. Information about success rates is essential for couples to make informed decisions. Many couples would prefer tubal surgery in the first instance so that they have the opportunity of natural conception, leaving open the option of IVF if there is no success after surgery. Tubal surgery is discussed at length in Chapter 9.

### Tubal surgery or IVF?

The relative merits of tubal surgery and assisted reproduction need careful comparison. *In vitro* fertilization is becoming more readily available, with a corresponding reduction in the incidence of tubal surgery. Crude figures indicate greater success with the new technology. Overall success with IVF is lower for patients with tubal factor infertility, although this is probably mainly related to patients with hydrosalpinges. In a study of 741 patients undergoing IVF, the 62 patients with ultrasound evidence of hydrosalpinges were found to have delivery rates per embryo transfer reduced from 22.8% to 6.6%[101] but tubal factor infertility without hydrosalpinges was found to carry similar success rates to other indications for IVF. Fleming and Hull[102] have found a 50% reduction of embryo implantation rate associated with hydrosalpinges and advocate distal salpingostomy or salpingectomy before IVF. Salpingectomy for hydrosalpinges has been confirmed to improve pregnancy outcome with IVF[103].

*In vitro* fertilization is associated with a higher incidence of multiple pregnancy[104]. Perinatal mortality rates following assisted conception procedures are treble those of spontaneous conception, although most of the increase is related to multiple pregnancies. There is a five-fold increase in perinatal mortality with triplets as compared with singletons. The predicted costs associated with delivery of each baby for a singleton pregnancy in the USA in 1991 were $9845, for a twin pregnancy $18 974 and for triplets $36 588[105]. Between 1986 and 1991, assisted reproduction techniques were found to be responsible for 35% of twins and 77% of higher order pregnancies[105].

In the National Health Service, only about 25% of purchasing authorities are supporting IVF treatment. There can be little doubt that, from a purely economic point of view, a greater number of pregnancies could be achieved with a given amount of funding using low-tech treatments. Many couples would prefer the opportunity to conceive naturally, and only resort to IVF if tubal surgery fails.

## FIBROIDS

Fibroids become more common in the latter years of reproductive life. The relationship between fibroids and infertility has been the subject of debate. Implantation and pregnancy rates have been found to be reduced only when the fibroids are distorting the endometrial cavity[106]. Until recently, the only treatment was myomectomy at laparotomy. Transcervical hysteroscopy with resection of submucous fibroids and subsequent successful pregnancies have been reported[107]. Hysteroscopic resection of intrauterine septae or adhesions has also been reported to increase pregnancy rates in infertile couples and reduce spontaneous pregnancy loss in patients with recurrent abortion difficulties[108]. Controlled trials are required to establish the benefits.

## INTRAUTERINE INSEMINATION

Artificial insemination of the partner's sperm has an obvious place when there is known to be a coital problem, either elucidated from the history or perhaps from repeated observation of absence of sperm on postcoital testing. Reduced male fertility, as recognized from semen analysis, and cervical hostility, demonstrated by postcoital testing or mucus penetration tests, have been further indications. Artificial insemination may also have a role to play when inferility is unexplained. At one time, untreated semen was used but adverse reactions sometimes occurred. Now, sperm for insemination are prepared by washing or swim-up to improve success rates and reduce possible complications. The swim-up preparation involves washing the sperm with culture medium, and, after centrifugation, removing the supernatant. The pellet of sperm is covered by 0.5 ml of medium. In the swim-up preparation, the sperm in the pellet are incubated at body temperature for 30–60 min. The supernatant subsequently carries a relatively high concentration of motile sperm and this is used for the insemination procedure. A variety of swim-up techniques and media such as Percoll[109] have been used in attempts to improve success rates.

Even when there is moderate-to-severe male subfertility, treatment using ovulation induction and intrauterine insemination (IUI) would seem to be a valuable initial treatment before contemplating more expensive and invasive assisted reproductive techniques[110]: a sample with more than 300 000 motile sperm and greater than 10% progressive motility is required[111].

Clearly, artificial insemination should be undertaken around the time of ovulation. Schwartz and his colleagues[112] assessed the relationship between the day of insemination and the last day of 'hypothermia' on the basal temperature chart and conception rates in a donor insemination protocol. The overall conception rate was 12% and the best results were obtained for insemination 3 days (20%) and 1 day (21%) before the last day of hypothermia.

Luteinizing hormone predictor tests can be used to indicate the fertile phase for a woman with irregular cycles, perhaps increasing the success rate for natural or artificial insemination. In a prospective randomized trial, however, urinary LH dipsticks used in a donor insemination programme did not increase the pregnancy rate compared to a group using basal temperature charts[113]. If LH urinary testing is employed, it is probably best performed in the evening rather than the morning. There is probably a relatively long lifespan for the gametes to achieve fertilization from between 8 and 31 h after detecting the LH surge[114]. On theoretical grounds, the administration of hCG 36–40 h before IUI might result in ovulation of immature ova, but in practice it does not diminish the pregnancy rate and may perhaps increase it[115].

When cervical factor infertility has been demonstrated, treatment seems to be similarly effective, whether or not there is evidence of antisperm antibodies in the female partner. Margalloth and co-workers[116] reported pregnancy rates with intrauterine insemination of 3% per cycle with unstimulated cycles, 7% per cycle with clomiphene citrate and 11% per cycle with hMG; 81% of the successes were achieved in the first two IUI treatment cycles. Success rates with artificial insemination are dependent on the age of the female partner and the total motile sperm count[117].

Artificial insemination with donor sperm has been the most successful treatment for male factor infertility although, not withstanding economic considerations, more modern treatments with IVF and intracytoplasmic sperm injection (ICSI) have an increasing role to play. Success rates in donor insemination programmes of 70% over six cycles have been reported. Frozen samples are now recommended to allow adequate testing of donors for human immunodeficiency virus although fresh donor samples have achieved pregnancy rates of 19% per cycle compared to frozen samples giving 5% per cycle[118]. Intrauterine insemination of donor sperm has been shown to be more effective than intracervical insemination[119]. A cervical cap with an intracervical reservoir does not increase pregnancy rates when compared to standard intracervical insemination[120].

Cervical mucus hostility can be associated with excessively acidic mucus with a periovulatory pH of < 6.0. Treatment with sodium bicarbonate (a level teaspoonful dissolved in half a pint of lukewarm water), by introducing 40 ml of the solution into the vagina with a syringe about 2 h before coitus, can significantly improve pregnancy rates[121]. Estrogens have been administered in the preovulatory phase for cervical mucus factor infertility[122].

## IMPLANTATION FAILURE

The majority of human embryos are lost as a result of implantation failure and any treatment that might reduce this problem would be a major advance in infertility treatment. Low-dose aspirin improves pregnancy rates in patients with antiphospholipid antibody[123,124]. Low-dose aspirin therapy has also been shown to improve pregnancy rates with impaired uterine perfusion, administered in addition to a standard HRT protocol[125].

## UNEXPLAINED INFERTILITY

In a summary of the available evidence, it was found that clomiphene, intrauterine insemination and hMG each double the chance of conception compared to no treatment[126].

In an early study, bromocriptine seemed an effective treatment for unexplained infertility[127]. However, the results of a double-blind controlled trial demonstrated no increase in pregnancy rate[28].

In a cross-over, randomized study of 26 couples with unexplained infertility, active management with clomiphene, ultrasound monitoring and hCG resulted in a higher pregnancy rate than unstimulated urinary LH-timed IUI-timed cycles[128].

*In vitro* fertilization and embryo transfer were originally developed for infertile women who had no Fallopian tubes or who had tubes that were irreversibly damaged. *In vitro* fertilization and gamete intrafallopian transfer (GIFT) increasingly found roles in other causes of infertility including male factor and unexplained infertility. *In vitro* fertilization and GIFT techniques include superovulation (increase in the number of oocytes available for fertilization) and an increase of the number of spermatozoa directly available for each oocyte. For women with no evidence of gross tubal pathology, superovulation and intrauterine insemination could provide some of the advantages of assisted conception techniques but with less invasive procedures and at lower cost.

In a retrospective study of 85 couples having IUI and hMG, 24 pregnancies were achieved[129]. In a prospective study of 62 women with unexplained infertility, 15 had timed IUI, 25 had hMG with superovulation and 22 had IUI and hMG[130]. The pregnancy rate for the combined therapy was 26.4% per cycle and 40.9% per couple; these results were significantly better than with either IUI or hMG alone. The authors recommended that IUI and hMG should be advised for couples with unexplained infertility before submitting them to high-tech assisted conception therapy. A successful outcome is more likely with four courses of IUI and hMG than one course of IVF or GIFT and this low-tech approach is also more cost-effective[131]. Melis and colleagues[132] randomized 200 couples with unexplained infertility or mild male factor problems into two groups. Both groups received gonadotrophin ovulation induction over three consecutive cycles. One group had IUI 30–36 h after hCG administration and the other group timed intercourse about 12 h after hCG. There were 35 pregnancies in the timed intercourse group and 33 pregnancies with IUI, suggesting in this study, at least, no advantage for IUI. Hurst and co-workers[133] and Chung and associates[134], however, found significantly better pregnancy rates with gonadotrophins and IUI compared to gonadotrophins and timed intercourse. The addition of down-regulation with GnRH analogues into IUI/gonadotrophin therapy regimens may increase pregnancy rates, possibly by reducing LH levels during the follicular phase and also by preventing a premature LH surge[135].

Patients with unexplained infertility, who fail to conceive with IUI and superovulation, prove to have a higher incidence of fertilization failure when they are introduced to IVF than patients with tubal factor infertility[136].

## SUCCESS RATES

In order to determine the success rate of a treatment programme, it is essential to know the prognosis without treatment. A prospective study of 2198 couples with infertility of greater than 1 year found an overall live birth rate of 14.3% after a further 12 months without treatment[137]. The relevant prognostic factors were duration of infertility, obstetric history, female partner's age, male factor, endometriosis and tubal pathology. This database might prove to be of value in determining any increase in pregnancy rates for a given treatment. There is a need to ensure that investigations and treatments recommended to couples have a reasonable chance of being in the patients' best interests[138].

Society and purchasers, in all walks of life, are being trained to believe in effectiveness measurements, often using arbitrary league tables. The success rates of infertility treatments are difficult to compare. There are a variety of causes with patients having a spectrum of severity. Often, there is a combination of factors. For example, age of each partner, duration of infertility and previous treatments all influence the likelihood of treatment success. There is a rapidly increasing number of treatments and a variety of protocols for each treatment. Finally, success may be reported in terms of biochemical pregnancy (a positive pregnancy test that may be performed between 9 and 21 days after the possible conception day), clinical pregnancy (evidence of a viable pregnancy on early ultrasound), ongoing pregnancy and livebirths. Livebirth rates may overstate success as this may include multiple births.

These problems are well recognized and useful attempts to satisfy the need for an overview have been made[139–141]. Whilst high-tech assisted conception techniques may provide higher success rates per cycle, they are completely unnatural and highly invasive. Furthermore, assisted conception has a high incidence of multiple pregnancies that are prone to obstetric and neonatal complications[142]. We believe that couples must be provided with unbiased information so that they can, as far as economic restrictions allow, follow the most appropriate treatment path of their choice. There is a need for better organisation and integration of resources to ensure that simple, less invasive and more economical investigations and treatments are fully utilized before resorting to high-tech interventions simply because these may be more modern and receive wider media coverage.

## LOW-TECH THERAPY GUIDELINES

Figure 1 in Chapter 7 provides a flow chart showing a simplified outline of infertility investigations and treatments. Some investigations may be delayed until after treatment has begun. For example, if it is apparent that there is anovulation and no obvious reason to suspect pelvic pathology, ovulation induction therapy may be provided for a few cycles before testing Fallopian tube patency.

Relevant patient information leaflets are provided for clarification. Each couple receives a leaflet relating to infertility investigation and treatment and also antenatal screening. Where appropriate, leaflets relating to polycystic ovary syndrome and recurrent miscarriage are also provided. By the end of the first consultation, ovulatory dysfunction and male factor infertility have usually been detected. Those factors identified which may be contributing to conception delay and proposed treatment are discussed with the couple. Obese patients are advised that weight loss may be all that is required to re-establish spontaneous ovulation[2]. In practice, the majority of our obese patients seem to resist advice in this area and we prefer not to pressurize them as this only achieves negative results.

Controlled trials have demonstrated the efficacy of reducing neural tube defects by folic acid administration in couples at high risk. It would probably be impossible to include sufficient patients to establish a prophylactic benefit for couples with no history of an affected fetus, but folic acid 5 mg daily for couples planning a pregnancy seems to be appropriate.

When there is evidence of ovulatory dysfunction from the history, preovulatory ultrasound scan or mid-luteal phase progesterone, oral ovulation induction is commenced. We do not investigate specifically to identify luteal phase deficiency or luteinized unruptured follicles, as we regard these as part of ovulatory dysfunction which is likely to respond to ovulation induction. If the ultrasound suggests polycystic ovaries or that the proliferative phase LH is elevated, we initially prescribe tamoxifen 20–40 mg daily from the 2nd to the 6th day, but otherwise clomiphene 50 mg daily from the 2nd to the 6th day has been our drug of first choice. Until recently, we did not monitor early treatment cycles. Current concerns about clomiphene, which effectively limit its use to six cycles, have encouraged us to monitor more rigorously. If the mid-luteal progesterone estimations are less than 30 nmol/l, we will increase the dose of clomiphene to 100 and then 150 mg.

Patients with irregular and infrequent menstruation have also received dydrogesterone (Duphaston®, Solvay) (Figure 1). In our pilot study, dydrogesterone 10 mg b.d. from days 21 to 26 of the menstrual cycle was prescribed[143]. Fifty-four normoprolactinaemic women received either tamoxifen, if there was evidence of polycystic ovaries on ultrasound and/or increased LH secretion, or otherwise clomiphene. Twenty-three women (42.6%) conceived (10.7% per cycle). Duphaston is licensed for the treatment of habitual abortion and also for cycle regulation in patients with amenorrhoea. In our experience, this progestogen helps to ensure a normal cycle until pregnancy occurs. In the 192 non-conception cycles, the average cycle length was 29.6 days. Since incorporating dydrogesterone into our protocols, failure to menstruate has been, almost invariably, associated with positive β-hCG pregnancy tests.

Patients with hyperprolactinaemia have been treated with bromocriptine. For patients who

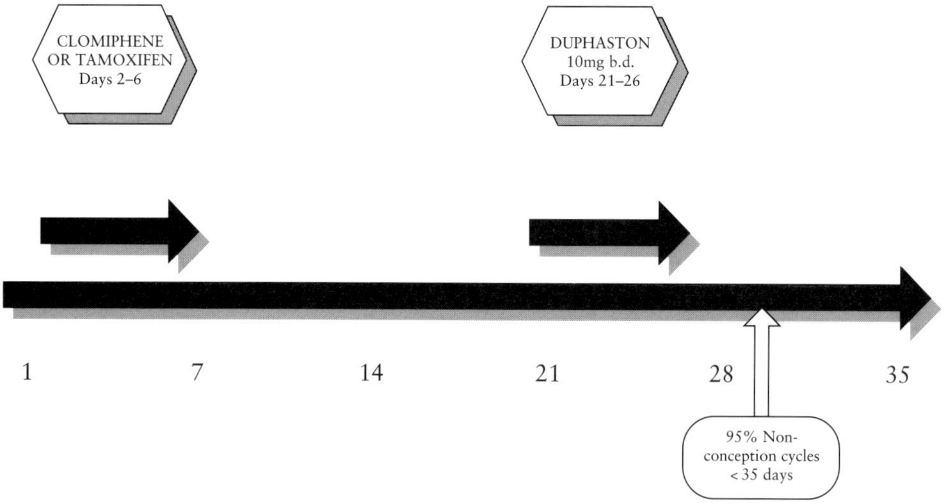


**Figure 1** Schedule of treatment with dydrogesterone (Duphaston®) for patients with irregular and infrequent menstruation

have difficulty tolerating bromocriptine, we have started to prescribe cabergoline. Failure to conceive after three cycles of ovulation induction is an indication to request hysterosalpingography and a postcoital test.

If there is a history of pelvic pain, or if there is significant tenderness at initial pelvic examination, we arrange laparoscopy with dye insufflation and take the opportunity to perform hysteroscopy and dilatation and curettage.

Borderline semen analysis is an indication for a repeat test and a postcoital test and, if a mild male factor infertility problem is diagnosed, our patients enter our IUI program. Patients with more severe male factor infertility are referred to our andrologist. Until the last few years, only donor sperm insemination was likely to be successful for these couples but modern techniques, including surgical sperm aspiration and intracytoplasmic sperm injection have revolutionized treatment options (Chapters 10, 13, 14).

When there is no apparent cause for the infertility identified at the first consultation, we arrange hysterosalpingography and a postcoital test. If these investigations are normal (unexplained infertility), we tend to prescribe clomiphene, or tamoxifen if the proliferative phase LH is elevated, and, if there is no success after a few cycles, IUI is offered. If there is no success within a few cycles, gonadotrophins are introduced.

Patients with tubal occlusion are counselled on the anticipated success rates of tubal surgery. We do not advocate surgery when there is severe disease or additional significant male factor problems. Patients should also appreciate that IVF could be successful when tubal surgery and other low-tech treatments fail. Patients with prolonged unexplained infertility should be considered for investigation as if they were prone to habitual abortion (Chapter 21). Women with elevated lupus anticoagulant or anticardiolipin may respond to low-dose aspirin. Should either partner have significant chromosome abnormality, donated gametes should be considered.

## REFERENCES

1. Knuth, U. A., Hull, M. G. and Jacobs, H. S. (1977). Amenorrhoea and loss of weight. *Br. J. Obstet. Gynaecol.*, **84**, 801–7
2. Clarke, A. M., Ledger, W., Galletly, C., Tomlinson, L., Blaney, F., Wang, X. and Norman, R.J. (1995). Weight loss results in significant improvement in pregnancy and ovulation rates in anovulatory obese women. *Hum. Reprod.*, **10**, 2705–12
3. Wu, C. H. and Winkel, C. A. (1989). The effect of therapy initiation day on clomiphene citrate therapy. *Fertil. Steril.*, **52**, 564–8

4. Lobo, R. A., Gysler, M., March, C. M., Goebelsmann, U. and Mishell, D. R. (1982). Clinical and laboratory predictors of clomiphene response. *Fertil. Steril., 37*, 168–74
5. Hurd, W. W., Randolph, J. F., Christman, G. M., Ansbacher, R. and Howe, D. M. (1994). Comparison of low intensity and high intensity monitoring of clomiphene citrate ovulation induction. In *Abstracts of the Scientific Oral and Poster Sessions of the American Society for Reproductive Medicine,* Programme Supplement, San Antonio, Texas, November 1994, S12
6. Gorlitsky, G. A., Kase, N. G. and Speroff, L. (1978). Ovulation and pregnancy rates with clomiphene citrate. *Obstet. Gynecol.*, **51**, 265–9
7. Gysler, M., March, C. M., Mishell, D. R. and Bailey, E. J. (1982). A decade's experience with an individualized clomiphene treatment regimen including its effect on the postcoital test. *Fertil. Steril.*, **37**, 161–7
8. Roumen, F. J., Doesburg, W. H. and Rolland, R. (1984). Treatment of infertile women with a deficient postcoital test with two antiestrogens: clomiphene and tamoxifen. *Fertil. Steril.*, **41**, 237–43
9. Taubert, H. D. and Dericks-Tan, J. S. (1976). High doses of estrogens do not interfere with the ovulation-inducing effect of clomiphene citrate. *Fertil. Steril.*, **27**, 375–82
10. Bateman, B. G., Nunley, W. C. and Kolp, L. A. (1990). Exogenous estrogen therapy of clomiphene citrate induced cervical mucus abnormalities: is it effective? *Fertil. Steril.*, **54**, 577–9
11. Shoham, Z., Zosmer, A. and Insler, V. (1991). Early miscarriage and fetal malformations after induction of ovulation (by clomiphene citrate and/or human menotropins), *in vitro* fertilization, and gamete intrafallopian transfer. *Fertil. Steril.*, **55**, 1–11
12. Nunley, W. C., Bateman, B. G. and Kitchin, F. D. (1985). Reproductive performance of patients teated with clomiphene citrate. *South. Med. J.*, **78**, 31–3
13. Rossing, M. A., Daling, J. R., Weiss, N. S., Moore, D. E. and Self, S. G. (1994). Ovarian tumors in a cohort of infertile women. *N. Engl. J. Med.*, **331**, 771–6
14. Anonymous (1995). Clomiphene (Clomid, Serophene): possible association with ovarian cancer. *Curr. Problems Pharmacovigilance*, **21**, 7
15. O'Herlihy, C., Pepperell, R. J. and Robinson, H. P. (1982). Ultrasound timing of human chorionic gonadotropin administration in clomiphene stimulation cycle. *Obstet. Gynecol.*, **59**, 40–5
16. Shaleve, E., Geslevich, Y., Matilsky, M. and Ben-Ami, M. (1995). Gonadotrophin-releasing hormone agonist compared with human chorionic gonadotrophin for ovulation induction after clomiphene citrate treatment. *Hum. Reprod.*, **10**, 2541–4
17. Fukushima, T. and Maeyama, M. (1983). Action of tamoxifen on folliculogenesis in the menstrual cycle of infertile patients. *Fertil. Steril.*, **40**, 210–14
18. Tajima, C. (1984). Luteotropic effects of tamoxifen in infertile women. *Fertil. Steril.*, **42**, 223–7
19. Messinis, I. E. and Nillius, S. J. (1982). Comparison between tamoxifen and clomiphene induction of ovulation. *Acta Obstet. Gynecol. Scand.*, **61**, 377–9
20. Buvat, J., Buvat-Herbaut, M., Marcolin, G. and Ardaens-Boulier, K. (1987). Antiestrogens as treatment of female and male infertilities. *Horm. Res.*, **28**, 219–29
21. Borenstein, R., Shoham, Z., Yemini, M., Barash, A., Fienstein, M. and Rozenman, D. (1989). Tamoxifen treatment in women with failure of clomiphene citrate therapy. *Aust. N.Z. J. Obstet. Gynaecol.*, **29**, 173–5
22. Elstein, M. and Fawcett, G. M. (1984). Effects of the anti-estrogens, clomiphene and tamoxifen, on the cervical factor in female infertility. *Ciba Found. Symp.*, **109**, 173–9
23. Gulekli, B., Ozaksit, G., Turhan, N. O., Senoz, S., Oral, H. and Gokmen, O. (1993). Tamoxifen: an alternative approach in clomiphene resistant polystic ovarian syndrome patients. *J. Pak. Med. Assoc.*, **43**, 89–90
24. Tan, S.-L. and Jacobs, H. S. (1991). *Infertility: Your Questions Answered*, p. 76. (Singapore: McGraw-Hill Book Co.)
25. Suginami, H., Kitagawa, H., Nakahashi, N., Yano, K. and Matsubara, K. (1993). A clomiphene citrate and tamoxifen citrate combination therapy: a novel therapy for ovulation induction. *Fertil. Steril.*, **59**, 976–9
26. Cook, L. S., Weiss, N. S., Schwartz, S. M., White, E., McKnight, B., Moore, D. E. and

Daling, J. R. (1995). Population-based study of tamoxifen therapy and subsequent ovarian, endometrial, and breast cancers. *J. Natl. Cancer Inst.*, **87**, 1359–64
27. Pepperell, R. J., McBain, J. C. and Healy, D. L. (1977). Ovulation induction with bromocriptine in patients with hyperprolactinaemia. *Aust. N.Z. J. Obstet. Gynaecol.*, **17**, 181–91
28. Wright, C. S., Steele, S. J. and Jacobs, H. S. (1979). Value of bromocriptine in unexplained primary infertility: a double-blind controlled trial. *Br. Med. J.*, **1**, 1037–9
29. Padilla, S. L., Person, G. K., McDonough, P. G. and Reindollar, R. H. (1985). The efficacy of bromocriptine in patients with ovulatory dysfunction and normoprolactinaemic galactorrhoea. *Fertil. Steril.*, **44**, 695–8
30. Falaschi, P., Rocco, A. and del Pozo, E. (1986). Inhibitory effect of bromocriptine treatment on luteinizing hormone secretion in polycystic ovary syndrome. *J. Clin. Endocrinol. Metab.*, **62**, 348
31. Weil, C. (1986). The safety of bromocriptine in hyperprolactinaemic female infertility: a literature review. *Curr. Med. Res. Opin.*, **10**, 172–95
32. Ferrari, C., Piscitelli, G. and Crosignani, P. G. (1995). Cabergoline: a new drug for the treatment of hyperprolactinaemia. *Hum. Reprod.*, **10**, 1647–52
33. Gemzell, C. A., Diczfalusy, E. and Tillinger, K. G. (1958). Clinical effect of human pituitary follicle-stimulating hormone (FSH). *J. Clin. Endocrinol. Metab.*, **18**, 1333
34. Loumaye, E., Campbell, R. and Salat-Baroux, J. (1995). Human follicle-stimulating hormone produced by recombinant DNA technology: a review for clinicians. *Hum. Reprod. Update*, **1**, 188–99
35. Caspi, E., Ronen, J., Schreyer, P. and Goldberg, M. D. (1976). The outcome of pregnancy after gonadotrophin therapy. *Br. J. Obstet. Gynaecol.*, **83**, 967–73
36. Rojas, F. J. (1995). Effects of ovulation induction with the gonadotrophins on the ovary and uterus and their implications for assisted reproduction. *Hum. Reprod.*, **10**, 2219–37
37. Butler, J. K. (1969). Time-course of urinary excretion after various schemes of therapy with human follicle-stimulating hormone (Pergonal). *Proc. R. Soc. Med.*, **62**, 34–7
38. Marshall, J. R. and Wider, J. A. (1971). Results of human menopausal gonadotropins (HMG). Therapy for anovulatory infertility using a non-variable treatment schedule: comparison with previous reports. *Fertil. Steril.*, **22**, 19–25
39. Ellis, J. D. and Williamson, J. G. (1975). Factors influencing the pregnancy and complication rates with human menopausal gonadotrophin therapy. *Br. J. Obstet. Gynaecol.*, **82**, 52–7
40. Shearman, R. P. (1969). Progress in the investigation and treatment of anovulation. *Am. J. Obstet. Gynecol.*, **103**, 444–63
41. Lunenfeld, B. and Insler, V. (1974). Classification of amenorrhoeic states and their treatment by ovulation induction. *Clin. Endocrinol. (Oxford)*, **3**, 223–37
42. van Santbrink, E. J. P., Donderwinkel, P. F. J., van Dessel, T. J. H. M. and Fauser, B. C. J. M. (1995). Gonadotrophin induction of ovulation using a step-down dose regimen: single-centre clinical experience in 82 patients. *Hum. Reprod.*, **10**, 1048–53
43. Smith, B. H. and Cooke, I. D. (1991). Ovarian hyperstimulation: actual and theoretical risks. *Br. Med. J.*, **302**, 127–8
44. Shoham, Z., Di Carlo, C., Patel, A., Conway, G. S. and Jacobs, H. S. (1991). Is it possible to run a successful ovulation induction program based solely on ultrasound monitoring. *Fertil. Steril.*, **56**, 836–41
45. Ritchie, W. G. (1985). Ultrasound in the evaluation of normal and induced ovulation. *Fertil. Steril.*, **43**, 167–81
46. Lavy, G., Diamond, M P., Nero, F., Schark, K. and DeCherney, A. H. (1987). Transvaginal and transabdominal ultrasound for monitoring of follicular development in an *in vitro* fertilization and embryo transfer program: patient response. *J. In Vitro Fertil. Embryo Transfer*, **4**, 293–5
47. Ron-el, R., Soffer, Y., Langer, R., Herman, A., Weintraub, Z. and Caspi, E. (1989). Low multiple pregnancy rate in combined clomiphene citrate–human menopausal gonadotrophin treatment for induction or enhancement. *Hum. Reprod.*, **4**, 495–500
48. Lu, P. Y., Chen, A. L. J., Atkinson, E. J., Lee, S. H., Erickson, L. D. and Ory, S. J. (1996). Minimal stimulation achieves pregnancy rates comparable to human menopausal gonadotropin in the treatment of infertility. *Fertil. Steril.*, **65**, 583–7
49. Whittemore, A. S., Harris, R. and Itnyre, J. (1992). Characteristics relating to ovarian cancer risk: collaborative analyis of 12 US

case–control studies. II. Invasive epithelial ovarian cancers in white women. *Am. J. Epidemiol.*, **136**, 1184–203
50. Shoham, Z. (1994). Epidemiology, etiology and fertility drugs in ovarian epithelial carcinoma: where are we today? *Fertil. Steril.*, **62**, 433–48
51 Shushan, A., Paltiel, O., Iscovich, J., Elchalal, U., Peretz, T. and Schenker, J. G. (1996). Human menopausal gonadotropin and the risk of epithelial ovarian cancer. *Fertil. Steril.*, **65**, 13–18
52. Mosgaard, B., Lidegaard, O. and Andersen, A. N. (1995). Use of fertility drugs in Denmark 1973–1993. An analysis based on sale statistics. *Acta Obstet. Gynecol. Scand.*, **74**, 614–18
53. Tarlatzis, B. C., Grimbizis, G., Bontis, J. and Mantalenakis, S. (1995). Ovarian stimulation and ovarian tumours: a critical reappraisal. *Hum. Reprod. Update*, **1**, 284–301
54. Bristow, R. E. and Karlan, B. Y. (1996). Ovulation induction, infertility, and ovarian cancer risk. *Fertil. Steril.*, **66**, 499–507
55. Goldstein, D. B., Sasaran, L., Shen, C., Rais, M. S., Zhang, J. J. and Acosta, C. D. (1995). Estrogen add-back therapy (EABT) in induction of ovulation. In *Abstracts of the Scientific Oral and Poster Sessions of the American Society for Reproductive Medicine,* Programme Supplement, Seattle, Washington, November 1995, S18
56. Ueno, J., Oehninger, S., Brzyski, R. G., Acosta, A. A., Philput, C. B. and Muasher, S. J. (1991). Ultrasonographic appearance of the endometrium in natural and stimulated *in vitro* fertilization cycles and its correlation with outcome. *Hum. Reprod.*, **6**, 901–4
57. Shapiro, H., Cowell, C. and Casper, R. F. (1993). The use of vaginal ultrasound for monitoring endometrial preparation in a donor oocyte program. *Fertil. Steril.*, **59**, 1055
58. Randall, J. M. and Templeton, A. (1991). Transvaginal sonographic assessment of follicular and endometrial growth in spontaneous and clomiphene citrate cycles. *Fertil. Steril.*, **56**, 208–12
59. Temmerman, M., Devroey, P., Naaktgeboren, N., Amy, J. J. and Van Steirteghem, A. C. (1984). Incidence, recurrence and treatment of the luteinized unruptured follicle syndrome. *Acta Eur. Fertil.*, **15**, 179–83
60. Balasch, J., Vanrell, J. A., Marquez, M., Burzaco, I. and Gonzalez-Merlo, J. (1982). Dehydrogesterone versus vaginal progesterone in the treatment of the endometrial luteal phase deficiency. *Fertil. Steril.*, **37**, 751–4
61. Balasch, J., Vanrell, J. A., Marquez, M. and Gonzalez-Merlo, J. (1983). Dehydrogesterone treatment of endometrial luteal phase deficiency after ovulation induced by clomiphene citrate and human chorionic gonadotropin. *Fertil. Steril.*, **40**, 469–71
62. Downs, K. A. and Gibson, M. (1983). Clomiphene citrate therapy for luteal phase defect. *Fertil. Steril.*, **39**, 34–8
63. Li, T. C., Warren, M. A. and Cooke, I. D. (1994). The artificial cycle as an effective treatment of persistently retarded endometrium in the luteal phase. *Hum. Reprod.*, **9**, 409–12
64. Lenton, E. A. (1984). The effect of dydrogesterone on the mid-cycle gonadotrophin surge in regularly cycling women. *Clin. Endocrinol. (Oxford)*, **20**, 129–35
65. Couzinet, B., Lestrat, N., Brailly, S., Brailly, S., Forest, M. and Schaison, G. (1988). Stimulation of ovarian follicular maturation with pure follicle stimulating hormone in women with gonadotropin deficiency. *J. Clin. Endocrinol. Metab.*, **66**, 552–6
66. Anderson, R. E., Cragun, J. M., Chang, R. J., Stanczyk, F. Z. and Lobo, R. A. (1989). A pharmacodynamic comparison of human urinary follicle-stimulating hormone and human menopausal gonadotropin in normal and polycystic ovary syndrome. *Fertil. Steril.*, **52**, 216–20
67. Bettendorf, G. (1990). Special preparations: pure FSH and desialo-hCG. *Baillieres Clin. Obstet. Gynaecol.*, **4**, 519–34
68. Fleming, R. and Coutts, J. R. T. (1986). Induction of multiple follicular growth in normal menstruating women with endogenous gonadotropin suppression. *Fertil. Steril.*, **45**, 226–30
69. Fleming, R., Haxton, M. J. Hamilton, M. P., McCune, G. S., Black, W. P., MacNaughton, M. C. and Coutts, J. R. (1985). Successful treatment of infertile women with oligomenorrhoea using a combination of an LHRH agonist and exogenous gonadotrophins. *Br. J. Obstet. Gynaecol.*, **92**, 369–73
70. Reissmann, Th., Felberbaum, R., Diedrich, K., Engel, J., Comaru-Schally, A. M. and Schally, A. V. (1995). Development and applications of luteinizing hormone-releasing hormone antagonists in the treatment of infertility: an overview. *Hum. Reprod.*, **10**, 1974–81

71. Mason, P., Adams, J., Morris, D. V., Tucker, M., Price, J., Voulgaris, Z., Van der Spuy, Z. M., Sutherland, I., Chambers, G. R., White, S., Wheeler, M. J. and Jacobs, H. S. (1984). Induction of ovulation with pulsatile luteinising hormone releasing hormone. *Br. Med. J.*, **288**, 181–5
72. Homberg, R., Eshel, A., Armar, N. A., Tucker, M., Masons, P. W., Adams, J., Kilborn, J., Sutherland, I. A. and Jacobs, H. S. (1989). One hundred pregnancies after treatment with pulsatile luteinising hormone releasing hormone to induce ovulation. *Br. Med. J.*, **298**, 809–12
73. Letterie, G. S., Coddington, C. C., Collins, R. L. and Merriam, G. R. (1996). Ovulation induction using s.c. pulsatile gonadotrophin-releasing hormone: effectiveness of different pulse frequencies. *Hum. Reprod.*, **11**, 19–22
74. Nakamura, Y., Yoshimura, Y., Tanabe, K. and Iizuki, R. (1986). Induction of ovulation with pulsatile subcutaneous administration of human menopausal gonadotropin in anovulatory infertile women. *Fertil. Steril.*, **46**, 46–53
75. Nakamura, Y., Yoshimura, Y., Yamada, H., Ubukata, Y., Yoshida, K., Tamaoka, Y. and Suzuki, M. (1989). Clinical experience in the induction of ovulation and pregnancy with pulsatile subcutaneous administration of human menopausal gonadotropin: a low incidence of multiple pregnancy. *Fertil. Steril.*, **51**, 423–9
76. Polson, D. W., Mason, H. D., Saldahna, M. B. Y. and Franks, S. (1987). Ovulation of a single dominant follicle during treatment with low-dose pulsatile follicle stimulating hormone in women with polycystic ovary syndrome. *Clin. Endocrinol.*, **26**, 205–12
77. Kuwahara, A., Matsuzaki, T., Kaji, H., Irahara, M. and Aono, T. (1995). Induction of single ovulation by sequential follicle-stimulating hormone and pulsatile gonadotropin-releasing hormone treatment. *Fertil. Steril.*, **64**, 267–72
78. Buckler, H. M., Evans, C. A. Mamtora, H., Burger, H. G. and Anderson, D. C. (1991). Gonadotropin, steroid, and inhibin levels in women with incipient ovarian failure during anovulatory and ovulatory rebound cycles. *J. Clin. Endocrinol. Metab.*, **72**, 116–24
79. Farhi, J., Soule, S. and Jacobs, H. S. (1995). Effect of laparoscopic ovarian electrocautery on ovarian response and outcome of treatment with gonadotropins in clomiphene citrate resistant patients with polycystic ovary syndrome. *Fertil. Steril.*, **64**, 930–5
80. Seibel, M. M., Berger, M. J., Weinstein, F. G. and Taymor, M. L. (1982). The effectiveness of danazol on subsequent fertility in minimal endometriosis. *Fertil. Steril.*, **38**, 534–7
81. Thomas, E. J. and Cooke, I. D. (1987). Successful treatment of asymptomatic endometriosis: does it benefit infertile women? *Br. Med. J.*, **294**, 1117–19
82. Telimaa, S. (1988). Danazol and medroxyprogesterone acetate inefficacious in the treatment of infertility in endometriosis. *Fertil. Steril.*, **50**, 872–5
83. Fedele, L., Parazzini, F., Radici, E., Bocciolone, L., Bianchi, S., Bianchi, C. and Candiani, G. B. (1992). Buserelin acetate versus expectant management in the treatment of infertility associated with minimal or mild endometriosis. *Am. J. Obstet. Gynecol.*, **166**, 1345–50
84. Shaw, R. (1995). Infertility associated with endometriosis. *Diplomate*, **2**, 188–94
85. Whitelaw, N. L., Haines, P., Ewen, S. P. and Sutton, C. J. G. (1993). Assessing the efficacy of laser laparoscopy in the treatment of endometriosis. *J. Obstet. Gynaecol.*, **13**, 486
86. Rock, J. A., Guziak, D. S., Sengos, C., Schweditsch, M., Sapp, K. C. and Jones, H. W. Jr (1981). The conservative surgical treatment of endometriosis: evaluation of pregnancy success with respect to the extent of disease as categorized using contemporary classification systems. *Fertil. Steril.*, **35**, 131–7
87. Sutton, C. (1993). Lasers in infertility. *Hum. Reprod.*, **8**, 133–46
88. Winston, R. M. and Margara, R. A. (1991). Microsurgical salpingostomy is not an obsolete procedure. *Br. J. Obstet. Gynaecol.*, **98**, 637–42
89. Singhal, V., Li, T. C. and Cooke, I. D. (1991). An analysis of factors influencing the outcome of 232 consecutive tubal microsurgery cases. *Br. J. Obstet. Gynaecol.*, **98**, 628–36
90. Reiss, H. (1991). Management of tubal infertility in the 1990s. *Br. J. Obstet. Gynaecol.*, **98**, 619–23
91. Lavy, G., Diamond, M. P. and De Cherney, A. H. (1987). Ectopic pregnancy: its relationship to tubal reconstructive surgery. *Fertil. Steril.*, **47**, 543–56
92. McComb, P. (1986). Microsurgical tubocornual anastomosis for occlusive cornual disease: reproducible results without the need for tubouterine implantation. *Fertil. Steril.*, **46**, 571–7

93. Gomel, V. (1978). Salpingostomy by microsurgery. *Fertil. Steril.*, **29**, 380–7
94. Xue, P. and Fa, Y. (1989). Microsurgical reversal of female sterilization. Long-term follow up of 117 cases. *J. Reprod. Med.*, **34**, 451–5
95. Fayez, J. A. and Suliman, S. O. (1982). Infertility surgery of the oviduct: comparison between macrosurgery and microsurgery. *Fertil. Steril.*, **37**, 73–8
96. Frantzen, C. and Scholosser, H. W. (1982). Microsurgery and post-infectious tubal infertility. *Fertil. Steril.*, **38**, 397–402
97. Cohen, B. M. (1978). Current status of fallopien tube transplantation. *Hosp. Pract.*, **13**, 87–94
98. Grant, A. and Robertson, S. (1966). Hydrotubation, a method treatment due to tubal damage: review of 327 cases. *Med. J. Aust.*, **2**, 847–50
99. Rock, J. A., Siegler, A. M., Meisel, M. B., Haney, A. F., Rosenwaks, Z., Pardo-Vargas, F. and Kimball, A. W. (1988). The efficacy of postoperative hydrotubation: a randomized prospective multicentre clinical trial. *Fertil. Steril.*, **42**, 373–6
100. Larsson, B., Lalos, O., Marsk, L., Tronstad, S. E., Bygdeman, M., Pehrson, S. and Joelsson, I. (1985). Effect of intraperitoneal instillation of 32% dextran 70 on postoperative adhesion formation after tubal surgery. *Acta Obstet. Gynecol. Scand.*, **64**, 437–41
101. Andersen, A. N., Yue, Z., Meng, F. J. and Petersen, K. (1994). Low implantation rate after *in vitro* fertilization in patients with hydrosalpinges diagnosed by ultrasonography. *Hum. Reprod.*, **9**, 1935–8
102. Fleming, C. and Hull, M. G. R. (1996). Imparied implantation after *in vitro* fertilisation treatment associated with hydrosalpinx. *Br. J. Obstet. Gynaecol.*, **103**, 268–72
103. Shelton, K. E., Butler, L., Toner, J. P., Oehninger, S. and Muasher, S. J. (1996). Salpingectomy improves the pregnancy rate in *in vitro* fertilization patients with hydrosalpinx. *Hum. Reprod.*, **11**, 523–5
104. Maloul, S., Manzur, A. and Asch, R. H. (1995). The obstetric outcome of assisted reproductive techniques. In Asch, R. and Studd, J. (eds.) *Progress in Reproductive Medicine,* Vol. 2, pp. 23–34. (Carnforth, UK: Parthenon Publishing)
105. Callahan, T. L., Hall, J. E., Ettner, S. L., Christiansen, C. L., Green, M. F. and Crowely, W. F. Jr (1994). The economic impact of multiple-gestation pregnancies and the contribution of assisted reproduction techniques to their incidence. *N. Engl. J. Med.*, **331**, 244–9
106. Farhi, J., Ashkenazi, J., Feldberg, D., Dicker, D., Orvieto, R. and Ben Rafael, Z. (1995). Effect of uterine leiomyomata on the results of *in vitro* fertilization treatment. *Hum. Reprod.*, **10**, 2576–8
107. Goldenberg, M., Sivan, E., Sharabi, Z., Bider, D., Rabinovici, J. and Seidman, D. S. (1995). Outcome of hysteroscopic resection of submucous myomas for infertility. *Fertil. Steril.*, **64**, 714–16
108. Goldenberg, M., Sivan, E., Sharabi, Z., Mashiach, S., Lipitz, S. and Seidman, D. S. (1995). Reproductive outcome following hysteroscopic management of intrauterine septum and adhesions. *Hum. Reprod.*, **10**, 2663–5
109. Ord, T., Patrizio, P., Marello, E., Balmaceda, J. P. and Asch, R. H. (1990). Mini-Percoll: a new method of semen preparation for IVF in severe male factor infertility. *Hum. Reprod.*, **5**, 987–9
110. Yovich, J. L. and Matson, P. L. (1988). The treatment of infertility by the high intrauterine insemination of husband's washed spermatozoa. *Hum. Reprod.*, **3**, 939–43
111. Ombelet, W., Puttemans, P. and Bosmans, E. (1995). Intrauterine insemination: a first-step procedure in the algorithm of male subfertility treatment. *Hum. Reprod.*, **10** (Suppl. 1), 90–102
112. Schwartz, D., Mayaux, M., Martin-Boyce, A., Czyglik, F. and David, G. (1979). Donor insemination: conception rate according to cycle day in a series of 821 cycles with a single insemination. *Fertil. Steril.*, **31**, 226–9
113. Barratt, C. L., Cooke, S., Chauhan, M. and Cooke, I. D. (1989). A prospective randomized controlled trial comparing urinary luteinizing hormone dipsticks and basal body temperature charts with timed donor insemination. *Fertil. Steril.*, **52**, 394–7
114. Martinez, A. R., Bernardus, R. E., Vermeiden, J. P. and Schoemaker, J. (1994). Time schedules of intrauterine insemination after urinary luteinizing surge detection and pregnancy results. *Gynecol. Endocrinol.*, **8**, 1–5
115. Check, J. H., Peymer, M. and Zaccardo, M. (1994). Evaluation of whether using hCG to stimulate oocyte release helps or decreases pregnancy rates following intrauterine insemination. *Gynecol. Obstet. Invest.*, **38**, 57–9

116. Margalloth, E. J., Sauter, E., Bronson, R. A., Rosenfeld, D. J., Scholl, G. M. and Cooper, G. W. (1988). Intrauterine insemination as treatment for antisperm antibodies in the female. *Fertil. Steril.*, **50**, 441–6
117. Campana, A., Sakkas, D., Stalberg, A., Bianchi, P. G., Comte, I., Pache, T. and Walker, D. (1996). Intrauterine insemination: evaluation of the results according to the woman's age, sperm quality, total sperm count per insemination and life table analysis. *Hum. Reprod.*, **11**, 732–6
118. Richter, M. A., Haning, R. V. Jr and Shapiro, S. S. (1984). Artificial donor insemination: fresh versus frozen semen: the patient as her own control. *Fertil. Steril.*, **41**, 277–80
119. Wainer, R., Merlet, F., Ducot, B., Bailly, M., Tribalat, S. and Lomboro, R. (1995). Prospective randomized comparison of intrauterine and intracervical insemination with donor spermatozoa. *Hum. Reprod.*, **10**, 2919–22
120. Coulson, C., McLaughlin, E. A., Harris, S., Ford, W. C. L. and Hull, M. G. R. (1996). Randomized controlled trial of cervical cap with intracervical reservoir versus standard intracervical injection by inseminate cryopreserved donor semen. *Hum. Reprod.*, **11**, 84–7
121. Jenkins, J. M., Anthony, F. W., Purdie, B., Gilbert, D., Noon, R. and Masson, G. M. (1989). Acidic endocervical mucus: a potentially reversible cause of subfertility. *Cont. Rev. Obstet. Gynaecol.*, **1**, 273–8
122. Harrison, R. F. (1980). Pregnancy successes in the infertile couple. *Int. J. Fertil.*, **25**, 81–7
123. Balasch, J., Carmona, F., Lopez-Soto, A., Font, J., Creus, M., Fabregues, F., Ingelmo, M. and Vanrell, J. A. (1993). Low-dose aspirin for prevention of pregnancy losses in women with primary antiphospholipid syndrome. *Hum. Reprod.*, **8**, 2234–9
124. Sher, G., Feinman, M., Zouves, C., Kuttner, G., Maassarani, G., Salem, R., Matzner, W., Ching, W. and Chong, P. (1994). High fecundity rates following *in vitro* fertilization and embryo transfer in antiphospholipid antibody seropositive women treated with heparin and aspirin. *Hum. Reprod.*, **12**, 2278–83
125. Wada, I., Hsu, C. C., Williams, G., Macnamee, M. C. and Brinsden, P. R. (1994). The benefits of low-dose aspirin in women with impaired uterine perfusion during assisted conception. *Hum. Reprod.*, **9**, 1954–7
126. Taylor, P. J. and Collins, J. A. (1992). *Unexplained Infertility*, p. 229. (Oxford: Oxford University Press)
127. Lenton, E. A., Sobowale, O. S. and Cooke, I. D. (1977). Prolactin concentrations in ovulatory but infertile women: treatment with bromocriptine. *Br. Med. J.*, **2**, 1179–81
128. Arici, A., Byrd, W., Bradshaw, K., Kutteh, W. H., Marshburn, P. and Carr, B. R. (1994). Evaluation of clomiphene citrate and human chorionic gonadotropin treatment: a prospective, randomized, crossover study during intrauterine insemination cycles. *Fertil. Steril.*, **61**, 314–18
129. Dodson, W. C., Whitesides, D. B., Hughes, C. L. Jr, Easley, H. A. and Haney, A. F. (1987). Superovulation with intrauterine insemination in the treatment of infertility: a possible alternative to gamete intrafallopian transfer and *in vitro* fertilization. *Fertil. Steril.*, **48**, 441–5
130. Serhal, P. F., Katz, M., Little, V. and Woronowski, H. (1988). Unexplained infertility – the value of Pergonal superovulation combined with intrauterine insemination. *Fertil. Steril.*, **49**, 602–6
131. Peterson, C. M., Hatsaka, H. H., Jones, K. P., Poulson, A. M. Jr, Carrell, D. T. and Urry, R. L. (1994). Ovulation induction with gonadotropins and intrauterine insemination compared with *in vitro* fertilization and no therapy: a prospective, nonrandomized, cohort study and meta-analysis. *Fertil. Steril.*, **62**, 535–44
132. Melis, G. B., Paoletti, A. M., Ajossa, S., Guerriero, S., Depau, G. F. and Mais, V. (1995). Ovulation induction with gonadotropins as sole treatment in infertile couples with open tubes: a randomized prospective comparison between intrauterine insemination and timed vaginal intercourse. *Fertil. Steril.*, **64**, 1088–93
133. Hurst, B. S., Tjaden, B. L., Kimball, A., Schlaff, W. D., Damewood, M. D. and Rock, J. A. (1992). Superovulation with or without intrauterine insemination for the treatment of infertility. *J. Reprod. Med.*, **37**, 237–41
134. Chung, C. C., Fleming, R., Jamieson, M. E., Yates, R. S. W. and Coutts, J. R. T. (1995). Randomized comparison of ovulation induction with and without intrauterine insemination in the treatment of unexplained infertility. *Hum. Reprod.*, **10**, 3139–41
135. Fanchin, R., Fernandez, H., Olivennes, F. and

Frydman, R. (1995). Ovulation induction in 1995: a new policy. *Hum. Reprod.*, **10**, 2224–5

136. Gurgan, T., Urman, B., Yarali, H. and Kisnisci, H. A. (1995). The results of *in vitro* fertilization – embryo transfer in couples with unexplained infertility failing to conceive with superovulation and intrauterine insemination. *Fertil. Steril.*, **64**, 93–7
137. Collins, J. A., Burrows, E. A. and Willan, A. R. (1995). The prognosis for live birth among untreated infertile couples. *Fertil. Steril.*, **64**, 22–8
138. Blackwell, R. E., Carr, B. R., Chang, R. J., De Cherney, A. H., Haney, A. F., Keye, W. R. Jr, Rebar, R. W., Rock, J. A., Rosenwaks, Z. and Seibel, M. M. (1987). Are we exploiting the infertile couple? *Fertil. Steril.*, **48**, 735–9
139. The management of subfertility. (1992). *Effective Health Care Number 3*, School of Public Health, University of Leeds
140. Hull, M. G. (1994). Effectiveness of infertility treatments: choice and comparative analysis. *Int. J. Gynaecol. Obstet.*, **47**, 99–108
141. Guzick, D. S. (1995). Design and analysis of infertility studies. In Asch, R. H. and Studd, J. W. W. (eds.) *Annual Progress in Reproductive Medicine*, Vol. 2, pp. 103–15. (Carnforth, UK: Parthenon Publishing)
142. Seoud, M. A., Toner, J. P., Kruithoff, C. and Muasher, S. J. (1992). Outcome of twin, triplet and quadruplet *in vitro* fertilization pregnancies: the Norfolk experience. *Fertil. Steril.*, **57**, 825–34
143. Viniker, D. A. (1996). Late luteal phase dydrogesterone in combination with clomiphene or tamoxifen in the treatment of infertility associated with irregular and infrequent menstruation: enhancing patient compliance. *Hum. Reprod.*, **11**, 1435–7

# Tubal surgery for infertility

# 9

*Timothy C. Rowe and Patrick J. Taylor*

## INTRODUCTION

Human life begins in the oviduct. When the meeting of the oocyte and the sperm is prevented by distortion or occlusion of the Fallopian tubes, conception cannot occur. Damage to the Fallopian tubes, resulting from sexually transmitted infections, is a tangible cause of infertility, and over the past three decades its management has been steadily refined. The ravages of pelvic infection continue to be a significant cause of infertility, although there has been a measurable reduction in the incidence of pelvic inflammatory disease since the early 1980s[1].

A single episode of pelvic inflammatory disease will leave a residue of tubal damage sufficient to cause infertility in nearly 20% of affected women[2]. Progress in both artificial reproduction and tubal surgical techniques means that restoration of fertility potential is possible. Helping couples to make a choice of treatment between these surgical and non-surgical options has become one of the major responsibilities of the fertility specialist. Both technical and non-technical considerations will have a bearing on this choice, and these will be discussed below.

The results of tubal surgery have improved enormously following the advent of microsurgical techniques. From the patient's perspective, the choice to undergo surgical treatment has become easier with the introduction of laparoscopic approaches to some procedures, particularly salpingoneostomy (salpingostomy). Each of these approaches – microsurgical and laparoscopic – represents an advance over older conventional techniques.

## MICROSURGICAL APPROACHES

The use of magnification in surgical treatment of distal tubal disease was first described by Swolin in 1975[3]. Magnification, the use of the operating microscope, and microsurgical techniques were subsequently further developed and applied to the correction of cornual and mid-tubal occlusion and in reversal of sterilization[4–6]. The best application of microsurgical techniques is actually in tubal anastomosis, since magnification enables the precise apposition of tubal segments using very fine suture material. Magnification also allows the recognition of subtle tubal abnormalities, even if the tube is shown to be patent.

The introduction of a microsurgical approach to the treatment of distal tubal disease resulted in a reduced incidence of postoperative adhesions and improved tubal patency rates, but viable pregnancy rates, disappointingly, were not significantly better than those following conventional surgical approaches. It is now apparent that the most important factor predicting outcome after surgery for distal tubal occlusion is the extent of tubal damage, not the surgical technique which is used. However, the application of microsurgical techniques to the management of proximal tubal obstruction (allowing tubocornual anastomosis to replace the cruder tubal implantation procedure) and to mid-tubal obstruction arising from sterilization procedures or pathological processes has greatly improved the outcome in these conditions.

The assimilation of microsurgical techniques into gynaecology has produced benefits beyond improved pregnancy rates. Microsurgery as a *concept*, and not just a collection of skills, has made gynaecologists much more conscious of the effects of peritoneal trauma and postoperative adhesions. The precise and minimally traumatic procedures involved in microsurgery have promoted the conservative approaches that are now considered standard care for women who are undergoing treatment for benign gynaecological disorders. To some extent, the expanded application of minimal access (endoscopic) surgery is a consequence of the application of microsurgical principles to the management of intra-abdominal lesions. Microsurgical principles, as applied to fertility-enhancing surgery, include gentle tissue handling, careful dissection, meticulous haemostasis, the use of delicate instruments and fine sutures, avoidance of tissue drying, and accurate approximation of tissues. The closed peritoneal cavity within which laparoscopic surgery is performed will largely prevent tissue drying, and eliminate the need to introduce abrasive packs. However, it can be argued that the other principles of microsurgery cannot be fulfilled as readily with laparoscopic surgery.

## LAPAROSCOPIC APPROACHES

While the laparoscopic approach to surgery is appealing to patients because of its minimally invasive character, microsurgery represents the gold standard of reproductive surgery. As far as possible, the principles of microsurgery must be applied to laparoscopic surgery. The closed peritoneal cavity of laparoscopy reduces the risk of tissue trauma by drying or abrasion and avoids the introduction of foreign material such as lint and talcum powder. A reasonable degree of magnification can be obtained laparoscopically by bringing the tip of the laparoscope close to the area of interest and by fitting a magnifying lens to the proximal lens. Haemostasis is enhanced by the pressure of the pneumoperitoneum on venous and capillary flow, and fine electrodes can be used for electrocautery.

However, laparoscopic instruments are, in the main, less sophisticated than are microsurgical instruments, and both the length of the laparoscopic instruments and the action of the abdominal wall as a fulcrum increase the force applied to tissue by the working end of the instruments. This increased force may generate undue trauma.

Laparoscopic suturing has, so far, been unable to match the ease and accuracy of microsurgical suturing. The use of very fine sutures in laparoscopic surgery is difficult, and as a result larger and fewer sutures are used. This will potentially compromise proper alignment and approximation of tissue planes, limiting the potential for anastomosis. In addition, the lack of stereoscopic vision with laparoscopic surgery compromises hand–eye coordination, although three-dimensional image systems for use with the video camera offer potential for better depth perception in the surgical field.

## INFERTILITY INVESTIGATION

Even in cases where the history clearly suggests a tubal or peritoneal factor, it is mandatory to assess other fertility factors. At a minimum, a semen analysis and confirmation of ovulation should be undertaken. Other factors (beyond tubal and peritoneal factors) should be assessed at the investigator's discretion.

In the assessment of tubal factors, hysterosalpingography (HSG) is the initial step. When properly performed, HSG allows evaluation of the uterine cavity and of intratubal architecture. Proximal tubal occlusion and non-occlusive lesions of the cornu can be identified. Hysterosalpingography also allows an assessment of the length, patency and architecture of the proximal segments where there is mid-tubal obstruction or in women seeking reversal of sterilization. It allows assessment of the intramural segment in proximal tubal occlusion and with non-occlusive cornual lesions. When the tubes are blocked distally, the presence of rugal markings in the ampullae is a favourable sign, suggesting a higher probability of pregnancy after reconstructive surgery; conversely, the presence of intratubal adhesions is an adverse prognostic sign (Figure 1), as is a complete absence of rugal markings. For optimal depiction of the tubal mucosa and tubal lesions, an

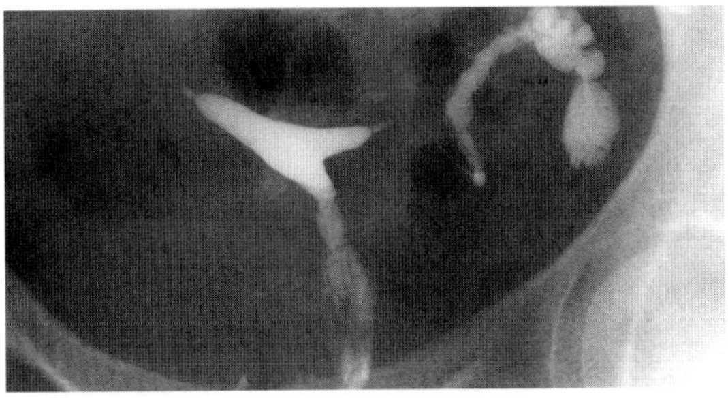

**Figure 1** Hysterosalpingogram showing the presence of intratubal adhesions in a hydrosalpinx

aqueous contrast medium (diatrizoate meglumine 60% (Hypaque M60)) is to be preferred over oil-soluble media.

In the evaluation of tubal or peritoneal factors, laparoscopy and HSG are complementary procedures. It is usually logical to perform laparoscopy *after* HSG, since the information provided by HSG about the status of the uterus and oviducts becomes important at the time of the subsequent laparoscopy, when it may be possible to perform reparative surgery. If this is being considered, the possibility must be discussed with the couple involved and an adequate length of time scheduled for the surgery. Furthermore, if the HSG has shown no abnormality in the uterine cavity, cornua, or tubal lumina, the surgeon who discovers unsuspected adnexal adhesions, tubal phimosis, or distal occlusion can undertake laparoscopic lysis of adhesions, fimbrioplasty or salpingostomy with confidence.

## SELECTION OF TREATMENT

Surgical skill includes both the technical aptitude for reconstruction and the judgement to decide when surgery is appropriate and when it is not. For the couple in whom there is a tuboperitoneal cause for infertility, or a previously performed tubal sterilization, the only options for achieving a pregnancy are through tubal reconstruction or *in vitro* fertilization (IVF). Depending on the nature and site of the damage, restoration of normal tubal function may be achieved microsurgically, by laparoscopically directed techniques, or by tubal cannulation. Making a choice of treatment will be influenced by both non-technical and technical considerations; these are discussed below. It must be emphasized that the choices are not necessarily mutually exclusive. Undergoing tubal reconstruction or tubal cannulation does not exclude the possibility of undergoing IVF subsequently, or vice versa.

### Non-technical considerations

Regardless of the potential for surgery or IVF, the choice of a particular form of treatment will depend upon the local expertise, the respective costs, the age of the woman, and the couple's perceptions of the various procedures.

*Costs of treatment*

The costs of undergoing one or another treatment for infertility may be considerable, and will be a significant factor if health insurance for these procedures is not available. If treatment (notably IVF) increases the potential for multiple pregnancy, the economic impact of this complication must be emphasized to the couple. The significance of issues of cost is an individual matter for each couple.

*Age of the woman*

The woman's age is a critical factor. There is general agreement, based on data from a number of sources, that fecundity begins to decline in women at about age 31. This tendency has been observed in both 'normal' couples[7] and in couples with unexplained infertility[8]. In women aged 40 or more who undergo reversal of sterilization, the live birth rate (approximately 14%) is significantly lower than that in women who are younger[9]. The results of IVF show a similar decline, with the live birth rate falling from 7.7% per treatment cycle in women aged 35–39 to a rate of 2.8% thereafter[10]. This dramatic decline in fecundity means that each cycle in which conception is attempted becomes increasingly precious. Couples with tubal factor infertility and a female partner aged 40 or older will logically undergo IVF as initial treatment, since there is likely to be a higher pregnancy rate per cycle with IVF and since success or failure is evident within the cycle of treatment. Tubal surgery does, however, offer the possibility of multiple cycles in which pregnancy may occur. If IVF is unsuccessful in a predetermined number of cycles, it may be reasonable to offer tubal surgery subsequently.

*Perceptions of the couple*

How the couple views assisted reproductive technologies and reproductive surgery will depend on numerous influences, including their own values and ethical views. Moreover, partners may not even agree with each other. The physician should aim to provide clear and accurate information to both partners, while at the same time refraining from interference with their decision-making except to identify and clarify misunderstandings and misinterpretations. Providing detailed descriptions of surgical techniques and procedures for gamete handling may be appropriate for some couples. The responsible physician will be cautious in dealing with couples desperate to undergo active treatment, since treatment with essentially no chance of success cannot be justified.

## Technical considerations

In counselling a couple with tubal factor infertility, it is essential to refer to results achieved in the local centre rather than results reported in the medical literature. This allows a factual basis for a decision about treatment; that is, the most obvious treatment would be that which provides the highest pregnancy rate in the centre in which the treatment is carried out. Since more than one factor may account for the couple's infertility, the choice of treatment should be made in the context of the individual couple.

In certain circumstances, any attempt at tubal repair is contraindicated, making IVF the only option for treatment (e.g. when both tubes have been removed, when there is a history of tuberculous salpingitis, or when there is severe tubal damage). In other instances, particularly in younger women, tubal reconstruction may be performed first and IVF undertaken subsequently if surgery proves unsuccessful.

In discussing the probability of success after either IVF or tubal surgery, it is important to compare the outcome of each procedure in a standard manner. It is a common perception that IVF offers a low chance of pregnancy, especially when compared with the results of tubal surgery; this perception is usually based on the understanding that quoted pregnancy rates for one IVF treatment cycle represent the highest rates of pregnancy that can be achieved. This is clearly not the case, since pregnancy rates remain constant through successive treatment cycles. Data from the Hallam Centre[10] show that after four IVF treatment cycles a cumulative conception rate of 44.6% and a live birth rate of 33.9% can be achieved. Comparative data from a normal United Kingdom population indicate a cumulative probability of pregnancy of 32% after 3 months and 54% after 6 months. *In vitro* fertilization can therefore be said to offer pregnancy rates that are comparable to those achieved by a normal population. However, the commonest expression of outcome of IVF is the pregnancy rate per embryo transfer, regardless of the outcome of the pregnancy. The outcome of tubal surgery, in comparison, is normally quoted either as a crude pregnancy rate (percentage of patients pregnant at 1, 2 or 3 years after surgery) or as a cumulative probability of pregnancy at a fixed point (usually 2 years after surgery) after life-table analysis. Comparisons of tubal surgery and IVF must take into account these potential differences in the expression of outcome.

The risks associated with any treatment option must be considered and the couple counselled appropriately. *In vitro* fertilization, with the accompanying stimulation of ovulation, is not without risk. The ovarian hyperstimulation syndrome may result from gonadotrophin therapy. Transvaginal oocyte retrieval may be followed by bleeding or infection of the gametes or the pelvis. Multiple pregnancies and their attendant complications represent a real risk of IVF; the twin pregnancy rate is approximately 20–25%, and triplets or higher-order multiple pregnancies account for approximately 4% of deliveries. The perinatal mortality associated with IVF is increased relative to national averages. Up to 20% of IVF pregnancies may abort, and 5–6% of clinical pregnancies are ectopic[11]. Couples considering IVF as treatment should be informed that this does not eliminate the possibility of miscarriage, ectopic pregnancy or other abnormal outcome.

The risks of procedures to restore tubal function, whether carried out by laparoscopy, laparotomy or tubal cannulation techniques, are small. Tubal cannulation is usually carried out under local anaesthetic and carries the risk of tubal perforation, but with no significant potential for morbidity. Laparoscopy carries a small (less than 1%) risk of damage to a viscus or major blood vessel. Laparoscopic surgery and laparotomy carry the risks common to many gynaecological procedures requiring general anaesthesia. Concerns regarding general anaesthesia may in most cases be resolved by a formal consultation between the patient and the anaesthetist. Patients who have no experience with major surgery should be advised about the transient effects on bladder and bowel that are a sequel to laparotomy.

Specific advantages of tubal surgery include the fact that the couple can attempt to become pregnant independent of any treatment facility, and can do so over multiple cycles. In addition, the abortion and multiple pregnancy rates in women who conceive after tubal surgery are not different from those of the normal population. The live birth and ectopic pregnancy rates will be governed by the specific nature of the tubal damage, the surgical techniques used, and whether or not the woman has one or both tubes present.

## RESULTS OF RECONSTRUCTIVE TUBAL SURGERY

Selection of the most appropriate approach is a critical part of the surgical management of tubal factor infertility. The results of surgery depend on the nature and extent of the tubal damage, but they also depend heavily on the expertise of the surgeon, both in the selection of cases and in technical skills. Selection directly affects outcome, in that results will be better if only patients with a good prognosis undergo surgery. Technical skills are obviously important, since the first surgical attempt is the most likely to be successful. If a second is needed, it must deal not only with the effects of the disease but also with the consequences of the initial surgical procedure.

Deciding whether or not surgical treatment is appropriate in an individual case is based on the projected probability of pregnancy after a particular procedure. Although series of patients undergoing specific procedures can provide an estimate of the probability, the individual case will have features that may alter the prognosis. These features include:

(1) The nature and extent of pelvic and adnexal adhesions;

(2) The severity of the disease affecting the tube;

(3) The length of tube affected by disease;

(4) The length of the reconstructed tube;

(5) The presence or absence of other pelvic disease; and

(6) The presence or absence of other factors affecting fertility, such as oligospermia, ovulatory disturbance or advanced age of the female partner.

An estimate of postsurgical prognosis must take each of these features into account.

The reporting of results must be based on the condition of the adnexa least affected by disease or residual damage. A review of the reported results from various reconstructive procedures is described below.

### Adnexal adhesions and fimbrial phimosis

The standard approach for treating adnexal adhesions or fimbrial phimosis is now by laparoscopy. It is not uncommon for unsuspected adnexal adhesions to be found at the time of diagnostic laparoscopy, so it is prudent to have instruments available at the time of diagnostic laparoscopy to allow simultaneous removal of adhesions. Laparoscopic salpingo-ovariolysis offers a cumulative live birth rate of 50–60% within 12 months, with a 5% ectopic pregnancy rate[12]. Laparoscopic fimbrioplasty, performed for fimbrial agglutination, phimosis, or prefimbrial phimosis, yields a cumulative live birth rate of 40–50% within 12–18 months[13–17]. The increased rate of ectopic pregnancies after salpingo-ovariolysis indicates that, in addition to the periadnexal disease noted, there must be damage to the tubal endothelium.

## Distal tubal obstruction

Surgical management of distal tubal obstruction may be performed laparoscopically or by microsurgery at laparotomy. Laparoscopic salpingostomy has evolved to become the procedure of choice, because pregnancy rates after laparoscopic surgery approach or equal those achieved after microsurgery. In individual cases, the outcome of surgery will depend on a number of variables. These factors include:

(1) Distal ampullary diameter;

(2) Thickness of the tubal wall;

(3) Status of the tubal endothelium;

(4) Extent of adhesions; and

(5) Nature of adhesions.

The American Fertility Society (now the American Society for Reproductive Medicine) developed a classification system for distal tubal occlusion based on these factors[18]. This and other scoring systems allow the surgeon to predict the outcome of surgery and, as a consequence, to provide appropriate pretreatment counselling for couples about the optimal approach.

The results of laparoscopic salpingostomy have been reported in relatively small series and suggest intrauterine pregnancy rates of 18–29%[14,17,19,20] with ectopic pregnancy rates of 3–11% over variable lengths of follow-up. After microsurgical salpingostomy, live birth rates range from 19 to 35% with ectopic pregnancy rates of up to 18% in periods of follow-up of 4 years and sometimes longer (Table 1). Although occasionally a microsurgical approach can be justified in distal tubal obstruction, it is clear that a laparoscopic approach can offer similar prospects for pregnancy but with reduced cost, operating time

**Table 1** Intrauterine and ectopic pregnancy rates after microsurgical or laparoscopic salpingostomy

| *Reference* | *Year* | *Number of patients* | *Pregnancy rate (%)* | |
|---|---|---|---|---|
| | | | *Intrauterine* | *Ectopic* |
| *Microsurgical salpingostomy* | | | | |
| Swolin[3] | 1975 | 33 | 27.3 | 18.2 |
| Gomel[5] | 1980 | 72 | 30.6 | 9.7 |
| Larsson[25] | 1982 | 54 | 38.9 | 0 |
| Verhoeven *et al.*[26] | 1983 | 143 | 23.8 | 2.1 |
| Tulandi and Vilos[27] | 1985 | 67 | 22.4 | 4.5 |
| Boer-Meisel *et al.*[28] | 1986 | 108 | 28.7 | 17.6 |
| Donnez and Casanas-Roux[29] | 1986 | 83 | 31.3 | 15.7 |
| Kosasa and Hale[30] | 1988 | 93 | 39.8 | 14.0 |
| *Laparoscopic salpingostomy* | | | | |
| Gomel[31] | 1977 | 9 | 44.4 | 0 |
| Daniell and Herbert[19] | 1984 | 22 | 18.2 | 4.5 |
| Dubuisson *et al.*[14] | 1990 | 34 | 29.4 | 2.9 |
| Canis *et al.*[17] | 1991 | 55 | 23.6 | 10.9 |
| McComb and Paleologou[20] | 1991 | 22 | 22.7 | 4.5 |
| Mecke *et al.*[32] | 1995 | 35 | 22.9 | 8.6 |

and with increased appeal to the patient. Repeat attempts at salpingostomy are almost never justifiable; in these cases, IVF is the preferred management.

### Proximal tubal obstruction

A diagnosis of proximal tubal obstruction is always provisional if made on the basis of hysterosalpingography or hydrotubation at laparoscopy. A tube may be patent despite failure of dye to pass; such failure may be due to cornual muscle spasm, an intraluminal mucus plug, synechiae obstructing the intramural or isthmic portion of the tube, or to poor technique. Selective salpingography or Fallopian tube cannulation under hysteroscopic, ultrasonographic or radiographic control will usually allow differentiation of these apparent obstructions from true pathological occlusion. After tubal cannulation, patency rates from 70 to 90% have been reported, and pregnancy rates of 30–50% are claimed when at least one tube remains open[21]. Nevertheless, because poor HSG technique will often lead to a specious diagnosis of tubal obstruction, the quoted high patency rates will include variable numbers of women whose tubes were never actually obstructed.

The value of tubal cannulation awaits clarification in the form of a randomized controlled study comparing cannulation with continued observation. Despite this, it is reasonable to attempt tubal cannulation in women whose initial test of tubal patency indicates proximal obstruction, because there appears to be minimal risk of morbidity associated with the procedure. True proximal tubal disease, such as salpingitis isthmica nodosa, extensive fibrosis or occlusive polyps, will be readily demonstrated in this way. If tubal patency cannot be established by means of cannulation, the choice for management is between microsurgery and IVF.

The live birth rate after microsurgical tubocornual anastomosis for proximal tubal occlusion ranges from 37% to 58%, with ectopic pregnancy rates of 5–7%[5,22,23].

### Reversal of sterilization

Microsurgical anastomosis of the tubal segments remains the primary treatment for reversal of tubal sterilization. The effectiveness of such a procedure will depend on the extent and location of the tubal destruction and the length and condition of the residual tubal segments. Provided that the reconstructed tube has a length of at least 4 cm with an ampullary length of at least 1 cm, live birth rates of 60–80% after surgery can be achieved. The reported rates of ectopic pregnancy after such surgery range from 2 to 5% (Table 2).

**Table 2** Intrauterine and ectopic pregnancy rates after microsurgical tubal re-anastomosis (reversal of sterilization)

| *Reference* | *Year* | *Number of patients* | *Pregnancy rate (%)* | |
|---|---|---|---|---|
| | | | *Intrauterine* | *Ectopic* |
| Winston[33] | 1980 | 105 | 60 | 2.9 |
| Gomel[34] | 1983 | 118 | 78.8 | 1.7 |
| DeCherney *et al.*[35] | 1983 | 124 | 58.1 | 6.5 |
| Henderson[36] | 1984 | 95 | 53.7 | 5.3 |
| Paterson[37] | 1985 | 147 | 59.2 | 3.4 |
| Rock *et al.*[38] | 1987 | 80 | 61.2 | 12.5 |
| Xue and Fa[39] | 1989 | 117 | 81.2 | 1.7 |
| Dubuisson *et al.*[40] | 1995 | 206 | 69.9 | ? |
| Rouzi et al.[41] | 1995 | 217 | 69 | 3.2 |

Sterilization by fimbriectomy has been deemed to be irreversible. However, this is not necessarily the case; if at least 50% of the ampulla has been preserved, performing ampullary salpingostomy can yield a subsequent live birth rate of approximately 30%[24].

## SURGICAL TECHNIQUES

### Instrumentation for microsurgery

Very few instruments are needed, the basic requirements being a microneedle-holder, platform microforceps (plain and toothed), and microscissors. The needle driver and forceps have rounded rather than pointed tips, and the needle-holder has a concave-convex jaw configuration for firm grasping of the needle. Iris-type scissors are usually used for tubal transection. Teflon-coated rods of different configuration and with rounded tips are used for retraction and elevation of tissues and adhesions.

Electromicrosurgery requires the use of a fine microelectrode. An insulated microelectrode with 100 μm shaft and conical pointed tip is used for both cutting (i.e. division of adhesions) and coagulation of bleeders. A microbipolar jeweller's forceps may also be used for electrodesiccation.

The ValleyLab electrosurgical unit (Valley Lab Inc., Boulder, Colorado) can be used in many commonly performed surgical and gynaecological procedures. It delivers steady current at low levels that allow use of a microelectrode for microsurgical procedures. The handle is equipped with a rocker switch that permits fingertip control of both cutting and coagulation modes.

Synthetic 8-0 sutures are best for gynaecological microsurgery; we use absorbable sutures except where a specific reason exists to use non-absorbable ones. It is essential that these sutures be armed with fine tapercut type needles; if not, the benefit of using fine sutures will be negated by needle trauma. A suture commonly used is 8-0 polyglactin on a 130 μm, 4 mm or 5 mm long tapercut needle.

### Instrumentation for laparoscopic procedures

As for microsurgical procedures, it is possible to perform laparoscopic tubal surgery with few instruments. A wide range of ancillary instruments is available, but the essential instruments are grasping forceps, hook scissors, needle-holders, and suction/irrigation cannulas. The instruments can vary in size from 3 to 12 mm diameter, but most will be of 5 mm diameter.

The grasping forceps are used to steady tissue. For grasping tissue which is to be removed, such as adhesions, the tips may be toothed to enable a firmer grasp. For manipulation or steadying of tissue for tuboplasty, the forceps must be able to hold the tissue precisely and firmly, yet atraumatically. A variety of such atraumatic instruments is available; the most commonly used are the Semm fenestrated forceps and the diamond-tip grasping forceps (Figure 2). For performing fimbrioplasty, an alligator or dolphin-nosed forceps with a tapered tip is required.

The hook scissors should have tips that, when closed, present a smooth rounded surface. Some hook scissors have sharp tips which overlap when closed. These scissors may damage intraperitoneal structures inadvertently. The scissors with a smooth surface may be used for manipulation in the closed position without fear of unexpected trauma.

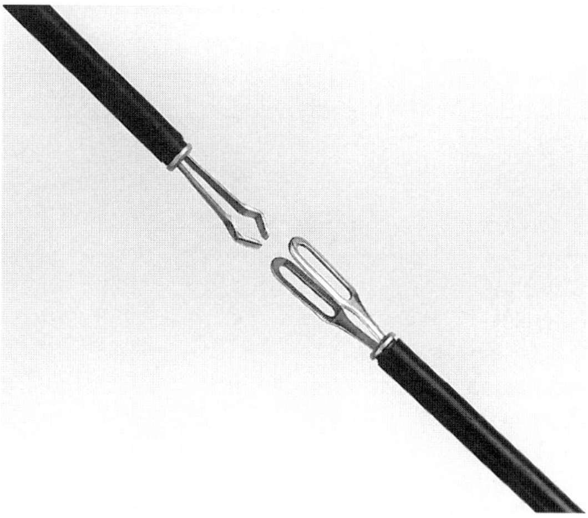

**Figure 2** Diamond-tip (left) and Semm fenestrated forceps for laparoscopic procedures

The needle-holder should be spring-loaded with the spring holding the jaws closed. The needles used may be straight or curved; the jaws of the needle-holder should be fashioned to hold either a straight or curved needle securely. Tissue placement of the suture is facilitated by the needle and needle-holder forming a rigid continuous instrument.

The suction/irrigation cannula must be capable of delivery of irrigating fluid and suction, and should have a finger-activated valve. This valve, when closed, permits neither inflow of fluid nor outflow of pneumoperitoneum. When opened in one direction, it permits suction and, in the other direction, irrigation occurs. The irrigating fluid can be instilled under pressure, by wrapping the intravenous (i.v.) bag containing the solution in an inflatable cuff or by using a specially designed pump. Pressures of up to 300 mmHg can be provided.

### Magnification

The use of an operating microscope provides a clear, highly magnified view, with coaxial illumination and an unchanging visual field. An objective lens with a focal length of 275 or 300 mm is recommended because it will leave an adequate working distance between the lens and the pelvic organs. The magnification, focus and attitude of the microscope may be altered during the procedure by hand or foot controls, depending on the type of microscope.

The use of magnifying loupes for tubal surgery is now an anachronism.

### Procedural set-up (microsurgery)

Proper attention to detail in setting up for infertility microsurgery facilitates the procedure itself and reduces unnecessary delays (and consequent surgical irritability). Steps that are taken before the induction of anaesthesia are as follows:

(1) The surgeon must ensure that all necessary instruments are available and in working order.

(2) The microscope is checked and adjusted for the surgeon's requirements.

(3) Any ancillary equipment (electrosurgical unit, television camera and monitor) is checked to ensure that it is in working order.

(4) The hysterosalpingogram films are placed on the viewing box, in the surgeon's field of view.

Once the patient is anaesthetized, a Foley catheter is inserted into the bladder. A paediatric Foley catheter is inserted into the uterine cavity for intraoperative chromopertubation. A sterile extension tubing is connected at one end to the catheter and at the other to a syringe filled with dilute dye solution. This enables the attendants to bring the syringe into the sterile field. The vagina may be packed to elevate the uterine fundus under the abdominal incision.

The surgeon and all attendants assisting at surgery wash their gloves thoroughly before the instruments are handled and the patient is draped. This reduces the introduction of starch into the peritoneal cavity.

A minilaparotomy incision is usually adequate for tubal reconstructive procedures. The site of the incision is infiltrated with 0.25% bupivacaine or 0.5% lidocaine solution before and after the operation. In the absence of contraindication, a suppository containing a non-steroidal anti-inflammatory agent (diclofenac sodium 100 mg) is inserted rectally. Because of these measures, and minimal bowel manipulation, the patients usually require only small amounts of systemic analgesics postoperatively. They are admitted to hospital on the day of surgery and discharged usually within 24 h of admission.

Good haemostasis of the abdominal wound is important to keep blood from dripping into the peritoneal cavity during the procedure. The gloves are rinsed once again before the peritoneal cavity is entered. The irrigation solution used throughout the procedure is a heparinized Ringer's lactate (Hartmann's) solution, with 5000 units of heparin being added to each litre. The irrigation solution, in an elevated i.v. bag, is connected by i.v. tubing to a hand-held irrigator. This arrangement allows periodic irrigation of the exposed peritoneal surfaces and ovaries, to prevent desiccation while the abdomen is open and to aid visualization of individual bleeders.

Once access to the peritoneal cavity is gained and the pelvic organs are examined, the operation goes forward:

(1) A wound protector is inserted and a modified Dennis-Brown retractor is put in place.

(2) Bowel is displaced into the upper peritoneal cavity and retained with a Kerlex pad soaked in heparinized lactated Ringer's (Hartmann's) solution. Manipulation of bowel is kept to an absolute minimum.

(3) The table is placed in a slight Trendelenburg position (10–15°); if desired, it may also be tilted towards the surgeon.

(4) The uterus and adnexae are elevated by packing the pouch of Douglas loosely with Kerlex pads washed in the irrigating solution.

(5) The microscope is then brought over the operative field and focused. The microscope need not be draped; it is cleansed before the procedure and sterile neoprene caps are applied to the controls.

### Procedural set-up (laparoscopic procedures)

Little preoperative preparation is needed. Bowel preparation is not required routinely, and shaving is also not done as a routine, although clipping of small areas of pubic hair may be advisable if ancillary instruments are to be inserted in these areas.

As with microsurgical preparation, the surgeon must ensure that all instruments and equipment are available and working normally. In particular, the standard assessment of gas supplies and gas insufflator, and of the compatibility of trochars, cannulae, laparoscopes and all ancillary instruments, must be carried out.

The configuration of the equipment and personnel within the operating theatre is an individual matter for each surgical suite. We have found it most convenient to arrange primary and secondary viewing monitors for video equipment so that they directly face the surgeon and assistant, respectively (Figure 3). The gas insufflator must, of necessity, be close to the patient, in order to minimize 'dead space' in the gas tubing and to avoid entanglement with other tubing and the light cable.

The technique of laparoscopy will not be further discussed here. For most laparoscopic surgical procedures, at least two and sometimes three ancillary portals will be required. These are placed suprapubically in the midline and at McBurney's points in either lower quadrant. Self-retaining cannulae are used in prolonged procedures to avoid slippage and the development of subcutaneous emphysema. The siting of these portals should be such that the mechanical advantage of the instruments is maximized but each instrument is able to move freely.

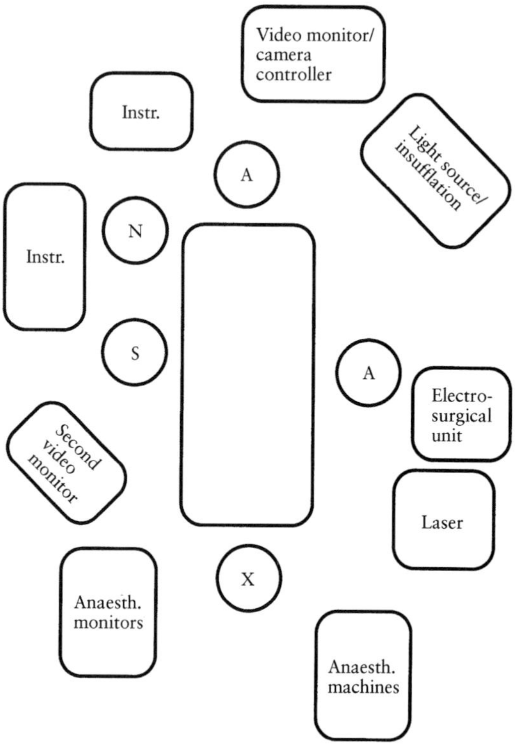


**Figure 3** Operating room set-up

## INDIVIDUAL PROCEDURES

If the tubes are patent, the primary approach to periadnexal disease is laparoscopic salpingo-ovariolysis, generally performed during the initial diagnostic laparoscopy. Laparotomy for this purpose is performed rarely and is usually part of a reconstructive tubal operation.

Periadnexal adhesions usually encapsulate parts or all of the tube and ovary and extend to the lateral pelvic wall, the posterior aspect of the broad ligaments, and the uterus. After the pelvic organs have been completely exposed, they are inspected thoroughly. The location, extent and nature of the adhesions are assessed. Chromopertubation is performed to confirm tubal patency. If this demonstrates tubal occlusion instead, salpingo-ovariolysis may be required to assess whether or not tubal reconstruction is feasible.

Clear identification and exposure of each adhesive layer is essential. The attachments of adhesions and what lies behind must be clearly identified before dissection begins. One adhesive layer must be divided at a time, bearing in mind that some adhesions that appear to be composed of a single layer are frequently composed of two layers.

To perform adhesiolysis, the adhesion is grasped with forceps at about its midpoint and gentle traction exerted, in order to expose one of its attachments. A small incision is made over a clear area to identify what lies behind the adhesion and whether it is composed of a single layer or double layers. The adhesion is divided parallel to the target organ, ensuring that large vessels are secured before transection. The line of division should be as close to the serosa of the structure anchoring the adhesion as is compatible with safety. Broad adhesions are dissected free of all attachments and removed through an ancillary portal. Narrower adhesions are simply divided.

We prefer the use of scissors for dissection to the use of a microelectrode or use of laser. Haemostasis is secured by desiccation of bleeders along the line of transection with a monopolar electrode or with microbipolar forceps. With cohesive adhesions, the dissection plane must be identified and developed by spreading the jaws of the scissors, by blunt dissection, or by hydrodissection.

Pelvic lavage is then carried out until the returning irrigation fluid (heparinized Ringer's lactate solution) is clear. Inspection of the dissected area after it has been flooded with irrigation solution, and the pneumoperitoneum has been partially released, will allow easy identification of any persisting bleeding points. These are then dealt with. Similarly, inspection of the fimbria when they are immersed in irrigation fluid allows for identification and correction of any interfimbrial adhesions.

### Fimbrioplasty

This term describes the reconstruction of the existing fimbria of a partially or totally occluded Fallopian tube. Tubal phimosis may be caused by the agglutination of the fimbria only. In this instance, chromopertubation will cause distension of the ampulla before dye passes into the peritoneal cavity. The agglutinated end of the tube may also be covered by a thin fibrous layer, leading to complete distal occlusion.

Usually, salpingo-ovariolysis must be performed before fimbrioplasty. Once the tube and ovary are free of adhesions, the condition of the tube can be assessed. When the distal end of the tube is covered by a fibrous layer, this is first either incised or removed to expose the agglutinated fimbria. A 3 mm alligator-jawed forceps is introduced (in the closed position) into the infundibulum of the tube while the tube is distended by chromopertubation. Once inserted, the jaws of the forceps are opened within the lumen of the tube, and gently withdrawn in the open position. It will be necessary to do this several times in different axes, in order to break down as many of the fimbrial adhesions as possible. There is usually very little bleeding; individual bleeding points can be spot desiccated.

### Salpingostomy (salpingoneostomy)

As with fimbrioplasty and salpingo-ovariolysis, our primary approach to the management of distal tubal occlusion has evolved to become a laparoscopic one. However, under some circumstances (for example, distal tubal occlusion in a patient with contralateral cornual occlusion) a microsurgical approach to salpingostomy is indicated.

Salpingostomy is the surgical creation of a new ostium in a tube whose fimbrial end is totally occluded, forming a hydrosalpinx or sactosalpinx. The prognosis for patients undergoing this procedure is heavily dependent on the structural and functional integrity of the tubal epithelium, and less dependent on the manner by which a new ostium is created.

A salpingostomy will often need to be preceded by salpingo-ovariolysis. When this has been completed, the tube is inspected thoroughly, with particular attention to the relationship between the distal tube and the ovary. If there is any adhesion, the distal tube must be dissected free from the ovary, continuing until the fimbria-ovarica is visualized. Further dissection may damage the vessels within this structure.

The surgical technique used laparoscopically is a modification of the technique used in microsurgery. The tube is distended by chromopertubation. This allows identification of the punctum in the centre of the distal end of the tube. There are usually radial avascular lines extending peripherally from the punctum, and the initial incision is placed in the axis of the fimbria ovarica, extending from the punctum towards the antimesosalpingeal surface of the tube. The hook scissors are used to make the incision. The superior margin of the incision is then grasped with the diamond-tip forceps, and, with the closed tip of the scissors inside the tubal lumen, the incision is gently stretched until the diameter approximates that of a normal distal tubal ostium.

There are two potential techniques for the creation of an everted stoma. If the mobility of the distal tube allows it, the simpler technique continues without a change of instruments. The diamond-tip forceps maintain a grasp of the incision at its superior margin, and the closed tip of the scissors prolapses the mucosa through the incision by pressing on the ampullary serosa (the 'intussusception' technique). The everted mucosa may be sutured in place (if tending to invert) by placement of one or more sutures, usually 6-0 polypropylene.

The second technique may be used if the mobility of the distal tube is limited. A second diamond-tip forceps grasps one lateral margin of the incision, and the forceps holding the superior margin changes its grasp to the opposing lateral margin. The two forceps are then rotated externally, rolling the margins of the incision simultaneously into eversion (Figure 4). The instruments then release their grip, and the everted margins, if tending to invert, are sutured to the ampullary serosa.

At the conclusion of the procedure, pelvic lavage is performed using the irrigation fluid to confirm haemostasis, and 300–500 ml of irrigation solution is left in the pelvis to allow organ flotation.

The microsurgical technique allows microscopic placement of incisions and sutures, although the practical importance of this is probably small. Once the normal anatomic relationships are restored, the tube is distended by transcervical chromopertubation. The occluded terminal end of the distended tube is examined through the microscope. The central punctum is entered first, and the incision is continued towards the ovary over an avascular line using the microelectrode and blend current. After the initial incision is made, additional radial incisions are made over avascular areas by everting the mucosa and working from within the tube. In this manner, it is possible to avoid cutting through the vascular mucosal folds, which will be shaped as neofimbria. This technique is associated with minimal bleeding. Bleeding points are coagulated individually with the microelectrode, using coagulating current. Once a satisfactory stoma has been fashioned, the mucosal edges are everted slightly and without tension and secured with interrupted 8-0 sutures (Figure 5).

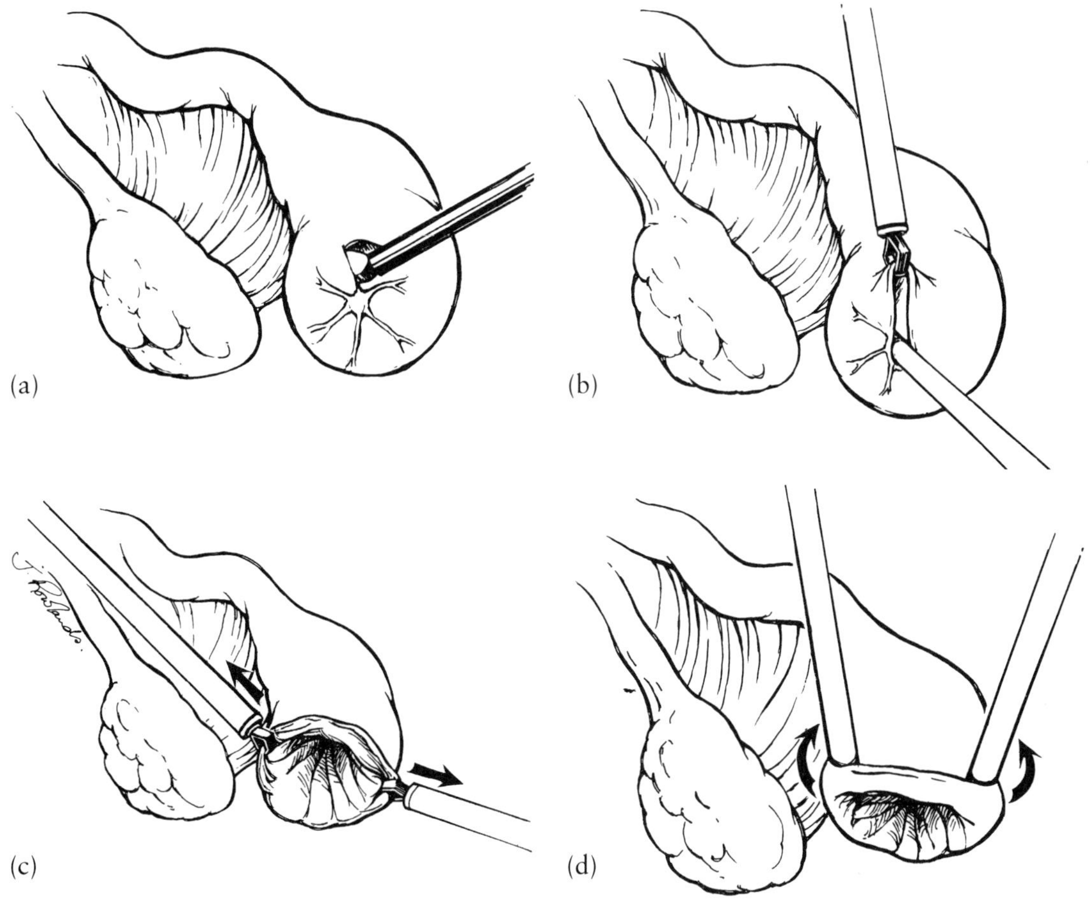


**Figure 4** Technique for performing salpingostomy by laparoscopy

## Tubocornual anastomosis for pathological cornual occlusion of the tubes

The traditional surgical approach to cornual occlusion associated with a variety of conditions (e.g. infection, salpingitis isthmica nodosa and endometriosis) has been tubo-uterine implantation. Microsurgical techniques and instrumentation allow anastomosis to be performed instead, after removal of the affected tubal segment. Selective salpingography and tubal cannulation are useful techniques in differentiating between true occlusion arising from a disease process and obstructions due to cornual spasm, mucus plug, or intratubal synechiae. However, the value of these techniques in the management of cornual occlusion associated with disease processes such as salpingitis isthmica nodosa remains to be determined. In such cases, microsurgical reconstruction remains the treatment of choice.

Initially, the cornual region of the uterus is injected superficially in a circular manner 1 cm proximal to the uterotubal junction with a dilute solution of vasopressin (10 units of vasopressin in 50 ml of normal saline). Care must be taken to avoid any intravascular injection. This approach minimizes bleeding and facilitates the procedures. The tube is incised adjacent to the uterus (at the uterotubal junction) (Figure 6), care being taken not to divide the arcade of artery and vein at the mesosalpingeal margin. The patency of the intramural portion of the tube is assessed by transcervical chromopertubation, and the cut surface is examined

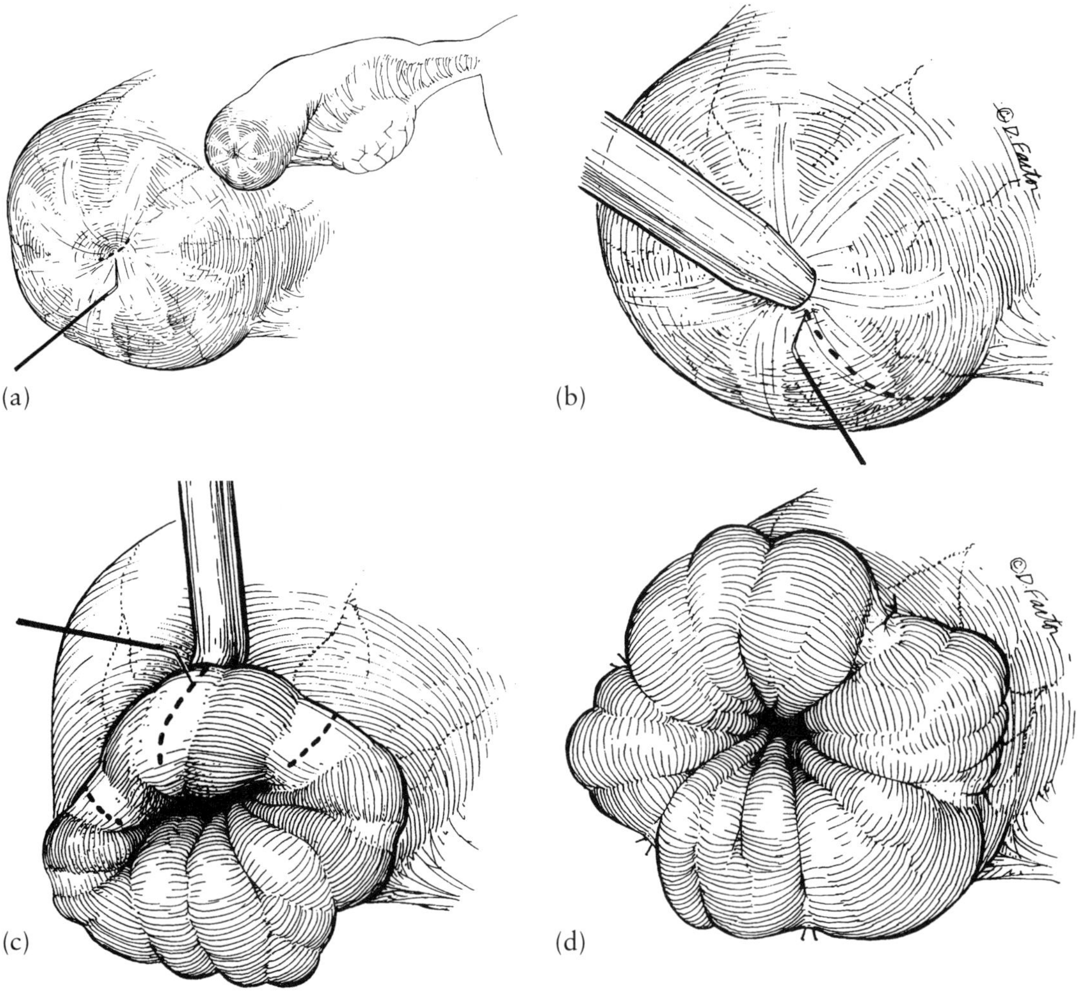

**Figure 5** Microsurgical salpingostomy. Reproduced from Gomel, V. and Rowe, T. C. (1988). Mastering reconstructive tubal microsurgery. In Sanz, L. (ed.) *Gynecologic Surgery*. (Oradell, NJ: Medical Economics). Original drawings © David Factor)

under the highest magnification for pathological changes. It may be necessary to excise varying lengths of the intramural tube until patent and normal oviduct is reached. With the uterus distended, the intramural tube is excised 1 or 2 mm at a time. The portion to be excised is first dissected free from the surrounding uterine musculature by means of the microelectrode (Figure 7). The tube is then grasped with a strong toothed microforceps and transected with the use of a curved blade or scissors (Figure 8). Excision is continued until the patent and normal intramural segment is reached. A normal tube is free of fibrosis; it has normal muscular architecture, and the mucosal folds are intact and exhibit a pristine vascular pattern.

The approach described prevents the creation of a large defect in the cornu. Depending on the extent of excision of the intramural segment, tubocornual anastomosis may be juxtamural, intramural, or juxtauterine.

The occluded or abnormal segment of isthmus is then excised. Serial incisions are placed with iris scissors on this segment of tube, starting at the uterotubal junction, until normal

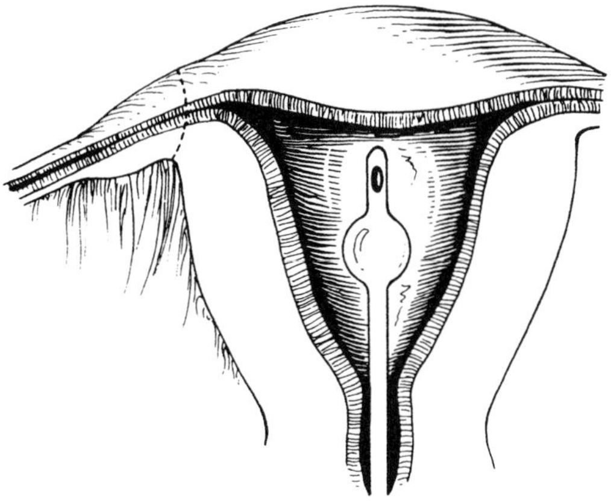

**Figure 6** Incision of the tube at the tubocornual junction. Reproduced with permission from Gomel, V. and Rowe, T. C. In DeCherney, A. H. and Pernoll, M. L. (eds.) *Current Obstetric and Gynaecologic Diagnosis and Treatment*, 8th edn. (Norwalk: Appleton & Lang)

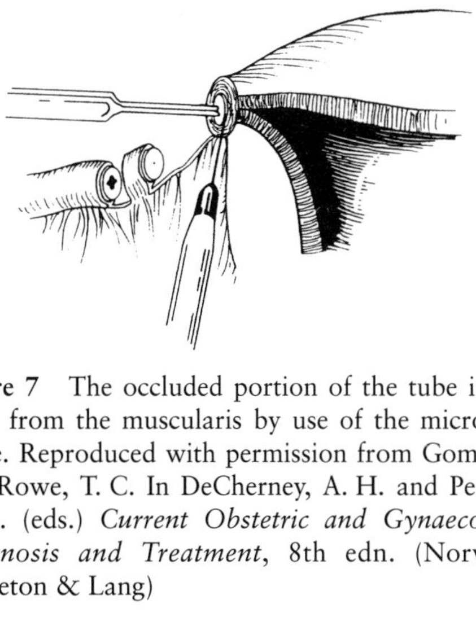

**Figure 7** The occluded portion of the tube is isolated from the muscularis by use of the microelectrode. Reproduced with permission from Gomel, V. and Rowe, T. C. In DeCherney, A. H. and Pernoll, M. L. (eds.) *Current Obstetric and Gynaecologic Diagnosis and Treatment*, 8th edn. (Norwalk: Appleton & Lang)

isthmus is reached. The patency of the distal segment of tube is confirmed by injecting irrigating solution through the fimbriated end (descending hydrotubation). The small transected segments of affected isthmus are excised from the mesosalpinx, remaining close to the tube in order to spare the tubal vessels. Haemostasis is achieved by desiccating only the more significant bleeders; over-zealous electrocauterization must be resisted to avoid devitalization of the anastomosis site.

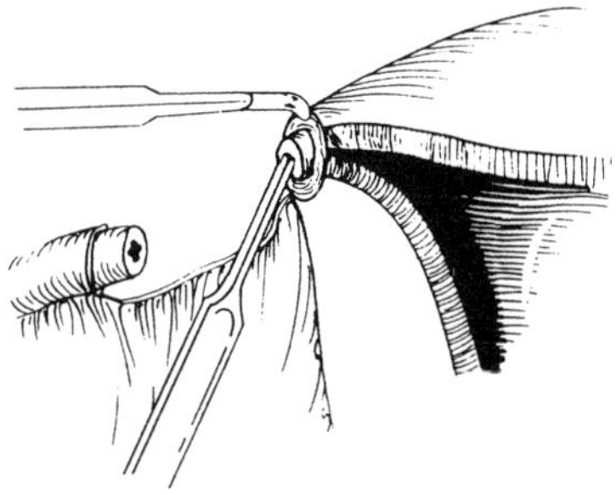

**Figure 8** The isolated segment of occluded tube is excised using a curved blade. Reproduced with permission from Gomel, V. and Rowe, T. C. In DeCherney, A. H. and Pernoll, M. L. (eds.) *Current Obstetric and Gynaecologic Diagnosis and Treatment*, 8th edn. (Norwalk: Appleton & Lang)

End-to-end anastomosis between the apparently healthy intramural and isthmic segments is then performed. The muscularis and epithelium are approximated with interrupted 8-0 polyglactin sutures placed at cardinal points in such a way that the knots remain external. Except in the case of juxtamural anastomosis, it is necessary to place all the sutures before they are tied. With anastomosis deeper in the cornu, tying the first suture would make placement of the subsequent sutures difficult or impossible.

The first muscular suture is placed at the '6 o'clock' position (Figure 9); it is not tied and is identified with a small Weck clip. The other sutures are placed using a single strand. This approach facilitates suture placement and prevents entanglement of sutures. The isthmus is held close to the intramural segment, and the '6 o'clock' suture is tied. Sutures must be tied without undue tension. It may be necessary to approximate the isthmic mesosalpinx to the uterus with a single 7-0 suture before tying the muscular sutures. Once the '6 o'clock' suture has been tied, further muscular sutures are tied individually after the loop between successive sutures has been divided. After apposition of the epithelium and muscularis, the seromuscularis of the cornu is approximated to the tubal serosa with 8-0 polyglactin sutures. The

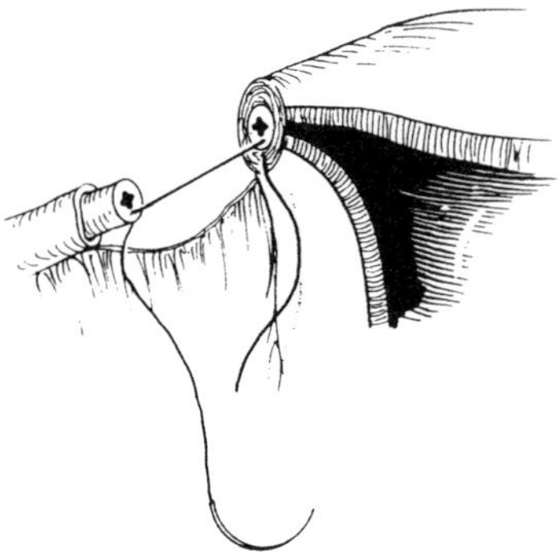

**Figure 9** The two segments are anastomosed at the mucosal level, the first suture being placed at the 6 o'clock position. Reproduced with permission from Gomel, V. and Rowe, T. C. In DeCherney, A. H. and Pernoll, M. L. (eds.) *Current Obstetric and Gynaecologic Diagnosis and Treatment*, 8th edn. (Norwalk: Appleton & Lang)

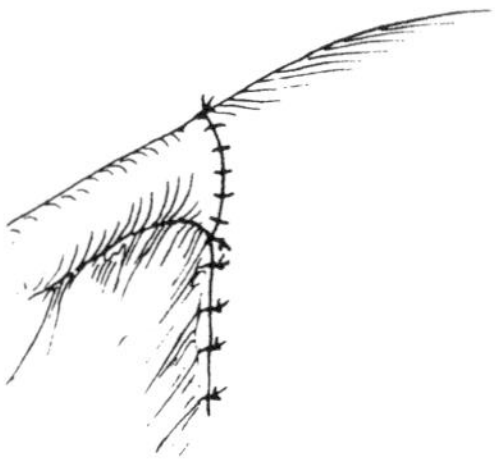

**Figure 10** The seromuscularis is closed, as is the defect in the mesosalpinx. Reproduced with permission from Gomel, V. and Rowe, T. C. In DeCherney, A. H. and Pernoll, M. L. (eds.) *Current Obstetric and Gynaecologic Diagnosis and Treatment*, 8th edn. (Norwalk: Appleton & Lang)

mesosalpinx is then joined to the uterus in a similar fashion (Figure 10).

Tubocornual anastomosis may also be performed for the purpose of sterilization reversal. Such cases commonly require juxtamural anastomosis, since the intramural segment of the tube is usually intact.

### Tubotubal anastomosis

Tubotubal anastomosis is performed most frequently for reversal of a prior sterilization procedure. Tubal occlusions associated with disease processes are rare at sites other than the cornu; they may be due to endometriosis or follicular salpingitis but are more frequently associated with tubal pregnancy which has arrested or has been treated conservatively.

The occluded segment is excised, or, in the previously sterilized group, the occluded ends are resected (Figure 11a). Transection of the tube is performed with iris scissors, and the occluded stump is excised from the mesosalpinx using the microelectrode. In this process, it is critical to stay close to the tube to avoid damaging the mesosalpingeal vessels. Patency of the proximal and distal tubal segments is confirmed (respectively) by transcervical chromopertubation and descending hydropertubation, and the cut surfaces are examined under high magnification.

End-to-end anastomosis of the tubal segments is performed in two layers using 8-0 suture material as described for tubocornual anastomosis. The first layer apposes the epithelium and muscularis, and the first suture is placed at the mesosalpingeal edge of the tube (6-o'clock position), and tied (Figure 11b). These sutures incorporate the muscularis and submucosa, avoiding the mucosa where possible. However, there is no evidence that inclusion of the epithelium adversely affects outcome. These sutures are placed so that the knots lie externally. Depending on the luminal calibre of the tubal segments, three or more additional sutures are placed to complete the approximation of the epithelial and muscular layers. The anastomosis is completed by apposition of the serosa and mesosalpinx using the same calibre of suture (Figures 11c–e).

## CONCLUSION

Infertility with an underlying tubal cause may be actively managed by tubal surgery or by *in vitro* fertilization. Couples so affected must be adequately investigated and counselled before a decision about management can be made. The non-technical considerations that apply to the decision-making process include the age of the woman, the costs of treatment, and the wishes

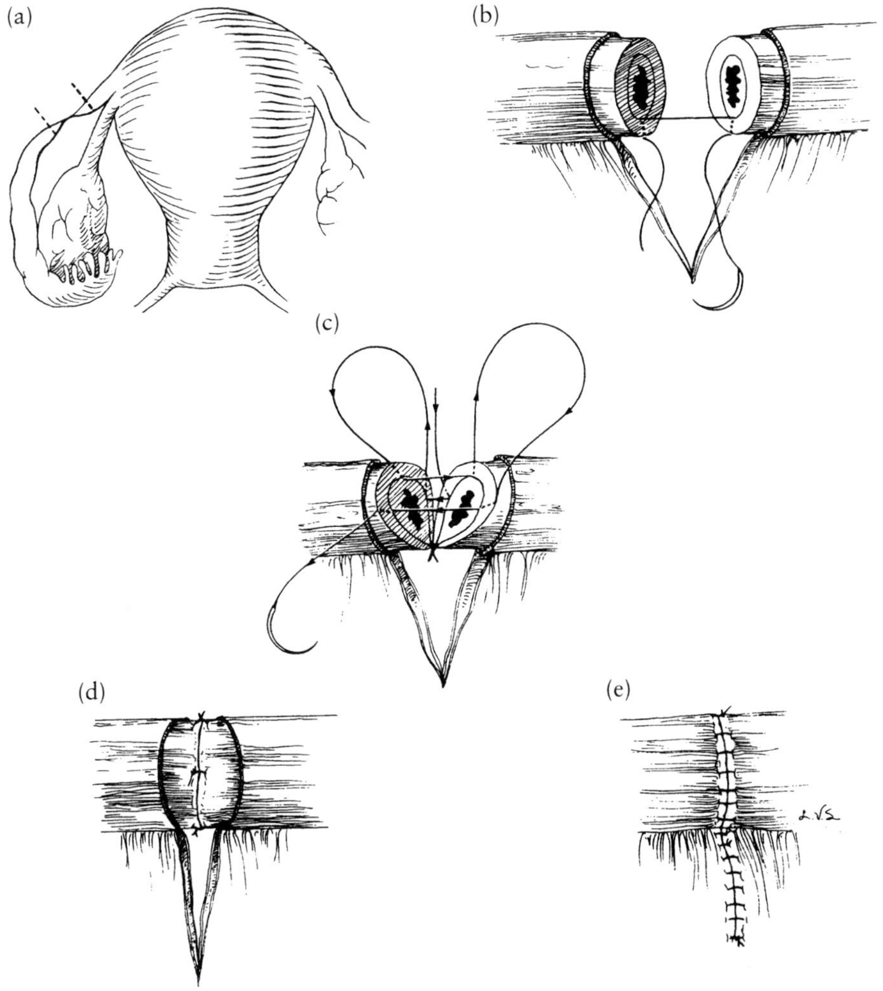


**Figure 11** (a) Tubotubal anastomosis: the ends of the occluded segments are transected; (b) the initial epithelial suture is placed at the 6 o'clock position and tied; (c) subsequent sutures are placed using a single strand; they are tied individually after division of the loop between successive sutures; (d) the muscularis has been closed; (e) the serosa and mesosalpinx are closed. Reproduced with permission from Gomel, V. and Rowe, T. C. In DeCherney, A. H. and Pernoll, M. L. (eds.) *Current Obstetric and Gynaecologic Diagnosis and Treatment*, 8th edn. (Norwalk: Appleton & Lang)

and values of the couple. Technical considerations include the potential risks of each method, complications, and estimated pregnancy rates; all of these considerations must be based on local experience. Counselled thus, most couples will reach a decision regarding management that is satisfactory both to them and to the physician involved.

## REFERENCES

1. Royal Commission on New Reproductive Technologies (1993). *Proceed With Care*, Final Report of the Royal Commission, p. 211. (Ottawa: Ministry of Government Services Canada)
2. Westrom, L. (1980). Incidence, prevalence and trends of pelvic inflammatory disease and its

consequences in industrialized countries. *Am. J. Obstet. Gynecol.*, **138**, 880–92

3. Swolin, K. (1975). Electromicrosurgery and salpingostomy: long-term results. *Am. J. Obstet. Gynecol.*, **121**, 418–19
4. Gomel, V. (1977). Reconstructive surgery of the oviduct. *J. Reprod. Med.*, **18**, 181–90
5. Gomel, V. (1980). Clinical results of microsurgery in female infertility. In Crosignani, P. G. and Rubin, B. L. (eds.) *Microsurgery in Female Infertility*, pp 77–94. (Orlando: Academic Press)
6. McComb, P. F. and Gomel, V. (1980). Cornual occlusion and its microsurgical reconstruction. *Clin. Obstet. Gynecol.*, **23**, 1229–41
7. van Noord-Zaadstra, B. M., Looman, C. W. N., Alsbach, H., Habbema, J. D. F., te Velde, E. R. and Karbaat, J. (1991). Delayed childbearing: effect of age on fecundity and outcome of pregnancy. *Br. Med. J.*, **302**, 1361–5
8. Collins, J. A. and Rowe, T. C. (1989). Age of the female partner is a prognostic factor in prolonged unexplained infertility: a multicenter study. *Fertil. Steril.*, **52**, 15–20
9. Glock, J. L., Kim, A. H., Hulka, J. F., Hunt, R. B., Trad, F. S. and Brumsted, J. R. (1996). Reproductive outcome after tubal reversal in women 40 years of age or older. *Fertil. Steril.*, **65**, 863–5
10. Tan, S. L., Royston, P., Campbell, S., Jacobs, H. S., Betts, J., Mason, B. and Edwards, R. G. (1992). Cumulative conception and livebirth rates after *in vitro* fertilisation. *Lancet*, **339**, 1390–4
11. FIVNAT (French *In Vitro* National) (1995). Pregnancies and births resulting from *in vitro* fertilization: French national registry, analysis of data 1986 to 1990. *Fertil. Steril.*, **64**, 746–56
12. Gomel, V. (1983). Salpingo-ovariolysis by laparoscopy in infertility. *Fertil. Steril.*, **34**, 607–11
13. Bruhat, M. A., Mage, G., Manhes, M. H., Soualhat, C., Ropert, J. F. and Pouly, J. L. (1983). Laparoscopy procedures to promote fertility: ovariolysis and salpingolysis: results of 93 selected cases. *Acta Eur. Fertil.*, **14**, 113–15
14. Dubuisson, J. B., Borquet de Joliniere, J. and Aubriot, F. X. (1990). Terminal tuboplasties by laparoscopy: 65 consecutive cases. *Fertil. Steril.*, **54**, 401–3
15. Fayez, J. A. (1983). An assessment of the role of operative laparoscopy in tuboplasty. *Fertil. Steril.*, **39**, 476–9
16. Gomel, V. (1975). Laparoscopic surgery in tubal infertility. *Obstet. Gynecol.*, **46**, 47–8
17. Canis, M., Mage, G., Pouly, J. L. *et al.* (1991). Laparoscopic distal tuboplasty: report of 87 cases and a 4-year experience. *Fertil. Steril.*, **56**, 616–21
18. Gomel, V. (1988). Distal tubal occlusion. *Fertil. Steril.*, **49**, 946–8
19. Daniell, J. F. and Herbert, C. M. (1984). Laparoscopic salpingostomy using the $CO_2$ laser. *Fertil. Steril.*, **41**, 558–63
20. McComb, P. F. and Paleologou, A. (1991). The intussusception salpingostomy technique for the therapy of distal oviductal occlusion at laparoscopy. *Obstet. Gynecol.*, **78**, 443–7
21. Simpson, C. W. (1991). Transcervical Fallopian tube catheterization. *J. Soc. Obstet. Gynaecol. Canada*, **13**, 37–42
22. Donnez, J. and Casanas-Roux, F. (1986). Prognostic factors influencing the pregnancy rate after microsurgical tubocornual anastomosis. *Fertil. Steril.*, **46**, 1089–92
23. McComb, P. (1986). Microsurgical tubocornual anastomosis for occlusive cornual disease: reproducible results without the need for tubouterine implantation. *Fertil. Steril.*, **46**, 571–7
24. Gomel, V. (1983). *Microsurgery in Female Infertility*, p. 233. (Boston: Little, Brown)
25. Larsson, B. (1982). Late results of salpingostomy combined with salpingolysis and ovariolysis by electromicrosurgery in 54 women. *Fertil. Steril.*, **37**, 156–60
26. Verhoeven, H. C., Berry, H., Frantzen, C. and Schlosser, H.-W. (1983). Surgical treatment for distal tubal occlusion: a review of 167 cases. *J. Reprod. Med.*, **28**, 293–304
27. Tulandi, T. and Vilos, G. A. (1985). A comparison between laser surgery and electrosurgery for bilateral hydrosalpinx: a two year followup. *Fertil. Steril.*, **44**, 846–8
28. Boer-Meisel, M. E., te Velde, E. R., Habbema, J. D. F. and Kardaun, J. W. P. F. (1986). Predicting the pregnancy outcome in patients treated for hydrosalpinx: a prospective study. *Fertil. Steril.*, **45**, 23–9
29. Donnez, J. and Casanas-Roux, F. (1986). Prognostic factors of fimbrial microsurgery. *Fertil. Steril.*, **46**, 200–4
30. Kosasa, T. S. and Hale, R. W. (1988). Treatment of hydrosalpinx using a single incision eversion procedure. *Int. J. Fertil.*, **33**, 319–23

31. Gomel, V. (1977). Salpingostomy by laparoscopy. *J. Reprod. Med.*, **18**, 265–7
32. Mecke, H., Semm, K., Lehmann-Willenbrock, E., Stojanov, M. and Freys, I. (1995). Pelviscopic salpingostomy with everted suture. *Zentralbl. Gynakol.*, **117**, 413–16
33. Winston, R. M. L. (1980). Reversal of sterilization. *Clin. Obstet. Gynecol.*, **23**, 1261–8
34. Gomel, V. (1983). *Microsurgery in Female Infertility*, pp. 237–42. (Boston: Little, Brown)
35. DeCherney, A. H., Mezer, H. C. and Naftolin, F. (1983). Analysis of failure of microsurgical anastomosis after mid-segment, non-coagulation tubal ligation. *Fertil. Steril.*, **39**, 618–22
36. Henderson, S. R. (1984). The reversibility of female sterilization with the use of microsurgery: a report on 102 patients with more than one year of follow-up. *Am. J. Obstet. Gynecol.*, **149**, 57–65
37. Paterson, P. J. (1985). Factors influencing the success of microsurgical tuboplasty for sterilization reversal. *Clin. Reprod. Fertil.*, **3**, 57–64
38. Rock, J. A., Guzick, D. S., Katz, E., Zacur, H. A. and King, T. M. (1987). Tubal anastomosis: pregnancy success following reversal of Falope ring or monopolar cautery sterilization. *Fertil. Steril.*, **48**, 13–17
39. Xue, P. and Fa, Y.-Y. (1989). Microsurgical reversal of female sterilization. *J. Reprod. Med.*, **34**, 451–5
40. Dubuisson, J. B., Chapron, C., Nos, C., Morice, P., Aubriot, F. X. and Garnier, P. (1995). Sterilization reversal: fertility results. *Hum. Reprod.*, **10**, 1145–51
41. Rouzi, A. A., Mackinnon, M. and McComb, P. F. (1995). Predictors of success of reversal of sterilization. *Fertil. Steril.*, **64**, 29–36

# Assisted reproductive technologies up to the year 2000

# 10

*Paul A. Rainsbury*

## INTRODUCTION

In 1968, a meeting was held at the Royal Society of Medicine in Wimpole Street, London at which Patrick Steptoe, a gynaecologist, showed laparoscopic slides of ovaries and follicles. After the lecture, Robert Edwards, a scientist from Cambridge, asked Patrick Steptoe if it would be feasible with laparoscopic technology to retrieve an egg from the ovary.

The treatment of infertility received a major boost in 1978 following the birth of Louise Brown. Steptoe and Edwards reported the birth of the world's first baby to be conceived through *in vitro* fertilization and embryo transfer (IVF–ET)[1]. Steptoe was quoted in *Time* magazine as saying 'this is the first time we've solved all the problems at once. We're at the end of the beginning – not the beginning of the end.'

The pioneers of IVF in humans applied technology which had been developed in animals. Walter Heap in the nineteenth century had already successfully transferred embryos flushed from the oviducts of one species of rabbit to another species of rabbit[2]. However, it was not until 1959 that Chang carried out successful *in vitro* fertilization with rabbit oocytes and sperm[3].

Steptoe and Edwards' meeting at the Royal Society of Medicine resulted in laparoscopic techniques being developed to successfully recover human oocytes[4]. It was fitting that Steptoe should develop this technique following his experience with a French gynaecologist, Raoul Palmer, in Paris in 1958, who taught him 'coelioscopy', the French equivalent of laparoscopy.

The first human pregnancy resulting from IVF treatment was achieved in 1976 by the two pioneers but sadly ended in an ectopic pregnancy[5]. Births from the USA and Australia quickly followed the UK's success. Despite some initial controversies[6,7], new assisted reproductive technologies (ART) – to coin a delightful American acronym – are now used by gynaecologists around the world in the management of infertile couples. We have come a long way from the original indication for IVF – damaged Fallopian tubes – in our use of this technology today.

Success rates from IVF–ET treatments have consistently improved internationally since 1978. Several groups have collected data on the pregnancy rates of IVF–ET clinics. The largest of these groups was the American Fertility Society (AFS), recently renamed the American Society for Reproductive Medicine (ASRM). The number of live deliveries per 100 ET procedures and the number of live deliveries per 100 oocyte recoveries (OCR) are among the most commonly used definitions of success.

It must be remembered that pregnancies resulting from ART are more complicated than spontaneous pregnancies (Chapter 8). There are higher rates of ectopic, heterotopic and high-order pregnancies. The numbers of spontaneous abortions, premature deliveries and Caesarean sections are increased. Perinatal mortality and morbidity rates are increased as a result of prematurity. There are higher rates of maternal morbidity associated with these pregnancies (pre-eclampsia, gestational diabetes, haemorrhage and anaemia) which all contribute to intrauterine growth retardation.

The complications associated with ovulation induction include ovarian hyperstimulation syndrome (OHSS) (see below and Chapter 8). Complications may arise from diagnostic laparoscopy (Chapter 7), anaesthesia or intravenous sedation associated with oocyte recovery procedures.

Pregnancy rates, even in the best clinics, are still low. A 20% take-home-baby rate is considered good. In the UK, the Human Fertilisation and Embryology Authority (HFEA) (Chapter 20) publishes yearly updated 'league tables' of IVF and donor insemination (DI) of the 53 clinics in the UK which offer these services. The current success rates are shown in a graphic figure in Chapter 19. Even here the best take-home-baby rates (live birth rates) are only 23%. One of the main contributing causes of poor pregnancy rates in ART has been the decreased viability of transferred embryos and the transfer of four-cell embryos into an environment that naturally would be receptive only to 5-day-old blastocysts. The ultimate aim of scientific research in this important area of implantation is to mimic *in vivo* conditions *in vitro*, so that at least the pregnancy rates of ART can parallel normal fecundity in the human. An attractive future concept includes the freezing of blastocysts generated from coculture, thawing them, and replacing them in natural cycles (Chapter 15).

Circumstantial evidence suggests that endometrial receptivity declines with increasing age and is adversely affected by ovarian superovulation and is also possibly affected by ovarian function. Future research must therefore focus on the molecular biology of the endometrium.

## IVF AND GAMETE INTRAFALLOPIAN TRANSFER

*In vitro* fertilization has now superseded gamete intrafallopian transfer (GIFT) as the method of choice in ART procedures. The GIFT technique is briefly described below.

### Gamete intrafallopian transfer

There are several stages involved in this process.

*Controlled ovarian hyperstimulation (COH): long LHRHa protocols (long regimen)*

Good rates of implantation are achieved throughout the UK using this protocol. The protocol is designed to suppress luteinizing hormone (LH) surges and also reduce the tonic LH level. The flow chart below (Figure 1) graphically demonstrates the various stages of the regimen.

Down-regulation may be achieved by several methods. At the BUPA Roding IVF unit, we commonly use buserelin subcutaneously (s.c.) starting with a dose of 500 µg for 2 weeks on either day 1 or day 21 of a classic 28-day cycle. An oestrogen assay is carried out on approximately day 14. This should be less than 100 pmol/l. Alternatively, Synarel nasal spray (Searle Pharmaceuticals, High Wycombe, Bucks, UK), Prostap 3.75 mg (Wyeth Laboratories, Maidenhead, Berks, UK) or Zoladex 3.6 mg (Zeneca Pharmaceuticals, Wilmslow, Cheshire, UK) may be used. The luteinizing hormone releasing hormone analogues (LHRHa) protocols are successful in obtaining a complete down-regulation of the pituitary gland and establishing basal conditions in the ovary. The long protocol also facilitates the programming of cycles which is useful when increasing numbers of patients are going through treatment.

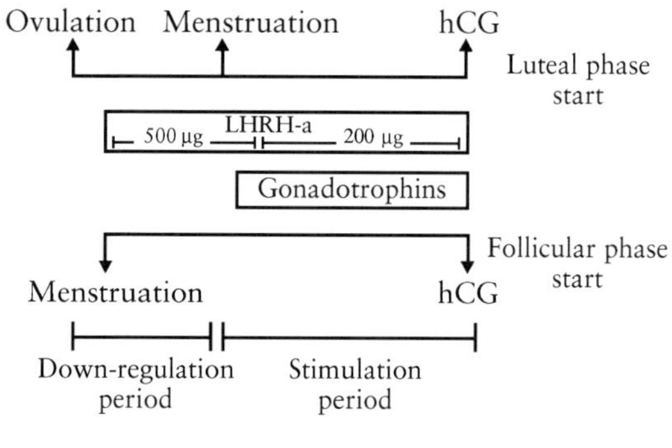


**Figure 1** Schematic diagram of long LHRHa protocol

Superovulation with gonadotrophins starts mid-week as shown. Puregon (Organon Laboratories Ltd, Milton, Cambridge, UK) at a normal starting dose of 150 IU (50 IU × 3 ampoules) is given intramuscularly daily. Transvaginal scans are carried out on days 6, 8 and 10 to monitor follicular growth rates, together with serum oestrogen assays on days 8 and 10. Follicular growth rates in the latter part of the cycle are approximately 1.5–2.0 mm per day and oestrogen levels normally rise from 5000 pmol/l on day 8 to 10 000 pmol/l on day 10. Ovarian hyperstimulation will be dealt with later in this chapter. Normally, by day 11 of stimulation, two leading follicles will have reached 18 mm in mean diameter.

The Siemens Sonoline Prima (Siemens plc, Siemens House, Swinbury-on-Thames, Middx, UK) is one of the most widely used follicular scanning machines in the UK (Figure 2). Dr Pat Thurley has covered transabdominal and transvaginal scanning in detail in Chapter 6 and highlighted their respective values as a tool in reproductive medicine. Suffice it to say that increasing resolution of ultrasound images has greatly facilitated oocyte recovery and embryo transfer. These will now be described in more detail.

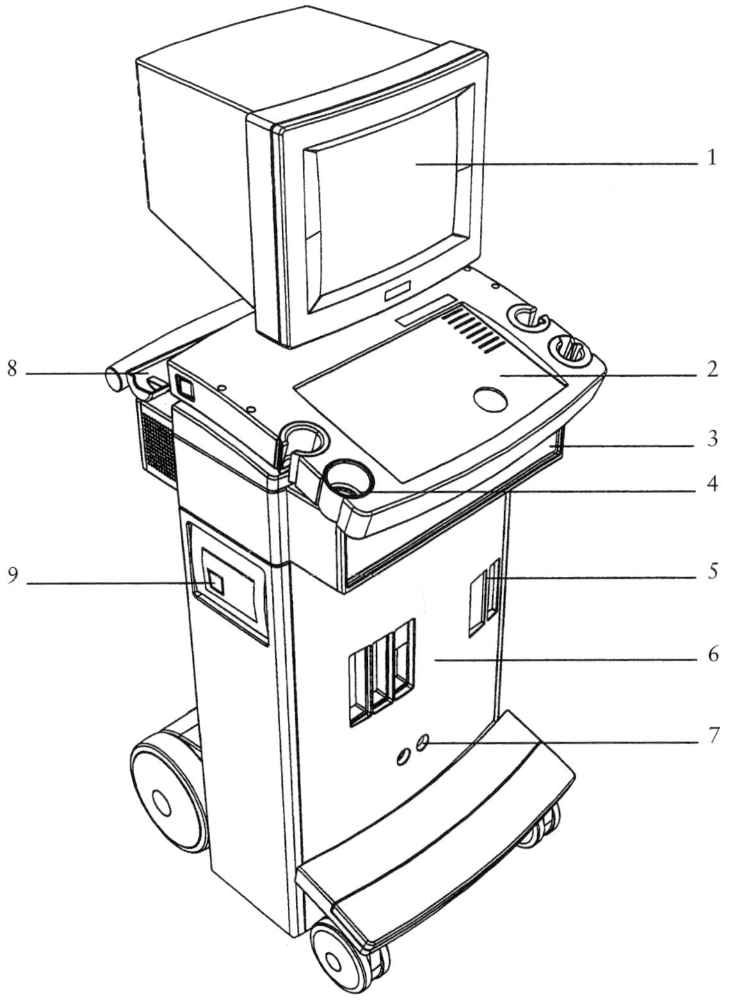


1 Monitor with imaging screen
2 Control panel
3 VCR bay (VCR is optional)
4 Transducer and gel holders
5 Floppy disk drive
6 Transducer ports
7 ECG and footswitch connections
8 Video printer
9 Endocavity transducer holder

**Figure 2** Siemens Sonoline Prima ultrasound imaging system

There are two methods of oocyte recovery laparoscopically-directed or ultrasound-directed. Laparoscopically directed recovery will be covered only briefly, as this technique has been largely superseded by ultrasound-directed oocyte recovery. The HFEA *Patient's Guide to DI and IVF Clinics* manual (1996 edition, p. 6) shows that nationally 19 983 patients were treated by IVF in a total of 25 730 cycles. The majority of these patients would have had their eggs collected by vaginal ultrasound. Patrick Steptoe in 1968[8] devised a method of aspirating oocytes laparoscopically from human preovulatory follicles (Figure 3). The world's first IVF pregnancy occurred in 1976 following laparoscopic egg recovery but unfortunately ended in an ectopic pregnancy[5]. It was a further 2 years before the pioneers Steptoe and Edwards achieved a live birth. The present technique of laparoscopic recovery has changed little since the early days, although, like ultrasound, the resolution of laparoscopic equipment has improved enormously (Figure 4).

Following controlled ovarian hyperstimulation (COH) and appropriately-timed human chorionic gonadotrophin (hCG), full general anaesthetic is induced, and the patient prepared, draped and placed in the Trendelenberg lithotomy position. The bladder is catheterized and emptied. A Verres needle connected to a $CO_2$ gas insufflater is inserted through a 1-cm subumbilical incision towards the pelvic cavity. A steady flow of $CO_2$ is delivered at a pressure not greater than 100 mmHg. Once an adequate pneumoperitoneum has been established, the $CO_2$ is changed to a mixture of 5% $O_2$, 5% $CO_2$ and 90% $N_2$, as 100% $CO_2$ could cause follicular fluid to become acidic[9–12].

Palmer grasping forceps are inserted in the midline 2.5 cm above the pubic symphysis. A trochar and cannula are passed into the

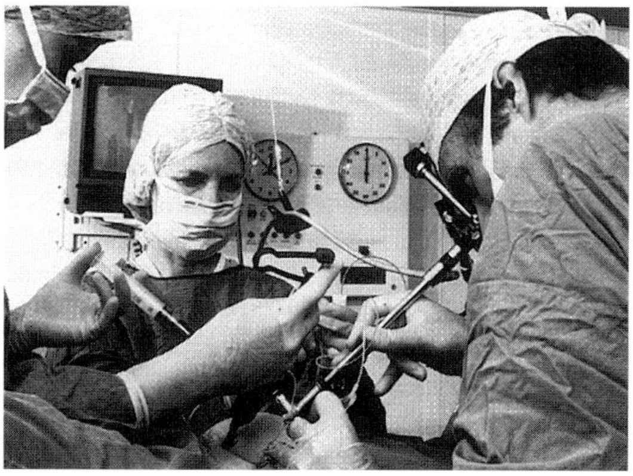

**Figure 3** Laparoscopic oocyte recovery

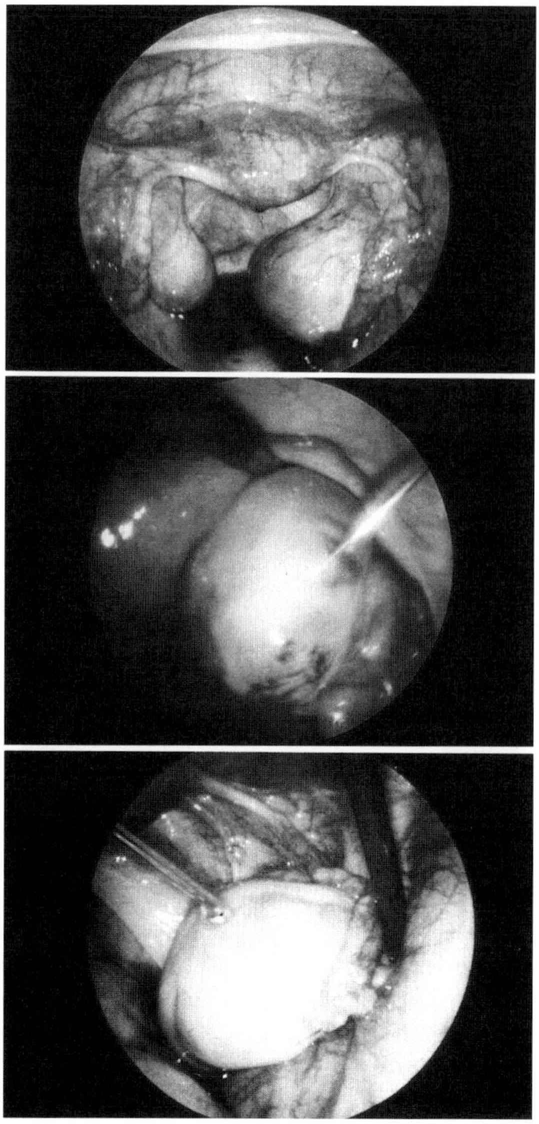

**Figure 4** (a) General view of the pelvis showing normal uterus and Fallopian tubes with stimulated ovaries; (b) left ovarian ligament grasped by forceps to steady ovary, with aspiration needle entering ovary; (c) as (b) but with left infundibulopelvic ligament grasped

peritoneal cavity through the left or right lower quadrant to access the left or right ovary and a double lumen follicle aspiration needle (Rocket, London, UK), designed by Professor Craft, is passed down after attaching it by a fine plastic tube to the collection pot and onto the Craft vacuum pump which is controlled by a foot pedal. It is essential to obtain a good view of the pelvic organs, especially the ovaries. Once this has been achieved by grasping the infundibulopelvic ligament (Figure 4), the needle and tubing are flushed through with Earle's medium (Chapter 13). The follicle is punctured by the needle and a vacuum applied up to 110 mmHg. Clear follicular fluid enters the collecting tube and this is passed through to the embryologist who identifies the egg. If no egg is found on the first aspirate, flushing continues and usually the egg is retrieved by the second or third flush. The scoring of the oocyte and its surrounding cumulus is described in Chapter 13. All available follicles are aspirated and, at the conclusion of the procedure, the pouch of Douglas is aspirated, as occasionally an oocyte may have been inadvertently dropped in the pouch.

The male partner has already produced a semen sample 2 h prior to the laparoscopy. This has been prepared according to standard sperm preparation techniques (Chapter 13). Poor specimens are prepared by the mini-Percoll method, whilst more normal specimens are prepared by layering. The final preparation of semen should contain between 50 000 and 100 000 motile spermatozoa for transfer into each Fallopian tube in a volume of 20–25 ml.

When the oocyte recovery is completed, the three best-quality oocytes are transferred to the Fallopian tubes, usually two into one tube and one into the other, together with appropriately prepared sperm. These oocytes are inseminated with the semen sample described above. The inseminated oocytes are drawn into a fine teflon catheter and transferred without delay from the embryology laboratory in order to prevent cooling, which can be harmful to the oocytes[13].

The surgeon, meanwhile, will have introduced a fine metal catheter through the abdominal wall, replacing the sharp obturator with a blunt obturator. The surgeon then introduces it gently into the ampullary end of the Fallopian tube to a depth of 2 cm. This process is made easier by grasping the antimesenteric border of the fimbriae with a specifically designed atraumatic forceps (Rocket, London, UK), and drawing the tube upwards so that the tubal ostium becomes visible. The blunt obturator is then removed and the catheter is introduced down the cannula and the oocyte/sperm mixture is expelled into the Fallopian tube. The catheter is withdrawn and returned to the laboratory to confirm that the oocytes have been transferred. The process is completed with the contralateral tube. When the procedure has been completed, the grasping forceps, needle, trochar and laparoscope are withdrawn from the peritoneal cavity and the abdomen is decompressed. Every effort is made to remove the remaining gas to prevent postoperative discomfort and shoulder-tip referred pain.

The major problems associated with the procedure are the unexpected finding of adhesions which may obscure the ovary, bleeding and endometriosis. Proper selection of patients can minimize the occurrence of such complications.

## *In vitro* fertilization

### *Controlled ovarian hyperstimulation: historical perspective*

Until the late 1980s, the most common ovarian stimulation regimen used in assisted conception was a combination of clomiphene citrate (an oestrogen antagonist, see Chapter 8) and exogenous gonadotrophin preparations. The rationale for this regimen is the defeat of oestrogen-driven negative feedback on endogenous gonadotrophin secretion. Acting at hypothalamic and pituitary levels, clomiphene citrate provokes a mild hypersecretion of pituitary gonadotrophins. If clomiphene citrate is given early in the cycle, it will stimulate the recruitment of a number of small follicles. The subsequent administration of exogenous gonadotrophins will then sustain the growth of this cohort of recruited follicles[14].

The inherent problem with this protocol is the unpredictability of the LH surge. One study showed that 20% of patients treated with clomiphene citrate and human menopausal gonadotrophin (hMG) had a pre-emptive endogenous LH surge, when using a leading follicular mean diameter of between 18 and 20 mm as the criterion for induction of ovulation[15]. Macnamee has shown, from elegant studies at Bourn Hall Clinic, that patients who established a clinical pregnancy had a significantly lower urinary LH output in the 2 days prior to ovulation induction (Figure 5).

A more detailed analysis has shown that a link exists between oocyte quality and the mean tonic urinary LH output in the late follicular phase. Failure of fertilization solely attributable to poor oocyte quality (as assessed by light microscopy) correlates with higher late follicular phase LH levels than those solely attributable to sperm factors (Table 1).

*GnRHa/FSH long protocol for controlled ovarian hyperstimulation*

It is clear that high levels of tonic LH can severely compromise oocyte quality and subsequent pregnancy rates. Conversely, low tonic LH levels result in better oocyte quality and higher fertilization/implantation rates.

A hypothalamic factor which controls the release of LH and follicle stimulating hormone (FSH) was first postulated in 1955[16]. Fifteen

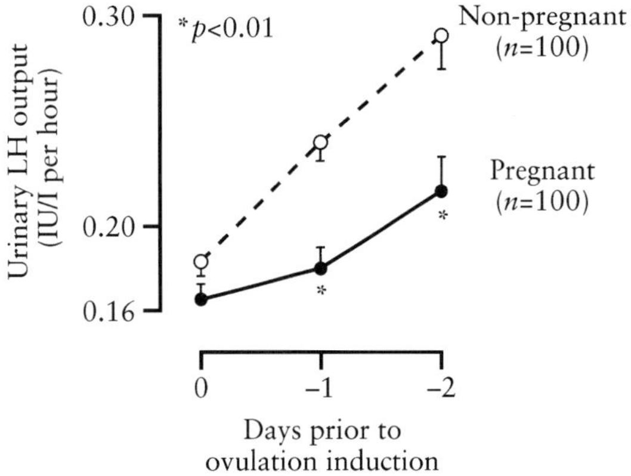


**Figure 5** Profiles of urinary LH output in pregnant and non-pregnant IVF patients

**Table 1** Mean (± SEM) late follicular phase LH levels (IU/l per hour) and ascribed reason for failure of fertilization

| *Ascribed cause* | *n* | *Urinary LH* |
|---|---|---|
| Poor oocyte quality | 25 | $0.31 \pm 0.04^{*\dagger}$ |
| Poor sperm quality | 25 | $0.20 \pm 0.03^{*}$ |
| Other non-oocyte problems | 10 | $0.22 \pm 0.03$ |
| Unknown | 25 | $0.21 \pm 0.04^{\dagger}$ |

$^{*}p < 0.01$; $^{\dagger}p < 0.01$

years later, the decapeptide luteinizing hormone releasing hormone (LHRH) was isolated and chemically characterized. LHRH (more recently known as GnRH (gonadotrophin releasing hormone)) and its analogues have become widely available for clinical use, and a number of applications have been described, including the induction of puberty with pulsatile GnRHa stimulation (see Chapter 3).

As GnRHa has become more widely available for clinical use, a number of therapeutic applications have been described. These include the treatment of hypothalamic hypogonadism and of course, by natural progression, in ovulation induction programmes as a down-regulating agent. One of the most commonly used GnRH agonists is buserelin (Suprefact, Hoechst UK Ltd, Hounslow, UK) given by s.c. injection starting on either day 1 or 21 of a 28-day cycle (Figure 6). Gonadotrophin releasing hormone agonists can also be administered as a nasal spray (Synarel) or as a long-acting depot injection (Prostap 3.75 mg) or in s.c. pellet form (goserelin 3.6 mg). All have the effect of desensitizing the pituitary gland. After initial administration of the analogue in whatever form it is given, there is a 400-fold rise in circulating levels of LH and a 40-fold rise in circulating FSH levels. As administration is continued, there follows a decrease in pituitary sensitivity to native LHRH, and a decrease in the synthesis and release of the gonadotrophins (Figure 7).

Once down-regulation has been accomplished by whatever method, oocyte recovery can be scheduled by delaying the administration of gonadotrophins. Normally 10–12 days of gonadotrophin administration is sufficient to reach the criteria for ovulation induction (at least three follicles with a mean diameter of 18 mm or greater) and also ensure adequate

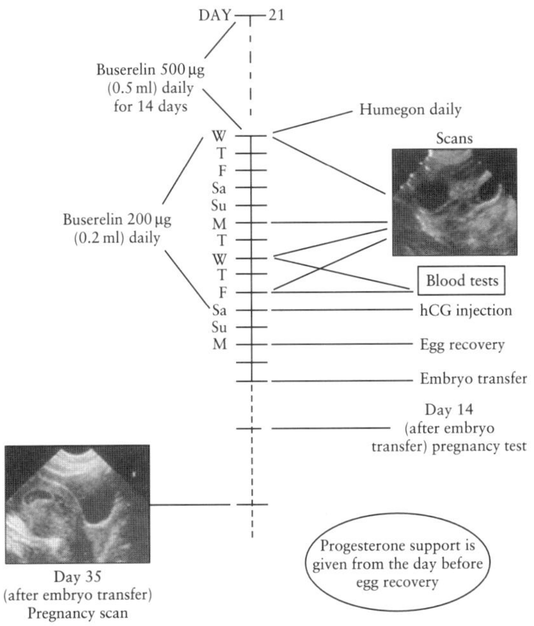


**Figure 6** Summary diagram of IVF protocol. The protocol may be adjusted to suit the response of individual patients

oestrogen priming for the endometrium. As the flow chart shows (Figure 6), Puregon (see Chapter 29) at a dose of 150 IU per day is started on a Wednesday. By the following Saturday week (day 11 of stimulation), the leading follicles will typically have reached 18 mm in diameter. Human chorionic gonadotrophin (Pregnyl, Organon Labs Ltd, Milton, Cambs, UK) is given by deep intramuscular injection on Saturday night. This is timed at 34.5 h before the oocyte retrieval on Monday morning at a dose of 5000–10 000 IU. Not every patient responds to gonadotrophin administration in the same way, so that some oocyte retrievals may have to be scheduled for Tuesday or Wednesday mornings, or occasionally brought forward to Sunday morning if follicular growth exceeds the normal 1.5–2.0 mm per day. The dose of hCG depends on day 10 oestrogen levels. These are serum measurements in pmol/l. As an approximation, 1000 pmol/l of oestrogen equates to one oocyte; therefore 10 000 pmol/l should equate to ten oocytes being recovered. As a rule of thumb this works well, but is not always accurate. If levels are greater than 10 000 pmol/l, then only 5000 IU of hCG are given (see below on oestradiol assays). The technique of transvaginal ultrasound-directed oocyte retrieval is described later in this chapter, and the detailed laboratory techniques of oocyte and sperm preparations are described in Chapter 13.

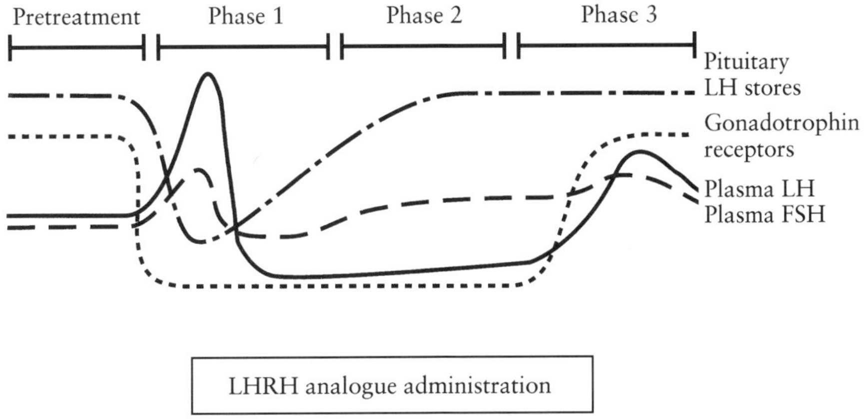


**Figure 7** The luteinizing hormone releasing hormone (LHRH) agonists and endogenous gonadotrophin levels

*Oestrogen assays*

The system used to assay serum oestrogen levels at BUPA Roding Hospital is the Mini Vidas (bioMerieux UK Ltd, Basingstoke, UK). This is a compact immunoanalyser with an integrated computer, screen, keyboard and printer (Figure 8). Oestrogen results are available within 20–60 min after the blood sample is received. Mini Vidas is equipped with a barcode reader (Figure 9), and the patient identification and the marker curve data are directly and easily entered. The advantage of this system can be summarized as follows:

(1) Compact and multiparametric;

(2) Completely automated;

(3) One-finger operation;

(4) Optimizes cost per patient;

(5) Same day results;

(6) Single or batch testing; and

(7) Constantly updated menu.

The Mini Vidas is also used for human immunodeficiency virus (HIV), hepatitis B and rubella assays (HIV and hepatitis B tests are mandatory for both partners going through IVF at the Roding). Because of the 60-min turn-around time, quick decisions can be made on the timing of hCG administration, for example, and patient waiting time is kept to a minimum.

*Ultrasound-directed oocyte recovery*

At the Roding, ultrasound-directed oocyte recovery (Figures 10 and 11) is performed under intravenous sedation (Fentanyl or Midazolam; doses 100 μg and 10 mg, respectively) administered by a consultant anaesthetist. The operating theatre set-up consists of monitoring equipment pulse oximeter and $pO_2$ monitor (it is vital to have a continuous readout of the patient's oxygen saturation when she is under intravenous sedation), emergency oxygen supply and face mask and cardiac resuscitation equipment. The patient is placed on the operating table in the lithotomy position and intravenous sedation is introduced through an intravenous catheter in the back of the hand. The vulva and vagina are rinsed with normal saline and drapes are applied.

Currently at the Roding, a Sonoline Prima with a variable two-frequency (5 and 7.5 MHz) vaginal probe is used (Figure 12). The transducer is covered with a Mates condom (Mates Healthcare Ltd, Surbiton, Surrey KT6 6AL) with about 2 ml of ultrasound gel placed on the end of the probe *before* fitting the condom. Suction and flushing is provided by the equipment shown in Figure 13 attached to the Pivet-Cook double lumen needle (Cook UK Ltd, Letchworth, Herts, UK). More details of this equipment are shown in Figures 14 and 15. Figure 16 shows the Cook test tube heater for sterile Falcon tubes prior to transfer through to the lab. Since the introduction of this system, oocytes are consistently retrieved from 90% of follicles aspirated[17].

The vaginal probe is introduced into the vagina with the needle guide (Rainsbury–Cook needle guide, Figure 17) attached. The pelvis is carefully scanned and the following noted: endometrial thickness, the position and accessibility of the ovaries and the number of follicles to be aspirated. The Pivet–Cook double lumen needle is inserted through the guide (Figure 18) and the probe is directed towards the posterolateral aspect of the vaginal fornix. Ideally only about 1 cm of tissue should separate the needle tip (which is ultrasound-opaque) and the ovarian capsule. The needle is thrust firmly through the lateral vaginal fornix into the ovarian stroma and into the nearest follicle, which is then aspirated until empty.

The clear follicular fluid is collected in a Falcon tube (Becton Dickinson UK Ltd, Falcon Labware, Cowley, Oxford, UK) and passed through the hatch into the embryology laboratory for identification of the oocyte (Figure 19) by the embryologist. If the embryologist fails to identify an oocyte in the first aspirate, the flushing continues using an equal volume of Earle's medium (Earle's with heparin, Chapter 13) up to a maximum of five to six flushes. Gentle curettage of the follicle by the needle tip may assist separation of the oocyte from the cumulus oophorus. Mobile ovaries can be stabilized by

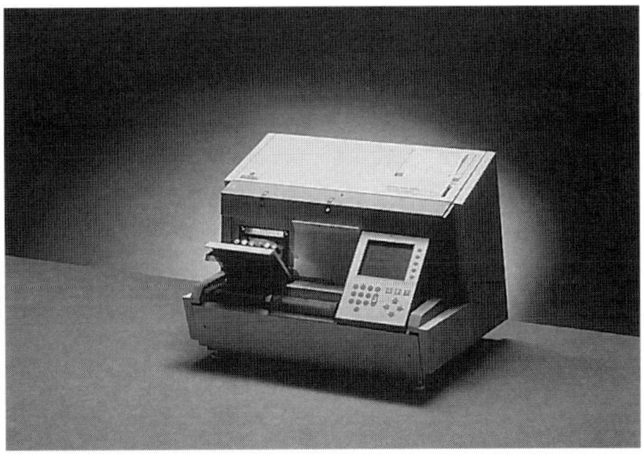

**Figure 8** Mini Vidas immunoanalyser

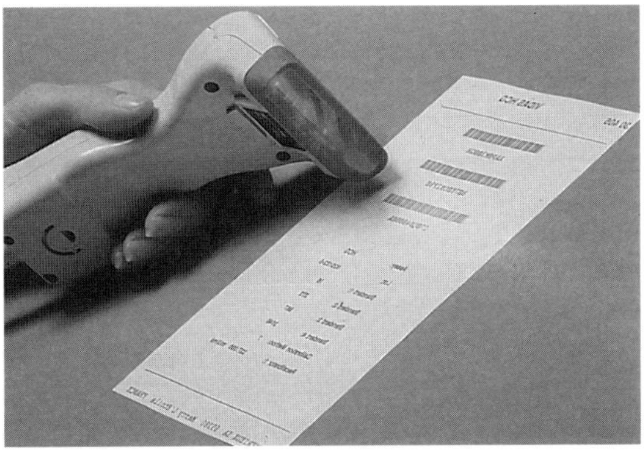

**Figure 9** Bar-code reader for Mini Vidas immunoanalyser

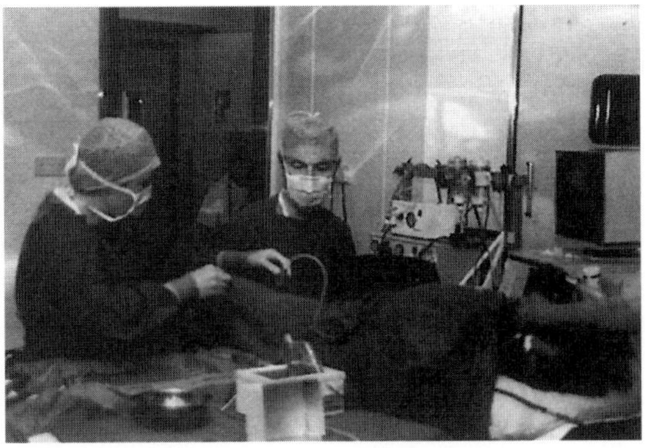

**Figure 10** Transvaginal oocyte recovery

the operator's assistant pressing on the left or right lower abdominal quadrant until the needle enters the ovarian stroma and accesses the follicles. When one ovary has been aspirated, the operator then turns his attention to the other. The author usually starts on the left side

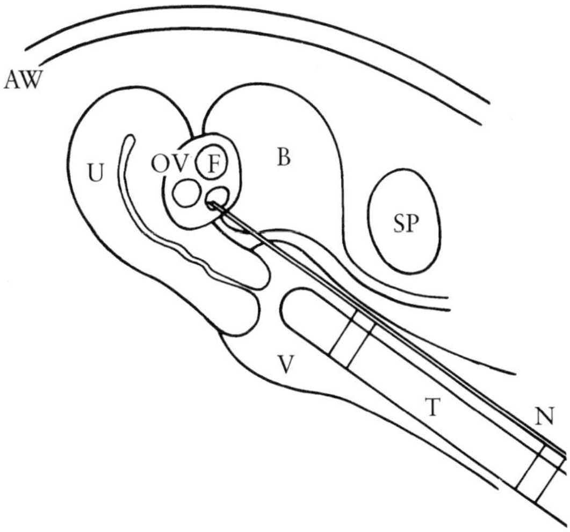


**Figure 11** Transvaginal oocyte recovery using a vaginal ultrasound probe with attached needle guide. T, transducer; AW, abdominal wall; B, bladder; SP, symphysis pubis; OV, ovary; F, follicles; U, uterus; V, vagina; N, needle

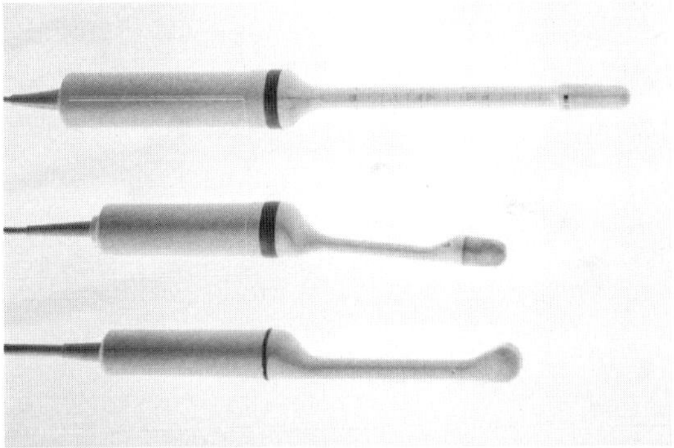

**Figure 12** Vaginal probes

(being right-handed) and then moves onto the right ovary. All visible oocytes are aspirated. The number of puncture sites in the vaginal vault is kept to a minimum to prevent bleeding. The probe is removed at the completion of the procedure. Any bleeding from the puncture sites will invariably stop by using steady pressure from a sponge-holding forceps loaded with a swab. The patient is returned to the ward and she may normally go home 2–3 h following the aspiration and after she has eaten. Two hours later, the male partner produces his sample by

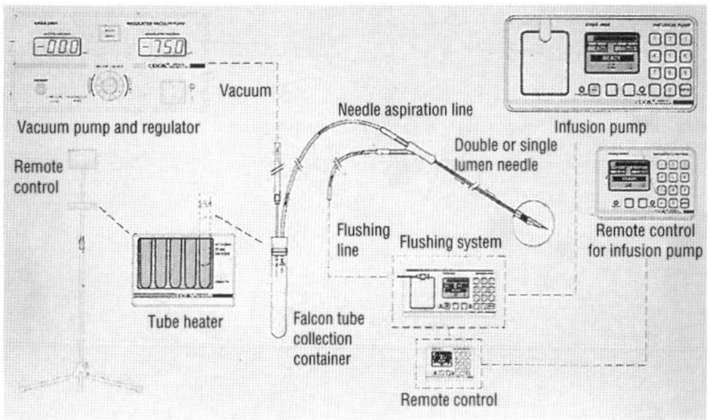


**Figure 13** Equipment for suction and flushing of oocytes

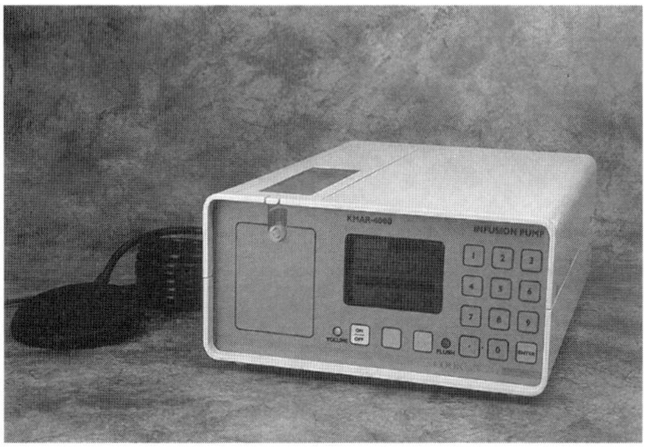


**Figure 14** Cook flushing system, K-MAR-4000 Series

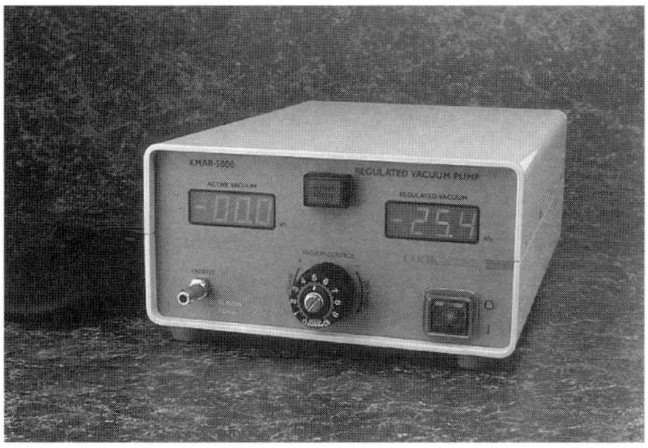


**Figure 15** Cook vacuum pump and regulator, K-MAR-5000 Series

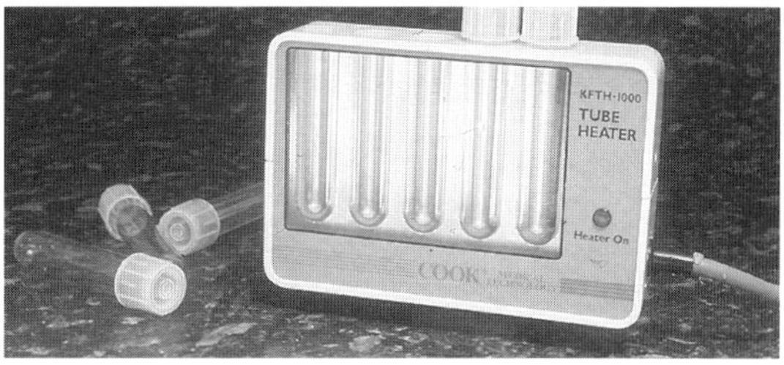


**Figure 16** Cook test tube heater, K-FTH-1000 Series

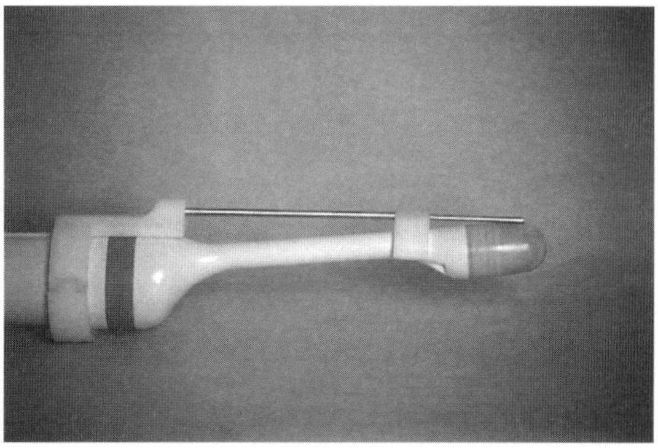

**Figure 17** Rainsbury–Cook needle guide

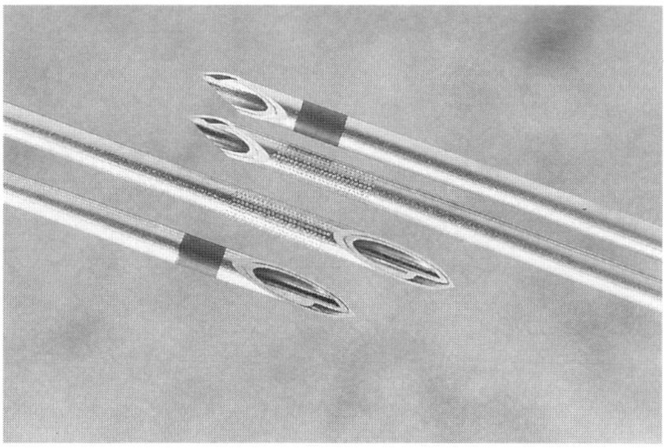

**Figure 18** Pivet–Cook double lumen needles

masturbation. This sample is carefully prepared as described in Chapter 13 and the oocytes are inseminated. The couple telephone the unit the next morning to confirm that fertilization has occurred. If there is none or the signs of fertilization are weak, then another semen sample may be required.

Vaginal ultrasound oocyte retrieval has the following advantages over the laparoscopic or transvesical methods[18]:

(1) The better image obtained with the vaginal probe, because of its closer proximity to the ovaries;

(2) Greater ease of use and shorter learning phase;

(3) Less pain, because the bladder wall is not pierced, thus necessitating less analgesia and sedation, with a consequently quicker return to normal activity;

(4) Because of the better visualization of the ovaries and of the smaller follicles, more oocytes are recovered, more embryos are available to transfer and freeze and therefore higher pregnancy rates have, in general, been reported;

(5) Because there is no need to catheterize the bladder or pass the aspirating needle through it, there is much less chance of dysuria, infection or haematuria than after transabdominal–transvesical ultrasound-directed oocyte recovery;

(6) Less risk of perforation of a viscus because of the proximity of the ovaries to the vaginal vault; and

(7) Much better patient acceptance, because it is less painful than laparoscopic oocyte recovery, both intraoperatively and post-operatively.

*Ultrasound-directed embryo transfer*

This technique has changed little since the early days of IVF. Figure 20 shows the Wallace embryo replacement catheter (Portex Ltd, Hythe, Kent, UK). This was originally designed by Professor R. Edwards and has been refined over the years.

Embryo transfer is carried out in the operating theatre under transabdominal ultrasound control, with a full bladder. The technique is shown in Figure 21 and the Edwards-Wallace catheter in Figure 20. Partners are encouraged to attend the embryo transfer mainly to provide the female partner with psychological support. The identity of the patient is checked on the name-tag by the accompanying nurse, and the gynaecologist and embryologist all counter-sign the case records to prevent any possible errors. The embryologist has a detailed discussion with the couple about the number and quality of fresh embryos being transferred to the uterus and the number, if any, which are of sufficient quality to freeze. The patient is placed in the lithotomy position in mild Trendelenberg. An appropriately-sized speculum is inserted into the vagina until a good view of the cervix is obtained. More recently the author has been carrying out a 'dummy-run' or trial catheterization on all patients on the conclusion of their oocyte recovery in order to assess the suitability of the cervix and endocervical canal for subsequent embryo transfer. The cervix is exposed and gently cleaned with swabs soaked in normal saline. The embryos are identified, scored and their details entered by the embryologist into a log (for further details see Chapter 13).

The author's preference is the Edwards/Wallace catheter (Figure 20). This has now been improved by using a stiff introducer for tight cervices. The catheter consists of a double-lumen system with a flexible outer sheath and a fine teflon inner catheter into which the embryos are loaded. A 1 ml tuberculin syringe is fitted to the catheter which is filled with medium. The embryos are then drawn up by the embryologist (Chapter 13) making a total volume of about 20 µl to be transferred. The catheter is passed through the hatch to the surgeon after dimming the theatre lights. Under abdominal ultrasound control the tip of the catheter is passed through the endocervical canal and into the endometrial cavity. It may sometimes be necessary to introduce the stiffer outer sheath first if the cervix is tight. If this fails, then a tenaculum forceps is applied to the cervix, particularly if this has been indicated in the previous 'dummy-run'. In very few cases it may be necessary to revert to sedation or general anaesthesia in order to cannulate the endocervical canal. Very occasionally it may prove necessary to 'freeze all embryos' and replace them in a frozen embryo transfer cycle[18] following cervical dilatation and hysteroscopy under general anaesthesia. After confirming that the tip of the catheter is approximately 1 cm from the uterine fundus, the embryologist

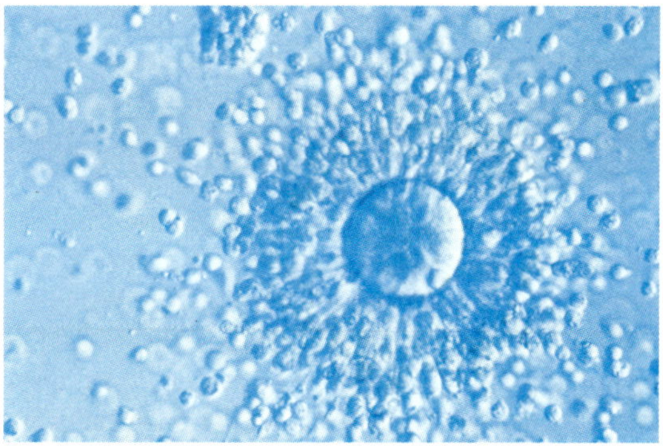

**Figure 19** Mature oocyte

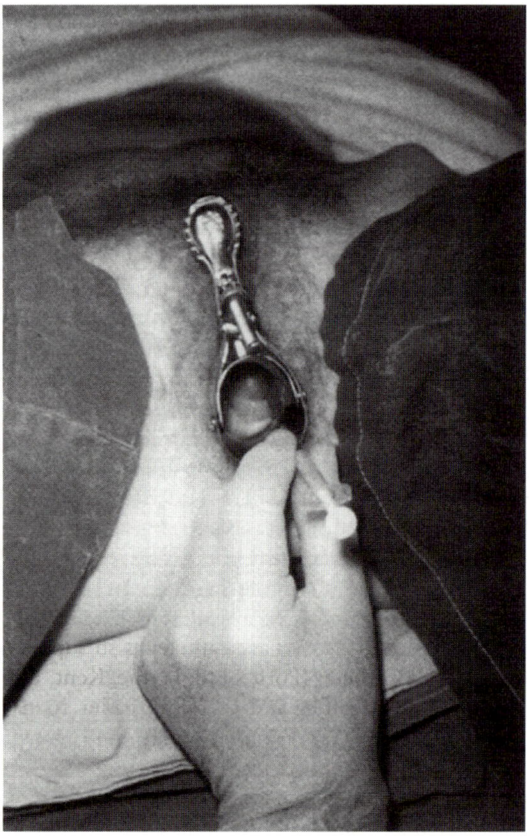

**Figure 21** Embryo transfer using a Bourn Hall catheter (Portex Ltd, Hythe, UK)

gently injects the embryo into the uterus. The ultrasound picture is frozen so that the patient can see the screen afterwards.

The empty catheter is returned to the laboratory to check that all the embryos have been

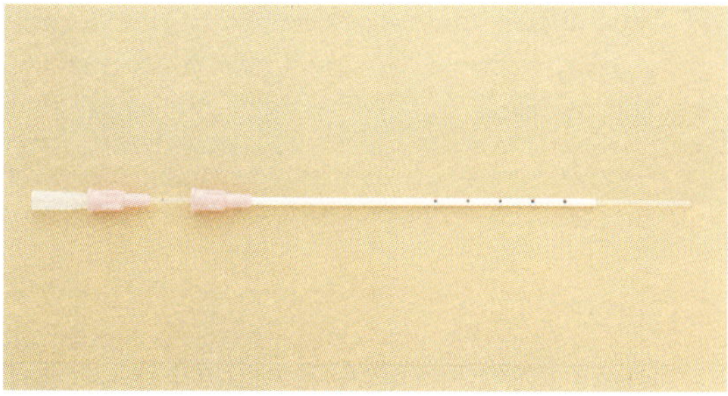

**Figure 20** Wallace embryo replacement catheter

discharged. Occasionally it may be necessary to repeat the procedure if one or more embryos are retained. The patient then lies flat on her back for 30 min before emptying her bladder and going home.

*Luteal support following administration of GnRHa, controlled ovarian hyperstimulation and IVF*

Gonadotropin releasing hormone agonists are now frequently used for pituitary desensitization during IVF treatment cycles in order to decrease the cancellation rate and increase the number of follicles being recruited following controlled ovarian hyperstimulation[19].

Luteal phase support is beneficial in terms of pregnancy rates but it is less clear what form this luteal phase support should take[20]. Progesterone is critical for implantation[21], because it induces secretory changes in the endometrium, thus allowing implantation to occur. However, serum progesterone levels do not always correlate well with histological findings[22]. Following GnRHa administration there is a fall in endogenous gonadotrophin levels which may then be insufficient to maintain the corpus luteum[23,24]. If there is no luteal support in down-regulated cycles there is a drop in both serum progesterone and oestrogen levels, and endometrial biopsies suggest defective luteal phases[23].

The main routes of administration of progesterone support, which is normally started on the day following hCG administration, are as follows:

(1) Oral;

(2) Vaginal;

(3) Rectal; and

(4) Intramuscular.

Oral medication consists of Utrogestan 100 mg (Besins Iscovesco, Paris, France), usually two tablets three times a day. Although this route is most acceptable to patients, poor bioavailability due to first pass metabolism makes oral medication impractical[25]. Serum levels of progesterone were similar when measured following rectal and vaginal administration, but patients required four times the dose by these routes when compared to intramuscular administration[26].

Cyclogest vaginal pessaries (Hoechst UK Ltd., Hounslow, UK), which can also be used rectally, are given in a dose of 400 mg twice daily. Gestone (Ferring Pharmaceuticals Ltd., Feltham, UK) is normally given in a dose of 50 mg intramuscularly daily, but this can be increased to 100 mg if endometrial response is unsatisfactory. Allergies to gestone are not uncommon, and so therefore the route of administration may have to be changed.

A pregnancy test on early morning urine is carried out 15 days later using the Clearview hCG kit. If the line turns blue, then a blood sample is taken to measure the β-hCG level. The author has seen a continuing pregnancy at a level as low as 18 U/l, but usually successful clinical pregnancies are associated with levels of β-hCG greater than 50 U/l. Higher levels (e.g. 200–300 or more) may indicate the presence of a multiple implantation. Following this, a day 35 scan (7 weeks gestational age) is carried out vaginally to confirm the presence of a clinical pregnancy. The crown–rump length measures around 10 mm at this stage; also the number of sacs are identified, and the presence of a fetal heart beat (see Chapter 5 for more details).

## OVARIAN HYPERSTIMULATION SYNDROME

Severe ovarian hyperstimulation syndrome (OHSS) is a life-threatening complication of gonadotrophin therapy[27–31]. An effort is made in all controlled ovarian hyperstimulation programmes to achieve a moderate number (usually eight to ten) of mature oocytes. Occasionally this gets out of control, and severe OHSS results. Fortunately, critical OHSS is uncommon. Asch and colleagues[32] reported an overall incidence of 1% for severe OHSS. However, when OHSS was accompanied by oestradiol levels of > 22 000 pmol/l, the incidence of severe OHSS rose to 38%. Navot and coworkers[33] suggested two degrees of OHSS, severe and critical, which, like any simple method of classification, is probably the best.

According to this classification, generalized oedema and liver dysfunction should be considered signs of severe OHSS, whereas adult respiratory distress syndrome, a tense ascitic situation combined with severe haemoconcentration, are signs of the most severe life-threatening form of critical OHSS.

The basic disturbance in OHSS is a shift of fluid from the intravascular into the extravascular space, creating a massive third space. This results in profuse ascites[33]. The pathophysiology of this shift is unclear but the following mechanisms have been postulated.

(1) Animal experiments have implicated a role for vasoactive substances such as histamine[34].

(2) Prostaglandins[35,36].

(3) Angiotensin.

(4) An intermediate factor, possibly released by hyperstimulated ovaries at ovulation, may be responsible for increased local capillary permeability, leading to leakage of fluid from the peritoneal capillaries. Human serum albumin (see below) used by the author to treat the condition may bind and inactivate this unknown factor, thus preventing the severe stages of OHSS developing[37]. The Royal College of Obstetricians and Gynaecologists take the condition of OHSS seriously enough to warrant issuing guidelines for its management and prevention. It is appropriate to quote part of these guidelines below.

**Management**

Continued management is supportive whilst waiting for the condition to resolve spontaneously. The main aims of management are to:

(1) Provide reassurance and symptomatic relief to the patient;

(2) Avoid haemoconcentration;

(3) Prevent thromboembolism; and

(4) Maintain cardiorespiratory and renal function.

Often patients are admitted to their nearest hospital and not the unit initiating treatment. Contact with the treating unit for exact details of drug regimens, etc. is advisable as soon as possible, followed by liaison with them on management.

Features to note on examination include:

(1) General state of hydration;

(2) Chest – difficulty in breathing, pleural or pericardial effusion;

(3) Abdomen – degree of distension; and

(4) Evidence of thromboembolism.

Initial investigations (and as necessary) include an ultrasound scan of the ovaries (dimensions), abdomen (ascites) and chest for pleural/pericardial effusions. A shielded chest X-ray (if dyspnoeic) should be carried out. In addition, haemoglobin and haematocrit, urea and electrolytes, albumin and LFTs should be investigated and a clotting factor screen carried out.

Nursing observations should include blood pressure, pulse, temperature (4-hourly), weight, abdominal girth (daily) and a strict fluid input/output chart should be kept. Urinary catheterization should be considered.

*Basic treatment*

Analgesia/antiemetics should be used as required. Preferred drugs would be paracetamol, paracetamol + codeine and/or diclofenac sodium. Indomethacin has been used by some workers in the treatment for OHSS with good results in order to block prostaglandin synthesis and prevent fluid shifts associated with OHSS; however, it is not recommended as a routine treatment. Metoclopramide or stemetil for nausea or vomiting are helpful (these can be given rectally). Full-length TED® (anti-embolism) stockings should be used to reduce venous thrombosis risk. Oral fluid intake should be encouraged if the patient is not vomiting. This may be sufficient in moderate cases if the patient is not significantly hypovolaemic, otherwise an intravenous drip should be erected. Human chorionic gonadotrophin support should be reduced if it is being given and changed to progesterone administration intramuscularly or Cyclogest per vaginum/per rectum.

*Maintenance of intravascular volume*

Initially, the aim is to replace fluids in the vascular compartment sufficiently to allow resumption of normal urine production (> 30 ml/h). Therefore, the intravenous infusion chosen depends on the type and extent of the intravascular disturbance. As a rough guide, if serum albumin is greater than 32 g/l and haemoglobin less than 14 g/dl, crystalloid solutions approximately 3 l in 24 h should be administered. Normal saline is the preferred crystalloid. Often patients become hyperkalaemic, and therefore potassium-containing fluids should be avoided.

If the serum albumin is less than 30 g/l, haemoglobin greater than 16 g/dl or serum urea greater than 6.0 mmol/l, solutions more effective at expanding the intravascular volume are preferred. Albumin 2 U followed by normal saline 2 l over 18–24 h should be given initially with future fluid replacement dependent upon response to the above and assessment of daily investigations. Other colloid solutions such as dextran or hydroxyethyl starch can be used (both have a small risk of anaphylactic reaction and need to be administered carefully with close monitoring).

*Diuretics*

These should be avoided as they remove fluid from the vascular compartment only.

*Surgery*
This should be avoided if at all possible but laparotomy may be necessary if there is marked haemorrhage or rupture of the cysts. These are difficult features to detect but a sudden fall in packed cell volume without a change in other indices of haemoconcentration indicates haemorrhage.

*Abdominal paracentesis*
Drainage of ascites or pleural effusions is symptomatically helpful if these are marked or in the presence of respiratory distress. Abdominal paracentesis should be performed under ultrasound control to avoid damage to the bowel or ovaries. Be aware that the ascites may rapidly reaccumulate and that paracentesis may accelerate protein loss, but this is rarely of clinical significance and should not deter the use of paracentesis in symptomatic relief when ascites is excessive.

*Anticoagulation*
This is of value if there is evidence of thromboembolism. Prophylactic subcutaneous heparin and TED stockings will be beneficial in severe forms of the disorder, even in the absence of thromboembolism.

*Termination of pregnancy*
Pregnancy has been terminated in extremely severe cases of OHSS to save the patient's life, but should rarely be necessary.

*Prevention of OHSS*
Several measures can be employed to prevent OHSS but there are numerous reasons why even the most careful and painstaking preventative measures cannot eliminate OHSS.

(1) There are no absolute criteria for the identification of the patient at risk but certain subgroups, as discussed, have a higher incidence.

(2) Careful monitoring of serum oestradiol and use of ultrasound screening to determine numbers of primary and secondary cohorts of follicles developing is essential (refer to RCOG Guideline No 2 on Ovulation Induction (April 1994)).

(3) Consideration must be given to cancellation of cycles (prior to hCG administration) if there are excessively high serum oestradiol values or large numbers of maturing follicles. Whilst regimens of oocyte collection and cryopreservation of all resultant embryos have been described, such an approach cannot be viewed as a complete prevention of OHSS.

(4) Education of patients towards recognition at an early stage of the symptoms of possible development of OHSS may be useful in identifying cases early. Provision of appropriate contact persons and telephone numbers is helpful should the patient or her general practitioner be concerned.

(5) Careful monitoring, in the luteal phase of presumed 'at risk' patients (e.g. multiple follicles, high oestradiol levels) may identify patients developing OHSS. Patients should be asked to weigh themselves daily. If weight increases by more than 5 kg, they should contact the unit.

(6) Consideration should be given to the use of progesterone in place of hCG for luteal phase support but particularly in 'at risk' patients.

'Coasting' is an effective method of preventing severe OHSS. When preovulatory peak oestradiol levels exceed 6000 pg/ml ($2.2 \times 10^4$ pmol/l) and more than 29 follicles are seen on the ultrasound scan, the subsequent risk of OHSS is greater than 80%[32]. Sher and associates in 1993[38] described an alternative approach to this problem which involved stopping gonadotrophin therapy, while continuing GnRHa therapy until oestradiol levels fell below 3000 pg/ml ($1.1 \times 10^4$ pmol/l) and then administering hCG when follicles had reached the appropriate size. This method avoided the need to cancel the IVF cycle, whilst eliminating the risk of OHSS subsequently developing. More recently, the same group, in a further study, confirmed that prolonged coasting prevents the occurrence of severe OHSS, or compromises IVF success rates[39].

## OOCYTE DONATION

The first human pregnancy using donated sperm was reported in 1884. Another century was to pass before a pregnancy using a donated embryo was reported[40].

Buster and co-workers[41] adopted a different approach by transferring embryos fertilized *in vivo* and obtained by uterine lavage of fertile donors after artificial insemination. Other centres subsequently developed alternative transfer techniques. For example, Asch extended his work on GIFT to include donated oocytes[42]. Yovich introduced the tubal transfer of zygotes (ZIFT)[43]. The first reported oocyte donation pregnancy was reported by Van Steirteghem[44] using the technique of frozen–thawed embryo transfer.

Serhal and Craft[45] described one of the most important advances in simplifying the steroid replacement regimen. Several different replacement protocols are now available. Brinsden and Avery have covered these in detail in Chapter 15.

Since that time, oocyte donation has become an established fertility treatment in women with ovarian failure, certain genetic disorders, advancing age, or previously failed IVF. The HFEA currently registers 46 IVF units to perform oocyte donation. This figure comprises 58% of all IVF units in the UK.

### Ethical and legal issues

Oocyte donation, when compared to other tissue donations, involves rather different considerations. If treatment is successful, the child born will be genetically that of the donor, and the child will pass these genes to the next and subsequent generations. These clinical and legal aspects are considered in Chapter 16. Oocyte donation is clearly different from sperm donation as the donor has to go through a 'mini-IVF' treatment cycle with all the associated risks of gonadotrophin therapy, as detailed earlier in this chapter.

A prospective donor should be counselled very carefully with regard to clinical risks and side-effects of treatment. She then signs a consent form in which she relinquishes any legal claims over any offspring which may result from her donation. The donor is then matched to a recipient in terms of physical characteristics and blood group. There is a natural shortage of egg donors, and often recipient waiting lists are years long[46]. The HFEA recommends that donors should be younger than 35 to reduce the incidence of fetal abnormality in the recipient.

Once the screening and consent procedure are completed, a conventional IVF cycle is started. At the BUPA Roding Hospital, this involves pituitary desensitization with the GnRHa from day 21 of the menstrual cycle. Once pituitary down-regulation has been achieved, gonadotrophin therapy is commenced. Serum oestradiol levels are closely monitored, together with serial vaginal ultrasound scans to monitor follicular growth to ensure adequate controlled ovarian hyperstimulation. Ultrasound-directed vaginal oocyte recovery is performed under intravenous sedation 34.5 h following appropriately timed administration of hCG. Despite all this inconvenience and discomfort, egg donors can only claim their legitimate travelling expenses as directed by the HFEA.

### Recipient screening

Oocyte recipients also need careful counselling prior to egg donation. In some instances, a trial cycle of hormone replacement therapy (HRT) is carried out in order to assess endometrial response. Menopausal women stop their HRT for 1 month, then begin Progynova (oestradiol valerate, Schering Health Care Ltd., Burgess Hill, UK) 2 mg three times daily for 16 days, adding in on day 16 gestone 50 mg for 2 days, increasing the strength to 100 mg on day 18 (which would equate to the day of embryo transfer in the actual donor/recipient cycle). Premenopausal women are put on the buserelin/HRT protocol 1 month prior to starting the treatment cycle. Measurement of endometrial response, in terms of thickness and 'halo effect', is performed, usually around day 18.

The treatment cycle starts when the donor begins the gonadotrophin stimulation stage, and on that day her recipient commences oestrogen. Progesterone is given to her the day after hCG is administered to the donor. At the BUPA Roding Hospital, we mainly carry out fresh embryo transfers. Recipients are carefully counselled regarding the risks of HIV infection from a fresh embryo transfer (as opposed to a frozen transfer, when repeat 6-monthly quarantine HIV testing can be carried out). Fresh embryo transfer follows 2 days after donor oocyte retrieval, and after the donor eggs have been exposed to the recipient's partner's appropriately-prepared sperm. Hormonal support continues until a pregnancy test 15 days following embryo transfer. If this later proves positive, then hormonal support is continued until the day 35 vaginal scan (equivalent to 7 weeks of gestational age). Intramuscular gestone can then be replaced by either oral, vaginal or rectal progesterone support (see earlier in this chapter).

Amenorrhoeic women are reported to have higher pregnancy rates in donor egg programmes when compared to normally menstruating women (48 vs. 20%[47]).

Donor oocyte programmes have allowed us to monitor pregnancies in groups of women who would not otherwise become pregnant. Many successful pregnancies in older postmenopausal women have been reported[48] without any significant increase in fetal complications, but with an increase in maternal complications such as pre-eclampsia.

### The future of oocyte donation

Oocyte donation has become a very successful means of treating many couples who would not otherwise achieve a pregnancy. The demand for donors is on the increase. In future, *in vivo* maturation of oocytes and possibly the use of fetal tissue may obviate the need for altruistic egg donors. Further research into the genetics of premature ovarian failure may also lead to new treatment strategies, making egg donation unnecessary.

## SURROGACY

This technique represents one of the most contentious treatments in the whole area of ART. It has been rightly described as a 'mine-field' of human emotion.

In this sector the author is primarily concerned with IVF surrogacy where embryos of the genetic couple are transferred to the uterus of the host (surrogate) as compared to 'commercial surrogacy' where the host is inseminated with the sperm of the commissioning couple's husband.

There are certain basic principles which need to be considered in any surrogacy arrangement.

(1) The clinical indication of host surrogacy must be clearly defined and presented to the ethics committee for approval.

(2) Independent legal advice should be taken by genetic and host couples.

(3) Careful and extensive counselling should be provided.

(4) Change in parentage of the resulting child by the commissioning couple (HFE Act, Section 30) or, if unmarried, not domiciled in the UK, or no genetic relationship adoption.

### Clinical indications

(1) *Absent uterus* This will include congenital absence of the uterus, blind or double uterus and hysterectomy. In such cases there is little or no chance that the woman can carry a child.

(2) *Recurrent miscarriage* Habitual abortion is a distressing condition and is an indication for carrying out surrogacy.

(3) *Pregnancy contraindications* These will include essential hypertension, severe

pre-eclampsia in a previous pregnancy, cardiac disease, renal impairment and severe blood dyscrasias.

(4) *Repeated failure of infertility treatment* At BUPA Roding this is the most common indication for surrogacy. The Ethics Committee applies an age restriction to this category – 37 years for the genetic woman and 35 years for the host.

(5) *Premature menopause* In certain circumstances, surrogacy would be indicated in women with premature menopause, in preference to oocyte donation. Occasionally the surrogate host can also act as an egg donor.

The following guidelines apply to all cases of surrogacy.

(1) Clinics who are considering surrogacy should not be involved in initiating or making arrangements between potential genetic parents and host couple.

(2) The relationship between genetic couple and host should be carefully considered. The British Medical Association's guideline No. 8[49] suggests that the two should not know each other. However, sister-to-sister surrogacy in the author's experience is very successful and would seem to refute this guideline. Counselling must be available to help families understand that future relationships within the family could be difficult; for example, reciprocity, where the commissioning genetic sister continually feels obliged to repay the debt.

(3) Independent counselling must be made available to both genetic and host couples. This is best done within the home setting so that all the issues and emotions can be explored in a natural setting. Advice should be taken from the general practitioners of both couples.

The counsellor should consider the following points with regard to surrogacy:

(1) The effect on the host;

(2) The effect on any existing children;

(3) The effect on family and friends;

(4) The hand-over of the child following delivery from host to genetic parents;

(5) The effect of any genetic abnormalities of the baby;

(6) The motives of the host;

(7) The risk of miscarriage in the host;

(8) Multiple pregnancies in the host; and

(9) Intercourse at the time of embryo transfer in the host during the early part of a subsequent pregnancy.

### Take-home-baby rates for BUPA Roding Hospital

Figure 22 is published in the 1996 edition of the HFEA's *The Patient's Guide to DI and IVF Clinics*, second edition. The same information is illustrated graphically in Chapter 19.

## THE ROLE OF THE HFEA

This is discussed in detail in Chapter 20 to which the author refers his readers. In the HFEA code of practice, reference is made to the welfare of the child in all licensed fertility treatments. 'A clinic must take account of the welfare of any child who may be born as a result of the treatment (including the need of that child for a father), and of any other child who may be affected by the birth'. A consent form (Figure 23) is given to all patients undergoing fertility treatment at the author's hospital.

The HFEA has now been in existence for 5 years having been established in 1991 by the Human Fertilisation and Embryology Act. It continues to be one of the few bodies in the world regulating the practice of reproductive technologies. The Authority keeps under constant review all relevant development and any new techniques (such as intracytoplasmic sperm injection (ICSI), see Chapters 14 and 30).

## In vitro fertilization treatments

**Adjusted live birth rates for stimulated fresh embryo IVF only***

| | |
|---|---|
| Per treatment cycle started | 17.9% ranging from 12.0% to 25.2% |
| Per egg collection | 18.8% ranging from 12.6% to 26.4% |
| Per embryo transfer | 21.6% ranging from 14.5% to 30.0% |

**The adjusted rates are calculated excluding micromanipulation cycles (such as ICSI), unstimulated cycles, frozen embryo transfers and treatments with donated eggs and embryos*

**Results for all IVF treatments†**

| | |
|---|---|
| Patients treated | 157 |
| Total number of treatment cycles | 211 |
| Number of stimulated treatment cycles | 135 |
| Number of treatment cycles where two embryos were transferred | 38 |
| Number of abandoned treatment cycles | 32 |

*†Includes micromanipulation cycles (such as ICSI), frozen embryo transfers and treatments with donated eggs and embryos*

| | |
|---|---|
| Number of singleton births | 26 |
| Number of sets of twin births | 10 |
| Number of sets of triplet births | 1 |

**Treatments with donated eggs or embryos**

| | |
|---|---|
| Number of treatment cycles with donated eggs | 23 |
| Number of treatment cycles with donated embryos | 13 |
| Number of live births | 7 |

**Frozen embryo transfers**

| | |
|---|---|
| Number of frozen embryo transfers | 43 |
| Number of live births | 5 |

## Donor insemination treatments (excluding GIFT)

Adjusted live birth rate per treatment cycle started‡

**All licensed DI treatments**

| | |
|---|---|
| Patients treated | 36 |
| Total number of treatment cycles | 92 |
| Number of stimulated treatment cycles | 56 |

| | |
|---|---|
| Number of singleton births | 11 |
| Number of sets of twin births | 0 |
| Number of sets of triplet births | 0 |

*‡A percentage rate is not given as there were too few treatments to make it meaningful*

**Figure 22** The take-home-baby rates for BUPA Roding Hospital, 1996 as published in *The Patient's Guide to DI and IVF Clinics*, 2nd edition, HFEA

### The background and history of the HFEA

The events that led to the setting up of the Human Fertilisation and Embryology Authority can be traced back to 1978 and the birth of the world's first 'test-tube' baby. Technological advances in assisted conception had raised important questions about their social and ethical implications, and the public and parliamentary debates which followed were well documented.

The notion of a statutory body to oversee the practice of certain advanced assisted conception techniques and of embryo research emerged with the publication in 1984 of the report of the Committee of Inquiry into Human Fertilisation and Embryology (the Warnock Report). After consultation and extensive debate in both Houses of Parliament, the Warnock Committee's proposals for such an Authority remained intact.

In 1985 the Medical Research Council and the Royal College of Obstetricians and Gynaecologists set up the Voluntary (later to become Interim) Licensing Authority for Human *In Vitro* Fertilisation and Embryology (ILA). It conducted an effective voluntary licensing system.

The passing of the Human Fertilisation and Embryology Act in 1990 meant that a statutory body was set up to oversee the area of assisted conception. It became the only national regulatory body in the world set up by statute to regulate fertility treatment. For the first time, an area of medicine, assisted reproduction, was to be controlled by an independent statutory body rather than by voluntary or self-regulation.

The Human Fertilisation and Embryology Authority (HFEA) took up its full powers on 1 August, 1991. It is an independent body, established by Parliament, and funded by income from its licensing of clinics and through a Government grant.

### The role of the HFEA

The principal task of the HFEA is to license and monitor those clinics that carry out *in vitro* fertilization (IVF), donor insemination (DI) and

**HFEA Register(96)1     CONFIDENTIAL     IVF TREATMENT CYCLE FORM**

1a.   HFEA centre ref. number  [ 0003 ]        1b.   Patient's clinic record number: [            ]

1c.   Name of centre where treatment started, if different: [            ]

2a.   Full name         SURNAME                                      No. [            ]
      of patient:       [            ]

                        FORENAME(S)
                        [            ]

2b.   Maiden name/or    [            ]              2c.   Date of birth:  [ 12-Dec-59 ]
      any other name:

                        2d.   UK resident:   YES ☐  NO ☒     2e.   UK postcode (first four characters) [        ]

3a.   Full name of      SURNAME
      husband/male      [            ]
      partner (if any):
                        FORENAME(S)
                        [            ]

3b.   Any other name:   [            ]              3c.   Date of birth:  [        ]

                        3d.   If male partner is named at 3a, did he attend the clinic with the patient:   YES ☐  NO ☐

4a.   Does treatment involve donated sperm:    YES ☐  NO ☒    donor's reference code: [        ]
4b.   Does treatment involve donated eggs:     YES ☐  NO ☒    donor's reference code: [        ]
4c.   Does treatment involve donated embryos:  YES ☐  NO ☐    If yes please complete 4a & 4b.
4d.   Donor(s) centre reference number(s) (if different from above) sperm donor [        ] egg donor [        ]

5.    Infertility:   Female  1^ ☐  2^ ☐      Male  1^ ☐  2^ ☐      Couple  1^ ☐  2^ ☐

6.    Female cause      Tubal disease ☐      Hydrosalpinx ☐      Anovulatory ☐      Polycystic Ovaries ☐
      of infertility:   Unexplained ☐        Other (describe) [            ]
                        Endometriosis:   Grade I ☐   Grade II ☐   Grade III ☐   Grade IV ☐

      Male cause of     Oligozoospermia ☐     Sperm concentration (×10^6/ml) [        ]
      infertility:      Asthenozoospermia ☐   % Progressively Motile [        ]
                        Teratozoospermia ☐    % Normal forms [        ]   (Criteria Kruger ☐   WHO ☐ )
                        Azoospermia ☐         Seminal antisperm antibodies [        ]
                        Other (describe) [            ]

7.    Previous obstetric history:   Total number of previous pregnancies [        ]   Total number of live births: [        ]
                        Total number of previous IVF pregnancies [ 0 ]   Total number of IVF live births: [ 0 ]
8.    Duration of infertility (unprotected intercourse (years)) [        ]   Since last pregnancy (years) [        ]
9.    Number of previous IVF treatments:   In total [        ]   At this clinic [        ]
10a.  Type of treatment   IVF ☐   ICSI ☐   Other micromanipulation (please specify) [            ]
                          Surrogacy ☐   FER ☐   Other (please specify) [            ]
10b.  Is treatment part of a clinical trial:   YES ☐  NO ☐    10c.  Does treatment involve transport IVF:  YES ☐  NO ☐
11.   Type of stimulation:   None ☐   Anti-oestrogens ☐   Gonadotrophins ☐   Other (please specify) ☐
12a.  Number eggs collected: [        ]              12b.  Number eggs exposed to sperm: [        ]
12c.  No. exposed to husband's/partner's sperm [        ]   No. embryos developed [        ]
      No. exposed to donor's sperm [        ]                No. embryos developed [        ]
      No. micro-injected [        ]                          No. embryos developed [        ]
13.   Treatment cycle abandoned prior to embryo replacement:   YES ☐  NO ☒
14.   Reason the cycle did not reach embryo replacement:   Poor response to stimulation ☐   No eggs collected ☐
      No embryos developed ☐   No viable embryos on thawing ☐   Risk of OHSS ☐   Other [        ]
15.   Date of embryos replacement or date when cycle was abandoned: [            ]
16.   Number of embryos transferred [        ]   Developed from: Frozen/thawing embryos ☐   ICSI ☐
      Partner's sperm ☐   Donor sperm ☐   Other micromanipulation ☐
17.   Total number of spare embryos after replacement [        ]   Number stored for treatment of patient [        ]
      Number stored for treatment of others [        ]   Number given for research [        ]   Number discarded [        ]
18.   Clinical pregnancy ☐   Ectopic pregnancy ☐   Miscarriage ☒

**Figure 23**   Human Fertilisation and Embryology Authority confidential *in vitro* fertilization treatment cycle form embryo research. The HFEA must ensure that treatment and research using human embryos are undertaken with the utmost respect and responsibility and that the vulnerability of infertile patients is not exploited.

The HFEA also regulates the storage of gametes (sperm and eggs) and embryos. In regulating treatment and research, the HFEA has to consider all relevant interests concerning patients, children and potential children, licensed clinics, the wider public and Parliament. It also needs to consider issues of safety, efficacy and ethics.

The HFEA's other main functions under the law are:

(1) To keep a formal register of information about donors, treatments and children born from those treatments. This is so that children born as a result of donated eggs or sperm can find out, if they wish, something about their genetic history.

(2) To produce a Code of Practice which gives guidelines to clinics about the proper conduct of licensed activities.

(3) To publicize its role and provide relevant advice and information to patients and donors and to clinics.

(4) 'To keep under review information about embryos and any subsequent development of embryos and about the provision of treatment services and activities by this (HFE) Act, and advise the Secretary of State, if he asks it to do so, about those matters'.

## CONCLUSION

We live in very exciting times globally in terms of rapidly advancing technology, but none more so than in the field of reproductive medicine. At the time of writing, Louise Brown has recently celebrated her 18th birthday, her birth being acknowledged as one of the greatest breakthroughs in medical history this century. The advent of intracytoplasmic sperm injection has revolutionized the management of male factor infertility (Chapter 14).

One area of intense interest is implantation of embryos. Until recently, studies on the implantation of human embryos were difficult and scarce. Patients could not be helped at this critical time except by various forms of luteal support. Today the emphasis is changing, as for example ultrasound increasingly becomes a valuable diagnostic tool. There are new insights into uterine cell populations, and the role of matrices, growth factors, cytokines and other factors involved in implantation. Techniques such as magnetic resonance imaging, angiography and spectroscopy are being used to enhance implantation rates. For example, the application of diffusion effect reduced echo imaging in magnetic resonance imaging has a resolution of 4 μm and can detect implantation sites and embryonic growth as early as day 7 in mice[60].

An enormous amount of human effort and research funds are being dedicated to improving the current low implantation rates. Unravelling the complexities of human embryo implantation will be one of the greatest challenges to confront clinicians and scientists alike as the year 2000 approaches.

## TRANSPORT OR SATELLITE *IN VITRO* FERTILIZATION

### Introduction

Transport or satellite IVF (T/S IVF) is an arrangement whereby IVF is carried out at a primary centre (which is HFEA licensed) but other parts of the treatment (e.g. ovulation induction or egg retrieval) are performed at a secondary centre (not necessarily HFEA licensed). The embryology and embryo transfer take place at a primary centre (or central unit).

Six years ago, in the Merseyside area, a system was established where IVF treatment could be carried out utilizing gynaecological expertise and resources in a District General Hospital (DGH) or satellite unit and embryological facilities available in a central unit. This was named transport IVF. The scheme, originally designed between the Royal Liverpool

University Hospital (RLUH) and two district general hospitals, proved to be a success and enabled a large number of infertile couples from the Merseyside region to be treated conveniently, successfully and cheaply.

This section on T/S IVF is intended to provide detailed help for clinicians wishing to set up a programme in a DGH or satellite unit. The methods described in subsequent parts of this section have been adopted specifically to suit the environment in the average DGH. The techniques have been greatly simplified and are based on current IVF practice. There are, of course, more sophisticated techniques available, but, bearing in mind the circumstances that exist in most DGHs, it is hoped that practitioners may glean sufficient information from this chapter to enable them to initiate their own programmes.

*We would strongly advise practitioners in participating centres to adhere to the recommendations outlined below as strictly as possible, especially with regard to patient selection and the ovulation induction regimen.* Experience has shown that inappropriate selection of patients, or the adoption of alternative induction regimens results in a sharp decrease in success rates. It is our belief that satisfactory results in IVF treatment in a DGH or satellite unit can be achieved only in a selected group of patients. Others, who require either complicated induction regimens or the use of sophisticated laboratory techniques, should have their treatment undertaken at the central unit.

**How does it work?**

(1) Patient selection and initial counselling are performed at the satellite unit.

(2) Ovarian stimulation is standard and incorporates GnRHa to facilitate programmed follicular aspiration on a routine operating list.

(3) Monitoring of follicular development is performed using ultrasound scanning together with estimation of serum oestradiol levels.

(4) The couple attend the central unit once prior to hCG administration for final counselling and to complete the paperwork.

(5) Follicular aspiration under vaginal ultrasound control is performed at the local hospital on a day care basis.

(6) Collected follicular aspirates are placed in a small 12 volt purpose-built incubator designed to plug into a car cigarette lighter socket and transported by the patient's partner to the embryological laboratory in the central unit.

(7) In the central unit oocyte identification and IVF is performed followed by ET 48 h later.

(8) Pregnancy testing is performed 14 days after embryo transfer at the satellite unit, as is subsequent day 35 scanning to confirm the number and site of the pregnancy or pregnancies.

**Patient selection**

*Initial investigations*

Standard infertility investigations including laparoscopy, hormonal profile and rubella status in the female partner and two semen analyses in the male partner, should be performed before the final consultation in the DGH or satellite unit. Patients who had cervical surgery (cone biopsy, cervical cautery, etc.) should have a catheter test performed.

Inclusion criteria are:

(1) Women 35 years of age or less;

(2) Tubal damage as a sole cause of subfertility; and

(3) Two normal recent semen analyses (count $> 20 \times 10^6$/ml, motility $> 50\%$, abnormal forms $< 30\%$ with no evidence of infection), or a satisfactory sperm migration test. The methodology of this is as follows:

   (a) Allow the semen sample to liquefy for 30 min at room temperature after production;

(b) Place 0.5 ml liquefied semen into a sterile 5 ml Falcon tube (Becton Dickinson);

(c) Layer 0.5 ml equilibrated culture medium onto the semen;

(d) Incubate for 90 min at 37°C in a 5% $CO_2$ incubator;

(e) Remove the upper 0.25 ml and assess the concentration of motile sperm; and

(f) A concentration of $< 1.0 \times 10^6$ motile sperm per ml is highly predictive of failed fertilization.

Suitable culture media are: Menezo B2; Medicult sperm preparation medium; Hams F10 with sodium bicarbonate; and Earles balanced salt solution (BSS) with sodium bicarbonate. Ideally a $CO_2$ incubator should be used but if unavailable the test may be performed using either Hams F10 or Earles BSS with 20 mol/l HEPES buffer in a 37°C oven or hot-block.

Patients who do not satisfy the above criteria can either be referred for specialized treatment in the central unit, or discharged from the infertility clinic. Exceptions may be considered if consultation is first made with the central unit. Exclusion criteria are:

(1) Women over 35 years of age;

(2) Patients with LH/FSH ratio higher than 3 : 1;

(3) Patients with laparoscopically proven moderate or severe endometriosis;

(4) Unexplained infertility;

(5) Male factor infertility;

(6) Patients whose ovaries are inaccessible for ultrasound-guided oocyte collection to be performed;

(7) Patients requiring oocyte donation or donor insemination; and

(8) Three previously unsuccessful IVF treatment cycles.

**Monitoring**

Ideally monitoring of T-IVF cycles should be achieved using a combination of hormonal assays and vaginal ultrasound scans.

*Preliminary scans*

The initial ultrasound is performed on a Thursday at least 5 days after the last menstrual period. Thickness of the endometrium is measured in the longitudinal section of uterus and both ovaries are checked for presence of ovarian cysts. If the endometrium is thicker than 4 mm or an ovarian cyst larger than 25 mm is detected the patient is advised to continue with her nasal spray and the treatment is delayed, and she is rescanned a week later (do not forget to inform the central unit, and to prescribe additional nasal spray). If hormonal assays are available, treatment should be delayed if serum oestradiol levels are higher than 200 pmol/l.

If a cyst persists 2 weeks later, drainage under ultrasound control should be considered. Patients who have endometriotic 'chocolate' cysts detected should be excluded from the treatment and referred to the central unit. Occasionally, an unexpected endometriotic cyst may be encountered, and in this situation a single dose of intravenous antibiotic should be administered (e.g. Augmentin).

*Day 8 scan (Friday, for collection on Tuesday)*

Follicular growth is monitored by ultrasound scan on day 8 of hMG injections. On this scan the number and diameter of follicles should be assessed. Follicles should have two diameters measured in two perpendicular planes. The presence of at least three follicles of a diameter of > 16 mm with corresponding serum oestradiol levels (700 pmol/l per follicle) indicates readiness for hCG injection. On rare occasions where these criteria are not achieved, if theatre time is available (and also time is available in the central unit), the treatment should be continued for an extra day and the sizes of follicles reassessed, otherwise the cycle should be cancelled.

*Day 10 scan (Monday, for collection on Wednesday)*
Follicular growth is monitored by ultrasound scans on day 10 of hMG injections. On this scan the number and diameter of follicles should be assessed. Follicles should have two diameters measured in two perpendicular planes. The presence of at least three follicles of a diameter of > 18 mm with corresponding serum oestradiol levels (1000 pmol/l per follicle) indicates readiness for hCG injection.

### The first visit to the central unit

The couple will first visit the central unit prior to the administration of the luteinizing hCG injection. This visit serves several purposes:

(1) It enables the couple to become familiar with the location of the unit;

(2) It allows them to meet the unit staff;

(3) The HFEA paperwork can be completed; and

(4) If required, blood can be obtained for culture medium preparation.

### Day of oocyte retrieval

On the morning of oocyte retrieval the couple report to the local hospital. Ultrasound guided follicular aspiration is carried out by the patient's gynaecologist in the DGH. The follicular aspirates are collected in sterile test tubes which must be filled as fully as possible, then tightly capped and placed in the incubator. The incubator is then locked and given to the male partner to transport to the central unit. During this journey the incubator is plugged into the car cigarette lighter. After arrival the male partner produces his semen sample which is then prepared.

*Follicular aspiration under vaginal ultrasound control*
This is carried out 36 h after hCG injection. It has been our practice to advise gynaecologists in participating centres to perform the procedure on a routine operating list under general anaesthesia. However, aspiration of follicles under vaginal ultrasound as a rule is a very simple and relatively pain-free procedure which in experienced hands lasts usually 5–10 min. Once sufficient expertise is acquired, it may be performed as an out-patient procedure.

*Preparation of instruments*
Cidex or any other chemical sterilising solutions are not acceptable in assisted conception procedures. Needle guides should be autoclaved before the procedure. Disposable single channel needles and tubing are recommended, but re-usable systems are best avoided. Having completed the procedure, the incubator is locked and handed to the male partner. Details regarding oocyte retrieval are entered into the appropriate section of the patient's T-IVF treatment book and sent together with incubator to the central unit. The patient may be discharged home a few hours after the procedure.

### Second visit to the central unit

At the central unit the follicular aspirates are examined and the oocytes are identified and inseminated. If fertilization takes place, the patient is informed, and 48 h after collection the embryos (a maximum of three) are replaced. This is a simple procedure requiring no sedation, and the patients are allowed home after about 20 min.

### Follow-up

This part of the treatment is carried out at the DGH. Luteal phase support with either hCG or progesterone vaginal pessaries is given to all patients. The choice of agent depends on the degree of ovarian stimulation. If more than ten follicles were present at oocyte retrieval, then progesterone pessaries (Cyclogest) are given, 200 mg twice daily for 2 weeks. If less than ten follicles were present at oocyte retrieval, hCG is given by deep intramuscular injection immediately following embryo transfer and repeated 72 h later. The patient reports the occurrence of any vaginal bleeding or other symptoms to the DGH. If the patient remains amenorrhoeic for

14 days after ET, a urinary pregnancy test (ICON, Hybritech, Nottingham, UK) is performed. If positive, an ultrasound scan is arranged 2 weeks later to confirm a pregnancy. Subsequent scans are arranged as necessary to check that the pregnancy is progressing normally. If a period occurs, the patient is seen in the next clinic for counselling and arranging another treatment if appropriate.

### Transport/satellite IVF and the HFEA

The HFEA is the governing body which grants licences to units to enable them to perform IVF procedures, and to which the centres are answerable. It is expected that individual transport centres (i.e. the DGHs) will be required to be licensed and inspected in the near future.

Our guidelines for practice are at present that the DGH is responsible for the following:

(1) Obtaining consent for the procedures involved in transport IVF;

(2) Providing implications counselling;

(3) Providing adequate information regarding hyperstimulation;

(4) Giving due consideration to the welfare of the child;

(5) Ensuring that the couple have been informed that they may seek further counselling. This can be provided by the DGH, or if this is unavailable, the couple should be referred to the central unit counsellor. This can be arranged by the transport IVF nursing co-ordinators; and

(6) Ensuring that all records pertaining to transport IVF patients are kept separately from the main notes and in a locked cabinet.

The HFEA Treatment Cycle form should be completed by the DGH in cases of cycles being abandoned prior to the central unit visit. All other Treatment Cycle forms will be completed by the central unit.

HFEA Research/Consent forms and information sheets are to be given to the couple by the DGH so that they have adequate time to consider their options. Completed forms must be returned to the central unit. HFEA outcome forms should be completed by the DGH and forwarded to the central unit. Please note that *all* pregnancies should have an outcome form, e.g. miscarriage, ectopic pregnancy, etc.

## ACKNOWLEDGEMENTS

I am indebted to Sue Howard for ensuring that the deadline for this particular manuscript was met.

I am also indebted for the section on transport or satellite IVF to Mr Charles Kingsland, Consultant Obstetrician and Gynaecologist, Reproductive Medicine Unit, Liverpool Woman's Hospital, Liverpool, UK.

## REFERENCES

1. Steptoe, P. C. and Edwards, R. G. (1978). Birth after reimplantation of a human embryo. *Lancet*, **2**, 366
2. Heap, W. (1891). Preliminary note on the transplantation and growth of mammalian ova within a uterine foster mother. *Proc. R. Soc.*, **48**, 457–8
3. Chang, M. C. (1959). Fertilization of rabbit ova *in vitro*. *Nature (London)*, **184**, 406
4. Steptoe, P. C. and Edwards, R. G. (1970). Laparoscopic recovery of pre-ovulatory human oocytes after priming of ovaries with gonadotrophins. *Lancet*, **1**, 683–9
5. Steptoe, P. C. and Edwards, R. G. (1976). Reimplantation of a human embryo with subsequent tubal pregnancy. *Lancet*, **1**, 880–2
6. Steptoe, P. C., Edwards, R. G. and Walters, D. E. (1986). Observations on 767 clinical pregnancies and 500 births after human *in vitro* fertilization. *Hum. Reprod.*, **1**, 89–94
7. Sharma, V., Riddle, A., Mason, B. A., Pampiglione, J. and Campbell, S. (1988). An analysis of factors influencing the establishment of a clinical pregnancy in an ultrasound based ambulatory *in vitro* fertilization programme. *Fertil. Steril.*, **49**, 468–78
8. Steptoe, P. C. (1968). Laparoscopy and ovulation. *Lancet*, **2**, 913

9. Steptoe, P. C. and Webster, J. (1985). Laparoscopy for oocyte recovery. *Ann. N.Y. Acad. Sci.*, **442**, 178–81
10. Edwards, R. G. and Steptoe, P. C. (1983). Current status of *in vitro* fertilization and implantation of human embryos. *Lancet*, **2**, 1265–9
11. Daya, S. (1988). Follicular fluid pH changes following intraperitoneal exposure of Graafian follicles to carbon dioxide: a comparative study with follicles exposed to ultrasound. *Hum. Reprod.*, **3**, 751–4
12. Verbessen, D., Camu, F., Devroey, P. and Van Steirteghem, A. (1988). Pneumoperitoneum induced pH changes in follicular and Douglas fluids during laparoscopic oocyte recovery in humans. *Hum. Reprod.*, **3**, 751–4
13. Pickering, S. J., Braude, P. R., Johnson, M. H., Cant, A. and Currie, J. (1990). Transient cooling at room temperature can cause irreversible disruption of the meiotic spindle in the human oocyte. *Fertil. Steril.*, **54**, 102–8
14. Macnamee, M. C. and Brinsden, P. R. (1992). Superovulation strategies in assisted conception. In Brinsden, P. R. and Rainsbury, P. A. (eds.) *A Textbook of In Vitro Fertilization and Assisted Reproduction*, p. 111. (Carnforth, UK: Parthenon Publishing)
15. Adams, J., Franks, S., Polson, D. W., Mason, H. D., Abdulwahid, N., Tucker, M., Morris, D. W., Price, J. and Jacobs, H. S. (1985). Multifollicular ovaries: clinical and endocrine features and response to pulsatile gonadotrophin releasing hormone. *Lancet*, **2**, 1375–9
16. Howles, C. M., Macnamee, M. C. and Edwards, R. G. (1987). Follicular development and early luteal function of conception and non-conceptual cycles after human *in vitro* fertilization. *Hum. Reprod.*, **2**, 17–21
17. Yovich, J. and Grudzinskas, G. (1990). *The Management of Infertility. A Manual of Gamete Handling Procedures*, 1st edn., p. 127. (London: Heinemann)
18. Brinsden, P. R. (1992). Oocyte recovery and embryo transfer technique for *in vitro* fertilization. In Brinsden, P. R. and Rainsbury, P. A. (eds.) *A Textbook of In Vitro Fertilization and Assisted Reproduction*, pp. 139–53. (Carnforth, UK: Parthenon Publishing)
19. Hughes, E. G., Fedorkow, D. M., Daya, S., Sagle, M. A., Van de Koppel, P. and Collins, J. A. (1992). The routine use of gonadotropin-releasing hormone agonists prior to *in vitro* fertilization and gamete intrafallopian transfer: a meta-analysis of randomized controlled trials. *Fertil. Steril.*, **58**, 888–96
20. Soliman, S., Daya, S., Collins, J. and Hughes, E. G. (1994). The role of luteal phase support in infertility treatment: a meta-analysis of randomized trials. *Fertil. Steril.*, **61**, 1068–76
21. Ghosh, D. and Sengupta, J. (1995). Another look at peri-implantation oestrogen. *Hum. Reprod.*, **18**, 1–2
22. Ben-Nun, I., Less, A. *et al.* (1992). Lack of correlation between hormonal blood levels and endometrial maturation in agonadal women with repeat implantation failure following embryo transfer from donated eggs. *J. Assist. Reprod. Genet.*, **9**, 102–5
23. Smitz, J., Devroey, P., Carnus, M. *et al.* (1988). The luteal phase and early pregnancy after combined GnRH-agonist/HMG treatment for superovulation in IVF or GIFT. *Hum. Reprod.*, **3**, 585–90
24. Smitz, J., Devroey, P., Braeckmans, P. *et al.* (1987). Management of failed IVF/GIFT programme with the combination of a GnRH-a analogue and hMG. *Hum. Reprod.*, **2**, 309–14
25. Buvat, J., Marcolin, G., Guittard, C., Herbaut, J., Louver, A. L. and Debaene, J. L. (1990). Luteal support after luteinizing hormone-releasing hormone agonist for *in vitro* fertilization: superiority of human chorionic gonadotropin over oral progesterone. *Fertil. Steril.*, **53**, 490–4
26. Nillius, S. J. and Johansson, E. D. B. (1971). Plasma levels of progesterone after vaginal, rectal, or intramuscular administration of progesterone. *Am. J. Obstet. Gynecol.*, **110**, 470–7
27. Zosmer, A., Katz, Z., Lancet, M., Konichezky, S. and Schwartz-Shohan, Z. (1987). Adult respiratory distress syndrome complicating ovarian hyperstimulation syndrome. *Fertil. Steril.*, **47**, 524–6
28. Rizk, B., Meagher, S. and Fisher, A. M. (1990). Ovarian hyperstimulation syndrome and cerebrovascular accidents. *Hum. Reprod.*, **5**, 697–8
29. Rizk, B. and Smitz, J. (1992). Ovarian hyperstimulation after superovulation for IVF and related procedures. *Hum. Reprod.*, **7**, in press
30. Waterstone, J., Parsons, J. and Bolton, V. (1992). *Lancet*, **337**, 975–6
31. Winkler, G. K., Ferguson, J. E., Takeichi, H. M. and Nuccitelli, R. (1992). *Dev. Biol.*, **127**, 143–56

32. Asch, R. H., Li, H.-P., Balmaceda, J. P. *et al.* (1991). *Hum. Reprod.*, **6**, 1395–9
33. Navot, D., Bergh, P. A. and Lafer, N. (1992). *Fertil. Steril.*, **58**, 249–61
34. Gregly, R. Z., Poldi, E., Enlik, Y. and Makler, A. (1976). Treatment of ovarian hyperstimulation by antihistamine. *Obstet. Gynecol.*, **47**, 83
35. Katz, Z., Lancet, M., Borenstein, R. and Cherke, J. (1984). Absence of teratogenicity of indomethacin in ovarian hyperstimulation syndrome. *Int. J. Fertil.*, **29**, 186
36. Borenstein, R., Elhalah, U., Lunenfeld, B. and Schwartz, Z. S. (1989). Severe ovarian hyperstimulation syndrome: a re-evaluated therapeutic approach. *Fertil. Steril.*, **51**, 791–5
37. Asch, R. H., Balmaceda, J. P., Ord, T. *et al.* (1993). *Fertil. Steril.*, **49**, 263–7
38. Sher, G., Feinman, M., Zouves, C. *et al.* (1993). *Hum. Reprod.*, **8**, 1487–90
39. Sher *et al.* (1995). *Hum. Reprod.*, **10**, 3107–9
40. Lutjen, P., Trounson, A., Leeton, J., Findlay, J., Wood, C. and Reron, P. (1984). The establishment and maintenance of pregnancy using *in vitro* fertilization and embryo donation in a patient with primary ovarian failure. *Nature (London)*, **307**, 174–5
41. Buster, J. E., Bustillo, M., Thorneycroft, I. H., Simon, J. A., Boyers, S. P., Marshall, J. R., Louw, J. A., Seed, R. W. and Seed, R. G. (1983). Non-surgical transfer of *in vivo* fertilized donated ova to five infertile women: report of two pregnancies. *Lancet*, **2**, 223–4
42. Asch, R., Balmaceda, J., Ord, T., Borrero, C., Cefalu, E., Gastaldi, C. and Rojas, F. (1987). Oocyte donation and gamete intrafallopian transfer as treatment for premature ovarian failure. *Lancet*, **1**, 687
43. Yovich, J. L., Blackledge, D. G., Richardson, P. A., Edirisinghe, W. R., Matson, P. L., Turner, S. R. and Draper, R. (1987). PROST for ovum donation. *Lancet*, **1**, 1209–10
44. Van Steirteghem, A. C., Van den Abbeel, E., Braeckmans, P., Camus, M., Khan, I., Smitz, J., Staessen, C., Van Waesberghe, L., Wisanto, A. and Devroey, P. (1987). Pregnancy with a frozen-thawed embryo in a woman with primary ovarian failure. *N. Engl. J. Med.*, **317**, 113
45. Serhal, P. F. and Craft, I. L. (1987). Ovum donation – a simplified approach. *Fertil. Steril.*, **48**, 265–9
46. *Ilford Recorder* (1996). 5th December
47. Edwards, R. G. *et al.* (1991). *Lancet*, **338**, 292–4
48. Antinori, S., Versaci, C., Gholami, G. H. *et al.* (1993). *Hum. Reprod.*, **8**, 1487–90
49. The British Medical Association (1990). *Surrogacy: Ethical Considerations.* (London: British Medical Association)
50. Panigez, M. (1994). *Proceedings 2nd International Conference on Early Human Pregnancy*, Atlantic City, USA

# A guide to the practice of andrology in the assisted conception unit

# 11

*Anthony V. Hirsh*

## INTRODUCTION

Andrology is a new field with relatively sparse scientific foundations, embracing disorders of male fertility, contraception and sexual function. Male infertility is due to an abnormality of the semen or a problem with its delivery to the female genital tract. There is no reliable treatment for most infertile men, but recent advances in assisted reproduction technology (ART) have reversed this dismal prognosis due to the advent of intracytoplasmic sperm injection (ICSI)[1]. ICSI has extended biological fatherhood because only one sperm cell for each egg is required. It has led to the discovery that many patients with azoospermia due to primary testicular failure produce at least some spermatozoa within the testes which are suitable for this technique. Consequently, donor insemination is required less frequently today. ICSI could revolutionize the practice of ART because the minimal sperm requirement means that postcoital sperm retrieval is feasible, thereby potentially negating the necessity for the male partner to provide a semen sample. All ART procedures could then be carried out on the female partner, thereby avoiding many of the personal, cultural and religious objections to masturbation and assisted conception[2].

Andrology is included in assisted conception units so that remediable male factor infertility can be diagnosed and treated in order to procure natural conceptions, with suitable irreversible cases selected for assisted reproduction. With the fertility team aware of the therapeutic possibilities in andrology, a fully comprehensive service for all infertile couples becomes available with appropriate cost-effective management for their individual and shared problems.

## APPLIED ANATOMY AND PHYSIOLOGY OF THE MALE REPRODUCTIVE SYSTEM

### The Y chromosome

The testis determining factor is a sequence of genes on the short arm of the Y chromosome, known as the SRY gene (sex determining region Y); genes on the long arm control spermatogenesis. Elaboration of the male phenotype depends on testosterone secretion by the fetal testis. Without testes an embryo, regardless of genetic sex, automatically develops as a female.

### Embryology

The testes arise from the medial ridges of the urogenital folds. From weeks 3 to 5, primordial germ cells migrate from the fetal yolk sac to the genital ridge epithelium, where sex cords with Sertoli cells and the germ cells proliferate into seminiferous tubules. The Sertoli cells and interstitial Leydig cells originate from the mesonephros. Placental gonadotrophins followed by pituitary luteinizing hormone (LH) stimulate Leydig cell secretion of testosterone which controls male development by a local effect, promoting and stabilizing the Wolffian (mesonephric) duct system. The testis also prevents development of a female system by secreting Müllerian inhibitory factor. Conversion of testosterone to 5α-dihydrotestosterone by 5α-reductase stimulates development of the penis from the genital tubercle, the scrotum from the labial folds of the cloaca, and the prostate gland and urethra from the wall of the urogenital sinus. Deficiency of androgen receptors or 5α-reductase may thus lead to female development, as in the testicular feminization syndrome.

### Anatomy[3]

The testis (Figure 1) is oval, normally 4.5–5.5 cm long (20–25 ml) in the adult, with its outer covering, the fibrous tunica albuginea, thickened posteriorly along the epididymal border, where it forms the mediastinum. Fibrous septa extend between the mediastinum and the tunica albuginea to divide each testis into 200–400 compartments enclosing one to four convoluted seminiferous tubules about 60 cm long. The seminiferous tubules straighten as the vasa recti, which converge and amalgamate to become the rete testis, a network of wide channels within the mediastinum from which 12–20 efferent ducts arise. The efferent ducts perforate the tunica albuginea at the upper pole of the testis to form a similar number of coni vasculosi which constitute the head (caput) of the epididymis. The efferent ducts then unite, forming the solitary, highly tortuous, 6 m long duct of the body (corpus) of the epididymis, which descends posteriorly, applied to the mediastinal margin of the testis. The junction between caput and corpus epididymis is the site where different embryological structures meet, the efferent ducts (originating from the testis) lined by a monolayer of ciliated cells, and the epididymal duct (arising from the Wolffian system) with a pseudostratified microvillous epithelium. The epididymal duct is initially narrow in the corpus, but develops a wide lumen in the tail (cauda) of the epididymis for sperm storage. The lumen then narrows and develops a muscular coat to become the convoluted portion of the vas deferens. This becomes the straight portion of the vas, which passes through the scrotum and inguinal canal, along the side wall of the pelvis towards the posterior aspect of the bladder anterior to the rectum. Here the vas hooks medially around the ureter, meets its fellow at the midline, enlarges to become the ampulla of the vas, and is then joined laterally by the seminal vesicle. The ampullae narrow as paired ejaculatory ducts which enter the prostate gland and open together on the verumontanum within the prostatic urethra (Figure 2).

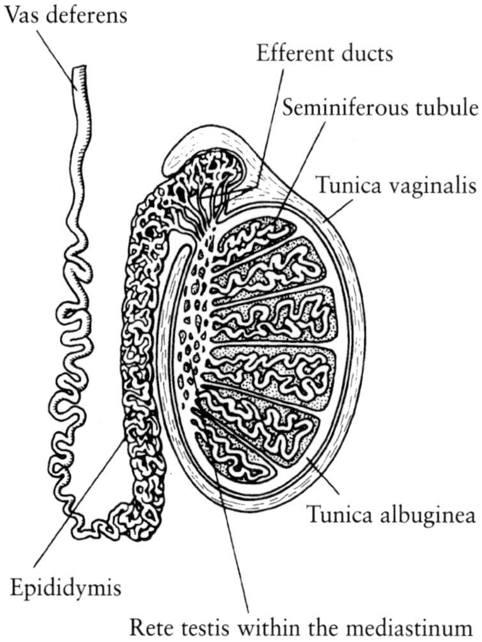


**Figure 1** The internal structure of the testis

### Spermatogenesis

The 70-day cycle of human spermatogenesis commences at puberty and continues throughout life. It is initiated and controlled from the hypothalamic–pituitary axis through secretion of gonadotrophin releasing hormone (GnRH), conveyed by its portal venous system, and is influenced by higher centres (Figure 3). GnRH (also known as LHRH) stimulates the anterior pituitary to secrete follicle stimulating hormone (FSH) and LH. The seminiferous tubules (Figure 4) are lined by Sertoli cells united by tight cell junctions, which form the blood–testis barrier, dividing them into basal and adluminal

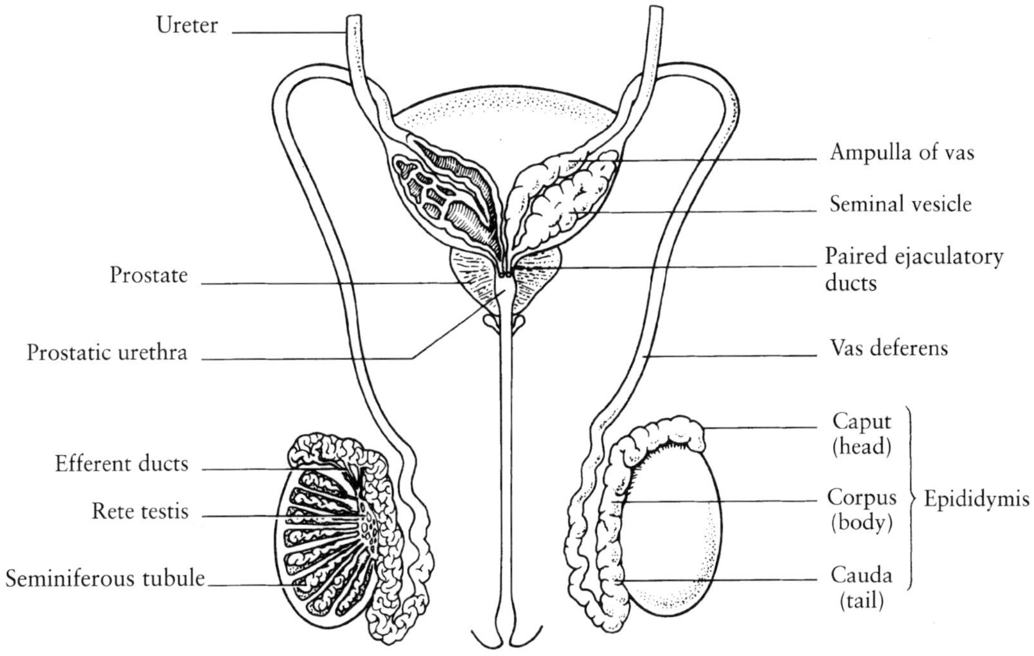


**Figure 2** The male reproductive system

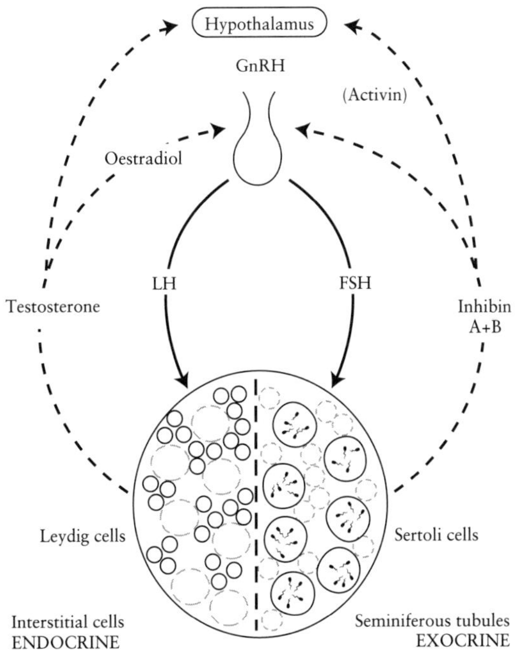


**Figure 3** Endocrine control of the testis

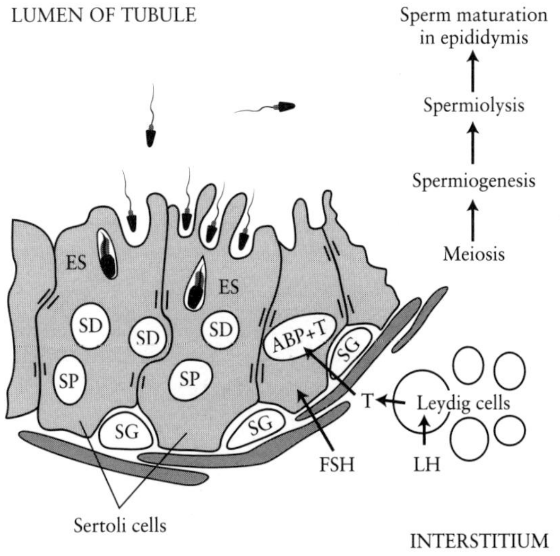


**Figure 4** Local endocrine control of spermatogenesis. SG, spermatogonia; SP, spermatocytes; SD, round spermatids; ES, elongated spermatids; T, testosterone

compartments. Sertoli cells respond to FSH by secreting androgen binding protein. The Leydig cells are stimulated by LH to produce testosterone, which regulates LH secretion by negative feedback through the bloodstream, acting via its conversion to oestradial by aromatase.

The androgen binding protein–testosterone complex ensures a high concentration of testosterone within the testis equivalent to about 100 times the circulating level.

The germ cells are nurtured through spermatogenesis by the Sertoli cells. Diploid stem cell 'dark type A spermatogonia' in the basal compartments of the seminiferous tubules give rise to 'clear type A spermatogonia' which enter the adluminal compartment to undergo meiosis. Proliferation through 'type B spermatogonia', then primary and secondary spermatocyte stages results in formation of haploid round spermatids. Spermatids undergo spermiogenesis, a process of metamorphosis, through which they elongate and develop acrosome caps and flagellae to become transformed into oval spermatozoa with tails. They are released from the surface of the Sertoli cells into the lumen of the seminiferous tubules, a process known as spermiolysis.

In response to meiosis, Sertoli cells secrete the A and B forms of the glycoprotein inhibin, which limit FSH secretion by negative feedback to the hypothalamus. Combination of inhibin A and B forms activin, which increases FSH secretion. Serum FSH is elevated if there is severe impairment of spermatogenesis, reflecting diminished inhibin secretion or increased activin. Sperm and androgen production decline with age, and the testis softens, leading to a gradual increase of LH and FSH. This may cause marginal subfertility and a reduced libido, but not usually erectile dysfunction or symptoms of androgen withdrawal.

## Testicular circulation

The testis is supplied by the internal spermatic artery, the artery to the vas deferens, and the cremasteric artery. Veins issuing from the testis unite to form the pampiniform plexus in the spermatic cord which has a close association with the helical spermatic artery, including microscopic arteriovenous anastomoses. The arrangement is a countercurrent mechanism for heat and metabolic exchange.

The internal spermatic vein is the principal vein draining the pampiniform plexus, commencing in or above the inguinal canal. Since additional (about 12) veins drain the testis to the external and internal iliac veins, and the arteries are narrow and long, blood flow through the testis is relatively slow. The left internal spermatic vein joins the left renal vein at a right angle, an arrangement less resistant to retrograde flow than the right internal spermatic vein, which drains by a narrow angle into the inferior vena cava. Venous flow from the left testis is further compromised by the 'compass' effect of the aorta and superior mesenteric artery compressing the left renal vein, and also pressure on the left common iliac vein by the right common iliac artery as it crosses the sacrum. This anomalous arrangement explains why varicoceles, which are caused by internal spermatic vein reflux, occur in 20% of normal men, predominantly on the left side (Figure 5).

Scrotal ventilation is required to maintain the testes 2° C below body temperature. The low testicular blood flow and efficiency of the pampiniform plexus establish the heat differential, and the dartos and cremateric muscles control the surface area of the scrotum by lowering and raising the testes. The countercurrent mechanism may also regulate the reduced $p\text{O}_2$ and high testosterone of the interior milieu of the testis. Retrograde venous flow in most varicoceles could thus affect the functions of testis and epididymis by increasing blood flow, thus elevating temperature[4], the $p\text{O}_2$, and the clearance of testosterone (Figure 6).

## The rete testis and epididymis

Spermatozoa from the seminiferous tubules traverse the rete testis and efferent ducts and are concentrated in the head of the epididymis, drawn by intense fluid absorption. After traversing the head and body of the epididymis in 2–14 days, they are stored in the tail of the epididymis, the seminal vesicles and vasal ampullae prior to ejaculation. Spermatozoa mature during their passage through the epididymis, where they acquire surface proteins which inhibit their motility and fertilizing ability until they disperse and activation occurs on ejaculation.

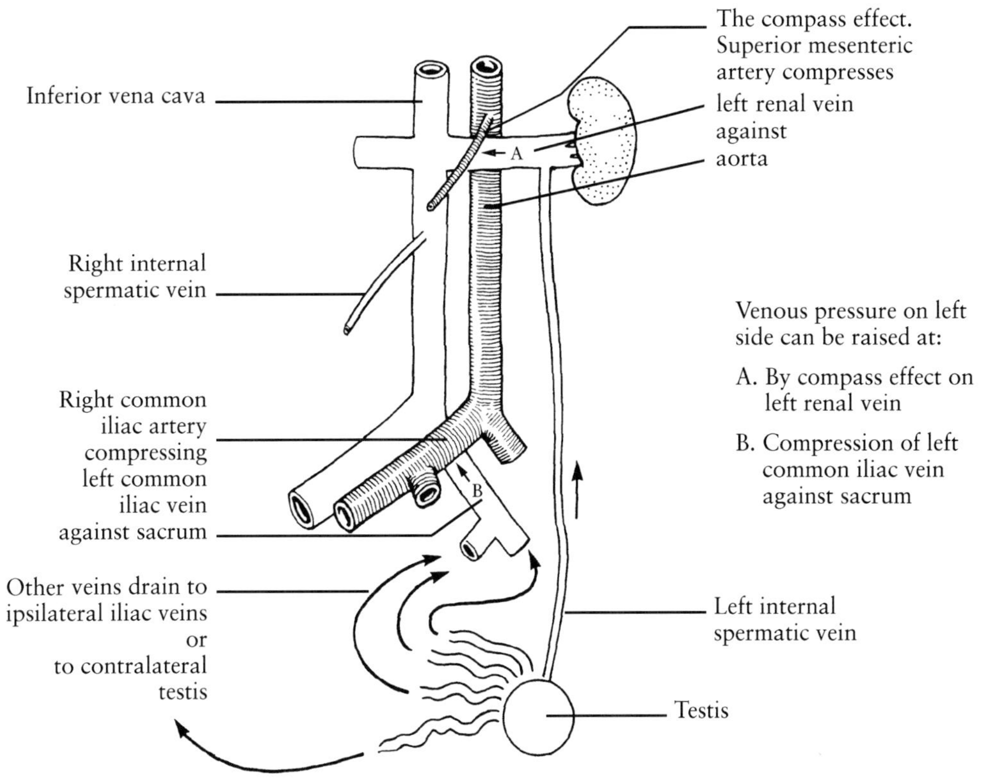


**Figure 5** The venous drainage of the left testis is doubly compromised, thereby predisposing to varicocele

Since the process of spermatogenesis (70 days) with passage through the epididymis (2–14 days) prior to ejaculation takes approximately 3 months, changes of sperm concentration in the semen in response to endogenous (fever) or exogenous factors (anabolic steroids) should be observed after about 12 weeks. Similarly, the effect of factors acting on the epididymis to influence sperm motility (ligation of a varicocele) should be observed within 2–3 weeks.

## Erectile function

The physiological mechanisms of erection are under the control of higher centres via the parasympathetic nervous system, with sacral outflow in roots S2, 3, 4 via the nervi erigentes. The rigidity of the penis depends on smooth muscle relaxation inside the corpora cavernosa, an intact nerve and arterial supply, and adequate venous closure. The most common conditions leading to impotence (erectile dysfunction) are psychological factors, diabetes mellitis, Peyronie's disease, venous leak impotence, arterial insufficiency, or a side-effect of medication, especially antihypertensive (β-blockers, thiazide diuretics) and antidepressant drugs. Less common causes are hyperprolactinaemia (pituitary microadenoma, spironolactone, cimetidine), spinal or pelvic injury, and androgen deficiency.

## Ejaculation

Ejaculation is a neurologically mediated sequence of events, distinctly separate from erection, and is controlled via the sympathetic nervous system at the level of T10–L2. During ejaculation, the internal (bladder neck) and external (membranous urethra) sphincters of the bladder tighten, thereby compressing the prostate, which discharges its secretion into the urethra (Figure 7). Emission of spermatozoa

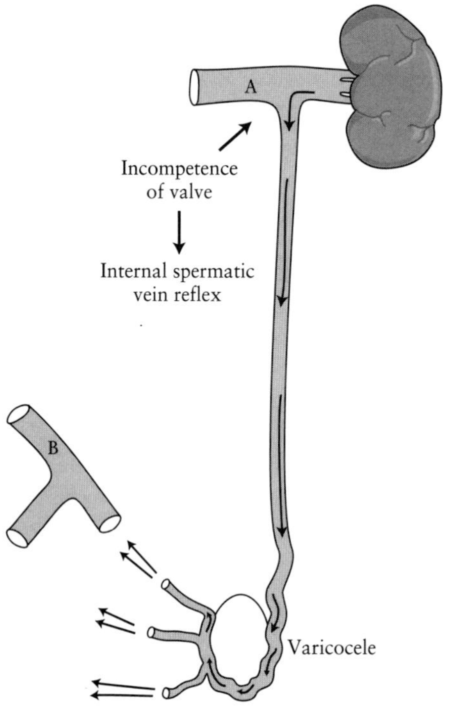


Figure 6 Aetiology of varicocele. Increased blood flow caused by internal spermatic vein reflux into a varicocele raises the temperature of the scrotum, and may impair spermatogenesis (testis) and sperm maturation (epididymis). A and B refer to Figure 5

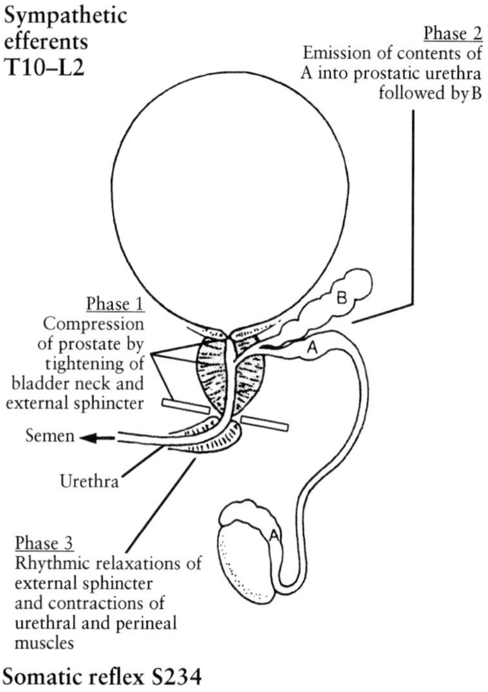


**Figure 7** The three phases of ejaculation

stored in the tail of the epididymis, vas deferens and vasal ampulla, through the ejaculatory duct into the prostatic urethra, is followed by seminal vesicle secretions. Pressure within the prostatic urethra increases, with the closed bladder neck preventing passage of the semen into the bladder. In the final phase of ejaculation, the seminal fluid, held under pressure, is released rhythmically through the penile urethra by a sequence of four to ten relaxations of the external urethral sphincter and bulbospongiosus muscles, a reflex mediated via the somatic sacral nerves, S2–4. Failure of ejaculation (aspermia) may occur after spinal cord or pelvic injury, multiple sclerosis, retroperitoneal or pelvic surgery, and with drugs, e.g. some antidepressants, phenothiazines, and antihypertensive agents.

Retrograde ejaculation occurs if the internal sphincter of the bladder fails to close, and the seminal emission into the prostatic urethra passes into the bladder at orgasm (Figure 8). There is either no external ejaculate or a small volume, depending on whether the retrograde ejaculation is partial or complete, although some urethral fluid usually appears from the bulbo-urthral glands. Retrograde ejaculation is diagnosed by the presence of spermatozoa in a postorgasmic urine sample, and may occur after bladder neck incision or transurethral resection of the prostate, sympathetic injury by retroperitoneal surgery, spinal injury, or diabetic neuropathy, and also occurs in congenitally wide bladder neck. Retrograde ejaculation may be a side-effect of phenothiazines, α-sympathomimetic and ganglion blockers.

## The seminal fluid, sperm hyperactivation, capacitation and fertilization

The seminal fluid functions as a transport medium for spermatozoa, forming a coagulum

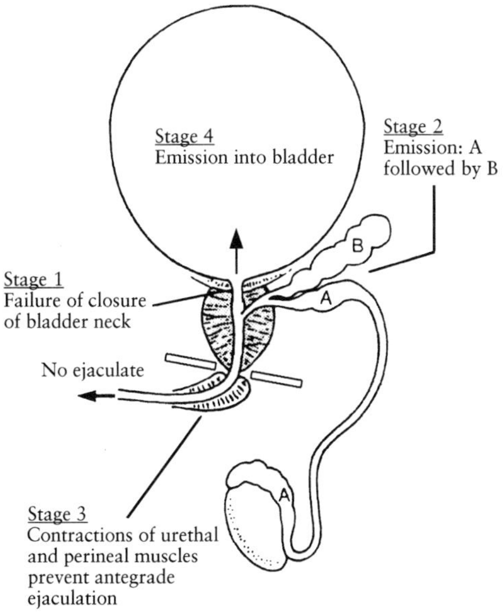


**Figure 8** Mechanism of retrograde ejaculation

on ejaculation which covers the cervix, acting as a physical shield and buffer against acid vaginal secretions. Normal semen is slightly alkaline (pH 7.2–8.0). The seminal vesicles contribute two-thirds of the volume of the semen, and secrete fructose and fibrin, with a higher pH than prostatic secretions. The prostate contribution is one-third of the semen volume, and contains citric acid, acid phosphatase and zinc. The volume component of sperm in seminal fluid is negligible. Semen is also rich in antioxidants, e.g. vitamins C and E, which protect sperm against the harmful effects of reactive oxygen species by a scavenger effect. Smoking may reduce seminal fluid vitamin C.

Having traversed the ovulatory mid-cycle cervical mucus due to their intrinsic motility, ejaculated spermatozoa are transported passively through the female tract, and a highly selected population appears in the oviducts within a few hours. Spermatozoa acquire the capacity to fertilize after 2–12 h in the female tract (or *in vitro*). Capacitated spermatozoa display hyperactivated motility, highly erratic movements due to increased lateral head displacement and diminished linear velocity, which may increase the number of sperm–egg collisions in the Fallopian tube. After capacitation, an influx of calcium ions leads to the acrosome reaction, the dissolution of the outer acrosomal membrane with release of hyaluronidase and acrosin. Low levels of reactive oxygen species may be important in the initiation of hyperactivation and the acrosome reaction. Hyaluronidase disperses the cells of the cumulus oophorus. Zona proteins ZP2 and ZP3 are receptors for sperm binding, which initiates oocyte activation and the extrusion of the second polar body, associated with a discharge of calcium ions. Hyperactivation probably provides the required thrust to allow one sperm, which is bound to the zona pellucida at the postacrosomal region, to penetrate through to achieve fertilization, and this is facilitated by the enzymic action of released acrosin. After the successful sperm has entered the oocyte, cortical granules below the vitelline surface fuse with the oolemma, commencing at the site of sperm penetration. This initiates the zona reaction, a hardening of its inner surface due to enzymes released into the perivitelline space, thereby obstructing further sperm penetration and preventing polyspermic fertilization.

## PATHOGENESIS OF MALE FACTOR INFERTILITY

From anatomical and physiological considerations, the fertility of a man depends on:

(1) Hypothalamic–pituitary axis function;

(2) The condition of spermatogenesis;

(3) Sperm storage, erectile and ejaculatory function;

(4) Semen quality and the fertilizing ability of spermatozoa.

These events result in the production of seminal fluid, but each process could be influenced by general or local, congenital or acquired disorders, acting individually, collectively or cumulatively. Although the seminal fluid analysis has been standardized by the World Health Organization (WHO)[5], it can vary considerably in normal subjects, and may have declined in some countries during the last 50 years due to possible environmental factors[6].

Male fertility also depends on the fertility of the female partner. Hargreave[7] showed that few wives had fertility problems where the husband had azoospermia, compared with a high incidence of female factors where the man was subfertile due to impaired semen quality. In individual gynaecological and urological based centres, referral patterns are biased by differing subspecialty interests and expertise. Baker and colleagues[8] arrived at no specific diagnosis in approximately 80% of cases, and Hull and colleagues[9], detecting sperm dysfunction in 24% (and azoospermia in 2%), found this was the largest defined cause of infertility in a large population. The diagnosis of unexplained infertility, where the semen is normal in up to 50% of couples, reflects the desirability of a standardized test of sperm function. In a multinational study of 8500 infertile couples, there was no male abnormality in 48.8%, with varicocele in 12.6%, idiopathic semen abnormalities in a total of 20.2%, accessory gland infection in 6.9%, suspected immunological factors in 3%, and sexual dysfunction in 1.3%; all other categories were less than 1%, including obstructive azoospermia, ejaculatory inadequacy, endocrine disease, and chromosome abnormality[10]. The situation was different in two urological studies where varicocele was diagnosed in 37–39%, endocrine abnormality in 4–9%, obstruction in 6–7%, with idiopathic male factor infertility in 5–25%[11,12].

## ANDROLOGICAL EVALUATION

Clinical evaluation of infertile men aims primarily to identify reversible causes of infertility. The assessment includes the exclusion of underlying medical disorders, the diagnosis of irreversible problems where ART is indicated, and an appraisal of the prognosis.

### History

The history begins with the duration of the infertility, any previous fertility, the frequency and effectiveness of coitus, with specific inquiry into ejaculatory function. More than 3 years' primary infertility suggests a male problem, but previous conceptions, including miscarriage, and optimistic signs from earlier treatment, including ART, are encouraging. The past history focuses on general illness, including recent fever, thyroid disease and diabetes mellitus, and also local conditions which might affect the testes, especially orchidopexy, torsion, herniorrhaphy, vasectomy, orchitis, urinary infection, and sexually transmitted disease. The inquiry concerning external agents which suppress testicular function includes tobacco, alcohol and marihuana intake, previous radiotherapy or chemotherapy (lymphoma, testicular tumour), and exposure to heat (welders, drivers), or chemicals (pesticides) at work. Common medications influencing male fertility include sulphasalazine, nifedipine, testosterone and illegal anabolic steroids for body building. Anosmia is indicative of Kallman's syndrome, sinusitis or bronchiectasis of Young's syndrome[13] or the Kartagener syndrome.

### Examination

Physical examination should be conducted away from the partner to allow the patient to volunteer any history of sexually transmitted disease or conception in a previous relationship. He is examined supine, and initial inspection may reveal gynaecomastia and the scanty facial, body or pubic hair of hypogonadism, or scars from inguinal or scrotal surgery. Examination of the penis and urethra may reveal hypospadius. Testis size should be assessed with a centimetre measure or orchidometer. Normal testes are 4.5–5.5 cm long (25 ml), firm and of equal size. In small testes (2–3 cm), spermatogenesis is impaired, but there are often some foci of normal spermatogenesis[14] useful for ICSI. The vas deferens is easily palpated at the neck of the scrotum, and the epididymis is applied above and behind the testis. Rectal examination is carried out to assess the prostate gland and seminal vesicles. Assessment of the spermatic cords for varicoceles is finally conducted with the patient standing in a well-illuminated warm area.

Varicoceles are classified as:

(1) Grade I, a palpable cough impulse in the spermatic cord;

(2) Grade II, dilated veins palpable in the spermatic cord or around the testis;

(3) Grade III, visible dilated veins within the scrotum.

Small varicoceles are best confirmed by scrotal ultrasound[15].

*Testicular or prostatic tumours*

Sometimes, gynaecomastia is the presenting symptom of a testicular tumour. Male infertility and cryptorchidism are risk factors in the aetiology of testicular cancer, and there should be no hesitation in referring a patient for a urological opinion if any palpable lesion is discovered within a testis, or there is an unexplained absent, ectopic or undescended testis. Similarly, any prostate nodule, or failure to identify the median prostatic groove on rectal examination, especially in men over 50, raises the possibility of prostate cancer, which should also prompt early urological referral.

## Investigations

Any medical reports or the results of previous investigation, at home or abroad, may give an indication of the nature of the fertility problem at the initial interview. Further investigations are helpful.

*Ultrasound of scrotum*

This is useful to confirm varicoceles, or identify spermatoceles or epididymal cysts in obstructive azoospermia. An occult testicular tumour will be detected occasionally. *Transrectal ultrasound* is used to evaluate men with low-volume ejaculates, to identify Müllerian prostatic cysts or dilated seminal vesicles in ejaculatory duct obstruction, or a wide bladder neck in retrograde ejaculation.

*Postcoital test (PCT)*

The postcoital test, often forgotten, will exclude a male fertility problem if there are adequate (> 50 per high-power field (HPF)) progressively motile spermatozoa in mid-cycle cervical mucus 9–24 h after coitus. A postcoital test is especially valuable in assessing problems of ejaculatory function and the significance of a low-volume ejaculate.

*Seminal fluid analysis*

The results of at least two analyses are required to assess the sperm parameters, since they vary widely even in fertile men. Semen is produced by masturbation after 3 days' abstinence. Normal semen variables are given in Table 1, and Table 2 describes the nomenclature of semen

**Table 1** Normal values in semen (*WHO Manual*, 1992[5])

| | |
|---|---|
| Volume | ≥ 2.0 ml |
| pH | 7.2–8.0 |
| Sperm concentration | $\geq 20 \times 10^6$/ml |
| Motility | ≥ 50% with forward progression within 60 min; or ≥ 25% with rapid progession within 60 min |
| Morphology | ≥ 30% with normal forms |
| White blood cells | $1 \times 10^6$/ml |
| Immunobead test | < 20% sperm bound to particles |
| MAR test | < 10% sperm bound to particles |

**Table 2** Nomenclature for semen variables (*WHO Manual*, 1992[5])

| | |
|---|---|
| Normozoospermia | normal ejaculate as defined in Table 1 |
| Oligozoospermia | sperm concentration $< 20 \times 10^6$/ml |
| Asthenozoospermia | < 50% spermatozoa with forward progression<br>< 25% spermatozoa with rapid progression |
| Teratozoospermia | < 30% spermatozoa with normal morphology |
| Oligoasthenoteratozoospermia | disturbance of all three variables |
| Azoospermia | no spermatozoa in the ejaculate |
| Aspermia | no ejaculate |

variables[5]. A *semen volume* persistently below 1.5 ml (hypospermia) may indicate ejaculatory dysfunction or ejaculatory duct obstruction, but is usually caused by difficulty in producing a sample. Increased viscosity may occur in accessory gland infection. The significance of a reduced *concentration of spermatozoa* (oligozoospermia) of $< 20 \times 10^6$/ml is undecided, but, if constant, the fertility may be abnormal. The most significant feature of sperm *motility* is the proportion of progressively motile spermatozoa (> 25%). *Sperm morphology* is the most subjective parameter, but is accepted as a valuable index of the fertilizing ability of sperm, since it is useful in predicting the outcome of *in vitro* fertilization (IVF), whether based on the WHO figure of < 30% or the strict Kruger criteria of < 4% normal forms[16,17].

*Sperm antibodies*
The mixed antiglobulin or MAR (> 10%) and direct Immunobead (> 20%) tests are useful screening tests on the semen for sperm coating antibodies. Male immunological infertility is confirmed in the serum by the tray agglutination test (TAT, titre > 1/32) or indirect Immunobead test (≥ 20%), and/or the seminal plasma by the TAT (titre > 1/2) or indirect Immunobead test (≥ 20%).

*Sperm preparation tests*
The swim-up, Percoll and Percoll gradient sperm preparation methods will provide a useful index of the fertility potential of the semen. The parameters acceptable for the various ART techniques vary between units, depending on their individual results. A total harvest of 5–8 million motile spermatozoa in the sperm preparation is suitable for homologous artificial insemination (AIH) by intrauterine insemination (IUI), and 1–2 million for IVF. Progressive sperm motility should be ≥ 90%, scoring at least 2–3 on a scale of 1–4. Twenty-four hour *in vitro* sperm survival of ≥ 40% with a progression score of 2 or more means there is a favourable prognosis for fertilization. ICSI is indicated if the sperm preparation parameters are below these levels, but the spermatozoa selected for microinjection must be viable, as verified by at least weak activity.

*Diagnostic andrology*
Sophisticated sperm function tests which can predict failure of fertilization during IVF are desirable, but the wider availability of ICSI has led to a decline in demand for such investigations. Most useful[18] are:

(1) Sperm morphology assessment[16,17];
(2) Reactive oxygen species (ROS) generated by active leukocytes, detected by luminometry[20];
(3) Motility parameters assessed by computer-assisted semen analysis (CASA), especially the presence of hyperactivation[19].

*Follicle stimulating hormone*
Where there is azoospermia, reduced testis size, or a sperm concentration $< 10 \times 10^6$/ml, an index of testicular function is given by the serum FSH level. In severely impaired spermatogenesis, the FSH level is more than twice the upper limit of the laboratory range, but, even with very high levels, for example in Sertoli cell and some cases of Klinefelter's syndromes, there are usually foci of normal sperm production[21], which are useful for ICSI.

*Testosterone*
The testosterone level has limited value in most infertile men since there is usually no demonstrable hormone deficiency[22]. If marginally reduced in hypogonadism, there may be a low libido, for example, Klinefelter's syndrome. In azoospermia, a low testosterone level with normal or low FSH level is suggestive of hypogonadotrophic hypogonadism. The testosterone level will be extraordinarily high in patients on anabolic steroids, in whom the FSH and LH levels will be virtually undetectable. Elevation of testosterone and LH together is indicative of a rare androgen insensitivity syndrome.

*Other hormone levels*
LH is raised in Leydig cell insufficiency, as in Klinefelter's syndrome, or in androgen

resistance. A constantly raised *prolactin* level is indicative of a pituitary microadenoma, which is confirmed by nuclear magnetic resonance imaging (MRI) of the pituitary, and is more often a cause of erectile dysfunction than infertility. *Dihydroepiandrosterone* (DHEA) reduction occurs in middle-aged men with asthenia, but is not linked to any male fertility disorder. *Inappropriate hormone levels*, for example low FSH or LH in bilateral cryptorchidism or Klinefelter's syndrome, may be due to an occult testicular tumour.

*Urine examination*
Microscopy of an initial urine sample after prostatic massage may reveal increased numbers of white or red blood cells in prostatitis, and occasionally a positive culture. Microscopic haematuria should be excluded by mid-stream urine analysis if any red cells are present. The presence of sperm in postorgasmic urine is indicative of retrograde ejaculation.

*Chlamydia*
This is confirmed by detection of chlamydia antigen in the urine, or by immunological studies: IgM indicates active infection, and IgG past infection.

*Genetic studies*
Screening for cystic fibrosis mutations is essential in men with congenital absence of the vas deferens presenting for ICSI. A buccal smear will identify chromatin-positive individuals with 47,XXY Klinefelter's syndrome, confirmed by full karyotyping. The karyotype may also identify other sex chromosome (e.g. XYY) or autosomal abnormalities in men with azoospermia or severe oligozoospermia, who have defective spermatogenesis[23]. Y chromosome microdeletions (azoospermia factor, AZF) found in 9% of such patients are not yet fully evaluated for routine clinical use[24].

*Testicular biopsy*
This is indicated in azoospermia due to primary testicular failure, and in cases of aspermia where the serum FSH level is elevated, to ascertain whether spermatozoa are available for ICSI. The Johnsen method[25] of scoring spermatogenesis is a useful index and is based on the most advanced stage of sperm production in the seminiferous tubules. Since the pathological appearances in testicular failure are patchy, multiple small biopsies (three to five per testis) provide more information. Foci of spermatogenesis are commonly present in the most severe forms of germ cell aplasia, and these could be missed during conventional single-site testicular biopsy procedure. Testicular tissue should also be cryopreserved for future ICSI cycles.

## A CLASSIFICATION OF MALE INFERTILITY (Table 3)

Seminal fluid analysis provides a useful basis on which to adopt a classification of male infertility, since methods are standard internationally[5] and infertile men are identified and clinically evaluated on the results. The following classification also considers sexual function, sperm coating and sperm function.

### Type I: mechanical (about 1%)

There is a physical problem with the delivery of seminal fluid to the external os at ovulation. This may be subclassified on the basis of ejaculatory function. Sperm function is normal in most patients, and pregnancies are achieved commonly by AIH. Other types of male infertility due to abnormal semen quality (types II–V) may co-exist:

(1) *Normal ejaculation*

- (a) Incorrect timing of coitus – separation due to travel or work shift;
- (b) Low semen volume – partial retrograde ejaculation or other dysfunction;
- (c) Limited vaginal penetration, e.g. physical disability due to hip contracture;
- (d) Anatomical abnormality – hypospadius, with sperm deposit low in the vagina;

**Table 3** A practical classification of male infertility[2]

| *Aetiology* | *Mechanism* | *Terminology* | *Sperm function* | *ART indicated* |
|---|---|---|---|---|
| *Type 1 Mechanical* | | | | |
| Low volume, hypospadius*, sexual* | ejaculation (i) normal | hypospermia | normal | AIH |
| Diabetes*, endoscopic resection | (ii) retrograde | cryptospermia | normal | AIH |
| Spinal cord injury, multiple sclerosis | (iii) failure | aspermia, anejaculation | normal | vibrator – AIH, electro-ejaculation, vas aspiration – IVF |
| *Type II Azoospermia* | | | | |
| Kallman's*, anabolic steroids* | (i) pre-testicular, FSH low | hypogonadrophic hypogonadism | normal | AIH – IVF |
| Cryptorchidism, radiotherapy, genetic | (ii) testicular, FSH high | primary testicular failure | immature | TESE – ICSI |
| Postinflammatory*, vasectomy* vas aplasia | (iii) post-testicular, FSH normal | obstructive azoospermia | immature | PESA – ICSI |
| *Type III Sperm coating* | | | | |
| Idiopathic antibodies*, unilateral obstruction*, infection | (i) sperm antibodies | immunological | normal (coated) | IVF |
| Nifedipine | (ii) pharmacological | calcium antagonists | ?normal | ?AIH – IVF |
| | (iii) non-specific | isoagglutination | normal (coated) | IVF |
| *Type IV Subnormal semen quality* | | †oligoasthenoteratozoospermia | | |
| Varicocele* | | oligozoospermia, asthenozoospermia | | |
| Salazopyrine*, alcohol | sperm preparation | | | |
| Idiopathic, genetic | (i) adequate | IVF fertilization | normal | IUI – IVF |
| Accessory gland infection | ($> 1 \times 10^6$ progressive) | IVF fertilization failure | dysfunction | ICSI |
| Unilateral obstruction* | (ii) inadequate ($< 1 \times 10^6$ progressive) | severe oligozoospermia | dysfunction | ICSI |
| *Type V Abnormal sperm function (normal concentration)* | | | | |
| Globozoospermia, immotile cilia syndrome | (i) overt absolute | tetatozoospermia | dysfunction | ICSI |
| Subnormal morphology | (WHO < 30%, Kruger < 4%) relative | strict morphology criteria | | ICSI |
| Absent motility | non-viable | necrozoospermia | | TESE – ICSI |
| Normal semen | (ii) occult – IVF no fertilization | normozoospermia | dysfunction | ICSI |
| ?Varicocele ?infection | diagnostic andrology | sperm dysfunction | | ICSI |

*Reversible male infertility where treatment often results in natural pregnancy; †also known as OAT syndrome or 'oligospermia'; ART, assisted reproduction technology; AIH, homologous artificial insemination; IVF, *in vitro* fertilization; TESE, testicular sperm extraction; ICSI, intracytoplasmic sperm injection; PESA, percutaneous epididymal aspiration; IUI, intrauterine insemination

 (e) Erectile dysfunction (impotence) – psychogenic or organic, normal ejaculation;
 (f) Psychogenic failure of intravaginal ejaculation.

(2) *Retrograde ejaculation*
 (a) Neurological – diabetes mellitus, multiple sclerosis;
 (b) Pharmacological – phenothiazines, sympathetic blockers;
 (c) Anatomical – congenital open bladder neck;
 (d) Iatrogenic – transurethral prostatectomy, bladder neck incision.

(3) *Ejaculatory failure (aspermia)*
 (a) Neurological – spinal cord injury, multiple sclerosis;
 (b) Pharmacological – antihypertensive or psychotropic medication;
 (c) Iatrogenic – retroperitoneal or pelvic surgery, sympathetic nerve injury.

**Type II: azoospermia (about 2%)**

This is defined as the absence of spermatozoa on at least two semen analyses. The subclassification depends on the state of spermatogenesis, which is inversely related to the serum FSH level and directly to testis size.

(1) *Pretesticular* – gonadotrophin deficiency with small prepubertal testes
 (a) Hypothalamic – Kallman's syndrome, craniopharyngioma, haemochromatosis;
 (b) Pituitary – trauma, ablation, tumours, isolated FSH deficiency, meningitis;
 (c) Secondary – anabolic steroids, testosterone injections.

(2) *Testicular* – grossly elevated FSH level, usually small atrophic testes
 (a) Congenital – Klinefelter's syndrome, congenital anorchia, cryptorchidism, AZF, myotonic dystrophy, XYY;
 (b) Acquired – radiotherapy, chemotherapy, mumps orchitis, castration.

(3) *Post-testicular* – obstructive azoospermia: normal FSH level, testis size, and spermatogenesis
 (a) Congenital – vas aplasia, cystic fibrosis, ? Young's syndrome, Müllerian cysts;
 (b) Acquired – gonorrhoea, chlamydia, tuberculosis, schistosomiasis, prostatitis;
 (c) Iatrogenic – vasectomy, hernia or hydrocele repair, pelvic surgery.

**Type III: immunological, sperm coating (about 5%)**

Spermatozoa are coated with antibodies or agents which hinder their normal function.

(1) *Immunological*
 (a) Idiopathic;
 (b) Acquired – unilateral obstruction, genitourinary infection, following reversal of vasectomy or obstruction.

(2) *Pharmacological* – calcium antagonists.

**Type IV: subnormal semen quality (80% of male infertility, and about 40% of all infertility)**

Sperm concentration is subnormal ($< 20 \times 10^6$/ml); motility and morphology vary. Testicular histology is also variable. Normal sperm function may result in delayed spontaneous conceptions. Therapy improves the situation in few men. IVF is indicated if the sperm preparation is adequate ($> 0.5 \times 10^6$ motile spermatozoa). ICSI is indicated if there are insufficient motile sperm, or sperm dysfunction is recognized by previous failure of fertilization, or by diagnostic andrology.

(1) *Idiopathic* – the majority;

(2) *Congenital* – unilateral cryptorchidism, or after bilateral orchidopexy;

(3) *Toxic* – alcohol, marihuana, cocaine, anabolic steroids (low dose);

(4) *Acquired* – varicocele, infection, unilateral obstruction, torsion, orchitis;

(5) *Genetic* – autosomal abnormalities, sex chromosome mosaics, azoospermia factor (AZF);

(6) *Iatrogenic* – salazopyrine, radiotherapy, chemotherapy, intramuscular testosterone.

### Type V: abnormal sperm function – normal concentration (about 10%)

The sperm count is normal ($20 \times 10^6$/ml or more), but there is total sperm dysfunction and ICSI is necessary to achieve fertilization. The problem is identified by either:

(i) Morphological abnormality of all spermatozoa – teratozoospermia;

(ii) Normal semen quality, but persistent failure of fertilization by IVF; or

(iii) Diagnostic andrology, strict morphology, computer-assisted semen analysis, or reactive oxygen species.

(1) *Overt sperm dysfunction*

   (a) Absolute – globozoospermia, Kartagener syndrome, immotile cilia syndrome, necrozoospermia;

   (b) Relative – idiopathic teratozoospermia, WHO < 30%, Kruger < 4%.

(2) *Occult sperm dysfunction*: normal semen parameters.

## MANAGEMENT OF MALE INFERTILITY

### The application of ART to the management of male infertility

Historical landmarks begin with the first recorded and successful case of homologous artificial insemination in 1776, by John Hunter, who advised a linen draper with hypospadius to use a warm syringe to introduce his semen into his wife[26]. A pregnancy achieved by AIH following aspiration of a natural spermatocele in vas aplasia[27] was the first successful surgical sperm retrieval.

Following its introduction, *in vitro* fertilization was utilized early for semen abnormalities[28], and then combined with surgical sperm retrieval to manage irreversible obstructive azoospermia using vasal[29] and epididymal[30,31] sperm. However, microassisted fertilization, epitomized by ICSI, improved the fertilization rate in severe oligozoospermia[1] and surgical sperm retrieval, which was extended to include testicular sperm[32,33]. Conceptions achieved with ICSI from round-headed acrosomeless sperm[34], spermatids from the testis or ejaculate in maturation arrest[35,36], and testicular sperm isolated from men with the Sertoli cell only[37] and Klinefelters syndromes[38] have further increased the scope of ART in male factor infertility.

### Overview

The principal conditions where treatment for male infertility is a realistic proposition with a *bona fide* chance of natural conception include (1) hypogonadotrophic hypogonadism, (2) obstructive azoospermia, (3) immunological infertility, (4) varicocele, and (5) some cases of ejaculatory or sexual dysfunction. Success can also be expected following cessation of (6) sulphasalazine therapy or (7) testosterone or anabolic steroid injections. Therapeutic agents which have been implicated in the aetiology of male infertility are listed in Table 4.

Most male infertility is ultimately managed by ART, with mechanical problems (type I) usually treated by AIH, azoospermia (type II) by reconstructive surgery or surgical sperm retrieval for ICSI, sperm antibodies (type III) and moderate semen abnormalities (type IV) by IVF, and severe semen abnormalities and sperm dysfunction (type V) by ICSI. The pregnancy rate of about 25%, and take-home-baby rate of 16–18% per cycle are similar following ART

**Table 4** Drugs which may affect male fertility

*Hypothalamic–pituitary–testicular axis*
Androgens – testosterone and anabolic steroid injections
High-dose corticosteroids
Progestogens, oestrogens
LHRH agonists
Antiandrogens – cyproterone, spironolactone, cimetidine

*Testis*
Cytotoxic agents, e.g. methotrexate for psoriasis
Colchicine
Nitrofurantoin, niridazole
Sulphasalazine
Gossypol

*Epididymis*
Amiodarone

*Spermatozoa*
(1) Acrosome – nifedipine
(2) Motility – lignocaine, procaine
propranolol
quinine
chlorpromazine

for all male factor problems, and are dependent on female age and fertility. The range of techniques available accommodates the wide variations in the quantity and quality of the sperm harvests derived from infertile men.

## Pretreatment counselling

Having identified the cause of the husband's infertility, both partners are counselled because a selection of treatments may be available for the specific male problem. The clinician should be aware of female factors which could influence the decision. IVF is already indicated where there are tubal problems, and ART should be considered early in a woman approaching 40 in order to establish if oocytes are still available and whether fertilization can be achieved with the spermatozoa of her partner. If she is below 35, the andrologist may be justified in trying to cure the husband, but natural pregnancy may not follow surgery for obstructive azoospermia or varicocele for 1–2 years, and most couples are anxious to commence families following prolonged infertility. The treatment indicated for each partner, the prognosis, details of which ART techniques apply, their limitations, success rates, and costs, are explained, with the alternative options of donor insemination or adoption. Some couples, unimpressed by the results, and possible genetic consequences (see below), and anticipating the expense and stress surrounding ART, prefer to remain childless, for few babies are available for adoption in the UK, especially for the relatively older infertile couples seen in most assisted conception units.

## Genetic anomalies and ART

In male factor infertility, the retrieval, selection and preparation of spermatozoa circumvent the natural events of sperm selection in both reproductive tracts. ICSI bypasses fertilization itself. There is no evidence that the routine procedures adopted for ART, especially ICSI, lead to fetal abnormality, and it appears that the uterus, by failing to permit implantation of a high proportion of transferred embryos, acts as an effective filter against the transmission of mutations.

In view of the power of ICSI, it is important to be aware that some male fertility problems are genetic and may thus be transmitted through ART[39]. The most common chromosome anomaly is 47,XXY, Klinefelter's syndrome, where spermatozoa are occasionally produced in 46,XY/47,XXY mosaicism. About 4% of men with azoospermia or oligozoospermia ($< 20 \times 10^6$/ml) are heterozygous for somatic chromosome aberrations, including reciprocal translocations, insertions, inversions or ring chromosomes. Such abnormalities could arise during defective spermatogenesis, which could also lead to a relatively high proportion of diploid spermatozoa. Deletions of DNA sequences from the long arm of the Y chromosome (AZF factor) are reported in 9% of azoospermic and severely oligozoospermic ($< 1 \times 10^6$/ml) men. In addition, about one in 25 individuals carry cystic fibrosis mutations. It is, therefore, important to advise that the male partner has a full chromosome analysis, and probably cystic fibrosis screening, before elaborate investigations or treatments are commenced, and to be prepared to refer the couple for *genetic counselling*.

## TYPE 1: MECHANICAL (OR PHYSICAL) INFERTILITY

Since the spermatozoa are essentially normal, therapy seeks to overcome the obstacles preventing transfer of semen to the cervix at ovulation. This is accomplished by:

(1) *Advice* on coitus to ensure semen is deposited intravaginally;

(2) *Treatment* of the male partner to improve sexual function; or

(3) *ART*, obtaining seminal fluid, usually for AIH.

If the semen is abnormal (Types II–V), IVF or ICSI may be indicated. The overall management depends on ejaculatory function. A postcoital test is helpful in identifying whether there is normal (antegrade) ejaculation, retrograde ejaculation (cryptospermia), or failure of ejaculation (aspermia), aided by microscopy of postejaculatory urine for sperm.

### Normal ejaculation

*Advice*
Advice on shift or travel schedules may help to synchronize coitus and ovulation. In physical disabilities, vaginal penetration may be improved by alternative positions for intercourse.

*Treatment*
Failure of intravaginal ejaculation may respond to *psychosexual counselling* or psychotropic medication. A low-volume ejaculate (hypospermia) due to partial retrograde ejaculation in prostatitis may respond to antibiotics (erythromycin, trimethoprim, doxycycline, ciprofloxacin) and/or ephedrine to tighten the bladder neck. Impotence is best managed in a specialist urological centre. Penile prostaglandin injections are effective for psychogenic impotence, but should be used cautiously since underlying marital problems could later affect the welfare of the child conceived.

*ART*
Timed AIH solves the physical and logistic problems separating sperm and egg, with semen cryopreservation if the husband travels frequently.

### Retrograde ejaculation

Retrograde ejaculation is diagnosed from the history and verified by finding sperm in postorgasmic urine. There is no ejaculate or a low semen volume.

*Advice*
Antegrade ejaculation can sometimes be induced during intercourse with a very full bladder, which improves bladder neck closure. Where the bladder neck is wide and lax, *intravaginal voiding* after orgasm may be possible. Urinary toxicity to sperm is minimized by alkalinizing the urine with oral sodium bicarbonate beforehand.

*Treatment*
Antegrade ejaculation can be induced in some patients with partial neurological lesions (e.g. diabetes mellitus) with ephedrine (15–30 mg) 30 min before coitus or desipramine, 50 mg alternate days. Surgical correction of the bladder neck is also feasible.

*ART*
Spermatozoa are retrieved from postorgasmic urine by voiding or through catheterization. Exposure to urine is limited by preliminary fluid restriction, oral sodium bicarbonate, or catheterization to instill a buffer solution. Spermatozoa are extracted and prepared for insemination, when intrauterine insemination (IUI) is usually effective. Urry and colleagues[40] achieved pregnancy in 16% of cycles using IUI with washed spermatozoa. If the yield is poor, IVF or ICSI is indicated. An alternative technique is to utilize rectal electroejaculation which can induce antegrade ejaculation in some cases of retrograde ejaculation.

## Ejaculation failure (aspermia)

Aspermia is usually incurable due to neurological damage from spinal cord or pelvic injury, multiple sclerosis, or retroperitoneal surgery. Most men with aspermia presenting for assisted conception have a spinal cord injury above T10, following motor cycle accidents. They are usually wheelchair-bound, with urinary drainage by condom device, indwelling or suprapubic catheter. They are otherwise healthy with young fertile wives dedicated to caring for them, often work and have a natural desire for a family. Spermatogenesis is usually normal, but testicular biopsy may be necessary if the testes are small or the FSH level elevated. Therapy for urine infection will minimize sperm contamination during ART.

*Advice*
Reflex ejaculation may occur with sexual activity, certain movements, or a penile vibrator (80 Hz) with home insemination by syringe, followed by IUI or IVF at the fertility unit, if this does not result in pregnancy.

*Treatment*
In some patients, the impotence can be managed by intracavernosal prostaglandin self-injection or a penile prosthesis, after which ejaculation may occur during intercourse.

*ART*
Rectal electroejaculation using a rectal probe to stimulate the seminal vesicles, is usually effective in providing semen for AIH or IVF (Chapter 12). If spinal dysreflexia is a risk, general anaesthesia is preferred; sublingual nifedipine may be used as prophylaxis against a hypertensive crisis. Sperm preparation medium instilled into the bladder is reaspirated with sperm after the procedure, since some retrograde flow occurs. Poor-quality semen improves with repeated ejaculations due to enhanced transit in the reproductive tract.

Vas deferens aspiration[41] is useful if electroejaculation fails to provide adequate semen, and is often the patient's first choice. A local anaesthetic spermatic cord block is necessary to avoid pain and spinal dysreflexia, as sympathetic sensory fibres from the testis are intact, but the scrotal skin is usually numb. The vas is exposed percutaneously. A minute transverse incision admits a fine 2 fg (umbilical) cannula, which is advanced towards the prostate or testis to aspirate vasal fluid (Figure 9). The vasotomy is repaired microsurgically. Adequate motile spermatozoa are usually obtained for IVF, cryopreservation, and often IUI. Vas aspiration can be repeated with little risk of obstruction. Sperm can also be retrieved by transperineal seminal vesicle aspiration under ultrasound control using local anaesthetic.

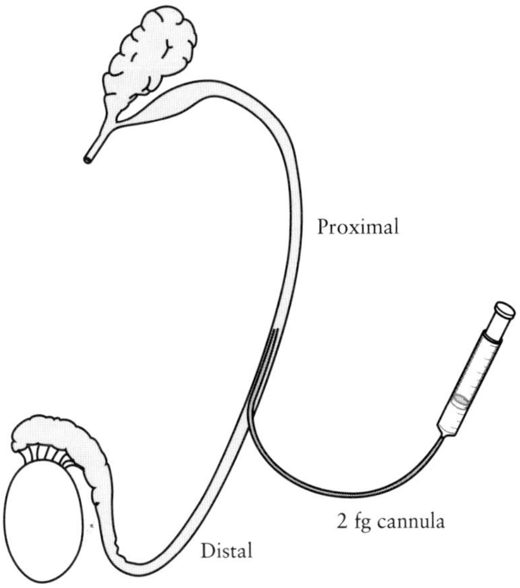


**Figure 9** Aspiration of the vas deferens in aspermia (vas aspiration)

Using a vibrator with home insemination for upper motor neuron lesions, and electroejaculation and IUI in lower lesions, Dahlberg[42] retrieved sperm from 29 of 35 spinal cord injured men, with vas aspiration required in six men. Pregnancy occurred in 51% of couples.

Aspermic men with testicular failure are diagnosed by the finding of small testes and elevation of the FSH level. Testicular sperm extraction for ICSI (see Figure 16 later) is indicated, and may be the only method available for aspermic patients in units without special equipment or expertise in the above procedures.

## TYPE 2: AZOOSPERMIA (Figure 10)

Azoospermia is diagnosed from two to three centrifuged semen samples. Low testosterone, FSH and LH levels suggest hypogonadotrophic hypogonadism. Small testes and a high FSH level indicate testicular failure. Normal-size testes and FSH level indicate obstructive azoospermia.

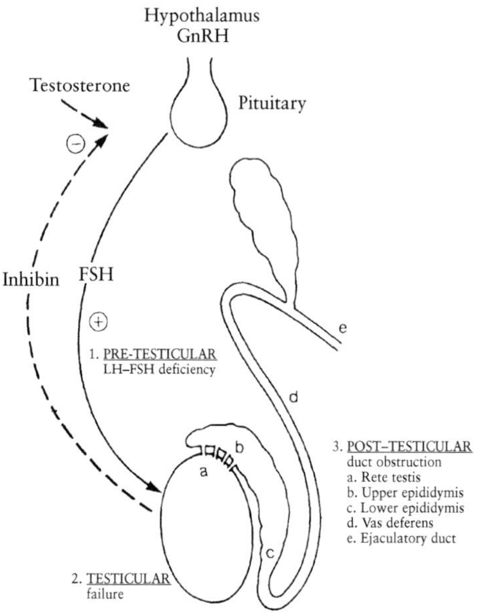


**Figure 10** The three types of azoospermia

### Pretesticular – gonadotrophin deficiency

Hypogonadotrophic hypogonadism is uncommon (< 1%). Primary hypogonadotrophic hypogonadism presenting as delayed puberty is treated by the paediatrician or endocrinologist. Adults with Kallman's syndrome have hypogonadism and anosmia due to a hypothalamic abnormality. Gonadotrophin deficiency may also be secondary to anabolic steroid or testosterone injections, cranial injury, meningitis, pituitary (prolactinoma) or hypothalamic tumour or haemochromatosis. A pituitary fossa X-ray, computed tomographic or magnetic resonance image scan is indicated if a cerebral tumour is suspected.

Hypogonadotrophic hypogonadism is treated with gonadotrophins. Leydig cells are first primed to generate testosterone using human chorionic gonadotrophin (hCG), Pregnyl or Profasi, 2000–5000 units intramuscularly twice weekly. The serum testosterone level should rise to normal within 6–12 weeks, and then FSH level, given as human menopausal gonadotrophin (hMG), Pergonal or Humegon, 75–150 units intramuscularly thrice weekly, stimulates the Sertoli cells. Spermatozoa may not appear in the semen for 1 year, but natural pregnancy occurs in over 50% of patients[43], even at a low count, because normal spermatozoa are produced. Pulsatile GnRH given by portable mini-pump may be successful if this regime fails[44].

Where hypogonadotrophic hypogonadism is due to testosterone or anabolic steroid injections, obtained illegally by sportsmen, gynaecomastia may arise from aromatization of testosterone to oestrogens. The serum testosterone level is extraordinarily high. If the androgens are withdrawn, the seminal fluid analysis is often normal within 6 months and natural pregnancy is usually established within 1 year.

### Testicular – primary testicular failure (testicular azoospermia)

Testicular azoospermia is also known as non-obstructive azoospermia, but this should also include hypogonadotrophic hypogonadism. The clinical features are atrophic testes with elevation of the FSH level. If testosterone output is reduced, hypogonadism may be present. Common causes are Klinefelter's syndrome, cryptorchidism, mumps orchitis and radiotherapy. In some cases (e.g. maturation arrest), the FSH level is normal and the diagnosis is established from biopsies taken during testicular exploration. In adults, orchidopexy rarely restores fertility.

Donor insemination was previously indicated, but the management has changed radically due to the success of ICSI using testicular spermatozoa (testicular sperm extraction, see later), which are present in isolated foci in 40–50% of patients. Preliminary diagnostic testicular biopsies are advisable, with cryopreservation, preferably by multiple sampling, in view of their patchy pathology. Karyotyping is desirable before diagnostic testicular biopsy since chromosome abnormalities may be present in some patients. AZF testing may be introduced in future if found to be clinically relevant.

Klinefelter's syndrome is a congenital disorder due to a 47,XXY karyotype occurring in one in 1000 men, caused by a meiotic non-dysjunction. Two X chromosomes remain in the oocyte, which is fertilized by a Y-bearing sperm. Buccal smears reveal Barr bodies. Patients are tall with eunuchoid features, female fat distribution, sparse body hair, small testes and gynaecomastia. They have azoospermia, but usually normal sexual function. Serum testosterone is often reduced due to defective Leydig cell function, with very high FSH and LH levels. Some men require androgen supplements in middle age if they experience sexual difficulty. Testicular histology reveals obliterated tubules or Sertoli cells only, and occasionally foci of spermatogenesis. In such cases, fertility is very rare (possibly due to XY/XXY mosaicism); however, a biochemical pregnancy has resulted from ICSI using testicular spermatozoa[38]. Most patients receive donor insemination as definitive therapy.

### Post-testicular (obstructive azoospermia)

Obstructive azoospermia is suspected where the testis size and FSH level are both normal. If either epididymis is distended, especially the caput, the diagnosis of obstruction is more certain.

*Low-volume fructose-negative ejaculate*

This is usually due to bilateral congenital absence of the vas deferens, which is confirmed by the clinical examination (surgical exploration is unnecessary). This can also be due to bilateral ejaculatory duct obstruction, where transrectal ultrasound may reveal seminal vesicle distension. Testicular exploration (see below) is indicated if the vasa are palpable in order to:

(1) Carry out reconstructive epididymal or vasal surgery, if feasible; or

(2) Obtain testicular biopsies which may detect spermatozoa useful for ICSI.

*Bilateral congenital absence of the vas deferens*

This condition occurs in one in 1000 men, and in 20% of men with obstructive azoospermia. It is linked with cystic fibrosis, since 98% of men with cystic fibrosis are sterile due to bilateral congenital absence of the vas deferens, and 66% of men with bilateral congenital absence of the vas deferens carry cystic fibrosis mutations, commonly DF508 or R117H in Europeans. Mutations in other races are different, but are absent if there is associated renal abnormality or unilateral vas aplasia.

Patients have normal andrological features, with normal-size testes. Neither vas is palpable. Bilateral congenital absence of the vas deferens is due to aplasia of the Wolffian (mesonephric) ducts. The head of the epididymis is usually present (engorged with sperm, Figure 11), because the efferent ducts arise from the testes. The body and tail of the epididymis are absent. The seminal vesicles and ejaculatory ducts fail to develop, explaining a low-volume fructose-negative ejaculate, but occasionally they persist and fructose is present. Spermatogenesis is usually normal, but testicular biopsy may be indicated if the FSH level is raised (rare). Treatment

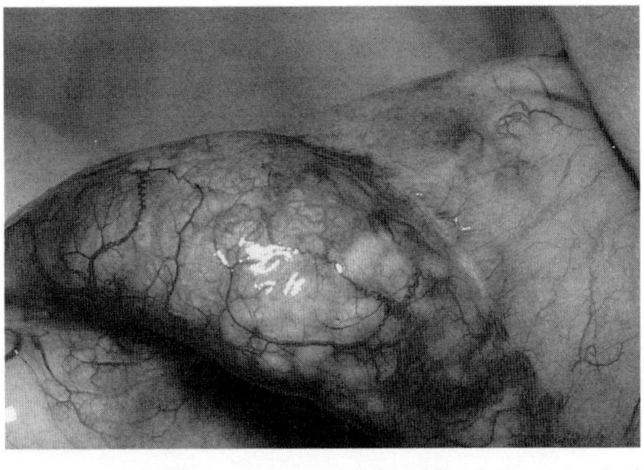

**Figure 11** The caput epididymidis in congenital absence of the vas deferens. Note the dilated tubules engorged with spermatozoa

is by epididymal sperm retrieval for ICSI (percutaneous epididymal aspiration, see Figure 16), but it is first essential to screen both partners for cystic fibrosis mutations. If one partner is positive, the risk of a child developing cystic fibrosis is one in 300, slightly above the normal incidence of one in 625 births, since one in 25 Europeans carry DF508. If both partners are carriers, the risk is one in four and assisted conception should only be undertaken after genetic counselling and if preimplantation diagnosis of embryos is available. Treatment is thus available for men with cystic fibrosis.

*Testicular exploration in azoospermia*

Under general anaesthetic, each testis is exposed through the tunica vaginalis and the epididymis is inspected for dilated tubules (Figure 11), which confirm the diagnosis of an obstruction. Vasography is then performed by injecting contrast medium through a fine 25-gauge needle into each vas, towards the bladder. The flow is usually unrestricted and X-ray screening will normally outline the seminal vesicles with contrast inside the bladder, signifying a patent proximal duct system (Figure 12). If the vasogram is normal, inspection of the epididymis through the operating microscope locates the site of the block and a suitable dilated tubule above this for epididymo–vasostomy. The tubule selected is incised and the fluid within aspirated and inspected for motile spermatozoa under a laboratory microscope. Higher incisions in the epididymis may be required until motile spermatozoa are found. The vas is divided at this level, mobilized without tension towards the epididymis, and a microsurgical epididymo–vasostomy is carried out in two layers (Figure 13b). Sperm appears in the ejaculate in 50% of patients within 6 months, but may not appear for 15 months. Good results are also achieved following non-microsurgical side-to-side epididymo-vasostomy if the block is at the tail of the epididymis, but not the caput[45]. If the vasogram reveals an obstruction of the vas, the block is resected and vaso–vasostomy (Figure 13a) is carried out to repair the defect[45].

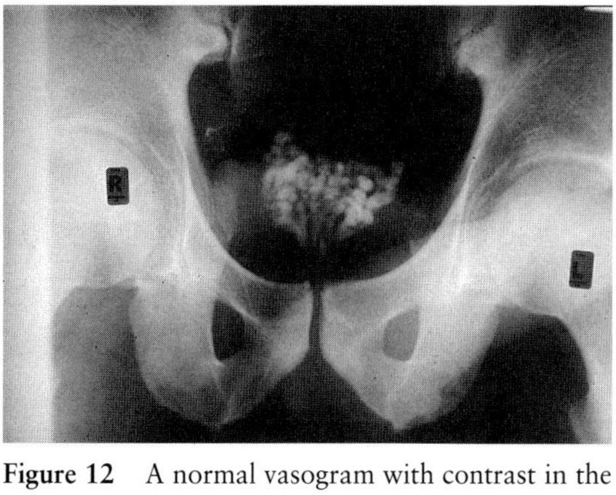

Figure 12 A normal vasogram with contrast in the bladder

Ejaculatory duct obstruction is diagnosed if the vasogram reveals dilated seminal vesicles with no contrast entering the bladder. This is often due to a Müllerian cyst. Endoscopic resection relieves the obstruction in about 50%[46].

*Results of testicular biopsy if there is no obstruction*

If there are no dilated epididymal tubules, testicular biopsies are obtained, preferably multiple since the pathological changes are often focal. If the biopsies reveal normal spermatogenesis (Figure 14a), the diagnosis is rete testis obstruction which is due to immune orchitis in about 50% of cases, confirmed by serum antisperm antibody testing (TAT or Immunobeads). Oral prednisolone 5 mg t.d.s. leads to sperm-positive ejaculates in half the patients in 3–6 months, with the possibility of natural conception or ART with ejaculated sperm. Alternatively, testicular sperm can be retrieved for ICSI (testicular sperm extraction, see Figure 16).

If the biopsies reveal impairment of spermatogenesis due to maturation arrest (spermatids, Figure 14b), spermatocytes, (Figure 14c), the Sertoli cell only syndrome (Figure 14d), or a mixed picture, ICSI is feasible using testicular sperm (testicular sperm extraction, see Figure 16) if foci of normal spermatogenesis (Figure 15) are identified in any of the biopsies. Spermatogonia or spermatocytes present in maturation arrest cannot be used for ICSI because they are diploid, and, since gonadotrophin therapy given to these patients almost invariably fails to induce sperm production, donor insemination is advised. Spermatids

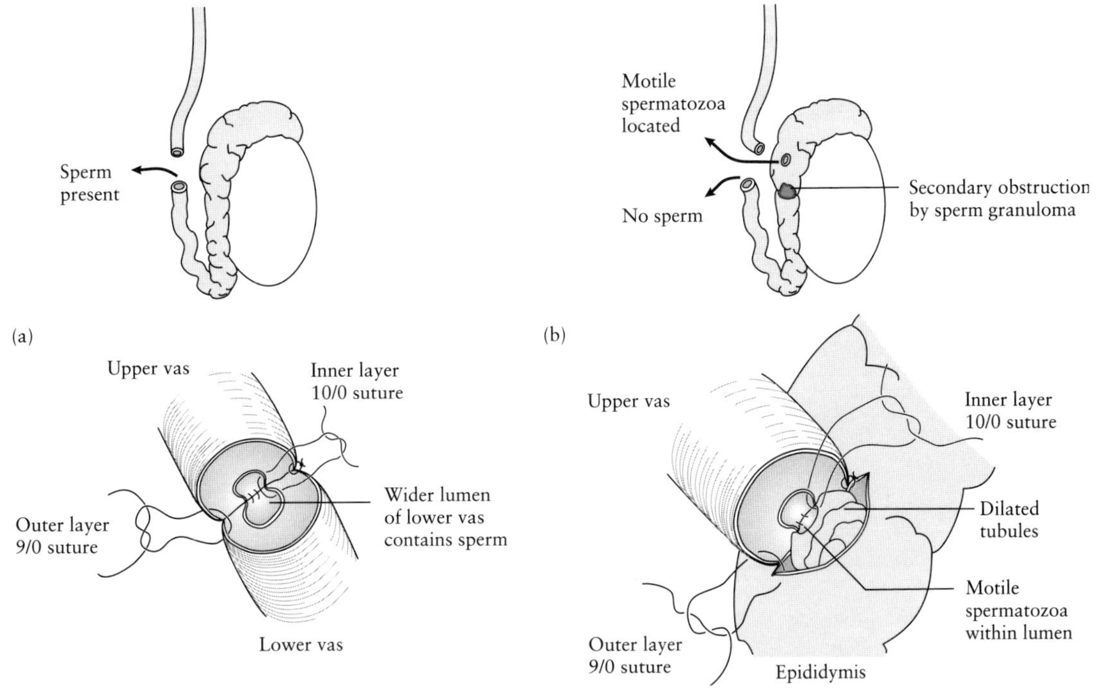


**Figure 13** Microsurgical two-layer anastomotic techniques used in vasectomy reversal and reconstructive microsurgery in obstructive azoospermia. (a) If sperm is identified in the lower (testis) segment of the vas, end-to-end vaso–vasostomy is carried out. The posterior layers are completed. (b) No spermatozoa are in the lower vas because there is a secondary block in the body of the epididymis due to a sperm granuloma. End (of vas)-to-side (of epididymal tubule) epididymo–vasostomy is performed at the site where spermatozoa have been identified in a specific epididymal tubule

present in the testis or semen in maturation arrest are haploid and can be utilized for ICSI[36]. Spermatid injection is not currently permitted in the UK; however, foci of spermatozoa may be present in these patients.

*Vasectomy reversal*

In view of the increasing divorce rate and popularity of vasectomy, men requesting vasectomy reversal in their second marriages are often seen in the infertility clinic. Reconstruction of the vas is more successful if little has been resected, and if carried out within 10 years of the original operation. End-to-end vaso–vasostomy by a one-layer non-microsurgical technique results in recanalization in 80–90% of patients within 3 months, with a 40% chance of spontaneous pregnancy[47]. Failure may be due to secondary epididymal obstruction from a sperm granuloma which may be bypassed by epididymo–vasostomy if recognized. 'Redo' vasectomy reversals are successful in about 50% of cases. Results are better with microsurgical techniques (Figure 13) in two layers, especially if microscopy is used to confirm the presence of spermatozoa in the vas (vaso–vasostomy), or the obstructed epididymal tubules (epididymo–vasostomy) at the site of the anastomosis[48–50].

## Surgical sperm retrieval in azoospermia (Figure 16)

Surgical sperm retrieval for ICSI is indicated in:

(1) Irreversible obstructive azoospermia, where spermatogenesis is normal. The three types of irreversible obstructive azoospermia commonly presenting for surgical sperm retrieval and ICSI are:

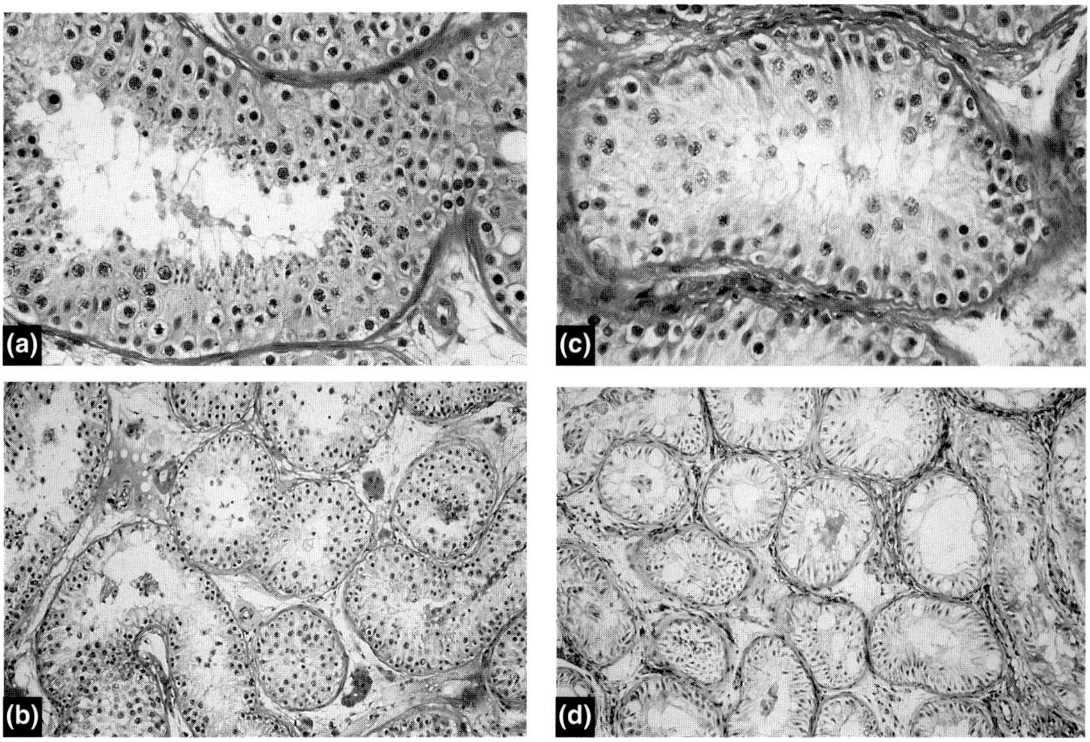


**Figure 14** Azoospermia: four examples of testicular histology. (a) Normal spermatogenesis. Formed spermatozoa are observed at the luminal borders of the Sertoli cells ready for release; (b) maturation arrest (at the spermatid stage); (c) maturation arrest (at the spermatocyte stage); (d) Sertoli cell only syndrome (germ cell aplasia or Del Castillo syndrome)

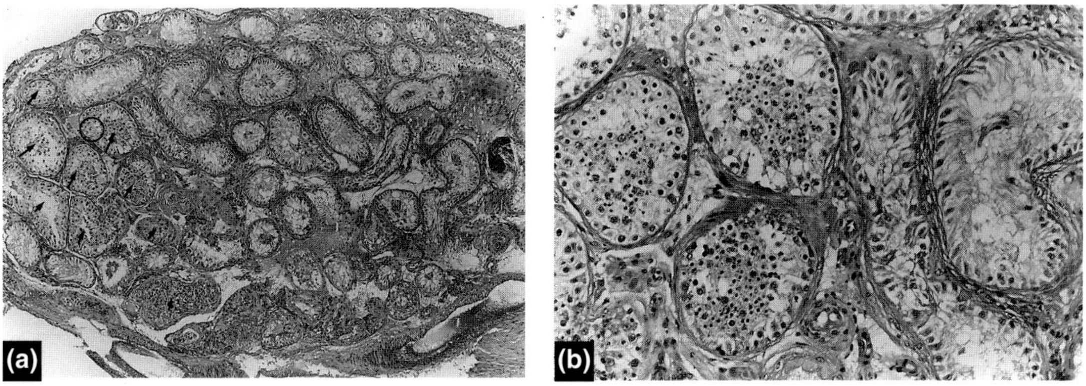


**Figure 15** Testicular histology of a man with primary testicular failure who had azoospermia, small testes (3 cm), high serum FSH level and a normal karyotype. (a) Low power (× 100): most seminiferous tubules contain Sertoli cells only, but there is a focus of tubules which exhibit spermatogenesis (arrows). In the entire biopsy, 2% of the seminiferous tubules had evidence of sperm production; (b) high power (× 400): a group of spermatozoa among Sertoli cells. (Courtesy of Dr Kishor Shah)

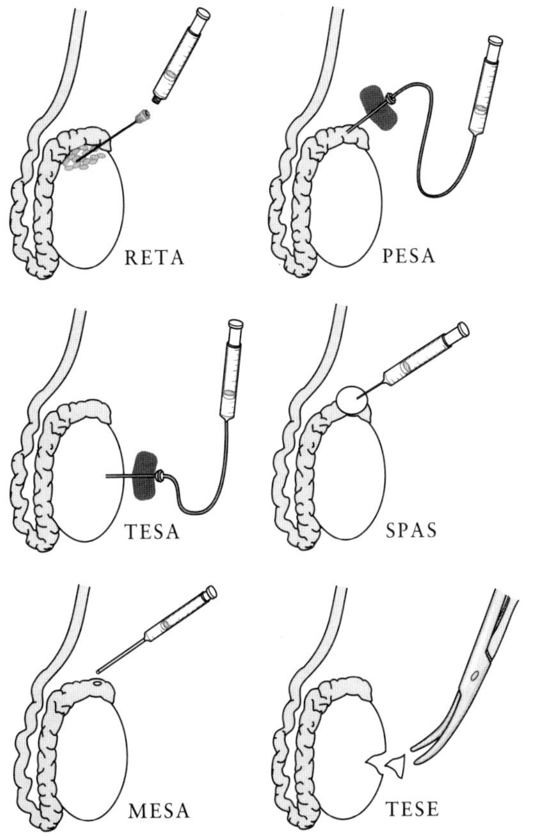


**Figure 16** Methods of surgical sperm retrieval utilized with ICSI in azoospermia. RETA, rete testis aspiration; PESA, percutaneous epididymal sperm aspiration; TESA, testicular sperm aspiration; SPAS, spermatocele aspiration; MESA, microsurgical epididymal sperm aspiration; TESE, testicular sperm extraction (from a biopsy)

(a) Bilateral congenital absence of the vas deferens;

(b) Irreversible vasectomy;

(c) Other cases of obstructive azoospermia, principally failed epididymo–vasostomy.

(2) Testicular azoospermia, where foci of normal spermatogenesis are identified on testicular biopsy. Genetic screening should be undertaken before considering surgical sperm retrieval in testicular azoospermia. If biopsy has not been carried out to confirm the presence of spermatozoa in the testis, some couples accept donor sperm back-up or the risk of abandoned egg collection if spermatozoa are not retrieved.

Since few spermatozoa are required for ICSI, minimally invasive techniques utilizing needle aspiration are usually effective in retrieving adequate spermatozoa[51]. In order to improve the acceptability of surgical sperm retrieval to patients, it is desirable to try to retrieve adequate spermatozoa for three ICSI cycles (cryopreservation for two additional cycles) from each surgical sperm retrieval procedure. The utilization of local anaesthesia avoids the risk, expense, and inconvenience of general anaesthesia, but in testicular azoospermia a general anaesthetic may be preferred, because multiple testicular biopsies are often required to accumulate adequate spermatozoa, especially where there are few minute foci of spermatogenesis. After selecting the least invasive procedures for surgical sperm retrieval and ICSI, spermatozoa were retrieved in all (100%) 27 cycles, with embryo transfer in 25 (93%) and conceptions in six (24%) couples[52]. Further experience has reaffirmed that ongoing pregnancies occur in one in six cycles and that most men prefer the convenience of sperm retrieval under local anaesthesia (unpublished results).

*Preliminary assessment*

Careful scrotal examination may locate minute cysts near the epididymis, since small natural spermatoceles, 1–2 cm diameter, occur in 4% of men with obstructive azoospermia. Spermatocele aspiration with a 25-gauge needle, generally without anaesthesia, usually yields viable spermatozoa (Figure 17), thereby avoiding a more invasive procedure[53]. The examination will also determine if the patient is a willing and suitable subject for sperm retrieval under local anaesthesia (see Figure 19). If either epididymis is engorged, percutaneous epididymal aspiration (Figure 16) is feasible, but, if collapsed, testicular sperm retrieval (testicular sperm aspiration or extraction, see Figure 16) may be required. Following recent epididymo–vasostomy (< 1 year), or where a man presenting for assisted conception is also considering future surgery for obstructive azoospermia, damage to the epididymis can be avoided by attempting rete testis aspiration under local anaesthesia with a 23-gauge needle (Figure 18). Rete testis aspiration is useful in one in six cases, but the sperm harvest is usually poor since rete testis fluid is a dilute concentration of spermatozoa. The epididymis can thus be intentionally avoided by retrieving testicular sperm (see Figure 16), leaving the epididymis intact.

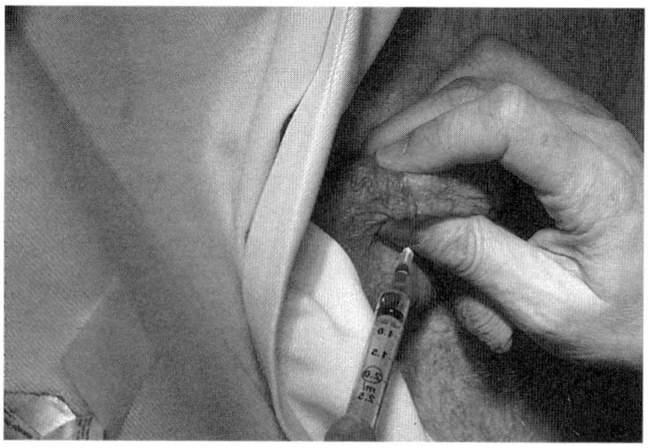

**Figure 17** Aspiration of a 1-cm diameter spermatocele in a patient with an irreversible vasectomy. The fluid contained viable spermatozoa. (Courtesy of Dr B. D. Stewart and Mr P. Bromwich, Midland Fertility Services)

*Percutaneous epididymal sperm aspiration (PESA)*

This procedure[54] can be carried out under general or local anaesthesia depending on the patient. A spermatic cord block can be achieved with a 1 : 1 mixture of 2% lignocaine and 0.5% bupivocaine plain, which will provide effective anaesthesia for over 1 h (Figure 19). The skin over the epididymis must also be infiltrated since the nerve supply is different. The testicular blood vessels are medial to the corpus epididymidis. Spermatozoa are retrieved by inserting a 21-gauge butterfly needle attached to a 10-ml syringe into the caput or upper corpus (Figure 20a). White fluid, often sanguinous, is

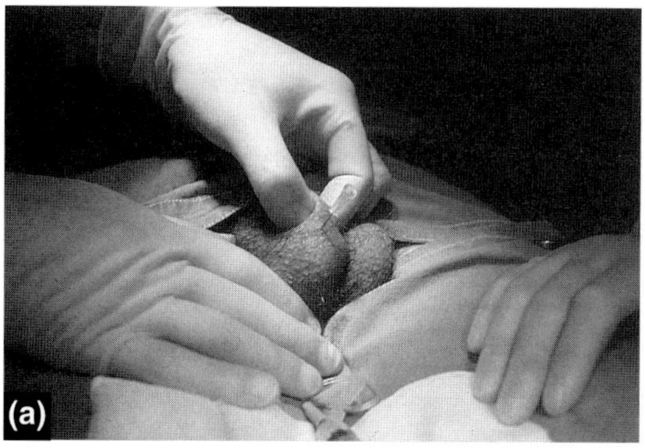


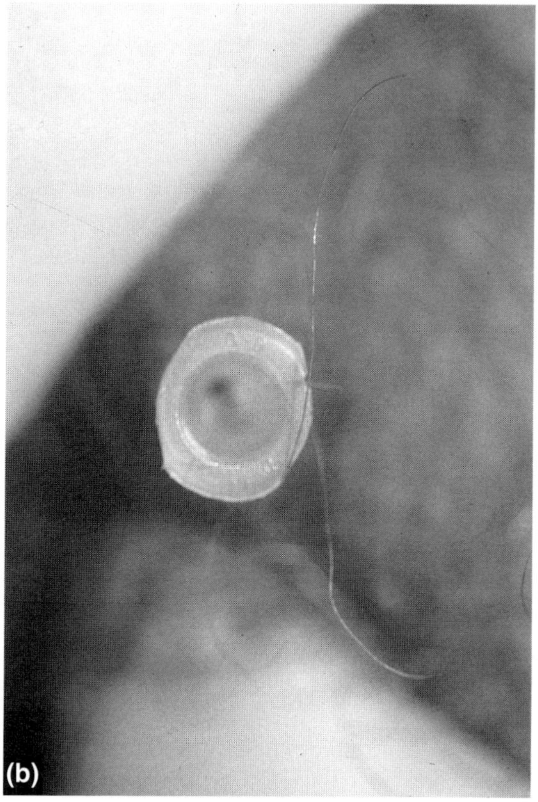


**Figure 18** Rete testis aspiration (RETA) under local anaesthesia. The caput epididymis is held between thumb and index finger. (a) A dry 23-gauge needle is inserted deeply into the mediastinum, then withdrawn slowly; (b) fluid appearing in the Luer fitting contains motile spermatozoa in one in six patients

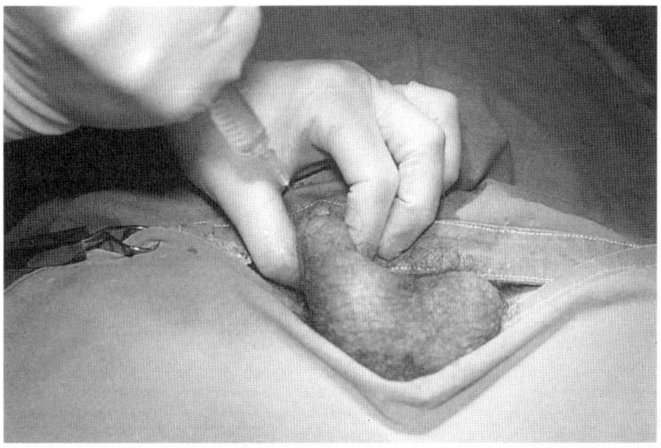

**Figure 19** Infiltration of the spermatic cord with local anaesthetic prior to minimally invasive surgical sperm retrieval in azoospermia

aspirated into the clear plastic tubing (Figure 20b). Microscopy usually reveals a high sperm concentration with some progressive motility, and a surfeit suitable for cryopreservation for future cycles. Patients return to work the next day. Postoperative pain is slight, with occasional haematoma or haematocele developing.

*Epididymal microaspiration (MESA)*

This procedure provides a better sperm harvest than percutaneous epididymal sperm aspiration, but this more invasive, often prolonged, microsurgical procedure under general anaesthesia[55] may no longer be justified in view of the convenience of minimally invasive surgical sperm retrieval for ICSI. Epididymal microaspiration is now probably only indicated where reconstructive surgery for obstructive azoospermia is carried out at the same time, when microsurgical repair of the incised epididymis preserves its continuity for coincidental epididymo–vasostomy or vaso–vasostomy. Epididymal microaspiration does, however, yield adequate spermatozoa for cryopreservation for many future cycles and may ensure that the patient will only ever have to undergo one surgical sperm retrieval procedure[55,56]. Epididymal microaspiration for IVF is no longer indicated due to inadequate fertilization[57].

*Testicular sperm aspiration (TESA) or testicular sperm extraction (TESE) in obstructive azoospermia*

Testicular spermatozoa can be retrieved under the same local anaesthesia if percutaneous epididymal sperm aspiration does not provide adequate viable spermatozoa. Testicular sperm aspiration[58] is carried out using a 19–21-gauge butterfly needle attached to a 20-ml syringe. With suction applied, the needle is inserted and re-inserted into the testicular parenchyma ten or more times before withdrawal. Testicular sperm aspiration is often unsuccessful, and a classical testicular biopsy by the 'window' technique through the scrotal skin and tunica vaginalis will enable a suitable 3–5-mm biopsy for testicular sperm extraction[59]. Spermatozoa with rudimentary activity are usually present in the first biopsy in obstructive azoospermia, but an additional sample may be necessary for cryopreservation. The scrotal wound is sutured in layers with fine (3/0) chromic catgut

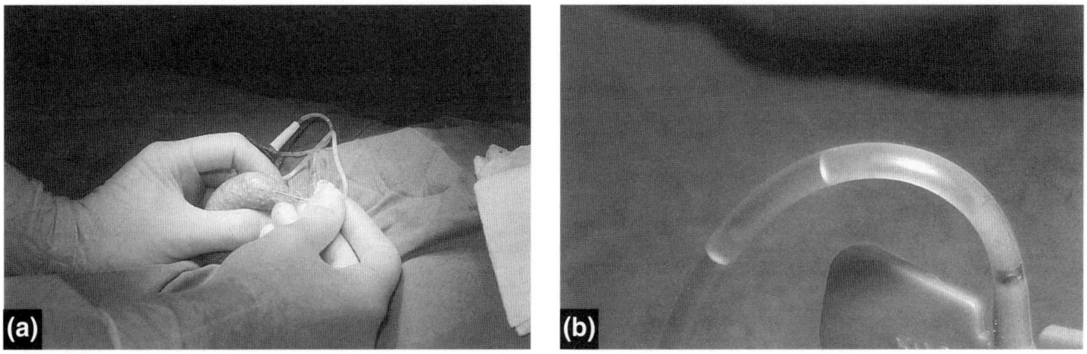


**Figure 20** (a) PESA, percutaneous epididymal sperm aspiration under local anaesthesia. The epididymis is held against the skin between the thumb and index finger. A 21-gauge butterfly needle is about to be plunged into the caput epididymidis; (b) white fluid appearing in the tubing usually contains motile spermatozoa

throughout, especially the dartos muscle to avoid a haematoma. The patient returns to work in 1–2 days, and complications are uncommon if a subcuticular suture (and prophylactic antibiotic) is used for the skin, as wound infection is then uncommon. Much embryological expertise is required to isolate spermatozoa from testicular tissue. They are often initially non-motile and their viability may not be established until activity is observed after 1–4 h in culture, or brief exposure to pentoxifylline, although normally formed inactive testicular spermatozoa are usually viable.

*Testicular sperm extraction (TESE) in testicular (non-obstructive) azoospermia*

It is now known that a single biopsy may not represent the entire testicular histology due to focal change. Multiple testicular sampling reveals focal spermatogenesis in 30–50% of the most severe cases of testicular failure, including the Sertoli cell only syndrome (Figure 15), and maturation arrest. Testicular sperm extraction under local or (preferably) general anaesthesia can provide spermatozoa for ICSI from such cases[37]. Multiple biopsies may be required in order to obtain sufficient spermatozoa for the retrieved oocytes, and this may involve the embryologist in a prolonged search for viable spermatozoa lasting many hours. Testicular aspiration, punch biopsy, or local anaesthesia may therefore limit the potential to obtain adequate spermatozoa in testicular azoospermia if there is patchy focal spermatogenesis. Testicular sperm extraction should not be repeated for 6 months to allow for testicular revascularization and recovery of spermatogenesis[60].

*Cryopreservation of surgically retrieved spermatozoa*

Surgical sperm retrieval is coordinated with oocyte retrieval when logistics permit, but there are often early or late responders to ovarian stimulation. Retrieved epididymal spermatozoa remain viable in the incubator for 12–24 h, and testicular spermatozoa for 2–3 days, thus allowing some flexibility in the timing of planned procedures for both partners. Advanced cryopreservation of sperm from epididymal microaspiration is also feasible, after which the alliquots may be thawed at will for future ICSI cycles, the male partner being required for only one occasion and the anxieties surrounding the timing of procedures thus being avoided[56]. Cryopreservation of a testicular tissue suspension or biopsy leads to improved sperm survival when compared with prepared spermatozoa[61], thereby adding a further dimension to surgical sperm retrieval.

## TYPE 3: IMMUNOLOGICAL INFERTILITY – SPERM COATING

Coating of the sperm surface by antibodies can interfere with sperm function. The significance of antisperm antibodies is not universally accepted, but antibodies to sperm occur in about 5% of men with primary infertility. Antibody-coated spermatozoa usually have subnormal motility and agglutinate in the seminal plasma. Penetration into cervical mucus and fertilization are both impaired. The MAR or Immunobead tests will detect antibodies attached to spermatozoa, which are significant if confirmed by TAT or Immunobead tests on serum or seminal plasma. IgA antibodies occur naturally and are most significant, and are sometimes due to associated genitourinary infection. IgG antibodies are often generated in obstructive azoospermia, and are present in the serum of 50% of men following vasectomy. However, even where high levels of IgG persist after successful vasectomy reversal, there is still a fair chance of natural conception, but, if persisting after recanalization in obstructive azoospermia, pregnancy is unusual. Treatment of a urinary infection may diminish the antibody level in some cases.

There are few proponents of steroids for sperm antibodies. This is because, although there is a one in three chance of a natural conception, pregnancies do not usually occur for 6–9 months[62], and the dose of steroid required is appreciable (prednisolone 20 mg b.d. for the first 10 days of the cycle, with 5 mg o.d. p.c. on days 11 and 12). Side-effects, for example, weight gain, insomnia, facial swelling, acne, diabetes mellitus, gastric irritation and peptic ulcer, are common, and aseptic necrosis of the hip has been reported. Sperm preparation techniques for IVF improve the fertilizing ability in male immunological infertility, with approximately a 30% chance of conception per cycle[63], but IUI does not give good results. The more direct approach of assisted conception is preferred by clinicians and patients, but economic considerations may deter some couples from seeking IVF. Some men accept the risks of steroids for the possibility of natural pregnancy through intercourse.

Unilateral testicular obstruction leads to a cell-mediated immune response which induces an immune orchitis. This leads to partial obstruction of the opposite rete testis, with a reduction of sperm flow from this unobstructed side. In addition, IgA antibodies secreted in the seminal plasma coat the sperm, further reducing the fertility potential of the ejaculate (Figure 21). The antibody production can be reduced by steroids and/or epididymo–vasostomy, which may both lead to an improvement in the ejaculate. IVF or ICSI are the most successful treatments. Removal of the obstructed testis leads to a one in ten chance of pregnancy, but remains an unpopular alternative option[64,65].

Calcium antagonists, such as nifedipine, used in hypertension and angina, bind to mannose ligands on the sperm acrosome and may thus be a cause of infertility by interfering with

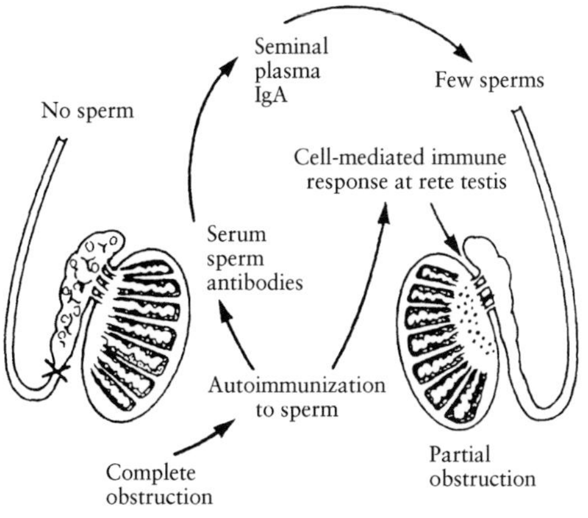


**Figure 21** Unilateral testicular obstruction leading to immunological infertility

the acrosome reaction and sperm zona binding[66]. Discontinuation of therapy can improve the chance of fertilization and conception by ART[67], but has not been shown to improve spontaneous conception. Sublingual nifedipine is often administered to spinal cord injured men, as prophylaxis against the hypertensive crisis of spinal dysreflexia induced during electroejaculation, but the excellent results from IVF and IUI appear to discount a significant antifertility effect in these patients.

## TYPE 4: OLIGOZOOSPERMIA (REDUCED SEMEN QUALITY)

The seminal fluid analysis is below the WHO standard, with usually $< 20 \times 10^6$/ml concentration, < 50% motility and < 25% progressive spermatozoa. This is usually associated with a reduction in the proportion of normal forms (< 30%), but teratozoospermia is considered under Type 5. For convenience, patients with a normal sperm concentration, but impaired (not absent) motility are included in Type 4 because there are similar features to oligozoospermia and many will undergo IVF.

Type 4 is probably a multifactorial group of problems which cannot be analysed succinctly due to lack of research, and includes wide ranges of the sperm parameters, from men with the occasional sperm in the ejaculate to those with a moderate count and impaired motility. There are usually more than 3 years' infertility with sperm dysfunction suggested by a poor postcoital test result. In some cases, there are features of testicular failure, e.g. previous orchitis, late orchidopexy, with small testes and raised FSH levels. There may be unilateral or incomplete obstruction with or without circulating sperm antibodies; 25% of men with ejaculatory duct obstruction present with oligozoospermia. In about 20–40% of cases, the problem is attributed to varicocele, accessory gland infection, or a genetic defect if the sperm count is $< 1 \times 10^6$/ml. The majority of patients have no abnormality on assessment or investigation, and the condition is diagnosed as 'idiopathic oligozoospermia', also known as 'oligospermia', '*o*ligo-*a*stheno-*t*eratozoospermia', or the 'OAT' syndrome. Idiopathic oligozoospermia is the largest single identified cause of infertility. Most couples are currently referred for ART directly and few are now seen by urologists or andrologists. Even with reduced semen quality, there is a one in three chance of normal fertility, and fertilization often occurs through IVF after improving the ejaculate by standard sperm preparation techniques.

Hargreave and Elton[68] showed that, in infertile couples, the chance of conception was not increased if the total motile sperm content in the ejaculate rose above $2 \times 10^6$, so there may be little justification in trying to increase the sperm count by therapy. This might simply increase the numbers of useless dysfunctional spermatozoa in the semen. Management of 'oligospermia' must be in conjunction with the female partner, as there is a high incidence of associated female infertility.

### Conservative treatment

A period of 3 months of conservative treatment enables accurate assessment of the fertility status of both partners, during which time the semen may show signs of recovery if the abnormality was due to transient suppression from a fever or other illness. Drugs known to impair fertility can be withdrawn, for example anabolic steroids or sulphasalzine, with alcohol consumption reduced to less than three units per day, or avoided completely with very low sperm concentrations. Although the value of boxer shorts and cold water baths to improve scrotal cooling may be debatable, this focuses the patient on his fertility problem and may help to alter a life or work style detrimental to fertility. Tobacco consumption may interfere with the acrosome reaction, and can decrease vitamin C in the ejaculate, thereby reducing an antioxidant and increasing the potential damage from leukocyte-generated reactive oxygen species.

### Medical treatment

The plethora of medical treatments which have been utilized in the management of oligozoospermia have not stood the test of clinical trials, probably because most are hormones and male infertility is only rarely due to a hormone deficiency. Once popular antioestrogens, principally clomiphene citrate and tamoxifen, mesterolone and gonadotrophin injections, although sometimes leading to improvement in sperm production, were not associated with increases in the conception rate. In rare cases with low testosterone levels, the effect of antioestrogens is more striking. Prednisolone has obvious side-effects and its use in the treatment of oligospermia remains empirical.

Subclinical prostatitis is common and suggested by a history of previous sexually transmitted disease, overt prostatitis, urinary or ejaculatory dysfunction, perineal discomfort, or tenderness of the caput epididymis or prostate. An initial urine sample after prostatic massage may reveal white or red blood cells, or there may be features of prostatitis on transrectal ultrasound. Prostatitis may be treated long term with one of four antibiotics known to penetrate the prostate (doxycycline, erythromycin, trimethoprim, quinolones). Leukocyte-generated reactive oxygen species, present in two-thirds of infertile men, impair sperm motility and its fertilizing ability, but chemiluminescence assessment of semen is not widely available[20]. Although the test is a good predictor of fertilization failure at IVF, reduction of seminal fluid reactive oxygen species with antibiotics and vitamin E led to only one conception in 90 patients (unpublished results). Long-term low-dose antibiotic therapy (e.g. doxycycline or erythromycin) with vitamin E or C, given empirically for suspected subclinical genitourinary infection, results in natural pregnancy occasionally.

### Surgical treatment

Due to the results of the recent WHO trial of varicocele ligation in male infertility, the varicocele is re-considered as an important cause of male infertility[69]. Although the incidence of varicocele is one in five, for example in fertile men requesting vasectomy, they also occur in up to 40% of subfertile men[15]. The aetiology of the infertility is unknown, but a temperature effect on the testis and/or epididymis is suspected (Figure 6). It is important to carefully examine oligozoospermic men for varicoceles, and to request scrotal ultrasound if there is any doubt. Spontaneous conception occurs after left internal spermatic vein ligation in 30–40% of couples in 1–2 years. The internal spermatic vein can also be obliterated with coils by interventional radiology (Figure 22). Transinguinal ligation is usually reserved for recurrences, which occur in 5% of patients following all methods.

Unilateral testicular obstruction[64], including ejaculatory duct obstruction[46] may present with oligozoospermia (Figure 21). There may be disparity in testicular sizes. The normal-size testis is usually obstructed with a swollen epididymis, and the smaller testis, with patent epididymis, is often defective and responsible for the poor quality sperm in the ejaculate. Sperm antibody levels reach significance in > 50% of cases, and ART is very effective, explaining why surgical reconstruction may be avoided. Removal of the obstructed testis leads to a diminution of antibody titres[65], but is not a popular option.

### Assisted conception

Whether IUI, IVF or ICSI is considered appropriate for couples with male factor infertility depends on the total motile sperm count (and progression) which can be prepared from the ejaculate, the age of the female partner and whether there are additional female infertility factors. Three cycles of IUI may lead to conception in 30% of couples with oligozoospermia, but a harvest of 5–8 million motile spermatozoa is required. In moderate oligozoospermia, IVF is feasible if 1–2 million or more progressive spermatozoa are obtained, and the motility and IVF performance may be enhanced by briefly exposing spermatozoa to pentoxifylline.

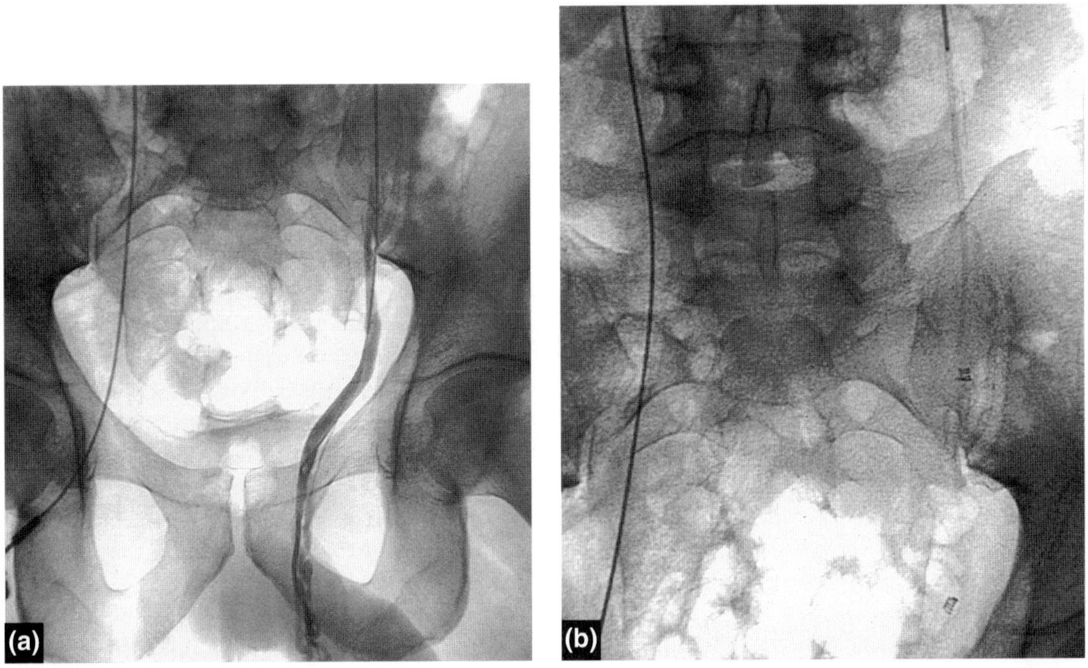


**Figure 22** Obliteration of a left varicocele by interventional radiology. (a) A cannula inserted into the right femoral vein is guided through the inferior vena cava and left renal vein into the left internal spermatic vein. Injection of contrast demonstrates the varicocele; (b) two coils have been positioned along the left internal spermatic vein to prevent further venous reflux. (Courtesy of Dr John Frank, Whipps Cross Hospital, London)

Empirical doxycycline therapy sometimes improves the fertilization rate during IVF. If there is failure of fertilization, there is a 50% chance that fertilization will be successful in a subsequent IVF cycle; however, ICSI is preferable as a more certain route to embryo transfer[28,70,71].

ICSI was developed for use where few spermatozoa are present in the ejaculate, especially in severe oligozoospermia. Success depends on the patience and skill of the embryologist, who may spend several hours isolating the few spermatozoa present in the ejaculate to accumulate sufficient for microinjection of all the retrieved oocytes. Genetic screening is desirable where the sperm concentration is $< 5 \times 10^6$/ml.

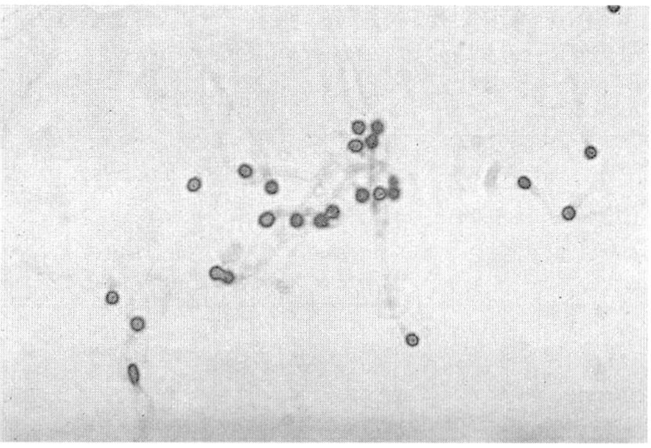

**Figure 23** Globozoospermia. The sperm heads are all round (marble-headed) due to failure of acrosome development (100% teratozoospermia). The sperm parameters are otherwise normal. Natural fertilization is impossible, but fertilization can be achieved by ICSI. (Courtesy of Dr Sue Avery, Bourn Hall)

## TYPE 5: NORMAL SPERM CONCENTRATION – SPERM DYSFUNCTION

Most couples in this group have a normal seminal fluid analysis, but failure of fertilization during IVF. This is due to *occult sperm dysfunction*, detectable by cervical mucus penetration tests, or more recent diagnostic andrology investigations. Fertilization may be improved if varicoceles or genitourinary infections, symptomatic or subclinical, are identified and treated. Idiopathic teratozoospermia may be used to define severe morphological abnormalities (WHO < 30% and Kruger < 5% normal spermatozoa in semen) which can be described as *overt sperm dysfunction*. Globozoospermia, necrospermia, and the immotile cilia syndrome including Kartagener's syndrome are absolute conditions which fit into this category. In these examples of type 5 infertility, fertilization is achieved only through ICSI, and is possible because the DNA of the sperm head remains intact.

The *immotile cilia syndrome* is an autosomal recessive disorder present in one in 20 000 individuals. Spermatozoa are either all immotile, or motility is severely impaired due to structural abnormalities of the sperm tails. This is due to the absence of dynein arms (muscular elements) from their axonemes (tails), which can be identified by electron microscopy, but the abnormality is present in all the cilia in the body. In half the cases, there is Kartagener's syndrome (associated situs inversus, bronchiectasis and chronic nasal sinusitis). *Globozoospermia* is also known as the round (or marble) headed (or acrosomeless) sperm syndrome. The patients are normal mature individuals with all parameters of the seminal fluid analysis satisfactory apart from 100% teratozoospermia due to failure of the acrosomal cap to develop. The bare sperm head is round (Figure 23) and cannot fertilize. During spermatogenesis, the acrosome develops separately from the sperm head, fails to unite and then disintegrates. In *necrozoospermia*, there is no sperm motility. Some activity may appear following prolonged empirical antibiotic and antioxidant therapy (erythromycin 250 mg b.d. with vitamin E 100 mg b.d.) or increased frequency of ejaculation. Other than this the above sperm abnormalities all fail to respond to any therapy, and ICSI is indicated.

It is preferable to select only viable spermatozoa for ICSI, and there is no problem with globozoospermia. If there is absolutely no sperm motility, some activity might be observed after pentoxifylline exposure, but, in practice, testicular sperm are viable, usually exhibiting rudimentary activity, and are suitable for ICSI.

## DONOR INSEMINATION

Due to the overwhelming success of ICSI in the management of male factor infertility, the indications for donor insemination are now few. Men with absolutely no sperm due to anorchia or total germ cell aplasia, have an absolute requirement for donor insemination. In an ideal society without economic constraints, this should be < 1% of infertile men. However, donor insemination is not yet relegated to the medical museum because it is relatively cheap, minimally invasive, and highly successful and remains a valuable option for infertile couples.

## CONCLUSIONS

In just a few years, ICSI has revolutionized the management of male infertility and conferred the opportunity of biological fatherhood on nearly every patient. At the dawn of the 21st century, andrologists still seek a true cure for male fertility disorders, and perhaps ART has paved the way. ICSI salvages available spermatozoa, and the outcome can be used to further advantage if we appreciate that, whatever the DNA content, spermatozoa from infertile men are usually capable of fertilization even if microassisted. Evidence so far suggests that the incidence of fetal abnormality in ICSI-conceived children is no greater than the normal fertile population, and this may be due to implantation selection by the uterus. Time, genetic advances and subsequent generations may modify this view, so we must continue to monitor the children and future developments in this field, especially as ICSI was introduced into routine clinical practice without extensive animal research.

Now that many of the dynamics of reproduction are understood, it could be a small step to understanding the abnormalities of the sperm cell envelope which cause most male infertility. The introduction of new therapies for the man is highly desirable because couples anticipate treatment to enable a natural conception when initially seeking medical advice for their infertility. Realigning their management around the procurement of a natural conception also reintroduces natural mechanisms of genetic selection into the treatment programme.

## FURTHER READING

Brinsden, P. R. and Rainsbury, P. A. (1992). *A Textbook of In Vitro Fertilization and Assisted Reproduction.* (Carnforth, UK: Parthenon Publishing)

Comhaire, F. H. (1996). *Male Infertility.* (London: Chapman and Hall Medical)

Edwards, R. G. and Brody, S. A. (1995). *Principles and Practice of Assisted Human Reproduction.* (Philadelphia: W. B. Saunders)

Glover, T. D., Barratt, C. L. R., Tyler, J. P. P. and Henessey, J. F. (1990). *Human Male Fertility and Semen Analysis.* (London: Academic Press)

Hargreave, T. B. (1994). *Male Infertility*, 2nd edn. (London: Springer-Verlag)

Schoysman, R. (1994). *Microsurgery of Male Infertility.* (Palermo: Fondazione per gli studi)

## REFERENCES

1. Palermo, G., Joris, H., Devroey, P. and Van Steirteghem, A. (1992). Pregnancies after intracytoplasmic sperm injection of single spermatozoon into an oocyte. *Lancet*, **340**, 17–18
2. Hirsh, A. V. (1996). Post-coital sperm retrieval could lead to the wider approval of assisted conception by some religions. *Hum. Reprod.*, **11**, 245–7
3. Hirsh, A. V. (1995). The anatomical preparations of the human testis and epididymis in the Glasgow Hunterian Anatomical Collection. *Hum. Reprod. Update*, **1**, 515–21
4. Hirsh, A. V., Kellet, M., Robertson, G. and Pryor, J. P. (1980). Doppler flow studies, venography and thermography in the evaluation of varicoceles of fertile and subfertile men. *Br. J. Urol.*, **52**, 560–5
5. World Health Organization (WHO) (1992). *WHO Laboratory Manual for the Examination of Human Semen and Sperm–Cervical Mucus Interaction*, 3rd edn. (Cambridge: Cambridge University Press)
6. Carlsen, E., Giwercman, A., Keiding, N. and Skakkebaeck, N. E. (1992). Evidence for

decreasing quality of semen during the past 50 years. *Br. Med. J.*, **305**, 609–13
7. Hargreave, T. B. (1994). Human infertility. In Hargreave, T. B. (ed.) *Male Infertility*, 2nd edn., pp. 1–16. (London: Springer Verlag)
8. Baker, G. H. W., Burger, H. G., de Kretser, D. M. and Hudson, B. (1986). Relative incidence of etiological disorders in male infertility. In Santen, R. J. and Swerdloff, R. S. (eds.) *Male Reproductive Dysfunction*, pp. 341–72. (New York: Marcel Dekker)
9. Hull, M. G. R., Glazener, C. M. A., Kelly, N. J. *et al.* (1985). Population study of causes, treatment, and outcome of infertility. *Br. Med. J.*, **291**, 1693–7
10. World Health Organization (WHO) (1987). Towards more objectivity in diagnosis and management of male infertility. *Int. J. Androl.*, Suppl 7
11. Dubin, L. and Amelar, R. D. (1971). Etiologic factors in 1294 consecutive cases of male infertility. *Fertil. Steril.*, **22**, 469–74
12. Greenberg, S. H., Lipschultz, L. I. and Wein, A. J. (1978). Experience with 425 subfertile male patients. *J. Urol.*, **119**, 507
13. Young, D. (1970). Surgical treatment of male infertility. *J. Reprod. Fertil.*, **23**, 541–2
14. Pryor, J. P., Hirsh, A. V., Fitzpatrick, J. *et al.* (1978). The correlation between testicular size and histology. Proceedings of *5th European Congress on Fertility and Sterility*, Rome, 371–2
15. Hirsh, A. V. (1995). Can we be more confident about identifying a varicocele by clinical examination or by ultrasound? *Ultrasound Obstet. Gynecol.*, **6**, 166–7
16. Kruger, T. F., Acosta, A. A., Simmons, K. F. *et al.* (1988). Predictive value of abnormal sperm morphology in in-vitro fertilisation. *Fertil. Steril.*, **49**, 112–17
17. Menkeveld, R., Stander, F. S. H., Kotze, T. J. W. *et al.* (1990). The evaluation of morphological characteristics of human spermatozoa according to strict criteria. *Hum. Reprod.*, **5**, 586–92
18. Sukcharoen, N., Keith, J., Irvine, D. S. and Aitken, R. J. (1996). Prediction of the *in-vitro* fertilization (IVF) potential of human spermatozoa using sperm function tests: the effect of the delay between testing and IVF. *Hum. Reprod.*, **11**, 1030–4
19. Burkman, L. J. (1991). Discrimination between nonhyperactivated and classical hyperactivated motility patterns in human spermatozoa using computerised analysis. *Fertil. Steril.*, **55**, 363–71
20. Aitken, R. J., Buckingham, D., West, K. M. *et al.* (1992). Differential contribution of leucocytes and spermatozoa to the generation of reactive oxygen species in the ejaculates of oligozoospermic patients and fertile donors. *J. Reprod. Fertil.*, **94**, 451–62
21. Pryor, J. P., Hirsh, A. V., Fitzpatrick, J. *et al.* (1978). The value of plasma FSH in the assessment of the infertile male. Proceedings of *5th European Congress on Fertility and Sterility*, Rome, 181–2
22. Hirsh, A. V., Tyler, J. P., Landon, L. *et al.* (1981). Testicular testosterone concentration, interstitial cell density and spermatogenesis in infertile men. *Int. J. Androl.*, **4**, 409–20
23. Chandley, A. C. (1994). Chromosomes. In Hargreave, T. B. (ed.) *Male Infertility*, 2nd edn., pp. 149–64. (London: Springer Verlag)
24. Vogt, P. H., Edelmann, A., Hirschmann, P. *et al.* (1996). The Y chromosome and (in)fertility in the male. *Hum. Reprod.*, **11**, abstract book 1, 32–3
25. Johnsen, S. G. (1970). Testicular biopsy score count. *Hormones*, **1**, 2–25
26. Poynter, F. N. L. (1968). Hunter, Spallanzani, and the history of artificial insemination. In Stevenson, L. G. and Multauf, R. P. (eds.) *Medicine, Science and Culture, Historical Essays in Honor of Owsei Temkin.* pp. 97–114. (Baltimore: John Hopkins)
27. Hanley, H. G. (1957). Pregnancy following artificial insemination from an epididymal cyst. *Proc. Soc. Study Fertil.*, **8**, 20–1
28. Cohen, J., Edwards, R., Fehilly, C. *et al.* (1985). *In-vitro* fertilisation: a treatment for male infertility. *Fertil. Steril.*, **43**, 422
29. Pryor, J. P. (1984). Surgical retrieval of epididymal spermatozoa. *Lancet*, **2**, 1341
30. Temple-Smith, P. D., Southwick, G. J., Yates, C. A. *et al.* (1985). Human pregnancy by *in vitro* fertilization (IVF) using sperm aspirated from the epididymis. *J. In Vitro Fertil. Embryo Transfer*, **2**, 119–22
31. Silber, S. J., Ord, T., Borrero, T. *et al.* (1987). New treatment for infertility due to congenital absence of the vas deferens. Lancet, 2, 850–1
32. Schoysman, R., Vanderzwalmen, P., Nijs, M. *et al.* (1993). Pregnancy after fertilisation with human testicular spermatozoa. *Lancet,* **342,** 1237

33. Craft, I., Bennett, V. and Nicholson, N. (1993). Fertilising ability of testicular spermatozoa, *Lancet,* **342**, 864
34. Bourne, H., Liu, D. Y., Clarke, G. N. and Gordon Baker, H. W. (1995). Normal fertilisation and embryo development by intracytoplasmic sperm injection of round-headed acrosomeless sperm. *Fertil. Steril.,* **63**, 1329–32
35. Silber, S. J. and Lenahan, K. (1995). Sertoli cell surgery: spermatid retrieval and ICSI in azoospermic patients with maturation arrest. *Hum. Reprod. Update,* 1, no. 6, CD-ROM, item 26 (video)
36. Tesarik, J. and Mendoza, C. (1996). Spermatid injection into human oocytes. I. Laboratory techniques and special features of zygote development. *Hum. Reprod.,* **11**, 772–6
37. Devroey, P., Liu, J., Nagy, Z. *et al.* (1995). Pregnancies after testicular sperm extraction and intracytoplasmic sperm injection in non-obstructive azoospermia. *Hum. Reprod.,* **10**, 1457–60
38. Tournaye, H., Liu, J., Nagy, P. Z. *et al.* (1996). Correlation between testicular histology and outcome after intracytoplasmic sperm injection using testicular spermatozoa. *Hum. Reprod.,* **11**, 127–32
39. Chandley, A. C. and Hargreave, T. B. (1996). Genetic anomaly and ICSI. *Hum. Reprod.,* **11**, 930–1
40. Urry, R. L., Middleton, R. G. and McGavin, S. (1986). A simple and effective technique for increasing pregnancy rates in couples with retrograde ejaculation. *Fertil. Steril.,* **46**, 1124–7
41. Hirsh, A. V., Mills, C., Tan, S. L., Bekir, J. and Rainsbury, P. (1993). Pregnancy using spermatozoa from the vas deferens in a patient with ejaculatory failure due to spinal injury. *Hum. Reprod.,* **8**, 89–90
42. Dahlberg, A., Ruutu, M. and Hovatta, O. (1995). Pregnancy results from a vibrator application, electroejaculation, and a vas aspiration programme in spinal-cord injured men. *Hum. Reprod.,* **10**, 2305–7
43. Ley, S. B. and Leonard, J. M. (1985). Male hypogonadotrophic hypogonadism: factors influencing response to human chorionic gonadotrophin and human menopausal gonadotrophin, including prior exogenous androgens. *J. Clin. Endocrinol. Metab.,* **61**, 746–52
44. Morris, D. V., Adeniyi Jones, R., Wheeler, M. *et al.* (1984). The treatment of hypogonadotrophic hypogonadism in men by the pulsatile infusion of luteinizing hormone-releasing hormone. *Clin. Endocrinol.,* **21**, 189–200
45. Hendry, W. F., Levison, D., Parkinson, C. M. *et al.* (1990). Testicular obstruction: clinicopathological studies. *Ann. R. Coll. Surg. Engl.,* **72**, 396–407
46. Pryor, J. P. and Hendry, W. F. (1991). Ejaculatory duct obstruction in subfertile males: analysis of 87 patients. *Fertil. Steril.,* **56** 725–30
47. Bagshaw, H. A., Masters, J. R. W. and Pryor, J. P. (1980). Factors influencing the outcome of vasectomy reversal. *Br. J. Urol.,* **52**, 57–9
48. Silber, S. J. (1977). Microscopic vasectomy reversal. *Fertil. Steril.,* **28**, 1191–202
49. Silber, S. J. (1978). Microscopic vasoepididymostomy, specific microanastomosis to the epididymal tubule. *Fertil. Steril.,* **30**, 565–76
50. Belker, A. M., Thomas, A. J., Fuchs, E. F. *et al.* (1991). Results of 1469 microsurgical vasectomy reversals by the Vasovasostomy Study Group. *J. Urol.,* **145**, 505–11
51. Tsirigotis, M. and Craft, I. (1995). Sperm retrieval methods and ICSI for obstructive azoospermia. *Hum. Reprod.,* **10**, 758–60
52. Hirsh, A. V., Dean, N. L., Mohan, P. J., Shaker, A. G. and Bekir, J. S. (1996). Sperm retrieval in azoospermia: natural spermatoceles, rete testis, epididymis (percutaneous or microsurgical), testis, local or general anaesthesia. *Hum. Reprod.,* **11**, abstract book 1, 103
53. Hirsh, A. V., Dean, N. L., Mohan, P. J., Shaker, A. G. and Bekir, J. S. (1996). Natural spermatoceles in irreversible obstructive azoospermia – reservoirs of viable spermatozoa for assisted conception. *Hum. Reprod.,* **11**, 1919–22
54. Shrivastav, P., Nadkarni, P., Wensvoort, S. and Craft, I. (1994). Percutaneous epididymal sperm aspiration for obstructive azoospermia. *Hum. Reprod.,* **9**, 2058–61
55. Silber, S. J., Devroey, P. and Van Steirteghem, A. C. (1994). Conventional *in-vitro* fertilisation versus intracytoplasmic sperm injection for patients requiring microsurgical sperm aspiration. *Hum. Reprod.,* **9**, 1705–9
56. Oates, R. D., Lobel, S. M., Harris, D. H. *et al.* (1996). Efficacy of intracytoplasmic sperm injection using intentionally cryopreserved epididymal spermatozoa. *Hum. Reprod.,* **11**, 133–8
57. Hirsh, A. V., Mills, C., Bekir, J., Dean, N., Yovich, J. L and Tan, S. L. (1994). Factors

influencing the outcome of in-vitro fertilization with epididymal sperm in irreversible obstructive azoospermia. *Hum. Reprod.,* **9**, 1710–16
58. Craft, I. and Tsirigotis, M. (1995). Simplified recovery, preparation and cryopreservation of testicular spermatozoa. *Hum. Reprod.,* **10**, 1623–6
59. Devroey, P., Liu, J. Nagy, Z. *et al.* (1994). Normal fertilization of human oocytes after testicular sperm extraction and intracytoplasmic sperm injection. *Fertil. Steril.,* **62**, 639–41
60. Schlegel, P. N. (1996). Physiological consequences of testicular sperm extraction. *Hum. Reprod.,* **11**, abstract book 1, 74
61. Stewart, B. D., Ward, S. A., Hirsh, A. V. *et al.* (1997). Twin pregnancy following use of cryopreserved testicular spermatozoa and intracytoplasmic sperm injection. *Hum. Reprod.,* in press
62. Hendry, W. F., Hughes, L., Scammel, G. *et al.* (1990). Comparison of prednisolone and placebo in subfertile men with antibodies to spermatozoa. *Lancet,* **335**, 85–8
63. Lahteenmaki, A., Rasanen, M. and Hovatta, O. (1995). Low-dose prednisolone does not improve the outcome of in-vitro fertilization in male immunological infertility. *Hum. Reprod.,* **10**, 3124–9
64. Hendry, W. F. (1986). The clinical significance of unilateral testicular obstruction in subfertile males. *Br. J. Urol.,* **58**, 709–14
65. Hendry, W. F., Parslow, J. M., Parkinson, M. C. and Lowe, D. G. (1994). Unilateral testicular obstruction: orchidectomy or reconstruction? *Hum. Reprod.,* **9**, 463–70
66. Benoff, S., Cooper, G. W., Hurley, I. *et al.* (1994). The effect of calcium channel blockers on sperm fertilization potential. *Fertil. Steril.,* **62**, 606–23
67. Hershlag, A., Rosenfeld, D. L., Scholl, G. M. and Benoff, S. (1996). The contraceptive effect of calcium channel blockers. *Hum. Reprod.,* **11**, abstract book 1, 55
68. Hargreave, T. B. and Elton, R. A. (1983). Is conventional sperm analysis of any use? *Br. J. Urol.,* **55**, 780–4
69. Hargreave, T. B. (1996). The World Health Organization Varicocele Trial. *Br. J. Urol.,* **77**, Suppl. 1, 39
70. Van Steirteghem, A., Liu, J., Joris, H. *et al.* (1993). Higher success rate of intracytoplasmic sperm injection than by subzonal insemination. *Hum. Reprod.,* **8**, 1055–60
71. Van Steirteghem, A., Nagy, Z., Joris, H. *et al.* (1993). High fertilization rates after intracytoplasmic sperm injection. *Hum. Reprod.,* **8**, 1061–6

# Treatment of anejaculatory infertility 12

## I Vibratory ejaculation for the treatment of anejaculation in men with spinal cord injuries

*Jens Sønksen, Dana A. Ohl and Paul A. Rainsbury*

### INTRODUCTION

Spinal cord injury (SCI) is a devastating medical condition. In an instant of time, an able-bodied individual becomes unable to move the limbs or control the bowel and urinary bladder normally, causing extreme changes in previously simple acts of daily living. Another function that is usually lost following SCI is the ability to procreate[1].

The impact of loss of ability to reproduce is amplified by the demographics of SCI. In the United States there are approximately 10 000 new SCI cases per year, but this is not a homogeneous population. Eighty-two per cent occur in males. Seventy-eight per cent of new SCI patients are 40 years of age or younger and 88% are 50 or younger[2]. Consequently, there are approximately 6400 new SCI men each year in the United States who are in their prime reproductive years (arbitrarily < 40), who become potentially infertile from SCI.

Male infertility following SCI is caused by erectile dysfunction[3] and absence of ejaculation[4]. Since there are ample methods to treat erectile dysfunction available for this patient population including vacuum erection devices[5], intracorporal injection therapy[6], and penile prostheses[7], the ejaculatory dysfunction is the prominent problem.

In this section we will focus on penile vibratory stimulation (PVS) to induce ejaculation combined with reproductive prospects in SCI men.

### PHYSIOLOGY OF EJACULATION

The ejaculatory reflex is a complex set of events, with many neurophysiological components[8].

The reflex is usually initiated by a combination of cerebral and genital input. Signals from visual, psychogenic and possible sleep-related erotic stimuli are sent through descending pathways to the thoracolumbar spinal cord where they are co-ordinated with input from the genital afferents in initiating the ejaculatory response. These cerebral factors are very poorly understood. Information from genital manipulation is carried into the sacral spinal cord via the dorsal nerves of the penis. The transmissions travel upward to the ejaculatory centre in the thoracolumbar segments of the spinal cord (Figure 1).

The ejaculatory reflex is co-ordinated in the thoracolumbar area. The efferents for seminal emission arise from spinal cord levels T11–L2. They course through the sympathetic chain and merge into the inferior mesenteric/hypogastric plexus. The hypogatric nerves carry the neural impulses to the ejaculatory organs, the prostate, epididymis and vasa deferentia, seminal vesicles and the urinary bladder neck. During

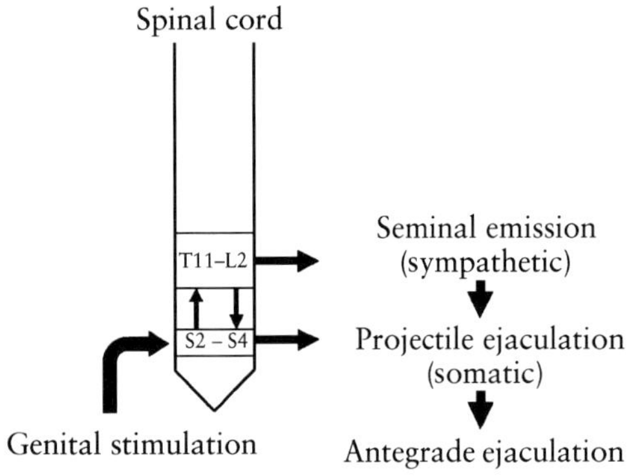


**Figure 1** The spinal cord and the afferent and efferent nerves involved in the ejaculatory reflex (for details see text)

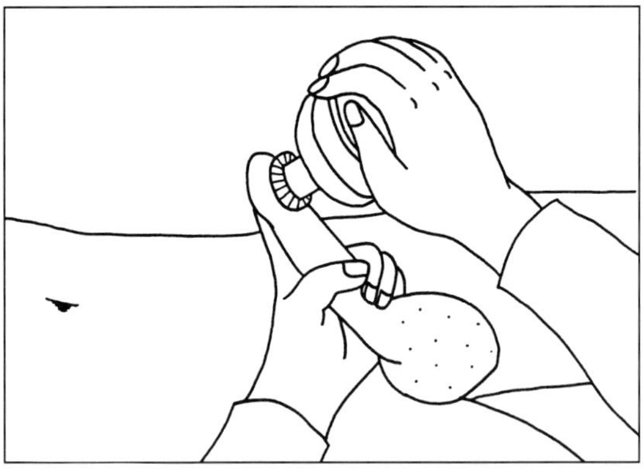

**Figure 2** Penile vibratory stimulation to induce ejaculation

seminal emission, sperm is transported through the ejaculatory ducts into the posterior urethra, where it becomes mixed with accessory gland secretions. The bladder neck is tightly closed to prevent retrograde ejaculation. At the time of seminal emission, the sensation of orgasm is appreciated. Immediately after seminal emission into the posterior urethra, rhythmic contractions of the bulbocavernosus and ischiocavernosus muscles and relaxation of the external urinary sphincter cause projectile ejaculation. These muscles are under the control of somatic fibres, not the sympathetic nervous system.

Even when the spinal cord is disconnected from the brain as in men with complete SCI, the neurological components of the ejaculatory centre in the spinal cord may respond to PVS and produce reflex ejaculation. However, no sensation of orgasm is appreciated in men with complete spinal cord lesion.

## TECHNIQUE OF PENILE VIBRATORY STIMULATION

The PVS procedure is performed with the patient placed in the supine position or in a sitting position in a wheelchair. The centre of the vibrator applicator is placed against the frenulum (Figure 2) for periods of 3 min or until antegrade ejaculation occurs. If no ejaculation has occurred, the stimulation periods are followed by a rest period of 1–2 min and stimulation begins again. The maximum number of stimulation cycles is usually six but may be less if the penis skin becomes bruised or abraded. The ejaculate is collected in a non-spermicidal container.

The required time to obtain ejaculation by PVS ranges from 10 seconds to 45 min[9–13]. During the PVS and ejaculation, a variety of reflex activities may be seen including abdominal contractions, leg spasms, penile erection, piloerection and scrotal wall contractions[10,12].

Ten to 15 min prior to PVS, 10–20 mg of nifedipine (a calcium channel blocker) is given sublingually in men with spinal cord lesion above T6 to prevent an episode of autonomic dysreflexia[14]. During the initial procedures, the blood pressure should be monitored until the right dose of nifedipine is established. In order to limit the risk of developing autonomic dysreflexia, the stimulation is stopped promptly when the rhythmic periurethral muscle contractions begin[15]. Using this technique, multiple ejaculations (more than three) may be obtained safely within several minutes, increasing the ejaculate volume[15].

In conclusion, PVS is a very easy, non-invasive method to induce ejaculation in SCI men and does not require extensive experience by the physician or the patient/partner to be successful. However, certain factors that influence the ejaculatory response are described in the following section.

## FACTORS THAT INFLUENCE EJACULATORY RESPONSE

It appears that, during PVS, a 'normal' ejaculatory reflex is induced. Successful ejaculation by PVS seems to require an intact ejaculatory reflex arc[9,10] which allows transmission of afferent stimuli to the sacral spinal cord (S2–S4), communication between the sacral and thoracolumbar regions (T11–L2) and neurogenic outflow from these spinal cord segments (Figure 1)[15]. Consequently, SCI men with the level of lesion at or above T10 will be the potential treatment group for PVS-induced ejaculation[16]. However, ejaculations induced by PVS have been reported in SCI men with a level of lesion below T10[11,12,16].

Brindley[17] reported that PVS always failed in SCI men with no hip flexion as a reflex response to scratching the soles of the feet. Failure of this reflex indicates damage of the L2–S1 spinal cord segments which are required to obtain reflex ejaculation. On the contrary, in the study by Sønksen and colleagues[12], ten out of 41 antegrade ejaculation responders had no hip flexion reflex.

The absence of the bulbocavernosus reflex indicates damage between the spinal cord segments of S2–S4 (afferent stimulation for the ejaculation reflex). This reflex is elicited by squeezing the glans penis between two fingers and the response is contraction of the external sphincter and the bulbocavernosus muscle. Szasz and Carpenter[10] indicated that absence of this reflex results in failure of PVS-induced ejaculation in SCI men. In two studies, the percentages of SCI men with an intact bulbocavernosus reflex who also exhibited antegrade ejaculation with PVS were 98% (40/41) and 78% (21/27), respectively[12,16].

Other patient characteristics such as patient age, duration of SCI and completeness of the SCI seem not to influence the ejaculatory response[10,12,16,17].

The vibratory amplitude is of great importance when inducing ejaculation by PVS. In a recent study, detailed measurements of the vibratory output demonstrated that a vibratory amplitude of 2.5 mm at a frequency of 100 Hz produced significantly higher ejaculation rates (96%) compared to much lower ejaculation rates (32%) with an amplitude of 1 mm[12]. This indicates that a high-amplitude vibration is essential to exceed an ejaculatory threshold to activate the reflex in the majority of SCI men. The efficacy of the high-amplitude vibration was verified in another group of 41 Danish SCI men (83% ejaculation rate)[12]. Furthermore, in a study from the University of Michigan, 65% of 34 SCI men obtained antegrade ejaculation when using a 2.5 mm vibratory amplitude at 100 Hz[16]. In the last study quoted, an ejaculation rate of 81% was noted in the men with spinal cord lesions above T10.

When examining the literature concerning PVS results, it becomes apparent that a wide range of ejaculation rates (19–91%) has been reported[4,10–12,16–27]. During the study by Sønksen and colleagues[12], measurements revealed that the manufacturers' specifications regarding the vibratory amplitudes were inaccurate and it was suggested that the previously low ejaculation rates seen in some centres are due to inadequate amplitudes of the vibratory equipment used. This concept was further supported by the fact that, when an adequate amplitude was used, ejaculation rates were identical whether the patients/partners were performing the PVS or an experienced physician.

Based on the results of the study by Sønksen and colleagues[12], vibrators for clinical (Figure 3) as well as home use (Figure 4) have been developed. Both vibrators meet the required frequency of 100 Hz and an amplitude of 2.5 mm.

An ongoing clinical test of the vibrators including 80 SCI men with spinal cord lesion above T10 (intact ejaculatory reflex) at the Universities of Copenhagen and Michigan shows that more than 80% of the men are able to obtain antegrade ejaculation (unpublished results).

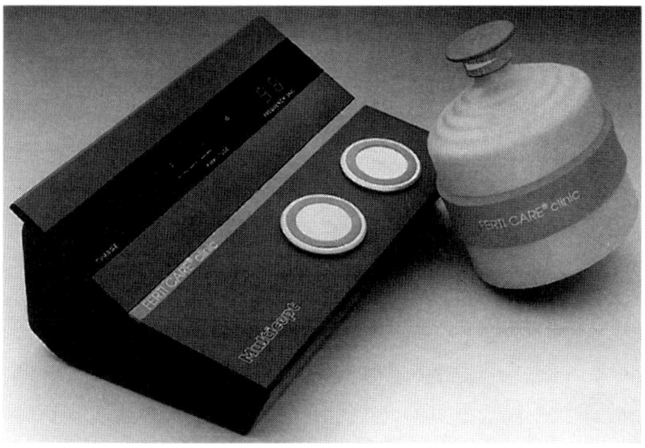

**Figure 3** FERTI CARE® *clinic* version (Osbon Medical, London, UK) (1996) developed to induce ejaculation in men with spinal cord injuries in the clinical setting. The amplitude, which varies with the applied pressure, can be read from the vibration unit during the procedures. The amplitude and frequency may be set at the recommended 2.5 mm and 100 Hz, or according to individual requirements. The options available include amplitudes between 0.1–5.0 mm and frequencies between 40–160 Hz

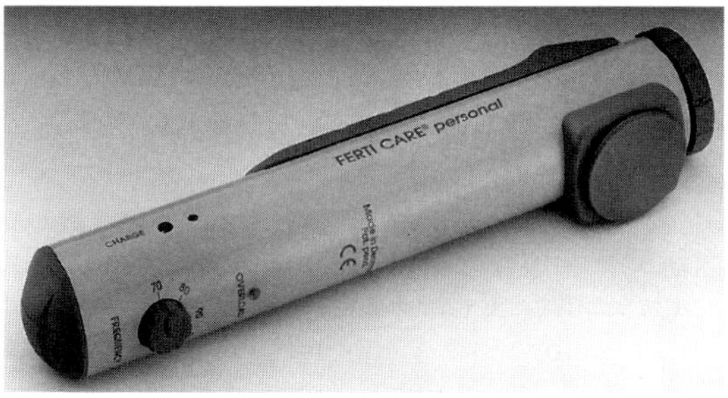

**Figure 4** FERTI CARE® *personal* version (Osbon Medical, London, UK) (1996) developed to induce ejaculation in men with spinal cord injuries in the home environment. The weight of the vibrator is approximately 350 g. The amplitude may be set between 1.0 and 3.5 mm and the frequency between 70 and 110 Hz. Furthermore, the vibrator has an overload indicator to avoid application of excessive pressure (to prevent skin injuries) and simultaneously indicate the recommended pressure

## ADVERSE EFFECTS FROM PENILE VIBRATORY STIMULATION

PVS is a safe method of sperm retrieval in SCI men and very few adverse effects have been reported. In a review of ten papers including 351 PVS-treated SCI men, minor problems were reported in 21 cases[28]. These included superficial penile skin bleeding or ulceration, but no treatment has been necessary other than a short rest period for skin healing.

Autonomic dysreflexia manifested by headache and rise in the arterial blood pressure have been reported in 14 of 329 SCI men during PVS and ejaculation[11,12,17,22,23,29]. None of the men received prophylactic medical treatment. In contrast, no episodes of autonomic dysreflexia were reported in four series including 188 SCI men when nifedipine was given prophylactically in men with lesions at or above T6 and/or a prior history of autonomic dysreflexia[12,16,26,27].

It is the authors' experience that autonomic dysreflexia can be controlled easily by nifedipine and, if the blood pressure rises to unacceptable levels, the procedure is immediately aborted with prompt return to baseline levels in nearly all cases. The nifedipine dose can be modified for the next procedure depending on the response to the drug.

## FACTORS THAT INFLUENCE SPERM QUALITY

In general, the sperm quality in SCI men is poor, as reported in several studies examining the ejaculates obtained by PVS or electroejaculation (EEJ)[10,11,16,17,21,23,26,27,30–32]. Specimens typically have a high sperm count with a low motility rate when compared to World Health Organization (WHO) standards[33]. Comparison of the sperm quality of ejaculates obtained by PVS and EEJ in 11 SCI men showed that antegrade ejaculates from PVS were superior to antegrade ejaculates from EEJ with regard to sperm motility (26% versus 11%), viability (25% versus 10%) and total motile sperm count (185 million versus 97 million)[34]. No significant difference between the sperm parameters from PVS and EEJ were seen when adding the spermatozoa isolated from the urinary bladder (retrograde ejaculation) into the sperm analysis following EEJ.

In a recent study of 51 SCI men examining PVS and prognostic factors which may affect sperm quality, a significantly better sperm motility was found in men with cervical lesions versus thoracic lesions (16% versus 7%) and incomplete versus complete lesions (19% versus 10%)[32]. This is in contrast to the EEJ study by Ohl and colleagues[30] where the sperm motility was highest in the thoracic lesions and the presence of motile sperm was more frequent with complete lesions.

It is well known that there is a high incidence of urinary tract infection in patients with SCI. Effects of urinary tract infections on sperm quality have been investigated in SCI men undergoing EEJ[35]. No significant effect on sperm quality was seen in ejaculates from SCI men with infected urine and semen compared to subjects without infections.

In two studies intermittent catheterization has been found to be superior to other methods of bladder management when looking at sperm motility[25,30]. Another study showed a trend toward a higher total number of motile sperm in SCI men performing reflex or Credé voiding[12].

It has been suggested that sperm antibodies in the seminal fluid may be a negative factor on the sperm function in SCI men[36]. However, in a series examining 32 semen samples for antibodies present on the sperm surface (direct immunobead test), only one test was positive[37].

Abnormal as well as normal testicular histology in SCI men have been reported[38–41]. Other factors that may affect the sperm quality in SCI men include elevated scrotal temperature, stasis of semen due to anejaculation, hormonal disturbances and various medications[42].

Further studies are needed to investigate the importance of the above factors' influence on sperm quality in SCI men since the results vary from normal to abnormal findings in different series.

## PREGNANCIES

### Home insemination

PVS and vaginal self-insemination performed by the couple at home is a viable option for those SCI men with adequate sperm quality. The SCI man and the partner should be carefully instructed in the use of PVS through supervised procedures at the hospital. Men with spinal cord lesion at or above T6 are instructed to self-administer nifedipine prophylactically to prevent autonomic dysreflexia. Those men whose autonomic dysreflexia is not well controlled by nifedipine are not candidates for home PVS. A non-spermicidal container is used for collection of the ejaculate and a 10-ml syringe is used for vaginal self-insemination.

In 1984, Brindley[17] reported seven home pregnancies following PVS and vaginal self-insemination with delivery of five healthy babies (one ongoing/one spontaneous abortion). Recently, several pregnancies have been reported from PVS procedures combined with self-insemination at home as shown in Table 1[26,27,43,44].

The unique advantage of PVS is the possibility of home use. Furthermore, it will allow the majority of SCI couples to perform the PVS procedure themselves at the hospital when a specimen is required in connection with assisted reproductive techniques.

**Table 1** Pregnancy results in SCI couples using penile vibratory stimulation and vaginal self-insemination at home

| *Reference* | *Number of couples attempting procreation* | *Number (%) of couples achieving pregnancy* |
|---|---|---|
| Dahlberg *et al.* (1995)[26] | 19 | 8 (42%) |
| Nehra *et al.* (1996)[27] | 8 | 5 (62%) |
| Elliot (1995)[43] | 22 | 10 (45%) |
| Sommer *et al.* (1995)[44] | 16 | 4 (25%) |

**Table 2** Pregnancy results in SCI couples using penile vibratory stimulation and intrauterine insemination (IUI) or *in vitro* fertilization (IVF)

| *Reference* | *Reproductive technique/ number of cycles* | *Number of couples attempting procreation* | *Number (%) of couples achieving pregnancy* |
|---|---|---|---|
| Pryor *et al.* (1995)[13] | IUI/12 | 6 | 5 (83%) |
| Sommer *et al.* (1995)[44] | IUI/16 | 3 | 3 (100%) |
| Dahlberg *et al.* (1995)[26] | IUI/— | 11 | 5 (45%) |
| | IVF/— | 1 | 1 (100%) |
| Nehra *et al.* (1996)[27]* | IUI/36 | 18 | 5 (28%) |
| | IVF/14 | 13 | 7 (54%) |

*No distinction between penile vibratory stimulation or electroejaculation

### Assisted reproductive techniques

The use of assisted reproductive techniques may increase the possibility of achieving pregnancy in SCI couples. Recently, several successful pregnancies have been reported using sperm obtained by PVS combined with assisted reproductive techniques such as intrauterine insemination (IUI) or *in vitro* fertilization (IVF) (Table 2)[13,26,27,44].

In general, IUI is recommended as the initial procedure in couples who are not candidates for self-insemination at home. IVF will be the next step for those couples failing IUI.

A relatively new method for assisted reproduction is intracytoplasmic sperm injection (ICSI) where one single spermatozoa is injected directly into the oocyte. Pregnancies achieved following ICSI procedures have been demonstrated utilizing spermatozoa from men with severe oligoasthenospermia[45]. The role of ICSI in SCI men with extremely poor sperm quality remains to be determined. However, SCI men with extremely poor sperm quality and SCI couples who fail to demonstrate fertilization during IVF ought to be appropriate candidates for ICSI.

## CONCLUSIONS

PVS is a low-cost, non-invasive and safe method of sperm retrieval. Ejaculation rates of 80–85% in SCI men with an intact ejaculatory reflex arc (above T10) have been demonstrated when using a vibratory amplitude of 2.5 mm at 100 Hz. Consequently, when using a medical grade vibrator, PVS ought to be the first choice of treatment in SCI men with anejaculation. EEJ will be an excellent option for PVS failures.

The spinal cord level of lesion (above T10) and the presence of the hip flexion and bulbocavernosus reflexes (alone or together) seem to be the best patient characteristics to predict PVS success in SCI men.

Despite the poor sperm quality in SCI men, acceptable pregnancy rates (25–62%) have been shown from home PVS and vaginal self-insemination. Together with assisted reproductive techniques for those couples who fail to achieve pregnancy at home, the reproduction prospects for SCI men and their partners look promising.

## REFERENCES

1. Amelar, R. D. and Dubin, L. (1982). Sexual function and fertility in paraplegic men. *Urology,* **20**, 62–5
2. National Spinal Cord Injury Statistics Center (1994). *Annual Report for the Model of the Spinal Cord Injury Care Systems.* (Birmingham, AL: National Spinal Cord Injury Statistical Center)
3. Biering-Sørensen, F. and Sønksen, J. (1992). Penile erection in men with spinal cord or cauda equina lesions. *Semin. Neurol.,* **12**, 98–105
4. Sønksen, J. and Biering-Sørensen, F. (1992). Fertility in men with spinal cord or cauda equina lesions. *Semin. Neurol.,* **12**, 106–14

5. Lloyd, E. E., Toth, L. L. and Perkash, I. (1989). Vacuum tumescence: an option for spinal cord injured males with erectile dysfunction. *SCI Nursing*, **6**, 25–8
6. Hirsch, I. H., Smith, R. L., Chancellor, M. B., Bagley, D. H., Carsello, J. and Staas, W. E. (1994). Use of intracavernous injection of prostaglandin E1 for neuropathic erectile dysfunction. *Paraplegia*, **32**, 661–4
7. Kimoto, Y. and Iwatsubo, E. (1994). Penile prostheses for the management of the neuropathic bladder and sexual dysfunction in spinal cord injury patients: long term follow up. *Paraplegia*, **32**, 336–9
8. Thomas, A. J. J. (1983). Ejaculatory dysfunction. *Fertil. Steril.*, **39**, 445–54
9. Brindley, G. S. (1981). Reflex ejaculation under vibratory stimulation in paraplegic men. *Paraplegia*, **19**, 299–302
10. Szasz, G. and Carpenter, C. (1989). Clinical observation in vibratory stimulation of the penis of men with spinal cord injury. *Arch. Sex. Behav.*, **18**, 461–74
11. Beretta, G., Chelo, E. and Zanollo, A. (1989). Reproductive aspects in spinal cord injured males. *Paraplegia*, **27**, 113–18
12. Sønksen, J., Biering-Sørensen, F. and Kvist Kristensen, J. (1994). Ejaculation induced by penile vibratory stimulation in men with spinal cord injuries. The importance of the vibratory amplitude. *Paraplegia*, **32**, 651–60
13. Pryor, J. L., LeRoy, S. C., Nagel, T. C. and Hensleigh, H. C. (1995). Vibratory stimulation for treatment of anejaculation in quadriplegic men. *Arch. Phys. Med. Rehab.*, **76**, 59–64
14. Steinberger, R. E., Ohl, D. A., Bennett, C. J., McCabe, M. and Wang, S. C. (1990). Nifedipine pretreatment for autonomic dysreflexia during electroejaculation. *Urology*, **36**, 228–31
15. Ohl, D. A. and Sønksen, J. (1996). Sperm collection for assisted reproduction in ejaculatory dysfunctions. In Acosta, A. A. and Kruger, T. F. (eds.) *Human Spermatozoa in Assisted Reproduction*, pp. 455–72. (Carnforth: Parthenon Publishing)
16. Ohl, D. A., Menge, A. C. and Sønksen, J. (1996). Penile vibratory stimulation in SCI males: optimized vibration parameters and prognostic factors. *Arch. Phys. Med. Rehab.*, in press
17. Brindley, G. S. (1984). The fertility of men with spinal injuries. *Paraplegia*, **22**, 337–48
18. Tarabulcy, E. (1972). Sexual function in the normal and in paraplegia. *Paraplegia*, **10**, 201–8
19. Piera, J. B. (1973). The establishment of a prognosis for genito-sexual function in the paraplegic and tetraplegic male. *Paraplegia*, **10**, 271–8
20. Francois, N., Jouannet, P. and Maury, M. (1983). La fonction génitosexuelle des paraplégiques. *J. Urol.*, **89**, 159–66
21. Sarkarati, M., Rossier, A. B. and Fam, B. A. (1987). Experience in vibratory and electroejaculation techniques in spinal cord injury patients: a preliminary report. *J. Urol.*, **138**, 59–63
22. Beilby, J. A. and Keogh, E. J. (1989). Spinal cord injuries and anejaculation. *Paraplegia*, **27**, 152
23. Siösteen, A., Forssman, L., Steen, Y., Sullivan, L. and Wickström, I. (1990). Quality of semen after repeated ejaculation treatment in spinal cord injury men. *Paraplegia*, **28**, 96–104
24. Rawicki, H. B. and Hill, S. (1991). Semen retrieval in spinal cord injured men. *Paraplegia*, **29**, 443–6
25. Rutkowski, S. B., Middleton, J. W., Truman, G., Hagen, D. L. and Ryan, J. P. (1995). The influence of bladder management on fertility in spinal cord injured males. *Paraplegia*, **33**, 263–6
26. Dahlberg, A., Ruutu, M. and Hovatta, O. (1995). Pregnancy results from a vibrator application, electroejaculation, and vas aspiration programme in spinal-cord injured men. *Hum. Reprod.*, **10**, 2305–7
27. Nehra, A., Werner, M. A., Bastuba, M., Title, C. and Oates, R. D. (1996). Vibratory stimulation and rectal probe electroejaculation as therapy for patients with spinal cord injury: semen parameters and pregnancy rates. *J. Urol.*, **155**, 554–9
28. Beckerman, H., Becher, J. and Lankhorst, G. J. (1993). The effectiveness of vibratory stimulation in anejaculatory men with spinal cord injury. Review article. *Paraplegia*, **31**, 689–99
29. Sønksen, J. O. R., Drewes, A. M., Biering-Sørensen, F. and Giwercman, J. (1991). Reflex ejaculation produced by penile vibration in patients with spinal cord lesions. *Ugeskr. Laeger.*, **153**, 2888–90
30. Ohl, D. A., Bennett, C. J., McCabe, M., Menge, A. C. and McGuire, E. J. (1989).

Predictors of success in electroejaculation of spinal cord injured men. *J. Urol.*, **142**, 1483–6

31. Buch, J. P. and Zorn, B. H. (1993). Evaluation and treatment of infertility in spinal cord injured men through rectal probe electroejaculation. *J. Urol.*, **149**, 1350–4
32. Sønksen, J., Ohl, D. A., Giwercman, A., Biering-Sørensen, F. and Kristensen, J. K. (1996). Quality of semen obtained by penile vibratory stimulation in men with spinal cord injuries: observations and predictors. *Urology,* in press
33. World Health Organisation (1987). *WHO Laboratory Manual for the Examination of Human Semen and Semen–Cervical Mucus Interaction.* (Cambridge: Cambridge Univeristy Press)
34. Ohl, D. A., Sønksen, J., Menge, A. C., McCabe, M. and Keller, L. M. (1996). Electroejacuation vs. vibratory ejaculation in SCI men: sperm quality and patient preference. *J. Urol.*, **155**, 231
35. Ohl, D. A., Denil, J., Fitzgerald-Shelton, K., McCabe, M., McGuire, E. J., Menge, A. C. and Randolph, J. F. (1992). Fertility in spinal cord injured males: effect of genitourinary infection and bladder management on result of electroejaculation. *J. Am. Paraplegia Soc.*, **15**, 53–9
36. Hirsch, I. H., Sedor, J., Callahan, H. J. and Staas, W. E. (1992). Antisperm antibodies in seminal plasma of spinal cord-injured men. *Urology,* **39**, 243–7
37. Menge, A. C., Ohl, D. A., Denil, J. Korte, M. K., Keller, L. and McCabe, M. (1990). Absence of antisperm antibodies in anejaculatory men. *J. Androl.*, **11**, 396–8
38. Stemmerman, G. N., Weiss, L., Averbach, O. and Friedman, M. (1950). A study of the germinal epithelium in male paraplegic. *Am. J. Clin. Pathol.*, **20**, 24–34
39. Bors, E., Engle, E. T., Rosenquist, R. C. and Holliger, V. H. (1950). Fertility in paraplegic males: a preliminary report of endocrine studies. *J. Clin. Endocrinol.*, **10**, 381–98
40. Perkash, I., Martin, D. E., Warner, H., Blank, M. S. and Collins, D. C. (1985). Reproductive biology of paraplegics: results of semen collection, testicular biopsy and serum hormone evaluation. *J. Urol.*, **134**, 284–8
41. Hirsch, I. H., McCue, P., Allen, J. and Staas, W. E. (1991). Quantitative testicular biopsy in spinal cord injured men: comparisons to fertile controls. *J. Urol.*, **146**, 337–41
42. Linsenmeyer, T. A. and Perkash, I. (1991). Infertility in men with spinal cord injury. *Arch. Phys. Med. Rehabil.*, **72**, 747–54
43. Elliot, S. (1995). Penile vibratory stimulation. State of the art lecture in American Society for Reproductive Medicine 51. Annual Meeting, Seattle, Washington, October 9, 1995
44. Sommer, P., Sønksen, J., Nyboe Anderson, A., Kristensen, J. K., Ziebe, S. and Biering-Sørensen, F. (1995). Fertility results from assisted ejaculation procedures in spinal cord injured men. Presented at the Electroejaculation Interest Group Meeting, Las Vegas, USA, April 22, 1995
45. Tournaye, H., Camus, M., Goossens, A., Liu, J., Nagy, P., Silber, S., Van-Steirteghem, A. C. and Devroey, P. (1995). Recent concepts in the management of infertility because of nonobstructive azoospermia. *Hum. Reprod.*, **10**, 115–19

# II The use of electroejaculation in the treatment of anejaculatory infertility

*Dana A. Ohl, Jens Sønksen, Stephen W. J. Seager and Paul A. Rainsbury*

## INTRODUCTION

Ejaculation dysfunction is an uncommon cause of male infertility in the general population[1]. There are certain clinical situations, however, such as men with spinal cord injury and other naturally occurring or iatrogenic neurological lesions, where ejaculatory dysfunction is the major cause of infertility. Historically, the record of treating such individuals has been quite poor. More recently, the development of procedures which can reliably induce ejaculation has changed the prospects for procreation of many men who are anejaculatory. Rectal probe electroejaculation (EEJ) has been the cornerstone in the treatment of anejaculatory infertility.

In this section, we will discuss the clinical conditions which lead to anejaculatory infertility and the EEJ procedure which may be used to treat the individuals suffering from these conditions.

## HISTORICAL PERSPECTIVE

EEJ was first performed in the ram by Gunn in 1936[2]. The procedure had been relatively well-defined in veterinary medicine for some time before its initial use in humans, most notably in animal husbandry and in animal fertility research[3,4]. Horne, Paull and Munro reported their results of a rather primitive form of EEJ in a group of spinal cord-injured (SCI) men in 1948[5]. The first human pregnancy achieved from the use of EEJ sperm was reported by Thomas and colleagues in 1975[6] and the first surviving live birth by Francois and co-workers in 1978[7]. In the United Kingdom, Brindley was instrumental in promoting the use of both penile vibratory stimulation and EEJ in spinal cord-injured men[8]. The first pregnancy in the United States was reported by Bennett and colleagues in 1987[9].

## CLASSIFICATION OF EJACULATORY DYSFUNCTION

Earlier in this chapter we reviewed the normal physiology of ejaculation and will not repeat this here.

### Premature ejaculation

Premature ejaculation is the inability to voluntarily delay ejaculation for a satisfactory period of time. The diagnosis of premature ejaculation cannot be assigned a definite *time* until climax occurs, as that which constitutes a satisfactory delay may vary from couple to couple[10].

Premature ejaculation is thought to be a psychogenic condition and responds very well to sex therapy[10]. The aim of therapy is to progressively increase ejaculatory delay via a series of exercises. A common method is the so-called 'start–stop' technique, where sexual activity is allowed to progress until just prior to climax, and then abruptly stopped until the man feels as if the urge to climax has abated. Sexual activity is then resumed. Occasionally, therapists will suggest that a painful stimulus is used to abort a seemingly inevitable climax, such as a sharp squeeze to the glans penis, but such painful techniques are probably unnecessary.

Sex therapy, in general, is quite successful but refractory cases may be treated with serotonin re-uptake inhibitors, such as fluoxetine; however, this treatment is still in its infancy and protocols are not yet well established[11].

Premature ejaculation is generally considered a sexual, and not a fertility problem. Infertility may result if ejaculation always occurs prior to intromission. However, in such extreme cases, the semen may still be collected in a specimen container and used for artificial insemination. It is not necessary, therefore, to contemplate the use of EEJ in men with premature ejaculation.

### Idiopathic anejaculation

This is another condition which is thought to be primarily psychogenic, and is also known by the synonyms primary anejaculation, psychogenic anejaculation, functional anejaculation, male anorgasmia, and retarded ejaculation.

These men have the inability to achieve both orgasm and ejaculation during sexual activity. It has usually been present throughout the patient's entire life. Evidence of a psychogenic source of the problem is found in the fact that nearly all these men have the ability to achieve climax and ejaculate during sleep. Many subjects have a conscious awareness of the sensation of orgasm, since they may abruptly awaken from sleep during a nocturnal emission and remember the associated feelings. There have also been associations to other psychological conditions[12].

In contradistinction to premature ejaculation, sex therapy is usually unsuccessful in helping men with idiopathic anejaculation, and infertility may remain an important problem. Patients may require procedures to extract sperm for the purpose of procreation. Men with refractory idiopathic anejaculation are candidates for EEJ procedures[12].

### Retrograde ejaculation

Retrograde ejaculation is caused by incomplete bladder neck closure during the process of seminal emission. Pharmacological and neurological conditions which cause retrograde ejaculation (see Table 1) may also cause absence of seminal emission and it may be only a matter of the degree of the neurological insult which differentiates these two conditions. Also, in addition to these causes of retrograde ejaculation, there may be anatomical causes of bladder neck incompetence. Because sperm are not ejaculated in an antegrade fashion, infertility results because sperm are not deposited in the vagina. The diagnosis of retrograde ejaculation is made by examining the postorgasmic urine.

**Table 1** Aetiologies of retrograde ejaculation and total absence of seminal emission

| |
|---|
| *Anatomical aetiologies* |
| TURP |
| Y-V plasty of bladder |
| Injury to bladder neck |
| Urethral stricture distal to ejaculatory ducts |
| *Pharmacological aetiologies** |
| Antihypertensives (e.g. prazosin) |
| BPH drugs (terazosin) |
| Anti-psychotics (trazodone) |
| *Neurogenic aetiologies** |
| Spinal cord injury |
| Myelodysplasia |
| Multiple sclerosis |
| Retroperitoneal surgery (RPLND or aortic surgery) |
| Diabetic neuropathy |
| Sympathectomy |

*Denotes causes of absence of seminal emission

α-Adrenergic neurons are responsible for bladder neck closure during seminal emission. This allows the possibility of pharmacological management. Some men with retrograde ejaculation may have bladder neck function restored by the administration of sympathomimetic agents, such as imipramine, ephedrine, and phenylpropanolamine[13,14]. A treatment period of 7 days is usually adequate to judge efficacy.

In the event that antegrade ejaculation does not result from this medication treatment, then sperm may be retrieved from the postejaculatory urine and used for artificial insemination. The suggested methodology for such a procedure varies in published reports[15–18]. Our bias is to prepare the patient with sodium bicarbonate, 1.5 g 12 and 2 h prior to the sperm retrieval procedure. This counteracts the acidity of the urine which may be damaging to sperm. Patients are instructed to fast on the day of the retrieval procedure. Some authors feel that the osmolality of the urine will be too high with this regimen, but we feel that, if one limits the amount of urine production, thereby limiting total urine contact, osmolality becomes less of a problem.

We also recommend catheterizing the patient with a plastic catheter to completely empty the bladder and to instill 30–40 ml of a sperm-friendly medium prior to ejaculation. The patient then masturbates to climax and is re-catheterized immediately to completely empty the bladder. Since the interval between catheterizations is a relatively short period of time, and since the patient is fluid-restricted, total urine production is limited and the contact of urine with the semen is minimized. The sperm is processed by normal laboratory techniques and used for artificial insemination. There are several reports of pregnancies in the literature from artificial insemination of retrograde ejaculates[15,17,19].

Since sperm specimens can be readily obtained in men with retrograde ejaculation, EEJ affords no advantage, and should not be used in this clinical setting.

## Absence of seminal emission/anejaculation

### *Spinal cord injury*

Men with spinal cord injury commonly suffer anejaculation. A relatively recent review of the literature, covering papers written on widely differing patient groups, suggests that the incidence of any retained ejaculatory function among spinal cord-injured men is between 0 and 55%, with most studies showing numbers which approach 0%[20]. Men with incomplete lesions, lower motor neuron lesions and lesions lower in the spinal cord have higher rates of spontaneous ejaculation[21], no doubt due to preservation of the sympathetic outflow from T11 to L2.

Approximately 70–80% of spinal cord-injured men can be managed with penile vibratory stimulation to induce a reflex ejaculation, but individuals who do not respond to the vibrator remain candidates for electroejaculation. Typically, people who do not respond to vibrator stimulation are those with lower motor neuron lesions, lower level lesions (below T9) and those with incomplete lesions[8,22].

### *Retroperitoneal lymph node dissection*

Men with testis cancer have excellent cure rates due to the combined medical/surgical approach to this condition. The retroperitoneal lymph node dissection is the integral part of the surgical management of low- and medium-stage testis cancer. Unfortunately, the classic operation removes the sympathetic nerves responsible for seminal emission and thus, although these men have normal sensation of orgasm, they commonly have ejaculatory dysfunction[23,24].

Fortunately, newer nerve-sparing modifications of the retroperitoneal lymph node dissection technique have resulted in preservation of ejaculation in nearly 100% of men with low-stage testis cancer[25,26]. However, men with high-stage testis cancer and those who require surgery following chemotherapy for large-volume disease still require the more radical operation.

Men with absence of antegrade ejaculation following this type of surgery require an examination for retrograde ejaculation, since some will suffer only bladder neck dysfunction. Most, however, will have total absence of seminal emission[24]. Prior to EEJ, treatment with sympathomimetics is indicated. Most men who have recovered from their surgery and have persistent anejaculation will not respond to medical management and will require EEJ to obtain semen specimens[27].

### *Diabetic neuropathy*

Patients with diabetic neuropathy occasionally suffer from peripheral neuropathy which may lead to anemission. They typically have other signs of neuropathy, including lower extremity pain and other autonomic problems, such as erectile dysfunction. Many diabetic men with ejaculatory dysfunction experience a relatively slow progression of their problem, with an initial phase of decreased ejaculate volume followed by retrograde ejaculation and then total absence of seminal emission. Some subjects can be 'rescued' with sympathomimetic agents in the initial phases of the dysfunction, but, once well-established, anemission will require EEJ to obtain a specimen. The EEJ technique has been demonstrated to be successful in both retrieval of sperm and in establishing pregnancies in this subpopulation[28].

*Multiple sclerosis*

Multiple sclerosis can also affect seminal emission through either a central or peripheral nerve malfunction, although the more common sexual dysfunction seen is erectile difficulty. In the authors' experiences, these men will not usually respond to penile vibratory stimulation, but it is reasonable to try such a course initially. Most will require EEJ, which has been successfully used to induce ejaculation and achieve pregnancy[29].

*Other neurological conditions*

Any other conditions which affect the ejaculatory mechanisms of the central nervous system or the peripheral sympathetic nerve outflow may also affect ejaculatory competence. Conditions in which the authors have successfully utilized EEJ to induce ejaculation include surgical nerve injury due to perirectal surgery, aortic grafting, and staging laparotomy for lymphoma, myelodysplasia, and brain death.

## THE ELECTROEJACULATION PROCEDURE

Electroejaculation is carried out with a transrectal electrical probe. We currently use the Seager equipment, as do most other centres throughout the world (Figure 1). Dr Seager was instrumental in bringing the practice of electroejaculation from its role in animal husbandry and adapting the equipment for use in humans. The probes used are generally 3 cm in diameter with either a transverse or a longitudinal arrangement. Alternating current is used to perform the electrical stimulation.

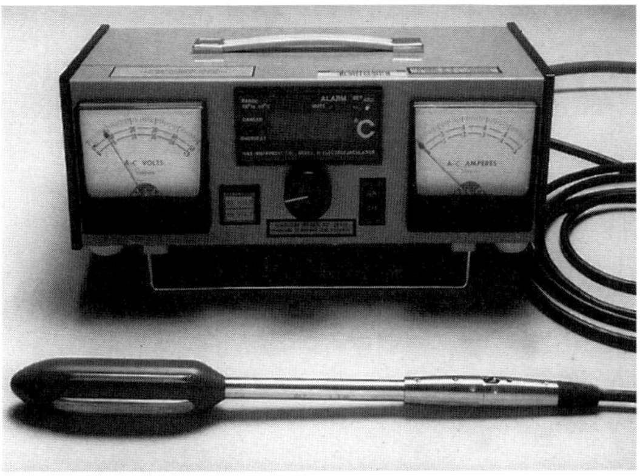

**Figure 1** Seager Model 11 Electroejaculator and 3 cm rectal probe (Dalzall USA Medical Systems, The Plains, VA, USA)

Prior to the procedure, the patient is catheterized to completely empty the bladder of urine. A sperm-friendly medium can be instilled, because most men undergoing EEJ will have at least some of the sperm ejaculated into the bladder (retrograde fraction)[27,30]. In spinal cord-injured men at risk for autonomic dysreflexia, nifedipine is given prior to the procedure to prevent dangerous increases in blood pressure induced by the electrical stimulation[31]. However, most men with autonomic dysreflexia have higher spinal lesions (above T6) and will respond to penile vibratory stimulation, circumventing the need for EEJ[22]. Spinal cord-injured men with sensation below T10 and all other individuals will require either a spinal or general anaesthetic to perform the procedure.

The appropriately sized rectal probe is inserted after sigmoidoscopy which confirms that there are no pre-existing rectal lesions. The electrical stimulus provides a wavelike pattern with the patient on his side (Figure 2). The power is progressively increased until ejaculation is completed. Ejaculation does not occur as an event, but, rather, intermittent release of semen occurs during the course of the procedure. After stimulation is terminated, repeat sigmoidoscopy is performed to exclude injury to the rectum. The bladder is then catheterized to empty the retrograde fraction. Both the antegrade and retrograde ejaculates are then examined, and processed separately, so that both fractions may be pooled and used for assisted reproductive technologies.

Complications to the procedure are rare but may include autonomic dysreflexia and rectal injury. The authors are aware of at least three rectal injuries in the United States from EEJ procedures. Changes in blood pressure are seen in the high spinal cord-injured patients, as

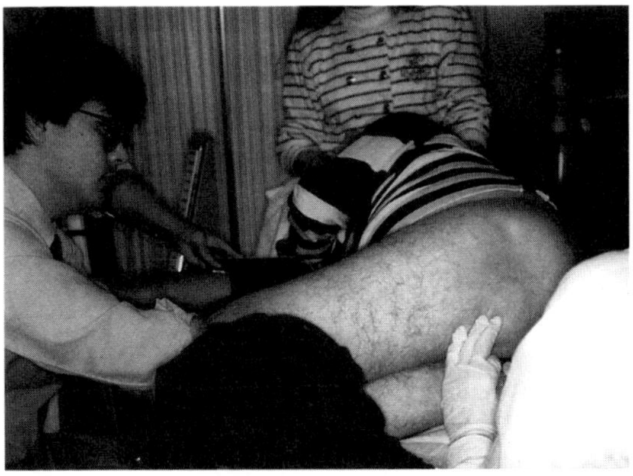

**Figure 2** During electroejaculation, the patient is positioned on his side. The operator places the rectal probe, and the assistant remains in the front to collect antegrade ejaculate. A third person is necessary to monitor the blood pressure in spinal cord-injured men who are prone to autonomic dysreflexia

noted above, and, for that reason, these individuals need continuous blood pressure monitoring. Anaesthetic complications are rare.

## RESULTS OF ELECTROEJACULATION

### Semen quality

Typically, electroejaculation procedures yield specimens of very high count but very poor motility[27,30,32,33]. This is similar to the quality seen with penile vibratory stimulation[34].

The functional capability of sperm may also be decreased. Studies by Denil and colleagues and Buch and colleagues were helpful in this area[32,33]. Electroejaculated specimens have poor sperm motility, poor sperm viability, decreased mucus penetration, decreased fertilizing capacity (by sperm penetration assay) and decreased motility longevity[32,35].

The reasons for poor sperm quality are not known at present, but there is evidence that denervation of the testis may cause abnormalities in epididymal sperm transport and epididymal maturation[36,37]. Although immunological infertility has been deemed by some investigators to be an important cause of poor sperm quality in spinal cord-injured patients[38], we have not found this to be an important issue[39]. The potential reasons for poor sperm quality in spinal cord-injured men are more numerous than in those with other aetiologies of anejaculation and have been reviewed elsewhere[40]. Men who are survivors of testicular cancer therapy have an additional set of risk factors which may impair fertility, including pretreatment subfertility, treatment-related subfertility and carcinoma *in situ* of the remaining testis[41].

### Pregnancies from electroejaculated sperm

Pregnancies from electroejaculated sperm are becoming more common. Table 2 lists several recent series regarding attempts at pregnancy with electroejaculated sperm[42–44]. The widely varying results are hard to explain. Of particular interest, in the series by Ohl and colleagues, is the achievement of more than 75% of the pregnancies by intrauterine insemination alone[42]. Lower success rates for intrauterine insemination have prompted Matthews and colleagues and Bar-Chama and colleagues to suggest that higher level assisted reproductive techniques should be used early in the treatment programme[43,44].

We believe that, in the case of men with spinal cord injury who are undergoing EEJ, intrauterine insemination is initially the procedure of choice. Many men in our experience are

**Table 2** Selected series of pregnancies achieved utilizing sperm obtained by electroejaculation

| *Series* | *n* | *Pregnancies from intrauterine insemination* | *Pregnancies from in vitro fertilization ± intracytoplasmic sperm injection* |
|---|---|---|---|
| Ohl *et al.*[42] | 120 | 41 | 12 |
| Matthews *et al.*[43] | 33 | 10 | 5 |
| Bar-Chama *et al.*[44] | 108 | 9 | not reported |

comfortable with this protocol, and the ease, safety and low cost of performing EEJ in the clinic setting, without an anaesthetic, allow multiple attempts to be made. Higher level assisted reproductive techniques such as *in vitro* fertilization, gamete or zygote intrafallopian transfer may be used in couples who fail to achieve a pregnancy after three to six cycles of intrauterine insemination[45].

In men who require an anaesthetic, the cost, effort and risk of retrieving a semen specimen by EEJ are substantially higher. Because of this, it seems to be prudent to proceed on to higher-level techniques immediately. Analysis of the programme results at the University of Michigan has indicated that it is cost-effective to perform high-level assisted reproductive techniques as the initial procedure in couples where the man requires an anaesthetic to undergo EEJ[42].

A special case exists, of course, for those uncommon individuals who have extremely poor semen quality, but who are not azoospermic. Such men are candidates for intracytoplasmic sperm injection (ICSI) of the electroejaculated sperm. Since the ICSI procedure requires so few sperm, one may argue that EEJ is not necessary, since percutaneous sperm retrieval with a needle or by local anaesthesia testis biopsy will usually give suitable numbers of sperm for the ICSI procedure. However, lingering uncertainties of the quality of sperm derived from the testis should favour obtaining sperm from the ejaculate for ICSI, even if the ejaculate is necessarily induced by EEJ.

## CONCLUSIONS

EEJ remains a cornerstone treatment in men who are unable to ejaculate. Although penile vibratory stimulation is an appropriate initial procedure for spinal cord-injured men, there is a 20% failure rate, and EEJ will be necessary. For all other aetiologies of anejaculation, EEJ is the only method available to induce seminal emission. Sperm quality and function in EEJ specimens are poor, and pregnancy rates are lower than with other patient populations undergoing assisted reproduction. When attempting to establish a pregnancy with EEJ sperm, we recommend initially using the technique of intrauterine insemination for men who do not require an anaesthetic for the EEJ procedure but moving on to IVF and other higher-level techniques for men who do require an anaesthetic for ejaculation induction.

## REFERENCES


1. Dubin, L. and Amelar, R. D. (1971). Etiologic factors in 1294 consecutive cases of male infertility. *Fertil. Steril.*, **22**, 469–74
2. Bennett, C. J., Seager, S. W., Vasher, E. A. and McGuire, E. J. (1988). Sexual dysfunction and electroejaculation in men with spinal cord injury: review. *J. Urol.*, **139**, 453–7
3. Howard, J. G., Bush, M., de Vos, V. and Wildt, D. E. (1984). Electroejaculation, semen characteristics and serum testosterone concentrations of free-ranging African elephants (*Loxodonta africana*). *J. Reprod. Fertil.*, **72**, 187–95
4. Platz, C. C., Wildt, D. E., Howard, J. G. and Bush, M. (1983). Electroejaculation and semen analysis and freezing in the giant panda (*Ailuropoda melanoleuca*). *J. Reprod. Fertil.*, **67**, 9–12
5. Horne, H. W., Paull, D. P. and Munro, D. (1948). Fertility studies in the human male with traumatic injuries of the spinal cord and cauda equina. *N. Engl. J. Med.*, **239**, 337–48
6. Thomas, R. J., McLeish, G. and McDonald, I. A. (1975). Electroejaculation of the paraplegic male followed by pregnancy. *Med. J. Aust.*, **2**, 789–90
7. Francois, N., Maury, M., Jouannet, D., David, G. and Vacant, J. (1978). Electroejaculation of a complete paraplegic followed by pregnancy. *Paraplegia*, **16**, 248–51
8. Brindley, G. S. (1984). The fertility of men with spinal injuries. *Paraplegia*, **22**, 337–48
9. Bennett, C. J., Ayers, J. W., Randolph, J. F., Seager, S. W., McCabe, M., Moinipanah, R. and McGuire, E. J. (1987). Electroejaculation of paraplegic males followed by pregnancies. *Fertil. Steril.*, **48**, 1070–2
10. Kaplan, H. S. (1989). *PE – how to Overcome Premature Ejaculation.* (New York: Brunner/Mazel)
11. Althof, S. E. (1995). Pharmacologic treatment of rapid ejaculation. *Psychiatr. Clin. North Am.*, **18**, 85–94

12. Stewart, D. E. and Ohl, D. A. (1989). Idiopathic anejaculation treated by electroejaculation. *Int. J. Psychiatr. Med.*, **19**, 263–8
13. Eppel, S. M. and Berzin, M. (1984). Pregnancy following treatment of retrograde ejaculation with clomipramine hydrochloride. A report of 3 cases. *S. Afr. Med. J.*, **66**, 889–91
14. Brooks, M. E., Berezin, M. and Braf, Z. (1980). Treatment of retrograde ejaculation with imipramine. *Urology*, **15**, 353–5
15. Shangold, G. A., Cantor, B. and Schreiber, J. R. (1990). Treatment of infertility due to retrograde ejaculation: a simple, cost-effective method. *Fertil. Steril.*, **54**, 175–7
16. Suominen, J. J., Kilkku, P. P., Taina, E. J. and Puntala, P. V. (1991). Successful treatment of infertility due to retrograde ejaculation by instillation of serum-containing medium into the bladder. A case report. *Int. J. Androl.*, **14**, 87–90
17. Urry, R. L., Middleton, R. G. and McGavin, S. (1986). A simple and effective technique for increasing pregnancy rates in couples with retrograde ejaculation. *Fertil. Steril.*, **46**, 1124–7
18. Volpe, A., Artini, P. G., Coukos, G., Uccelli, E., Marchini, E. and Genazzani, A. R. (1992). Sperm retrieval for direct intraperitoneal insemination in a diabetic with retrograde ejaculation. A case report. *J. Reprod. Med.*, **37**, 219–20
19. van der Linden, P. J., Nan, P. M., te Velde, E. R. and van Kooy, R. J. (1992). Retrograde ejaculation: successful treatment with artificial insemination. *Obstet. Gynecol.*, **79**, 126–8
20. Sønksen, J. and Biering-Sørensen, F. (1992). Fertility in men with spinal cord or cauda equina lesions. *Semin. Neurol.*, **12**, 106–14
21. Griffith, E. R., Tomko, M. A. and Timms, R. J. (1973). Sexual function in spinal cord-injured patients: a review. *Arch. Phys. Med. Rehabil.*, **54**, 539–43
22. Sønksen, J., Biering-Sørensen, F. and Kristensen, J. K. (1994). Ejaculation induced by penile vibratory stimulation in men with spinal cord lesion. The importance of the vibratory amplitude. *Paraplegia*, **32**, 651–60
23. Fossa, S., Ous, S., Abyholm, T., Norman, N. and Loeb, M. (1985). Post-treatment fertility in patients with testicular cancer. II. Influence of *cis*-platin-based combination chemotherapy and of retroperitoneal surgery on hormone and sperm cell production. *Br. J. Urol.*, **57**, 210–14
24. Kedia, K., Markland, C. and Fraley, E. (1975). Sexual function following high retroperitoneal lymphadenectomy. *J. Urol.*, **114**, 237–9
25. Jewett, M. A. S., Kong, Y. S., Goldberg, S. D., Sturgeon, J. F., Thomas, G. M., Alison, R. E. and Gospodarowicz, M. K. (1988). Retroperitoneal lymphadenectomy for testis tumor with nerve sparing for ejaculation. *J. Urol.*, **139**, 1220–4
26. Donohue, J. P., Foster, R. S., Rowland, R. G., Bihrle, R., Jones, J. and Geier, G. (1990). Nerve-sparing retroperitoneal lymphadenectomy with preservation of ejaculation. *J. Urol.*, **36**, 287–91
27. Ohl, D. A., Denil, J., Bennett, C. J., Randolph, J. F., Menge, A. C. and McCabe, M. (1991). Electroejaculation following retroperitoneal lymphadenectomy. *J. Urol.*, **145**, 980–3
28. Gerig, N. E., Meacham, R. B. and Ohl, D. A. (1996). The use of electroejaculation in the treatment of ejaculatory failure secondary to diabetes mellitus. *Urology*, in press
29. Ohl, D. A., Grainger, R., Bennett, C. J., Randolph, J. F., Seager, S. W. J. and McCabe, M. (1989). Successful use of electroejaculation in two multiple sclerosis patients including a report of a pregnancy utilizing intrauterine insemination. *Neurourol. Urodynamics*, **8**, 195–8
30. Ohl, D. A., Bennett, C. J., McCabe, M., Menge, A. C. and McGuire, E. J. (1989). Predictors of success in electroejaculation of spinal cord injured men. *J. Urol.*, **142**, 1483–6
31. Steinberger, R. E., Ohl, D. A., Bennett, C. J., McCabe, M. and Wang, S. C. (1990). Nifedipine pretreatment for autonomic dysreflexia during electroejaculation. *Urology*, **36**, 228–31
32. Denil, J., Ohl, D. A., Menge, A. C., Keller, L. M. and McCabe, M. (1992). Functional characteristics of sperm obtained by electroejaculation. *J. Urol.*, **147**, 69–72
33. Buch, J. P. and Zorn, B. H. (1993). Evaluation and treatment of infertility in spinal cord injured men through rectal probe electroejaculation. *J. Urol.*, **149**, 1350–4
34. Szasz, G. and Carpenter, C. (1989). Clinical observations in vibratory stimulation of the penis of men with spinal cord injury. *Arch. Sex. Behav.*, **18**, 461–74
35. Denil, J., Ohl., D. A., Hurd, W. W., Menge, A. C. and Hiner, M. R. (1992). Motility longevity of sperm samples processed for

intrauterine insemination. *Fertil. Steril.*, **58**, 436–8

36. Billups, K. L., Tillman, S. L. and Chang, T. S. (1990). Reduction of epididymal sperm motility after ablation of the inferior mesenteric plexus in the rat. *Fertil. Steril.*, **53**, 1076–82
37. Billups, K. L., Tillman, S. and Chang, T. S. (1990). Ablation of the inferior mesenteric plexus in the rat: alteration of sperm storage in the epididymis and vas deferens. *J. Urol.*, **143**, 625–9
38. Beretta, G., Zanollo, A., Chelo, E., Livi, C. and Scarselli, G. (1987). Seminal parameters and auto-immunity in paraplegic/quadraplegic men. *Acta Eur. Fertil.*, **18**, 203–5
39. Menge, A. C., Ohl, D. A., Denil, J., Korte, M. K., Keller, L. and McCabe, M. (1990). Absence of antisperm antibodies in anejaculatory men. *J. Androl.*, **11**, 396–8
40. Linsenmeyer, T. A. and Perkash, I. (1991). Infertility in men with spinal cord injury. *Arch. Phys. Med., Rehabil.*, **72**, 747–54
41. Ohl, D. A. and Sønksen, J. (1996). What are the chances of infertility and should sperm be banked? *Sem. Urol. Onc.*, **14**, 36–44
42. Ohl, D. A., Hurd, W. W., Wolf, L. J., Menge, A. C., Ansbacher, R., Christman, G. and Randolph, J. F. (1995). Electroejaculation and assisted reproductive technologies. *Fertil. Steril.*, **64** (Suppl.), S138
43. Matthews, G. J., Gardner, T. A. and Eid, J. F. (1996). *In vitro* fertilization improves pregnancy rates for sperm obtained by rectal probe ejaculation. *J. Urol.*, **155**, 1934–7
44. Bar-Chama, N., Ozkan, S., Lipshultz, L. I. and Lamb, D. J. (1994). Pregnancy in patients undergoing electroejaculation. *J. Urol.*, **151**, 302A
45. Randolph, J. F., Ohl, D. A., Bennett, C. J., Ayers, J. W. and Menge, A. C. (1990). Combined electroejaculation and *in vitro* fertilization in the evaluation and treatment of anejaculatory infertility. *J. In Vitro Fertil. Embryo Transf.*, **7**, 58–62

# Laboratory techniques 13

*Marie Hayes*

## AN INTRODUCTION TO EMBRYOLOGY

During development of the embryo, the germ plasm is set aside from the rest of the embryo, the soma, to produce what will become the next generation. The soma goes on to form all of the adult structures whilst the germ plasm is thought to produce the germ cells which will become sperm or eggs.

The early precursors of the germ cells, known as primordial germ cells, appear early in development at 24 days after fertilization. At this time, like all other cells in the body, they are diploid (that is, they possess a double set of chromosomes). They arise in a site remote from the sexual organs and migrate by an amoeboid-type movement through the gut mesentery to populate the sex organs.

The numbers of primordial germ cells are initially small; there are as few as 100 in the yolk sac. During migration, they multiply and, by the time they reach the gonad, there are several thousand. In the female fetus, the primordial germ cell is differentiated into oogonia, whilst in the male fetus they will form spermatogonia, but only at puberty.

The number of oogonia in a 5-month fetus is approximately 7 million; these degenerate so that by birth there may be only a million or fewer functional germ cells present. These oogonia form oocytes; they have commenced meiotic division which will lead to them becoming haploid (that is, possessing one full set of chromosomes). Spermatogonia, however, replace themselves by continued mitotic division, so the number of sperm that can be produced is vast. Spermatogonia, however, remain diploid only as they enter terminal differentiation.

### Mitosis and meiosis

In mitosis, the single chromosomes double, and then double chromosomes separate to give twice the number of single chromosomes. One set of 46 single chromosomes goes to each daughter of the associated cell division.

In meiosis, the single chromosomes must double as in mitosis, but then each chromosome pairs up with its corresponding partner. At the first division, one of each pair of double chromosomes goes to each daughter, giving each daughter 23 double chromosomes. This is followed by a second division in which each daughter cell acquires a single chromosome from each of the double ones, so that it has 23 single ones. While the chromosomes are paired, gene recombination occurs, leading to a unique set of genes.

### Oocyte development

At birth, all oocytes are arrested in the primary oocyte stage where the first meiotic division and exchange of genetic material has taken place but before the daughter cells separate. Each primary oocyte is surrounded by flattened cells derived from the ovarian tissue, and these together are referred to as a primordial follicle.

At puberty, these primordial follicles undergo hormonally induced changes causing the primary oocyte to enlarge, and an acellular matrix layer (zona pellucida) is deposited around the oocyte.

The first meiotic division of the oocyte is completed, producing two daughter cells; one inherits all the cytoplasm and is known as the secondary oocyte, the other is known as the first polar body. The first stage of the second meiotic division is now completed rapidly followed by another pause. The oocyte is now ready for ovulation.

### Spermatogenesis

The primordial germ cells in the male migrate to the primary sex cords where they remain until puberty, at which time the sex cords become tubular and the germ cells, now known as spermatogonia, live along the inner surface.

At this stage they can re-enter mitotic division, resulting in the generation of haploid spermatids. Spermatids are round cells which undergo dramatic differentiation to form spermatazoa.

### Fertilization

The oocyte is a large cell approximately 80 µm in diameter. A layer of cortical granules lies in its cytoplasm beneath the oocyte membrane. The first polar body lies in the perivitelline space inside the zona pellucida. Outside the zona is a cloud of cells derived from the follicle walls, known as corona radiata (Figure 1).

The spermatozoon is much smaller than the oocyte. The genetic material is contained in the posterior part of the head, while the acrosome containing digestive enzymes is in the anterior section. The long tail provides motive force (Figure 2).

Normal fertilization occurs in the ampulla of the uterine tube. Newly ejaculated sperm cannot fertilize an egg, as they must first undergo maturation, known as capicitation, whereby proteins are removed from the head of the sperm to reveal specific binding molecules underneath. Once binding of the sperm with the egg has occurred, the acrosome membrane fuses with the outer sperm membrane and the digestive enzymes break down the zona. Several sperm may bind to one egg and a race proceeds to digest their way through the zona. Once inside the perivitelline space, the sperm is engulfed by the oocyte.

When a sperm binds to an egg, the cortical granules fuse with the egg membrane and release ZP3 into the perivitelline space where they alter the zona pellucida so that no more sperm can penetrate. This is called 'slow block', and it is thought that, as in the invertebrates, 'fast block' may also occur where binding causes a membrane depolarization in a second which prevents polyspermy (more than one sperm fertilizing the sperm).

Fusion causes the oocyte to complete the second meiotic division and extrudes the second polar body into the perivitelline space. The two pronuclei then fuse to form a single nucleus approximately 12 h later. Fusion marks the conclusion of fertilization and produces a zygote.

The zygote then divides 24–36 h after fertilization, the resulting daughter cells or blastomeres being half the size of the zygote. After 4 days, there will be approximately 32 cells forming a cluster (the morula). At this point, a space is created by the cells moving apart and pump-

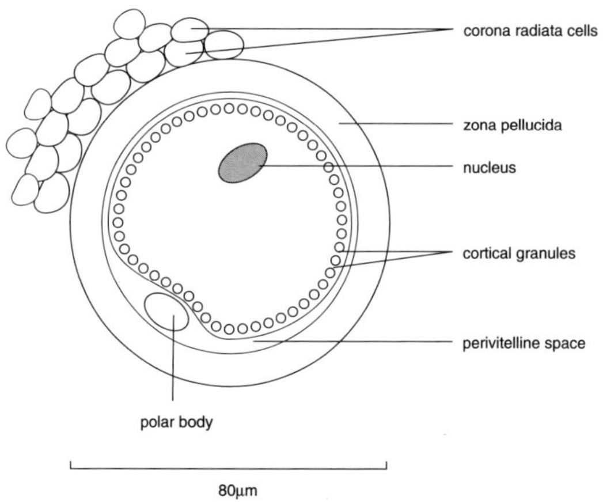


**Figure 1** The human oocyte

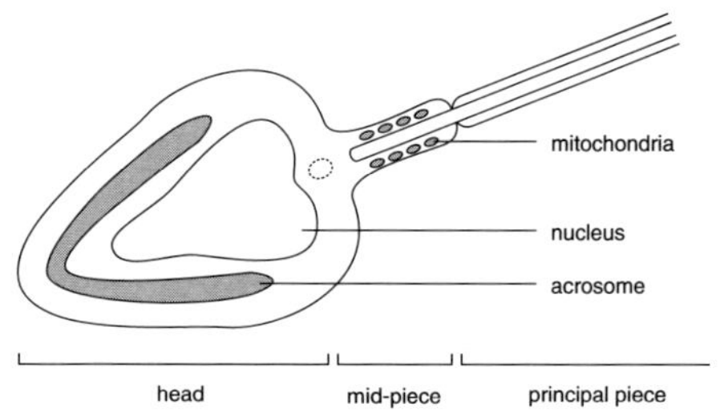


**Figure 2** The human sperm

ing fluid into the cavity. This stage is known as the blastocyst, and, as this enlarges, it begins to 'hatch' from the zona pellucida.

At around 6 days after the blastocyst has emerged from the zona, it begins to adhere to the uterine wall (implantation). At the end of the 2nd week after fertilization, the main body axis begins to become apparent (gastrulation) and is referred to as the gastrula. The existence of the main body axis is confirmed by the development of the neural tube and a process known as neurulation. Damage during this period to the conceptus has a good chance of being repaired completely as many cells can change their nature to compensate for any damage.

The period from fertilization to neurulation is known as the pre-embryonic period. The period from neurulation until 9 weeks is known as the embryonic period, when all the main body organs are laid down. This period is sometimes known as the critical period as the embryo is very susceptible to environmental damage. From 9 weeks to birth is known as the fetal period when the fetus grows in size and maturity.

## THE EMBRYOLOGY LABORATORY

In the past decade the face of the embryology laboratory has changed significantly, with the introduction of many new techniques, more accurate and sensitive equipment and an increase in the skills required by the clinical embryologist.

The introduction of the HFEA (The Human Fertilisation and Embryology Authority) in 1991 meant the introduction of regular inspections of fertility units, and in particular the embryology laboratory. A successful assisted conception unit depends not only on appropriate patient selection, ovarian stimulation, monitoring, timing and expertise of oocyte retrieval and embryo transfer by the clinicians but also on a fully functioning laboratory with protocols which are rigorously adhered to by the embryologists.

Handling oocytes and embryos on a daily basis could potentially lead to their delicacy being overlooked. Removed from their natural environment within the body, oocytes and embryos are subject to many non-physiological conditions that may be detrimental to their viability[1,2] and the developmental potential of cultured embryos is markedly reduced compared with that of embryos *in vivo*[3].

The objective of the embryology laboratory is the production of viable embryos for replacement in a suitably primed woman's uterus. A viable embryo is one that is capable of producing an ongoing pregnancy.

Full sterile precautions are adopted in the operating theatre and the laboratories at all times. The entire complex is air-conditioned with filtered air under positive pressure ventilation and access is restricted to the appropriate personnel wearing theatre clothes, hats and shoes.

### Laboratory cleaning

The laboratory is deep cleaned once a week. This consists of the floor being cleaned using an industrial floor scrubber using PF-7X detergent. It is then thoroughly rinsed and buffed. All surfaces are damp dusted using PF-7X detergent followed by water. Bench surfaces and laminar flow surfaces are cleaned using PF-7X followed by rinsing, then wiping areas with 70% ethanol, using disposable tissue at all times.

Incubators are cleaned once a month (for humidified incubator) or immediately after treatment of a patient with a potentially contagious condition.

### Daily cleaning

Bench surfaces and the laminar flow cabinet are cleaned every morning before use using 70% ethanol. Following each oocyte retrieval, the yellow bags (for incineration only) containing waste from ovarian follicle aspirations are removed from the laboratory, double bagged and sealed ready for collection and disposal. During the course of the day, any spillages are dealt with appropriately depending on the source of the spillage and the area is cleaned immediately.

At the end of each day all rubbish bags are removed and double bagged for disposal. Benches, flow hood, microscopes and all equipment are wiped with tissue soaked in 70% ethanol.

### Incubator cleaning

(1) The incubator has its $CO_2$ flow turned off.

(2) Water is removed from the incubator (humidified incubator) and the shelves removed.

(3) The shelves are washed in PF-7X and thoroughly rinsed. They are then sterilized in a hot air oven at 180°C for 4 h.

(4) The incubator is rinsed and drained several times using sterile water, then dried completely using sterile swabs.

(5) The incubator is rinsed and dried again.

(6) If the incubator is capable of heating to high temperatures it is heated for 4 h.

(7) Once cooled, sterile water is placed in the bottom (humidified incubator) and the set-up process for the incubator is undertaken (see manufacturer's instructions).

(8) The shelves are replaced. Most set-up procedures take at least 24 h, so this should be undertaken at a time when the incubator is not required for at least 2 days.

### Pipette cleaning

Pasteur pipettes are rinsed in sterile water overnight then shaken dry and put into sterilizing containers. They are then sterilized at 180°C for 4 h.

## MEDIA PREPARATION

Aseptic techniques are used throughout and all media preparation takes place in a laminar flow cabinet.

### Stock medium

Basic stock media are used to produce 8% serum media and 15% serum media for tissue culture. The composition is as follows:

500 ml Minimal Essential Medium (MEM) with Earles salts and L-glutamine (Gibco)
30 mg Penicillin
25 mg Streptomycin

The osmolarity is adjusted using sterile water to 280–285 mosmol (approximately 25 ml of water needed). This is filtered using a 0.22 μm filter (with filling bell). This medium can be stored for 1 week at +4°C.

### Flushing medium

This is used to flush the ovarian follicles to aspirate oocytes. The composition is as follows:

500 ml Minimal Essential Medium (MEM) with Earles salts and L-glutamine (Gibco)
30 mg Penicillin
25 mg Streptomycin
1.1925 g HEPES
0.9 ml Heparin (1000 U/ml)

The penicillin, streptomycin and HEPES are added to the MEM and the osmolarity altered to 280–285 mosmol using sterile water. Then 25 ml can be removed and used for freeze thaw medium. This is filtered with a 0.22 μm filter and 0.9 ml of heparin is added to the 500 ml of medium and filtered using a 0.22 μm filter (with filling bell). This can be stored at +4°C for up to 3 weeks or stored in the incubator for up to 1 week.

### 8% serum medium

This is used for oocytes at the time of oocyte retrieval, culture of oocytes for 24 h and sperm preparations. It is prepared by adding 0.8 ml of patient's serum to 9.2 ml of stock medium.

Patient's own serum is taken and filtered using a 0.22 μm filter and then heat-inactivated in a water bath at 56°C for 35 min. This can be prepared and stored in advance for up to 5 days.

Media are generally prepared and filtered the day before use and incubated overnight with a loose cap to allow equilibration.

### 15% serum medium

This is used for 24–48 h embryo culture and culture of embryos post-thawing. It is prepared by adding 0.45 ml of patient's serum to 2.55 ml of stock medium.

Medium is prepared and then filtered using a 0.22 μm filter the day before use and incubated overnight to allow equilibration.

### Medium for embryo freezing and thawing

The composition of the basic freeze/thaw medium is:

500 ml MEM with Earles salts and L-glutamine (Gibco)
30 mg Penicillin
25 mg Streptomycin
1.1925 g HEPES

The medium is prepared, the osmolarity is adjusted to 280–285 mosmol with sterile water and it is then filtered with a 0.22 μm filter. This can be stored at +4°C for 2–3 weeks.

### Embryo cryoprotectant medium

This is prepared by adding 1.0 ml patient's serum to 4.0 ml basic freeze/thaw medium. These are mixed together, then 0.6 ml is discarded and 0.6 ml of propylene glycol is added drop by drop and gently mixed, and this is filtered with a 0.22 μm filter. This must be used within 2–3 days.

### Embryo thawing medium

This has the following composition:

2.55 ml Basic freeze/thaw medium
0.45 ml Patient's serum
1.045 g Sucrose

These ingredients are mixed until the sucrose is fully dissolved and then filtered using a 0.22 μm filter. This must be used within 2–3 days.

### Cryoprotectant for sperm

This has the following composition:

850 ml Sterile water
150 ml Glycerol
5.8 g Sodium chloride
0.4 g Potassium chloride
0.76 g Calcium lactate
0.12 g Magnesium sulphate
0.05 g Sodium dihydrogen phosphate (V)
2.60 g Sodium hydrogen carbonate
4.77 g HEPES
8.59 g Glucose
8.59 g Fructose
10.00 g Glycine
0.05 g Streptomycin
0.05 g Penicillin
4.00 g Human serum albumin (Fraction V No. 1 – 1653)

These ingredients are mixed in a sterile roller bottle (Falcon) and then filtered using a 0.22 μm filter.

If the medium is to be frozen for storage the glycerol must not be added. The medium can then be aliquoted into the appropriate amounts and frozen. The relevant amount of glycerol can then be added on defrosting ready for use.

## OOCYTE RECOVERY AND CULTURE

Prior to the patient's treatment, the medical history is studied with particular attention given to previous *in vitro* fertilization (IVF) treatment cycles, especially any allergies, oocyte quality, sperm quality, any problems in producing the sperm sample, fertilization rates and embryo quality. Comments should be documented in the notes if any recommendations are made for particular use of media or for techniques relevant to the particular patient.

Preparation begins the day prior to oocyte recovery with the setting up of the oocyte collection dishes with 0.9 ml of 8% serum medium in the inner well of four Falcon dishes and 5 ml basic medium in the outside well. Four dishes are prepared for each patient and labelled and these are incubated overnight. If the incubator is not humidified, liquid paraffin must be overlaid in the centre well.

The flushing medium is also incubated overnight with approximately 250 ml allowed per patient. If the patient has a high number of follicles or there were problems in recovery of the oocytes in previous collections, then an extra 250 ml of flushing medium should be prepared. The caps of Falcon bottles should remain loose whilst in the incubator to allow circulation of the gases.

### Oocyte collection

Half an hour prior to oocyte collection the laminar flow cabinet and the relevant heated equipment are switched on and wiped with 70% ethanol.

The patient's clinical notes are reviewed to prepare laboratory notes and permanent adhesive labels for the oocyte collection dishes. The labels indicate the patient's name, hospital number and dish number. The laboratory notes are completed with the patient's name, hospital number, date of birth, treatment number, cause of infertility and number and size of follicles at last ultrasound scan.

The flushings from the oocyte collection are collected into 15 ml Falcon test tubes and placed into a heated test tube rack at 37°C in the laboratory. The contents of the tubes are examined using a stereo dissecting microscope with transmitted illumination base and heated stage (37°C) which is located in the laminar flow cabinet. As each follicle is flushed, the contents are poured carefully into 60 mm Petri dishes (Falcon) which have been warmed on a dish warmer (37°C), so that they may be viewed through the microscope. All tubes, dishes and fluids must be kept at 37°C throughout. Cooling of the oocytes can cause irreversible disruption of the meiotic spindle[4].

Each dish is scanned carefully in order to locate the oocyte and each tube is checked before discarding to ensure no loss of oocytes. When an oocyte is identified, the oocyte collection dish is taken from the incubator or mini bench top incubator. The oocyte is carefully washed in the outer well, gently aspirating in and out of the Pasteur pipette in the medium until all traces of blood are removed. It is then placed in the centre well. The quality of the oocyte is assessed and graded and these details are entered in the laboratory notes. The oocyte collection dish is replaced in the incubator as soon as possible. The oocytes are distributed among the four dishes as they are collected.

## GRADING OF OOCYTE–CUMULUS COMPLEX

The oocytes are graded according to their maturity, assessing the amount of cumulus, expansion and distribution of the cumulus cells and the appearance of the oocyte itself. Both the oocyte and the cumulus are given a scoring as shown in Table 1 and Figure 3.

**Table 1** Scoring of the oocyte and cumulus

| *Oocyte quality* | *Cumulus quality* | *Description* |
|---|---|---|
| A | a | The egg can be seen clearly inside the cumulus mass, the cytoplasm is visible through the corona radiata, the cumulus has expanded to a fluffy mass and is evenly dispersed. |
| B | b | Oocyte–cumulus mass is slightly smaller. Cumulus is less dispersed, cytoplasm may have an uneven coloration and is possibly mature. |
| C | c | Is immature, the cumulus mass is condensed, there is a tightly opposed layer of corona cells around the oocyte, and it is much smaller than the mature oocyte–cumulus complex. |
| D | d | The oocyte is totally devoid of cumulus, the cytoplasm is dark and the germinal vesicle may be viewed. The oocyte seldom matures and would not fertilize with IVF. |
| Post-mature luteinized oocyte | | Perhaps due to oocyte collection being delayed a day or two. The egg is very pale and the cumulus mass has broken down and looks almost lace-like with areas of agglutination. These oocytes should be inseminated without delay. |

## INSEMINATION OF OOCYTES

The oocytes are incubated for 3–6 h prior to insemination. Approximately 2½ h postoocyte collection, the husband produces his semen sample or the appropriate donor sperm is defrosted.

The specimen is prepared by one of the semen preparation techniques and diluted to a concentration of 1–3 million per ml and a volume of 100 μl injected into each centre well of each dish.

If the semen preparation is below the minimum concentration, then the eggs can be placed in microdroplets of medium overlaid with oil and the insemination of this lower number of sperm into the microdroplet gives a higher concentration of sperm surrounding the egg. This method has now been superseded with the advent of the intracytoplasmic sperm injection (ICSI) technique, whereby patients with semen preparations of below $1 \times 10^6$/ml are now almost invariably advised to enrol in the ICSI programme.

The eggs and sperm are incubated overnight along with two 15% serum dishes for culture after dissection.

## DISSECTION OF THE EMBRYOS

Tools required depend on the preference of technique.

### Mouth pipetting

The mouth pipette consists of a mouthpiece in a length of silicon tubing (approximately 25 cm long) attached to a 0.22 mm filter with another piece of silicon tubing attached to this. A standard Pasteur pipette will fit comfortably into the end of this tubing.

A standard Pasteur pipette is pulled to varying sizes by heating the pipette on a Bunsen burner until the glass is malleable and then quickly pulling so as to reduce the diameter of the pipette. A clean break is then achieved by slowly stroking the length of the pulled section of the pipette until it breaks. A clean unjagged edge must be achieved otherwise damage to the embryo will result. The embryos are gently taken in and expelled from the pulled pipette until the cumulus cells are removed.

### Needle dissection

Two 23 g needles and two insulin needles are used to gently shave the cells that surround the zona pellucida.

Between 16 and 22 h after insemination of the eggs, the coronal cumulus cells are removed and signs of fertilization can be visualized. Normal fertilization results in the production of two pronucleates in the cytoplasm of the embryo (Figure 4). Those eggs showing signs of normal fertilization are transferred to the 15% serum dish and cultured overnight ready for transfer the following day. If there is in excess of two pronucleates, this usually indicates polyspermy and such embryos are never replaced into the patient (Figure 5). Embryos showing only one pronucleate are also abnormal and are not transferred.

Those found to be unfertilized remain in the dish containing the sperm for a further 24 h when they are re-inspected. Alternatively, they may be placed in a fresh dish and a fresh semen sample prepared and re-insemination undertaken.

If six or more oocytes show clear signs of fertilization, then embryo freezing at the pronucleate stage may be considered. The patient's previous history regarding fertilization rates, embryo quality and post-thaw quality is also considered when deciding how many zygotes are to be frozen at this stage.

## EMBRYO GRADING

On day 2 (approximately 48 h postoocyte collection), the embryos are examined and graded (Figures 6 and 7).

*Grade 1* These embryos have even, regular shaped, spherical blastomeres with clear nongranular cytoplasm and intact zona. No fragmentation is seen.

*Grade 2* These embryos have even-sized blastomeres with negligible fragmentation.

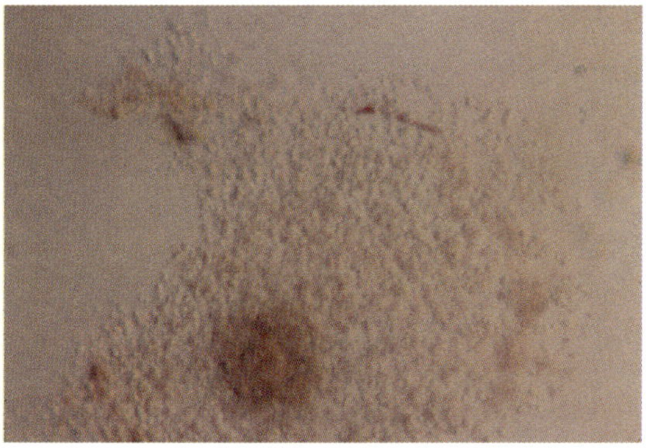

**Figure 3** Good quality oocyte

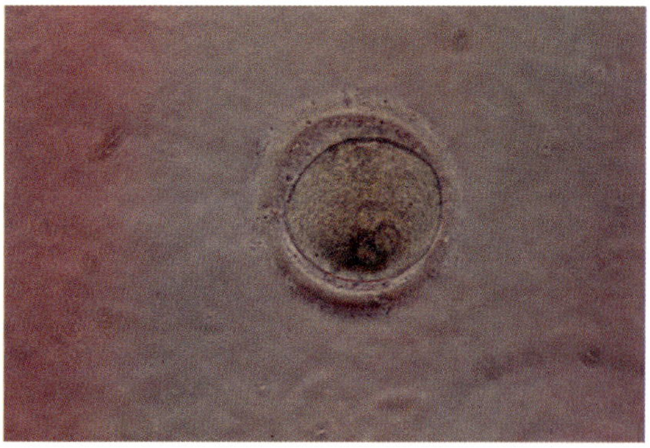

**Figure 5** Triploid embryo, unsuitable for transfer

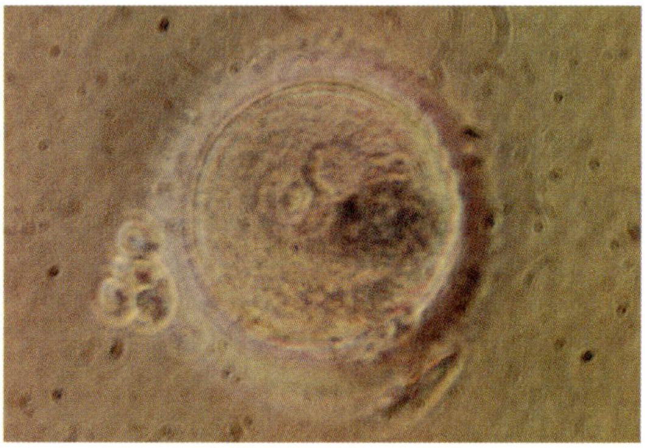

**Figure 4** Bipronucleate embryo

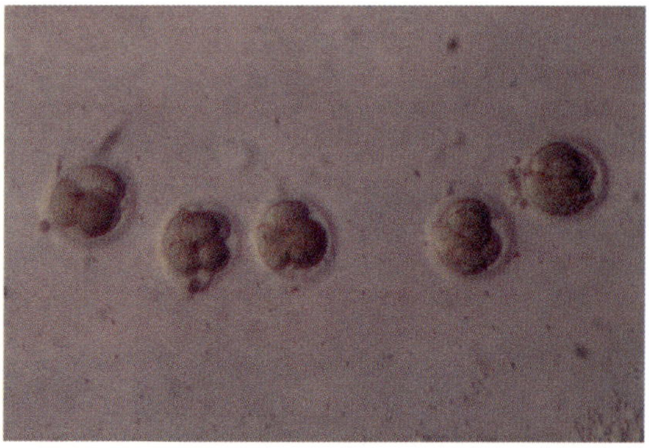

**Figure 6** Selection of good quality embryos

*Grade 3* Clear signs of division can be seen, but up to 50% fragmentation is visible and the cytoplasm may be slightly dark.

*Grade 4* In excess of 50% fragmentation can be seen. The cytoplasm is usually dark and signs of remaining blastomeres are clearly visible.

*Grade 5* Total fragmentation of the embryo has occurred. This is not viable and would not be replaced.

## ASSESSMENT AND SELECTION OF EMBRYOS FOR TRANSFER

A decision is made on the number of embryos for transfer. This will take into account the woman's age, previous obstetric history, cause of infertility, the age of the woman or woman who donated the eggs (if applicable), the quality and number of the embryos and of course the couple's personal wishes. In the UK, HFEA regulations state that the maximum number of embryos allowed to be replaced in any one cycle is three. This obviously leads to the slim possibility of triplets but a very real possibility of having twins. The chance of multiple pregnancy and the associated risks has to be discussed in detail with the couple.

In general, those embryos at later stages[5] and of higher quality should be selected for transfer. Remaining embryos are graded and the question of freezing suitable embryos has to be addressed with the couple.

## EMBRYO TRANSFER

The selected embryos are transferred to a 15% patient's serum dish and labelled for transfer.

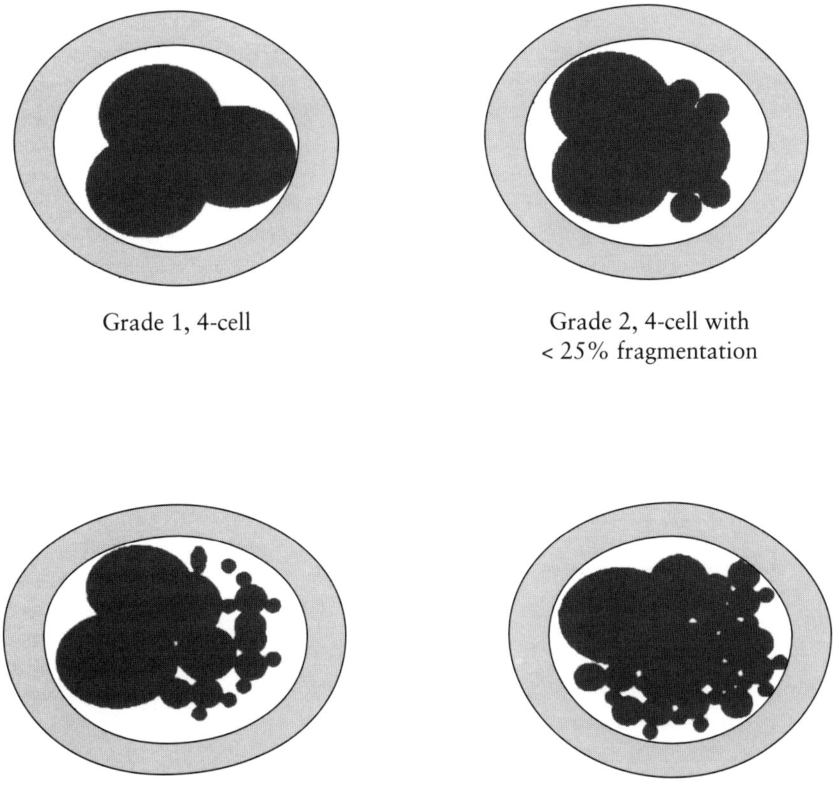

Grade 1, 4-cell

Grade 2, 4-cell with < 25% fragmentation

Grade 3, 4-cell with 25–50% fragmentation

Grade 4, 4-cell with > 50% fragmentation

**Figure 7** Embryo quality and fragmentation

An embryo transfer catheter is selected and placed on the warming tray (37°C). Usually a trial transcervical catheterization is undertaken following oocyte recovery and, depending on the ease with which this was achieved, together with records of any previous embryo transfers, a suitable catheter is chosen.

Unless there are expected to be any problems, our preference is the 23 cm Wallace Embryo Replacement Catheter. A 1 ml sterile syringe is also placed on the warming tray.

The patient is taken into the treatment room which is adjacent to the embryology laboratory and positioned on the couch in the lithotomy position. A Cusco's speculum is inserted into the vagina and positioned for a clear view of the cervix. The cervix is wiped using sterile water and sterile cotton balls (using a sponge holder).

Once the clinician is ready, the embryologist again checks the patient's identity, takes the embryos for transfer out of the incubator and views them under the dissecting microscope. Then using powder-free, sterile gloves of the correct size, the catheter is attached to the syringe (remaining sterile at all times) and 30 µl of air is taken up. The embryos are viewed through the microscope and are taken up into the catheter in approximately 30 µl of medium in the catheter. A further 10 µl of air is taken up so that the medium containing the embryos is visibly clear at the end of the catheter. The catheter is then held steady at the top and the syringe end is gently flexed up and down. The position of the medium should be maintained during this process. If it is not, the system is not air-tight and a new syringe and catheter must be used.

The loaded catheter is then passed to the clinician who gently introduces it through the cervix into the uterus. Once in position the catheter can be viewed in the uterus using the abdominal ultrasound. When this is clearly visible and the position within the uterus is confirmed, the embryos are slowly discharged from the catheter. This is visible on the ultrasound screen and the picture can be frozen and explained to the couple after the transfer.

The catheter is gently removed and checked in a tissue culture dish with medium to make sure that all of the embryos have been expelled and none remain in any mucus or fluid which may be on the outside of the catheter.

Following embryo transfer, the patient then remains in a slightly inclined position (head down) for 30 min before emptying her bladder and travelling home.

## EMBRYO CRYOPRESERVATION

Freezing of spare embryos or, occasionally all embryos, allows replacement of embryos at a later stage, in a cycle much less pressurized for the patient and at a much reduced cost in comparison to a full IVF embryo transfer (IVF-ET) package.

Usually only embryos with a quality of 1, 2 or sometimes 3 will be frozen and the expected recovery rate after thawing is approximately 75%. For some 100% recovery may be achieved but others may find that their embryos repeatedly fail to recover after freezing. Embryos are preferably frozen on day 2 or day 3 (pronucleate or 2–4 cell stage), although on exception they can be frozen on day 4.

### Preparation

Embryo freezing medium is prepared and is used at room temperature. The heated base plate on the microscope is turned off. Coloured plugs for the embryo crystal straws (both Rocket) are labelled with the patient's name, hospital number, date of egg collections and number of straws. The cryocanes are labelled with the patient's initials and a goblet with the same information as the plug.

The Planar freezing machine is prepared as per the manufacturer's instructions and the programme required entered. Embryo freezing medium (0.9 ml) is pipetted into the centre well of a Falcon culture dish and the embryos are carefully placed into the medium, watching carefully through the microscope as they may migrate to the outside of the well. A timer set at 30 min is started immediately. The microscope light is turned off and the dish left undisturbed.

After approximately 25 min (this will depend on the number of embryos to be loaded into straws), the embryos are organized in the dish in groups of three, two and singly depending on the number, for ease of loading. A 1 ml or 2 ml syringe is attached to the end of the straw containing the coloured sealant and approximately 2.0 cm of the length of the straw of medium is taken up, followed by a small amount of air. The embryos are then taken up in approximately 0.8 cm of medium. The remainder of the straw is air. Air is drawn into the straw until the medium touches the sealant, thereby sealing that end of the straw. The coloured, labelled plug is dipped into medium and inserted into the other end of the straw in order to seal it. The syringe is removed and the position of the embryos is checked by rolling the straw and viewing under the microscope.

At exactly 30 min the straws are loaded into the freezing machine and the programme is started.

### Embryo freezing programme

A planar embryo freezing machine is used with the programmes indicated in Table 2. After completion of the programme, the straws, together with the holding carriage, are removed from the freezing machine and plunged into liquid nitrogen. The straws are removed from the holding carriage taking care not to break off the coloured handles nor to remove them from the liquid nitrogen for longer than is necessary.

The straws are placed into the labelled goblets which are attached to the canes and a 2 ml

**Table 2** Embryo freezing programme

| *Ramp no.* | *Programme description* |
|---|---|
| 1 | –1°C per min to 20°C |
| 2 | Hold for 30 min at 20°C (during which time embryos are loaded into cryoprotectant at start of ramp) |
| 3 | –2°C per min to –7°C |
| 4 | Hold for 5 min at –7°C; buzzer sounds for manual seeding*, then holds for a further 15 min |
| 5 | –0.3°C per min to –30°C |
| 6 | –10°C per min to –150°C |

*Seeding consists of holding a small pair of pointed scissors or forceps in liquid nitrogen until cool then touching the meniscus of the medium containing the embryos. A change in the medium is immediately visible, when it becomes opaque

vial placed over the top of them to ensure that they cannot float out of the goblet. The cane is stored in the embryo bank. All information is recorded into the embryo freezing book along with any problems which may have occurred.

## EMBRYO THAWING

At the beginning of the patient's frozen embryo replacement cycle, we discuss with the couple the number of embryos frozen, the quality and the expected thaw-out rate. We inform them that we will not know how many embryos have been thawed successfully until the day of replacement.

The day prior to thawing the embryos, two 15% patient serum dishes are prepared and incubated overnight.

### Method

(1) 1 ml of thawing medium is placed in the centre well of a Falcon tissue culture dish.

(2) A plunger which fits snugly into the straw and a pair of scissors are cleaned with 70% ethanol and allowed to dry.

(3) A jug of water at 37°C is made ready.

(4) The patient's embryo straw is removed from the embryo bank, checking all the details thoroughly.

(5) The straw is held at room temperature for 40 s then plunged into the 37°C water until defrosted (3–4 s).

(6) The embryos are viewed inside the straw using the microscope whilst gently rolling the straw on the microscope base plate.

(7) The plastic labelled plug is cut off the straw and the plunger inserted into the other end. The embryos are slowly expelled into the thawing medium. The embryos are kept in the thawing medium for exactly 5 min.

(8) The embryos will float and migrate to the outside of the well. Using a mouth pipette they are returned to the centre of the dish where they are more visible.

(9) After 5 min, shrinkage will be observed in those embryos which have survived the freezing process and these are transferred into a 15% patient serum dish and replaced into the incubator.

(10) After 10 min the embryos should be inspected for normal expansion and transferred to another 15% patient serum dish.

The thawed embryos are transferred to the patient's uterus in the same way as for a fresh embryo replacement.

## SEMENOLOGY

Semen analysis is the most commonly used method for assessing male fertility. Normal semen consists of a mixture of spermatozoa and secretions from the testis and epididymis, in addition to secretions from the prostate, seminal vesicles and bulbourethral glands, which are mixed at the time of ejaculation.

### Semen collection

Semen samples are routinely produced on the premises, particularly for the initial analysis. This is important as, if there is a problem in producing a semen sample in the hospital, this should be discovered prior to egg collection and appropriate arrangements made. It would be a tragedy to find that, once the egg collection has taken place, the partner has problems producing in the hospital environment. It can be arranged for the sample to be brought with the couple immediately prior to egg collection or a seminal collection device can be used (a special non-spermicidal condom).

The usual method for seminal collection is as follows:

(1) The patient is provided with clearly written or oral instruction as appropriate to the collection of the specimen and if needed the transport of the specimen.

(2) Ideally the patient should have abstained from intercourse for approximately 3 days but no longer than 7 days.

(3) If there are any special requirements for production which are made apparent during previous analysis these should be adhered to. An example would be producing the sample into medium if there are sperm antibodies present.

(4) The sample is collected in the privacy of a specially allocated room close to the laboratory. If this is not possible it should be delivered to the laboratory within 1 h of production.

(5) Unless otherwise arranged, the sample should be produced by masturbation without the use of lubricants into a wide-mouthed sterile container provided by the hospital.

(6) Samples must not be produced by coitus interruptus.

(7) Incomplete samples should not be taken as a true analysis.

(8) Samples should be protected from extremes of temperature during transport to the laboratory.

(9) The container should be labelled with full name, date and time of collection and number of days abstinence.

**Preliminary macroscopic examinations**

*Liquefication*

A normal semen sample liquefies completely within 30 min. In some cases complete liquefication does not occur within 60 min and should be recorded. The sample should be mixed well in the original container before proceeding with analysis.

*Appearance*

The semen sample should be examined immediately after liquefication. A normal semen sample has an homogeneous grey opalescent appearance. The more oligozoospermic the sample, the less opaque it will be.

*Volume and consistency*

The volume can be measured using a graduated test tube or syringe. The consistency or viscosity can be estimated by allowing the semen to drop via gravity from a 5ml pipette and observing the length of the thread. A sample with normal viscosity will fall in discrete drops, whereas a sample which is viscous will form a thread of more than 2 cm in length.

*pH*

pH paper with a range of 6.1 to 10.0 should be used and the change due to the semen should be measured against a calibration strip. The pH should be in the range of 7.2 to 8.0. If the pH is less than 7.0 in an azoospermic sample then dysgenesis of the vas deferens, seminal vesicles or epididymis may be present.

*Assessment of sperm density and motility*

A phase contrast microscope is recommended for all examinations of unstained preparations of fresh or washed spermatozoa. A counting chamber should be used, either Makler or Horwell, for assessing the density and the motility (see manufacturer's instructions for use).

The preparation is examined at a magnification of ×400 and the number of sperm in a particular number of squares is counted (the number depends on the chamber used). The motile sperm only are then counted in the same squares.

$$\text{Percentage motility} = \frac{\text{Number of motile sperm}}{\text{Total number of sperm}} \times 100$$

Sperm density is measured in $10^6$/ml. Motility is given as a percentage.

*Progression*
Progression is measured on a scale of 0–4 (the Macleod Scale) where 0 indicates motility without forward progression and 4 indicates very rapid regular forward progression. This assessment is based on personal judgement, therefore vast experience of the semenologist is required for an accurate and consistent result. Other observations should be noted, such as excessive lateral head movement or unusual swimming patterns.

*Morphology*
Spermatozoa can be classified using either bright field microscope optics on fixed, stained specimens or high quality phase–contrast optics on wet preparations. The following categories of defects should be counted:

(1) Head shape/size and number of heads;

(2) Neck and midpiece defects;

(3) Tail defects; and

(4) Cytoplasmic droplets.

The percentage of abnormal sperm is calculated.

### Sperm antibody tests

*Mixed antiglobulin test*
The Ortho MAR kit is used (Ortho Diagnostics).

(1) Add one drop of latex beads to one drop of semen and mix.

(2) Add one drop of anti-immunoglobulin G (IgG) and mix thoroughly.

(3) Place coverslip over mixture and leave for 1min and then read the test.

(4) Re-read after 5 min. There should be a count of more than $5 \times 10^6$ motile sperm per ml in order for a clear result to be obtained.

**Table 3** Normal semen parameters

| *Test* | *Normal values* |
|---|---|
| Volume | ≥ 2.0 ml |
| pH | 7.2–8.0 |
| Sperm concentration | $\geq 20 \times 10^6$/ml |
| Total sperm count | $40 \times 10^6$ per ejaculate or more |
| Motility | 50% or more with good forward progression (grades 3 or 4) |
| Morphology | 30% or more with normal forms (Kruger scale will be much lower) |
| White blood cells | $< 1 \times 10^6$/ml |
| MAR test (Ortho) | less than 30% of sperm with adherent particles |

A negative result is shown when less than 30% of sperm are bound. A positive result is shown when more than 30% of sperm are bound.

The normal values of sperm variables as described by the WHO (World Health Organization) are shown in Table 3.

The WHO laboratory manual for the examination of human semen and sperm–cervical mucus interaction published by Cambridge University Press[6] is a suitable reference book for all aspects of semenology including biochemical analysis of semen, sperm function tests, various staining techniques for morphology and evaluation of cervical mucus.

### Determination of reactive oxygen species

It has been observed that excessive generation of reactive oxygen species by the washed human sperm is associated with functional competence[7]. The excessive generation of reactive oxygen species results in peroxidation of the unsaturated fatty acids in the sperm plasma membrane and by reducing membrane fluidity, impairs the ability of affected cells to engage in the membrane fusion events associated with fertilization. Diagnosis of the presence of oxygen free radicals must be treated appropriately by the andrologist.

**Sperm preparation techniques**

The purpose of sperm preparation techniques is the extraction of the sperm from the seminal plasma which is known to contain substances which inhibit capacitation and longevity of the sperm, thereby preventing fertilization[8]. The method of sperm preparation will be dependent upon the motile count, the volume, the presence of sperm antibodies and the viscosity.

*Direct migration*

(1) The patient produces a sample into a sterile container and this is allowed to liquefy for 30 min.

(2) Semen analysis is undertaken.

(3) Very gently layer 3 ml of 8% serum medium above the semen sample (do not mix) and incubate at 37°C in 5% $CO_2$ for 1 h.

(4) Using a pipette, 1 ml of the 8% serum medium is drawn off taking care not to disturb the underlying semen. Note the pipette tip should go no further than half-way into the medium.

(5) Semen analysis of this medium is completed.

(6) If the sample is to be used for IVF then a washing step is included here. This consists of adding 1 ml of 8% serum medium and centrifuging for 5 min at 200 g. The supernatant is removed carefully and discarded and the pellet is resuspended in 1.0 ml of 8% serum medium and then a sperm count is undertaken.

*Wash and swim-up technique*

(1) Sample is produced into a sterile container, allowed to liquefy and a semen analysis undertaken.

(2) 2 ml of semen is pipetted into a 5 ml test tube (Falcon) and 2 ml of 8% serum medium is added and mixed.

(3) This is centrifuged for 5 min at 1400 rpm.

(4) The supernatant is discarded and 1 ml of 8% serum medium added and resuspended. Again this is centrifuged for 5 min at 1400 rpm.

(5) The supernatant is very gently pipetted off without disturbing the pellet.

(6) 0.7 ml of serum medium is gently overlayed on the pellet by running the medium down the side of the test tube.

(7) This is incubated at 37°C, with 5% $CO_2$ for 30–45 min.

(8) The supernatant is carefully removed and a sperm count undertaken. This is then ready for intrauterine insemination or IVF insemination.

If this is a first consultation sample then it is cultured overnight and the percentage motility calculated after 24 h. The results of the 24-h survival rate and initial semen analysis will determine the route of treatment the patient will be advised to follow.

*Discontinuous Percoll gradient*

*Isotonic Percoll* This has the following composition:

10 ml 10 × Concentrated EBS
9 ml serum (or Albuminar 5, Armour Pharmaceuticals)
3 mg Sodium lactate
2 ml 1 mol/l HEPES

This is filtered through a 0.22 μm filter and 90 ml of Percoll (Sigma) added. This can be stored at +4°C for up to 1 week.

Using 100% isotonic Percoll, 80% and 40% dilutions are made.

(1) 2.0 ml of 80% Percoll are pipetted into 10 ml conical test tubes and these are overlayed gently with 40% Percoll.

(2) Up to 2 ml of semen can be layered onto each of these layers in each tube and these are centrifuged at 600 *g* for 20 min. During this process cells, debris, dead and abnormal sperm accumulate at the interfaces of the two Percoll concentrations. The pellet should contain functionally normal sperm.

(3) The pellet is carefully removed and suspended in 1 ml 8% serum medium, then a semen analysis is undertaken.

This sample can then be spun and layered for swim-up preparation or can be washed and resuspended in fresh medium for use.

In normal semen, a discontinuous Percoll density gradient selects spermatozoa with better motion characteristics, more hyperactivity and improved longevity compared with the direct swim-up technique, and the three-layer technique (mini Percoll) gives better sperm motility characteristics, shows improved fertilization capability and is generally adopted as the preferred technique[9].

*Mini Percoll preparation* This method is usually used for oligoasthozoospermia[10].

(1) 95%, 70% and 50% Percoll concentrations are prepared.

(2) Into 5.0 ml test tubes, 0.3 ml of 95%, followed by 0.3 ml 70%, followed by 0.3 ml 50% Percoll is gently pipetted, ensuring the layers do not mix.

(3) 0.3–0.5 ml of semen is layered over the Percoll gradient very slowly. Several gradients for each sample may be required.

(4) This is centrifuged for 20 minutes at 1500 rpm.

(5) The pellets are removed from each of the tubes, taking care not to disturb the layers and transferred to a 5 ml tube containing 2.0 ml 8% serum medium.

(6) This is centrifuged for 10min at 900 rpm.

(7) The supernatant is discarded and the pellet is resuspended in 0.1 ml. A semen analysis is undertaken and the sample diluted to the required concentration.

### Sperm enhancers

*Pentoxifylline*

Pentoxifylline (Sigma product no. P-1784) is a methylxanthine derivative and acts as an inhibitor of cyclic 3′5′ adenosine monophosphate (cAMP) phosphodiesterase activity[11,12]. As a result of treatment of semen with pentoxifylline, the intracellular cAMP concentration increases and this leads to an increase in sperm motility, enhancement of acrosome reaction[13] and protection of the sperm plasma membrane through an antioxidant action[14].

*Patient selection for pentoxifylline use* The following criteria are used:

(1) Oligozoospermic – less than $5 \times 10^6$/ml sperm.

(2) Moderately oligozoospermic – less than $20 \times 10^6$/ml sperm.

(3) Normospermic count with asthenzoospermia – greater than $20 \times 10^6$ sperm per ml but with a poor motile count or reduced progression.

(4) Previous poor fertilization rates.

Patients are selected for pentoxifylline on the basis of their semen analysis performed in-house and with consideration of previous IVF attempts. Patients will receive counselling on the use of pentoxifylline and will be required to provide written consent for its use.

*Method*

(1) Pentoxifylline is made up in 8% patient serum medium to a concentration of 2 mg per ml. This is then filtered with a 0.22 μm filter.

(2) The sperm is then prepared by the IVF sperm preparation techniques.

(3) An equal volume of pentoxifylline solution is added to the sperm preparation and incubated at 37°C and in 5% $CO_2$ for 30 min.

(4) After 30 min, add approximately 2 ml 8% serum medium and centrifuge for 10 min at 1500 rpm.

(5) Remove the pellet with a Pasteur pipette and add to approximately 2 ml of 8% serum medium. Centrifuge once more at 1500 rpm for 10 min.

(6) The supernatant is removed and the pellet resuspended in 8% serum medium to the desired concentration.

It has been calculated that, using this method, the fertilizing sperm will have been exposed to 1–2 pmol of pentoxifylline. The preparation of the sample is timed so that when the final sample is ready, insemination of the eggs can be carried out immediately.

### Semen cryopreservation

Cryopreserved semen has several advantages over the use of fresh semen, the most important being the quarantining of donor sperm until it can be deemed free of infectious diseases. Other uses of cryopreservation include freezing due to inconsistent semen quality, inability of the man to produce samples under times of stress, a sample pre-frozen will avoid unnecessary pressure to produce on the day, and the possibility that the partner may be unavailable on the day of insemination or IVF.

However, these advantages have to be balanced against the fact that fewer pregnancies have been reported using cryopreserved semen as compared to fresh semen[15], along with decreased post-thaw survival[16] and motility[17].

Cryoprotectants are universally used to aid in the removal of cellular water and the protection from damage due to ice formation. Cryoprotectants can be classified into either penetrating (glycerol and dimethylsulphoxide, DMSO) and non-penetrating (lactose and trehalose) based on their ability to enter cells. Glycerol is the most widely used cryoprotectant in spite of the fact that part of the observed reduction in sperm motility is due to the glycerol toxicity[18].

The majority of sperm banks use glycerol alone[20], but there is an increase in the use of 'extenders' in addition to glycerol which utilize a zwitterion buffer system. Others contain glycerol, glycine and either sucrose or egg yolk, citrate, dextrose and glycine as cryoprotectant agents.

*Methodology of sperm cryopreservation*

(1) Cryoprotectant is removed from the fridge and allowed to equilibrate to room temperature.

(2) Semen sample is produced using the guidelines applicable for the semen analysis.

(3) Semen analysis is undertaken and the results recorded in the relevant semen freezing book.

(4) The cryoprotectant is added on a 1 : 1 equal volume basis, slowly over 10 min, mixing regularly.

(5) Cryovials are labelled with the patient's name, hospital number and date of freezing, or, if a donor, with the donor's code number, date and ethnic origin.

(6) 0.7 ml of semen–cryoprotectant is aliquoted into each cryovial and the top securely tightened.

(7) The cryovials containing the semen–cryoprotectant are placed in the vapour phase of the sperm bank (liquid nitrogen vapour at −70°C) for freezing[20].

(8) Once frozen, the specimens are stored in liquid nitrogen (−196°C) in the sperm bank and their storage position recorded in the appropriate semen freezing book.

## DISCUSSION

Many factors influence the outcome of assisted conception, from patient selection and stimulation protocols to embryo replacement techniques. Clinical procedures, however, would fail to produce the required result without an efficient and expertly run embryology laboratory. Procedures from laboratory to laboratory may vary slightly along with the use of different tissue culture media, but the basic principles of embryology are applied in all laboratories.

Undoubtedly, new procedures will be continuously introduced, but each new technique must be carefully evaluated and compared to existing proven methods before becoming standard practice.

With each new development, problems once untreatable are now being treated and success rates which were initially low are now increasing to give infertile couples a realistic chance of achieving a pregnancy.

## REFERENCES


1. Byatt-Smith, J. G., Leese, H. J. and Gosden, R. G. (1991). An investigation by mathematical modelling of whether mouse and human preimplantation embryos in static culture can satisfy their demands for oxygen by diffusion. *Hum. Reprod.*, **6**, 52–7
2. Reiger D. (1992). Relationships between energy metabolism and development of early mammalian embryos. *Theriogenology*, **37**, 75–91
3. Peek, J. (1991). Assessment of embryos from *in vitro* fertilization. *Fertil. Dev.*, **3**, 113–17
4. Pickering, S. J., Braude, P. R., Johnson, M. H., Cant, A. and Currie, J. (1990). Transient cooling to room temperature can cause irreversible disruption of the meiotic spindle in the human oocyte. *Fertil. Steril.*, **54**, 102–8
5. Lewin, A., Schenker, J. G., Safran, A., Zigelena, N., Avrech, O., Abramov, Y., Friedler, S. and Reubinoff, B. E. (1994). Embryo growth rate *in vitro* as an indicator of embryo quality in IVF cycles. *J. Assist. Reprod. Genet.*, **11**, 500–3
6. World Health Organization Laboratory Manual for the Examination of Human Sperm and Sperm–Cervical Mucus Interaction. (Cambridge University Press)
7. Aitken, R. J., Clarkson, J. S., Husing, G. F. and Irvine, D. S. (1987). Cell biology of defective sperm function. In Mohin, H. (ed.) *New Horizons in Sperm Cell Research,* pp. 75–89. (New York: Gordon and Breads)
8. Van der Ven, H., Bhattacharyya, A. K., Binor, Z., Leto, S. and Zaneveld, L. J. D. (1982). Inhibition of human sperm capacitation by a high molecular weight factor from human seminal plasma. *Fertil. Steril.,* **41**, 227–80
9. Moohan, J. M. and Lindsay, K. S. (1995). Spermatozoa selected by a discontinuous Percoll gradient exhibit better motion characteristics, more hyperactivation and longer survival than direct swim up. *Fertil. Steril.,* **64**, 160–5
10. Ord, T., Patrizio, P., Marello, E., Balmaceda, J. P. and Asch, R. H. (1990). Mini-Percoll: a new method of semen preparation for IVF in severe male factor infertility. *Hum. Reprod.,* **5**, 987–9
11. Schoenfeld, C., Amelar, R. D. and Dubin, L. (1975). Stimulation of ejaculated human spermatozoa by caffine. *Fertil. Steril.*, **26**, 158–61
12. Aitken, R. J., Mattei, A. and Irvine, S. (1986). Paradoxical stimulation of human sperm motility by 2-deoxyadenosine. *J. Reprod. Fertil.,* **78**, 515–27
13. Cummins, J. M., Pember, S. M., Jequier, A. M. *et al.* (1991). A test of the human sperm acrosome reaction following challenge (ARIC). Relationship of fertility and the semen parameters. *J. Androl.,* **12**, 98–103
14. Garella, M., Lipovae, V. and Mariott, T. (1991). Effect of pentoxifylline on superoxide anion production by human sperm. *Int. J. Androl.,* **14**, 320–7
15. Richter, M. A., Hanning, R. V. and Shapiro, S. S. (1984). Artificial donor insemination: fresh versus frozen semen; the patient as her own control. *Fertil. Steril.,* **41**, 277–80
16. Keel, B. A. and Black, J. B. (1980). Reduced motility lone levity in thawed human spermatozoa. *Arch. Androl.,* **4**, 213–15
17. Keel, B. A. and Webster, B. W. (1989). Semen analysis data from fresh and cryopreserved donor ejaculates; comparison of cryoprotectants and pregnancy rates. *Fertil. Steril.,* **52**, 100–5
18. Critser, J. D., Huse-Benda, A. R., Aaker, D. V., Arneson, B. W. and Ball, G. D. (1988). Cryopreservation of human spermatozoa. III. The effect of cryoprotectants on motility. *Fertil. Steril.,* **50**, 314–20
19. Sherman, J. K. (1990). Cryopreservation of human semen. In Keel, B. A. and Webster, B. W. (eds.) *Handbook of the Laboratory Diagnosis and Treatment of Infertility,* pp. 229–60. (Boca Raton: CRC Press, Inc.)

# Intracytoplasmic sperm injection 14

*Terry Leonard*

## INTRODUCTION

The use of intracytoplasmic sperm injection (ICSI) for assisted fertilization in infertile couples is arguably the most significant advancement in assisted reproductive technology (ART) since the development of *in vitro* fertilization and embryo transfer (IVF-ET). In the late 1970s and early 1980s IVF-ET was developed initially to bypass blockage in the Fallopian tubes. In this process, relatively small numbers of sperm (in the order of $10^5$) are mixed with oocytes. The concentration of sperm in a normal human ejaculate is in the order of $10^7$–$10^8$/ml. Therefore IVF can be applied in patients with a diminished number of sperm[1]. The treatment of male factor infertility with IVF is successful up to a point. There were still couples who had a failure of fertilization *in vitro* and others with too few sperm to attempt IVF; therefore there was a need to develop further techniques to assist fertilization. The first technique developed was partial zona dissection (PZD)[2] which was superseded by subzonal insemination (SUZI)[3,4] which in turn was replaced by ICSI[5]. Each of these techniques brought the sperm continually closer to the eggs until finally, with ICSI, a single sperm is injected into the oocyte cytoplasm.

In PZD a hole is punctured in the zona pellucida (zona) so that sperm can swim through this hole into the perivitelline space instead of penetrating the zona. This is performed by piercing the zona with a microneedle (Figure 1), passing it into the perivitelline space and out through the other side of the zona without touching the vitelline membrane, and then making the needle rip through the zona resulting in a small tear.

In SUZI one or more sperm are picked up in the microinjection pipette. The oocyte is held, the microinjection pipette is passed through the zona, and the sperm are injected into the perivitelline space (Figure 1). This brought sperm

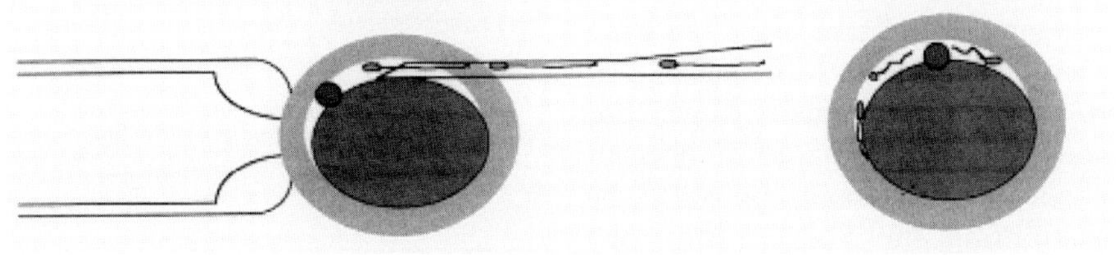

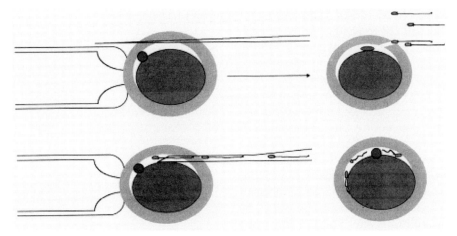

**Figure 1** Top panel: partial zona dissection followed by insemination of sperm; lower panel: subzonal insemination

into contact with the vitelline membrane. Although SUZI helped a great many patients achieve fertilization, ICSI was shown to be a more effective procedure[6,7].

## WHEN IS ICSI REQUIRED?

With the availability of the ICSI technique in a large number of units the question which most often arises is which patients require ICSI. The answer is simple: those who have a high chance of fertilization failure when their sperm and oocytes are mixed together *in vitro* (*in vitro* insemination). The difficulty is deciding when probability of fertilization is low.

The groups of patients likely to fail or to have low fertilization rates are as follows:

(1) Those who did not achieve *in vitro* fertilization in a previous IVF treatment cycle;

(2) Those who had a low fertilization rate ($\leq 10\%$) in a previous IVF treatment cycle;

(3) Those who have sperm surgically removed from the epididymis or testes;

(4) Those with extremely poor semen parameters; and

(5) Those with poor semen parameters.

### Low or no fertilization (groups 1 and 2)

It has been observed that there is a subgroup of patients who will fail to achieve *in vitro* fertilization on one occasion but who will achieve fertilization on another occasion. Because of this, some workers have suggested that ICSI should only be performed on couples who fail to achieve fertilization twice with conventional IVF. However, patients are reluctant to undergo a cycle of conventional IVF treatment following a failure of fertilization when ICSI is available. It has therefore become the practice to perform ICSI after one failure. If a large number of oocytes are collected then a compromise can be reached by splitting the oocytes into two groups and performing ICSI in one group and *in vitro* insemination with the other.

Occasionally a failure of fertilization is due to abnormal or immature oocytes or even a very low number of oocytes. This is not an indication for ICSI, but an indication that there is a problem with the ovarian stimulation regimen or with oogenesis.

There is an interesting group of men who have 'normal' sperm parameters but fail to fertilize oocytes *in vitro*. In Table 1 the data show that in 139 out of 1930 (7.2%) treatment cycles there was a failure to fertilize *in vitro* (conventional IVF) in normal spermic men. Very few of these will have failed to fertilize due to immaturity or poor morphology of the oocyte. This will be evident on microscopy. The majority of patients who have a failure to fertilize will have at least one fertilized oocyte when they are subsequently mixed with donor sperm 1 day after insemination of the husband's sperm. This suggests that failure of fertilization is more frequently due to a sperm factor.

These motile sperm are said to have a functional problem, i.e. the sperm cannot achieve one or more of the events leading to fertilization. The reasons for this could be because all, or the majority, of the sperm fail to:

(1) Capacitate;

(2) Acrosome react;

**Table 1** A comparison of complete failure of fertilization rates in IVF treatment cycles in different sperm parameter groups

| *Sperm category* | *Number of CFTF/ treatment cycles* | % |
|---|---|---|
| Normal parameters | 139/1930 | 7.2 |
| Oligozoospermic only | 34/141 | 24.1 |
| Asthenozoospermic only | 33/125 | 26.4 |
| Teratozoospermic only | 30/373 | 8 |
| Oligoasthenozoospermic | 25/49 | 51 |
| Oligoteratozoospermic | 17/55 | 30.9 |
| Asthenoteratozoospermic | 31/75 | 41 |
| Oligoasthenoteratozoospermic | 44/71 | 62 |
| Total | 353/2819 | 12.5 |

IVF, *in vitro* fertilization; CFTF, complete failure to fertilize

(3) Bind to the zona pellucida;

(4) Penetrate the zona pellucida;

(5) Fuse with the vitelline membrane; or

(6) Undergo nuclear decondensation.

Although there has been some progress in identification and measuring these factors, it is still impossible to identify which sperm are capable of fertilization.

### Surgical sperm aspiration (group 3)

The number of sperm obtained from testicular biopsy are too few to perform any other technique than ICSI. Epididymal sperm obtained by microsurgical epididymal sperm aspiration (MESA) although plentiful on most occasions invariably have low numbers of motile sperm with poor progression. Table 2 compares the fertilization rate of epididymal sperm when conventional insemination is used (10.7%) to that with ICSI (49%). These results are compatible with those of Silber[8] (IVF-MESA, 6.9%; ICSI MESA, 41%).

### Extreme semen parameters (group 4)

Patients with sperm parameters which are extreme will need ICSI. These are:

(1) Those with < 100 000 sperm per ml;

(2) Those with < 1% motility;

(3) Those with > 95% abnormal sperm; and

(4) Those with a sperm progression of 1 on a scale of 1–4.

**Table 2** A comparison of fertilization rates with epididymal sperm using different assisted reproductive techniques

| | *Fertilization rate (no. 2 Pn/no. oocytes)** | |
|---|---|---|
| *Technique* | *Ratio* | *%* |
| *In vitro* fertilization | 19/177 | 10.7 |
| Subzonal insemination | 15/70 | 21 |
| Intracytoplasmic sperm injection | 370/758 | 49 |

*no. 2 Pn, number of two-pronuclear zygotes (normal fertilization)

### Poor semen parameters (group 5)

Patients with previous failure of fertilization, those with extreme semen parameters and those whose sperm are obtained surgically from the epididymis or testes need ICSI. There is no difficulty in this decision.

However, the largest group of patients seeking treatment will be those in a 'grey' area. These are men whose sperm parameters are lower than 'normal', but not extreme, and who have not had an IVF attempt in the past. The difficulty is deciding between conventional IVF and ICSI. One way to attempt to answer this question is to look at individual clinic records and see what fertilization rates were achieved with men with similar semen profiles.

Table 1 shows the number of IVF attempts that had a complete failure of fertilization in various sperm categories. This is a series of 2819 treatment cycles between 1988 and 1993 at the Lister Hospital, London. In all of the 2819 cycles two or more oocytes have been inseminated with husband's (ejaculated) sperm only and they exclude SUZI cases. Table 1 shows the percentage of complete failures to fertilize (CFTF) in patients with 'normal' sperm parameters, and those with one, two, or three factors which deviate from 'normal'. Having a high number of abnormal forms alone does not increase the chance of CFTF. Only one in four patients with oligozoospermia or asthenozoospermia had CFTF. Table 3 shows that there was no correlation between sperm concentration and CFTF when the oligozoospermic group was subdivided. Table 4 shows that this was also true for motility.

Table 1 also shows that there is a higher chance of CFTF if there are two factors; with the combination of oligoasthenozoospermia (low sperm count and motility), half the patients had CFTF. In patients with three factors CFTF was again higher compared to patients with only two.

To examine the oligoasthenozoospermic and oligoasthenoteratozoospermic groups, we looked at the motile concentration (low sperm count and motility and poor morphology). Table 5 shows that only when the motile concentration of sperm is higher than 5 million/ml is there a reasonable chance of fertilization; if the motile concentration is less than 5 million/ml the chance of CFTF is greater than 50%.

**Table 3** A comparison of complete failure of fertilization rates in *in vitro* fertilization treatment cycles in subgroups of oligozoospermic men

| *Sperm concentration* ($\times 10^6$/ml) | *Number of CFTF/ treatment cycles* | % |
|---|---|---|
| < 5 | 8/27 | 29.7 |
| 5–9 | 5/23 | 21.7 |
| 10–14 | 11/41 | 26.8 |
| 15–19 | 10/50 | 20 |

CFTF, complete failure to fertilize

**Table 4** A comparison of complete failure of fertilization rates in *in vitro* fertilization treatment cycles in subgroups of asthenozoospermic men

| *Motility percentage* | *Number of CFTF/ treatment cycles* | % |
|---|---|---|
| < 11 | 1/6 | 16.7 |
| 11–20 | 7/19 | 36.8 |
| 21–30 | 10/61 | 16.4 |
| 31–40 | 11/39 | 28.2 |

CFTF, complete failure to fertilize

The only semen parameters which correlate well with fertilization rates are sperm progression in unprepared semen and the percentage survival of prepared sperm after overnight incubation in IVF medium at 37°C with 5% $CO_2$. Table 6 compares the rate of CFTF in a group of 2114 IVF treatment cycles with sperm progression and sperm survival. This is a series of 2114 treatment cycles between 1988 and 1993 at the Lister Hospital, London. Each of these cycles have two or more oocytes and were inseminated with husband's ejaculated sperm. Sperm survival is expressed as a percentage of moving sperm, and sperm progression is expressed on a nominal scale: 1 = non-progressive sperm, 2 = sluggish sperm, 3+ = good forward movement, 1.5 = a mixture of 1 and 2, 2.5 = a mixture of 2 and 3. Table 6 shows that, as the sperm progression decreases, there is an increase in CFTF, and patients with a progression less than or equal to 2 should have ICSI treatment. Table 6 also shows that, as the overnight incubation sperm survival decreases, there is an increase in CFTF. Patients with a sperm survival of less than 35% should be treated with ICSI. The risk of CFTF is particularly high when there is a combination of progression ≤ 2 and < 35% sperm[9].

## EQUIPMENT

The additional equipment required to perform the ICSI technique in an IVF laboratory (Figure 2) is as follows:

**Table 5** A comparison of complete failure of fertilization rates in *in vitro* fertilization treatment cycles and motile sperm concentration in subgroups of oligoasthenozoospermic and oligoasthenoteratozoospermic men

| *Motile sperm concentration* ($\times 10^6$/ml) | *Oligoasthenozoospermic* | | *Oligoasthenoteratozoospermic* | | *Both* | |
|---|---|---|---|---|---|---|
| | *CFTF rate* | % | *CFTF rate* | % | *CFTF rate* | % |
| < 1 | 9/12 | 75 | 24/30 | 80 | 33/42 | 78.6 |
| 1–5 | 12/23 | 52 | 20/38 | 52.6 | 32/61 | 52.4 |
| 5–7 | 4/14 | 29 | 0/3 | 0 | 4/17 | 23.5 |

CFTF, complete failure to fertilize

**Table 6** A comparison of complete failure of fertilization rates in *in vitro* fertilization treatment cycles with sperm progression and prepared sperm survival after overnight incubation

| | *Sperm survival* | | | | | | | |
|---|---|---|---|---|---|---|---|---|
| | *< 35%* | | *35–50%* | | *> 50%* | | *Total* | |
| *Progression (scale of 1–4)* | *CFTF rate* | *%* | *CFTF rate* | *%* | *CFTF rate* | *%* | *CFTF rate* | *%* |
| 1.5 | 11/14 | 79 | 2/8 | 25 | 0/3 | 0 | 13/25 | 52 |
| 2.0 | 15/22 | 68 | 8/26 | 30 | 2/14 | 14 | 25/62 | 40 |
| 2.5 | 35/77 | 45 | 64/525 | 12 | 25/691 | 4 | 124/1298 | 10 |
| ≥ 3.0 | 11/18 | 61 | 16/237 | 7 | 15/479 | 3 | 42/734 | 6 |
| Total | 72/131 | 55 | 90/796 | 11 | 42/1187 | 4 | 204/2114 | 9.6 |

CFTF, complete failure to fertilize

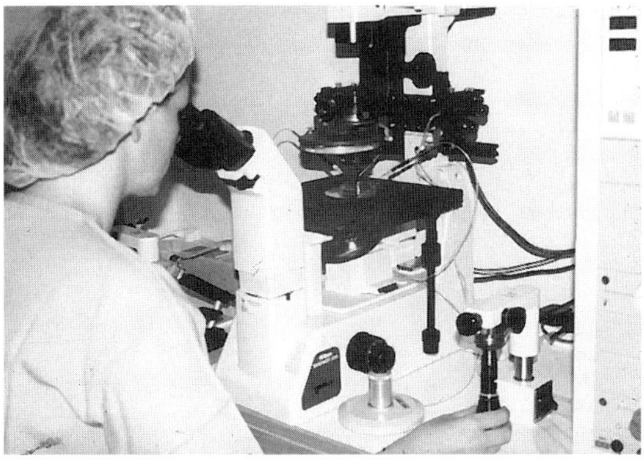

**Figure 2** Equipment required for intracytoplasmic sperm injection

(1) A sturdy inverted microscope;

(2) Heated stage for microscope;

(3) Two sets of micromanipulators;

(4) Microtools or microtool manufacturing equipment;

(5) Vibration-free bench (required in some locations); and

(6) Video and VDU (optional).

A sturdy microscope is required to minimize movement of the microscope during operation. The inverted type is required because it has a much greater working space between the objective and the light source for working in Petri dishes. A good optical system designed for working with non-stained material is required. The Hoffman modulation system is recommended as most workers use plastic Petri dishes. Visualization is a very important factor in performing this technique. A low-power objective, e.g. × 4 will be required for scanning the Petri dish, and × 10, × 20 and possibly × 40 will be required when performing the ICSI. As the microscope stage needs to be moved during the ICSI technique it should not be of a fixed type. The stage should be heated in order to reduce heat loss in the Petri dish.

The fine movements required by the ICSI technique cannot be achieved by hand. The movements are controlled by two sets of micromanipulators. These consist of robot arms which hold the microtools, a three-dimensional coarse manipulator and a three-dimensional fine manipulator. The fine movements of these manipulators are controlled by joysticks. The movement made on the joystick controlling the fine manipulator is scaled down so that small movements of the joystick become the microscopic movements of the microtool. It is very important that all three-dimensional movements for the fine control can be achieved by a single joystick.

Microtools are manufactured from borosilicate glass capillary tubes. In the ICSI technique two microtools are required. The holding pipette which keeps the oocyte still during the injection procedure and the injection needle which is used to pick up the sperm and then inject the sperm into the oocyte. The microtools fit into a holding arm at the micromanipulator and therefore the movement of the microtools is controlled by the micromanipulator.

The microtools can be manufactured in the laboratory or purchased. Three major pieces of equipment are required to make ICSI microtools. These are a capillary puller, a microbeveller and a microforge. The manufacture of the tools requires considerable skill. The size and the shape of the tools have a great effect on the percentage of oocyte survival and fertilization. There are a number of companies supplying these tools commercially: Hunter Scientific Leonard Microtools manufacture in the UK, Cook in Australia and Humagen in the USA.

Vibrations in the walls and floor will travel through benches and microscopes. These vibrations may be small but when one is working at a microscopic level they can be significant. Many buildings do vibrate, especially tall ones. Some workers have built their ICSI table up from the floor without touching the walls and use a very heavy substance such as marble as a table top. Vibration may still be present even after building such tables. One way to dampen this vibration is to stand the microscope on top of four tennis balls. These balls must be cut in half and the cut edge placed down on the bench surface. Vibration-free tables are available but are very expensive. As general advice, budget for a vibration-free table but try putting the microscope on a wide, well-supported bench first.

Video controls and a VDU are essential for teaching and training in ICSI.

## THE ICSI TECHNIQUE

The ICSI technique can be split up into the following stages:

(1) The removal of cumulus and corona radii cells;

(2) Selection of oocytes;

(3) Sperm preparation;

(4) Alignment of the ICSI needles;

(5) Immobilization of sperm;

(6) Moving and positioning of oocytes;

(7) Picking up sperm; and

(8) Intracytoplasmic injection.

This is only a small part of the overall treatment cycle. These steps take place between oocyte collection and examination for evidence of fertilization. The other processes that need to be carried out in an ICSI treatment cycle are covered in other chapters.

### Removal of cumulus and corona radii cells

When oocytes are collected from the ovaries they are attached to a surrounding layer of dense corona radii cells, plus a much larger cumulus mass. These must be removed in order to visualize and manipulate the oocyte during the ICSI technique. The method used is a combination of an enzymatic digestion of cell–cell bonds and mechanical removal of the cells.

*Method*

Prepare the following: an organ culture dish (Falcon 3027) with 1 ml medium (medi-cult 10310060) containing 0.01% hyaluronidase (Sigma H4272) in the central well; a Petri dish (Falcon 3001) with 6 × 30 μl microdrops of IVF medium covered with mineral oil (Sigma M8410); and capillary tubes or pulled Pasteur pipettes 200–250 μm and 160 μm.

(1) Place up to six oocytes in the hyaluronidase solution – wait 30–60 seconds;

(2) Using the larger pulled pipette agitate the cumulus masses, and draw oocytes up and down the pipette until the majority of cumulus cells fall off (Figure 3);

(3) Transfer them to one of the six IVF medium droplets;

(4) Take the thinner pipette, draw the oocytes up and down until the remaining cumulus and the corona radii cells fall off;

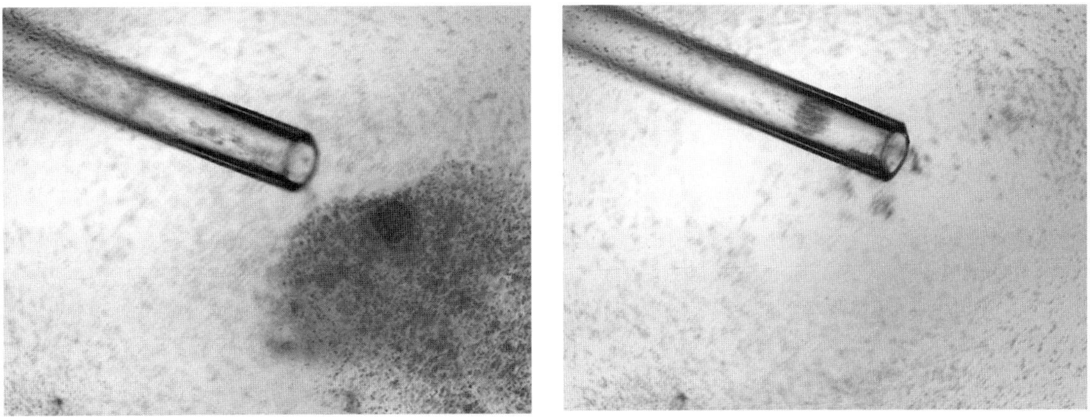

**Figure 3** Removal of cumulus tissue from an oocyte with a micropipette

(5) Transfer the oocytes to a clean droplet, move them around the droplet and then into the next droplet (this is repeated until the oocytes have been washed in all the droplets); and

(6) The morphology and maturity of the oocytes is then assessed.

When looking at a non-stained oocyte the only indications of maturity are the presence or absence of polar bodies and germinal vesicles (Figure 4). This is because the internal structures cannot be seen. An oocyte with one polar body is at arrested metaphase awaiting a sperm to trigger the second meiotic division. These oocytes can therefore be injected. Oocytes without a polar body or germinal vesicle are at an uncertain stage in meiosis. They are often said to be in metaphase I but they are somewhere between germinal vesicle breakdown and metaphase II. These oocytes should be left in culture to see if they extrude the first polar body, and then later injected with sperm.

The morphology of mature oocytes shows some variations. The polar body itself can appear very flat against the vitelline membrane, or can be almost completely spherical. It is thought that flatter polar bodies suggest an earlier stage of extrusion. The polar body also can be fragmented or have divided into two polar bodies.

The ooplasm can vary in granularity and colour. Oocytes with darker granular centres behave, when injected with sperm, like aged

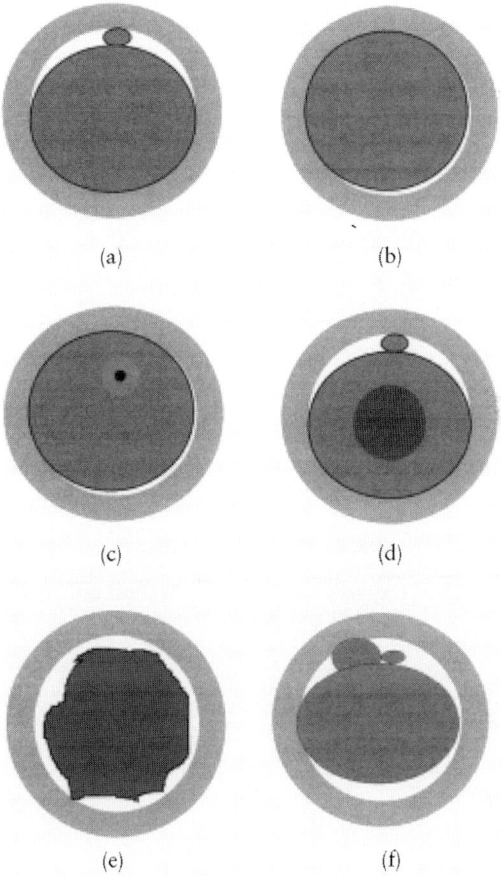


**Figure 4** Maturity and morphology of oocytes: (a) mature (metaphase II) oocyte; (b) oocyte at metaphase I; (c) germinal vesicle stage; (d) over-mature oocyte showing signs of ageing; (e) atrophied oocyte; and (f) fragmented oocyte

oocytes; the ICSI needle penetrates the vitelline membrane with ease and the cytoplasm does not need to be disrupted. The death rate is more than twice that of other oocytes.

Other morphological variations are elongated oocytes, those with vacuoles and giant oocytes which can be twice the normal size.

There is variation in the shape and thickness of the zona pellucida. Often, elongated pieces of zona can be seen; this occurs both when the ooplasm is also elongated and when it is normal in shape.

### Sperm preparation techniques

*Percoll separation technique*[10] *for ICSI*

To make the Percoll solution, add 0.3 g $NaHCO_3$ to 25 ml minimum essential medium–Earle's balanced salt solution (MEM–EBSS) × 10 concentration and filter. Add 6 ml of this solution to 54 ml Percoll (Sigma P1644). This is then considered to be the 90% Percoll solution. Take 20 ml of the 90% solution and add 20 ml of IVF medium to make a 45% solution.

*Method*

(1) Perform semen analysis.

(2) Set up the Percoll gradients:

  (a) Place 1 ml of 90% Percoll in a 15 ml conical tube (2099 Falcon),

  (b) Layer 1 ml of 45% Percoll on top of the 90% solution.

(3) Layer 1–3 ml of semen onto the Percoll gradient; if the volume of semen is greater than 5 ml and the concentration low then make more than one tube.

(4) Centrifuge at 2000 rpm (400 **g**) for 10 min.

(5) Remove supernatant and resuspend pellet in 1–2 ml of IVF medium. Place in a clean conical tube. If there are two or more tubes for one patient, pool the pellets at this point. Wash by centrifugation (5 min at 1300 rpm/170 **g**).

(6) Remove supernatant and resuspend the pellet accordingly:

  (a) If there is a large pellet and the semen analysis indicates there will be a large number of sperm, resuspend in 0.5 ml of IVF medium. Analyse and adjust the sperm concentration to 500 000/ml;

  (b) If there are likely to be very few sperm or few active sperm in the pellet, or the pellet cannot be seen, resuspend just in the medium left in the tube after removing the supernatant (about 10–20 μl); or

  (c) Take the pellet and place in a Petri dish under oil and examine.

A conventional Percoll preparation technique can be used to separate sperm in ICSI cases when the concentration of mobile sperm is greater than 500 000/ml. When the motile concentration of sperm falls below 500 000/ml additional techniques will need to be applied.

One microlitre of a 500 000/ml sperm preparation (see point 6(a) above) is placed in one 10-μl microdroplet. Sperm is then picked up from this droplet when performing ICSI. This microdroplet could contain IVF medium or 10% polyvinylpyrrolidone (PVP) in IVF medium (medi-cult). The sperm are allowed to migrate to the other side of the Petri dish.

If there are very few sperm seen in the ejaculate (< 100 000/ml) then the Percoll preparation can still be used but without the 45% Percoll layer.

Depending on what is found in the microdroplet following the Percoll preparation, different methods can be applied. If there are large numbers of active sperm, but debris or other cells in the preparation, a cleaner preparation can be made by sedimentation. The microdroplet is incubated for 1–2 h and then the top part of the microdroplet is aspirated and placed under oil.

If there is a low motility (15 to 1%) in the preparation then a sperm migration technique could be used to separate them. In this technique 5 μl of the Percoll preparation is carefully placed in the centre of a 10-μl droplet and incubated. Sperm will migrate from the central part of the Petri dish towards the interface. The sperm can then be picked up with the ICSI needle for injection. If there is not enough room for the immobilization of sperm then the sperm can be transferred to a clean droplet (either medium or 10% PVP) and immobilized first.

When the motility is still extremely low in the preparation (less than 1%) or the sperm movement is non-progressive, a fishing technique can be used. In this technique an ICSI-like needle is used to pick up motile sperm and place them into an adjacent microdroplet. This needle is 10 μl in diameter without a bevelled tip, but it is angled like an ICSI needle. The tip is first placed in a microdroplet containing medium only and a small amount of medium is drawn into it. The tip is then moved into the oil next to the sperm-containing drop, the microsyringe is then drawn up creating an upwards pressure in the needle, but not enough to draw up oil. The stage control is used to scan the droplet for a motile sperm. When one is found the needle tip is lowered into the sperm drop and the motile sperm is drawn into the needle. This is repeated until several sperm are found which are then transferred into a clean microdroplet. Some dead sperm and debris may be taken into the needle in this manner but the free swimming sperm will often move away from them. If very low sperm concentration is seen in the Percoll preparation, then the whole drop is used for sperm pick-up.

*Epididymal sperm*
The samples obtained from epididymal aspiration often have very high numbers of sperm, but they rarely have a motility of more than 20%, and poor progression. Epididymal sperm can be prepared in the same manner as ejaculated sperm with poor motility. The volumes aspirated are small and therefore mini Percoll preparation should be used[11].

The only difference when performing ICSI and a combination of MESA or percutaneous epididymal sperm aspiration (PESA) is the emphasis on saving as much sperm as you can for future treatments (Figure 5).

Epididymal sperm do not freeze well[12]. It is expected that thawed specimens will have a motility of less than 1%. The best way to deal with these specimens is to perform mini Percoll separation; resuspend in four to six microdroplets under oil and then fish out the motile sperm into a clean microdroplet before intracytoplasmic injection.

*Testicular biopsies*
Testicular biopsies are collected into IVF medium and kept at 37°C, 5% $CO_2$ until processed. The biopsies are then placed in a Petri dish (Falcon F3001) and teased (pulled) apart with sterile microscope slides[13]. The tissues are macerated until the surrounding medium becomes cloudy. Everything is then put into a conical tube and the pieces of tissue are allowed to settle.

The fluid is then removed and either washed by centrifugation in IVF medium (170 **g** for 5 min, twice) or put on a mini Percoll gradient. The remaining tissue is kept in case no sperm are seen in the preparations. If the fluid is examined before washing and sperm are seen, then a Percoll preparation rather than a wash can be performed. The advantage of the Percoll is that other cells, of which there are many, can be selected against and this will concentrate motile sperm. The disadvantage is that after a while the sperm start to stick to other sperm or cells and are difficult to pick up. They therefore need to be picked out and put into a clean microdroplet before ICSI (see fishing technique) (Figure 6). Verheyen and colleagues[14] compared four mechanical methods of preparing testicular sperm. They were (1) rough shredding with microscope slide; (2) as in method 1, then fine mincing; (3) as in method 2, then vortexing; and (4) as in method 3, then crushing (electrically). They concluded that there was little difference between the methods but the mincing and Percoll preparation yielded a higher number of motile sperm.

It is likely that in some testicular biopsies, especially those taken from men with spermatozoa dysfunction, there will be too few sperm to perform Percoll preparations. The fluid from macerated biopsy could be directly examined

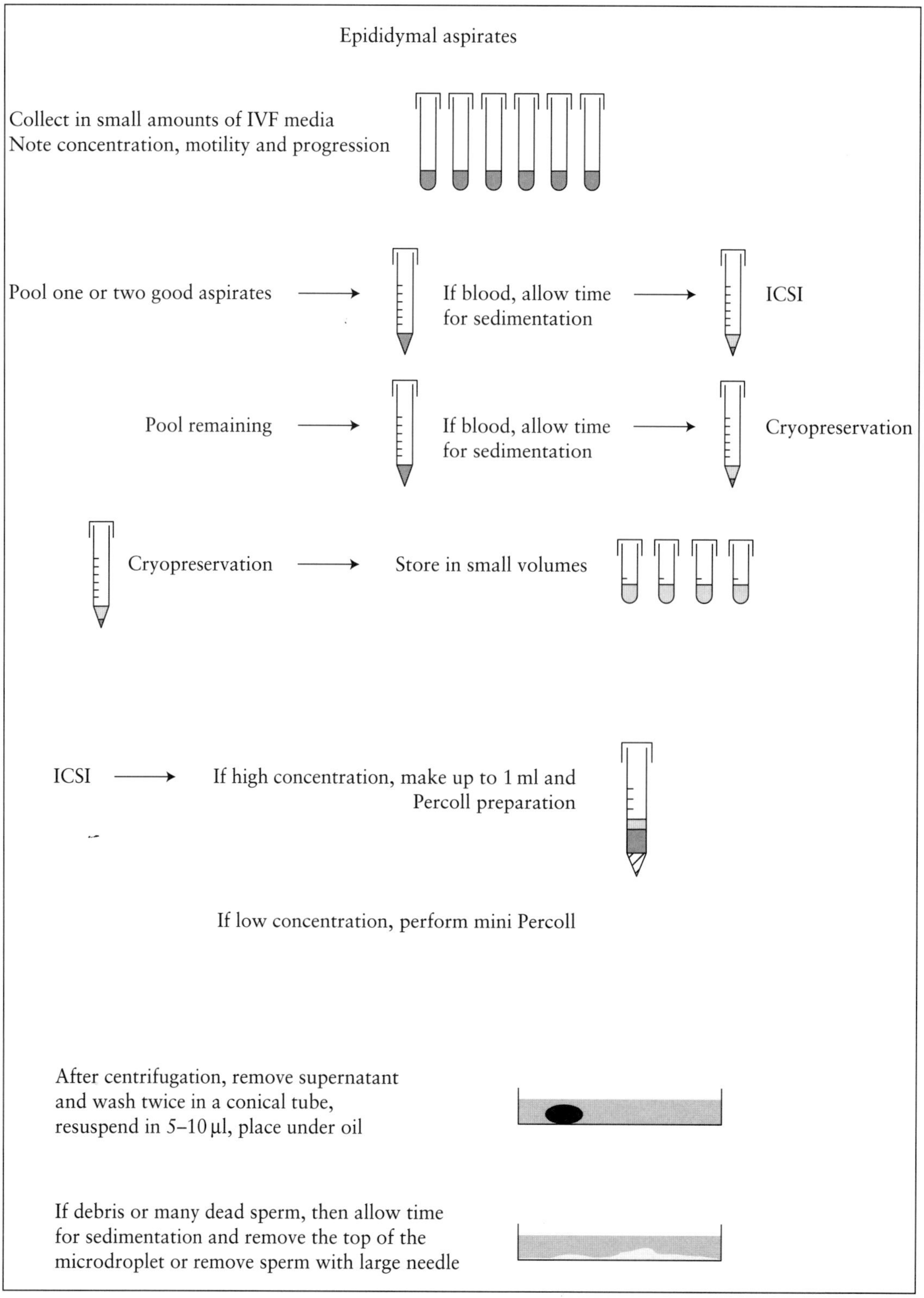


**Figure 5** Sequence of events in preparing epididymal sperm

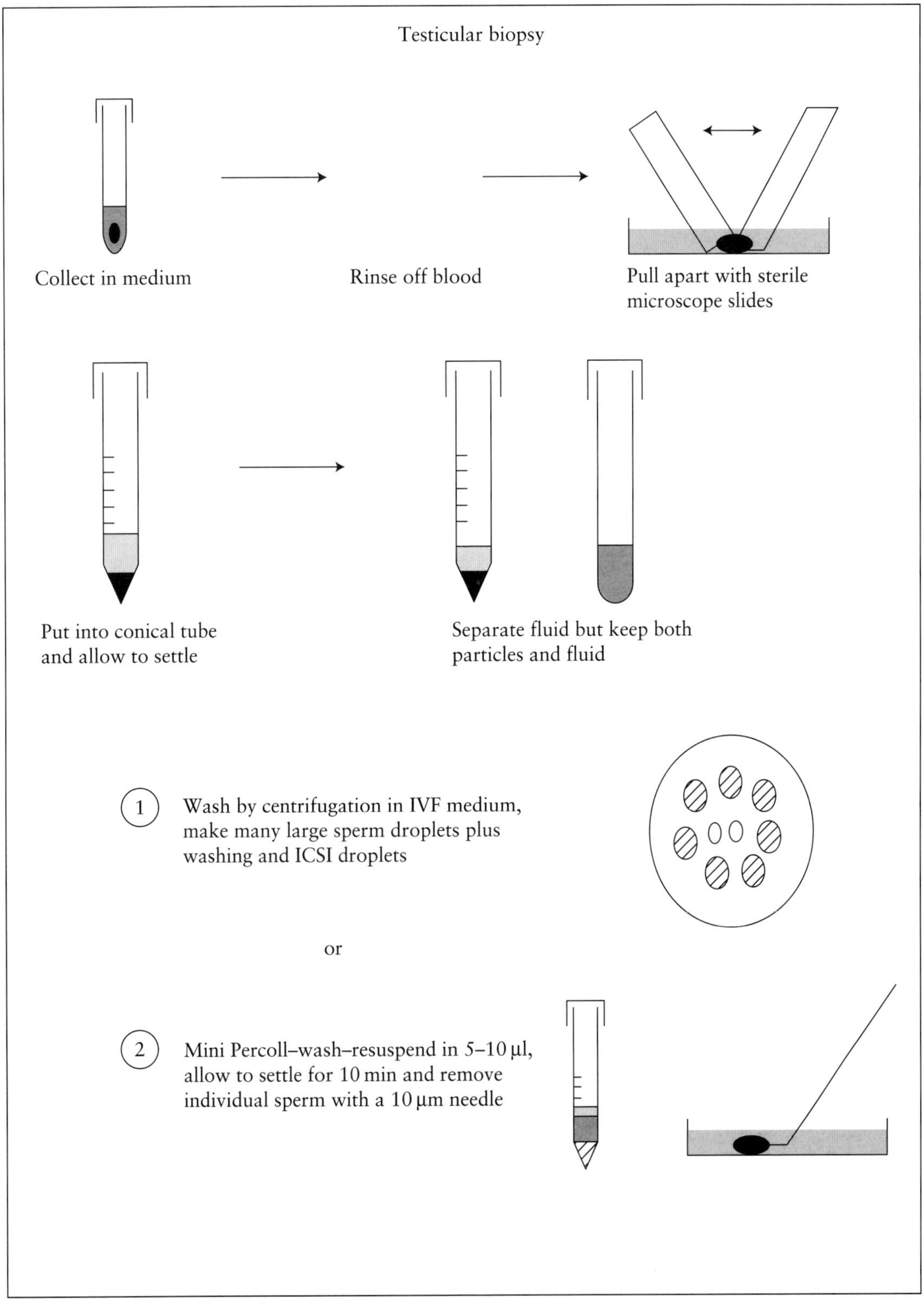
Testicular biopsy
Collect in medium
Rinse off blood
Pull apart with sterile microscope slides
Put into conical tube and allow to settle
Separate fluid but keep both particles and fluid
1
Wash by centrifugation in IVF medium, make many large sperm droplets plus washing and ICSI droplets
or
2
Mini Percoll–wash–resuspend in 5–10 µl, allow to settle for 10 min and remove individual sperm with a 10 µm needle

**Figure 6** Sequence of events in preparing testicular sperm

for sperm, but it may also be necessary to physically separate with microneedles those sperm which are bound to Sertoli cells.

### Alignment of ICSI needles in the manipulator

The ICSI needle is put into the tool holder (Research Instruments) up to its maximum depth and then brought forward 1 cm; the holder screw mechanism is then tightened. When using a Narishige tool holder push the needle in so that 4–5 cm of the needle are outside the holder. Place the tool holder in the right hand micromanipulator with the needle-tip over the light source. The angle at which the tool holder is held should then be such that the angled tip of the needle is parallel with the stage of the microscope, e.g. our ICSI needles are angled at 30° from the plane of the needle, therefore the angle of the tool holder must be at 60° on the manipulator.

Put the tip of the ICSI needle in the microscopic field of vision under a very low power (e.g. × 4 objective). Loosen the tool holder and rotate it on the manipulator so that the bent portion of the needle looks as if it is straight.

Make sure that you can focus on a good portion of the needle (from the tip); the portion of the needle after the bend will be out of focus. If there is a graticule in the microscope make sure that the movement of the needle from right to left does not wander. The needle then needs to be aligned so that the tip is parallel with the microscope stage. This is done in two stages, first by looking through the centre of the two eye pieces at the tip of the needle in the light source and adjusting the angle of the tool holder. The second adjustment is made later when the needle is in the sperm-containing droplet. This is done by focusing on a non-moving sperm and bringing the tip of the needle in to the same optical plane. Raise the needle up slightly and bring it down on top of the sperm. If the tip of the needle will not touch the sperm, then it is 'elbow down' and the tool holder needs to be moved in an anti-clockwise direction. If the needle can touch the sperm but you cannot focus along a good portion of the needle, then it is 'tip down' and the tool holder needs to be moved in a clockwise direction.

Put the ICSI needle along the middle of the microscope field with the tip almost in the centre. Align the holding pipette in the same manner (the last part of the alignment can be done by eye only) so that the tips of the needle and pipette are facing each other and then raise them up away from the stage.

*Equilibration*

The Research Instruments SAS10/2 microinjector is an air-filled system with a 10-ml syringe capacity. This allows good control for large movements of media within the holding pipette. This requires no equilibration and is excellent for moving, rotating and holding oocytes or embryos.

The microinjector for the ICSI needle must have a much lower syringe capacity (less than 1 ml) and be oil-filled for the greater control of small volumes.

One method to equilibrate the needle is to, after alignment, inject oil through the tool holder and into the back of the ICSI needle until the oil can be seen 3–5 mm from the tip of the tool holder. This is left to settle for a few minutes. There should be a corresponding movement of the oil in the ICSI needle when the injector is rotated in and out. If this does not happen there will be no control of the movement of media and sperm in and out of the ICSI needle. The other method of equilibration of the ICSI needle will give finer control. A Petri dish containing microdroplets under oil is placed on the stage. Focus on a droplet. The ICSI needle is lowered into the oil and is left there for 5 s and then lowered further into the microdroplet. Due to capillary action a small amount of oil and then medium is drawn into the needle. Under a low power (e.g. × 4 objective) focus on the oil in the needle. Draw it further up the needle with the microinjector so that it sits in the portion of the ICSI needle beyond the bend (unparalleled portion). There should be a corresponding movement of this oil in the ICSI needle when the injector is rotated in and out. The oil acts as a buffer and movements are slowed down.

The flow rate will increase if the oil is higher up the needle and decrease if nearer the tip. Therefore this arrangement can be further used to control the speed of picking up and injecting sperm. Maintaining this control is an extremely important aspect of the ICSI procedure. There will be a reduced flow rate within the ICSI needle if sperm are slowed down in polyvinylpyrrolidone (PVP) solutions because of its viscous nature.

The ICSI procedure is performed in the lid of a 60 × 15 mm Nunc Petri dish (150288). The dish is set up in the following way. Place six 5-μl droplets of IVF medium around the centre of the Petri dish in a 2 × 3 pattern, then cover with mineral oil. A small volume (1–5 μl) of sperm suspension is added to the left central droplet and examined for sperm density. Ideally there should be two to eight sperm per × 200 magnification field of view. The oocytes to be injected are placed in the adjacent microdroplet (central right).

## Immobilization of sperm

After alignment, focus on the sperm-containing droplet. Sperm are immobilized with the ICSI needle prior to picking them up. This is performed by a combination of a downwards movement of the needle on to the sperm and a sideways movement from left to right across the sperm. This causes damage to the tail or mid-piece. If this movement (swipe) is too heavy it will result in an angled sperm tail or the sperm tail becoming partly embedded in the surface of the Petri dish. Sperm tails with angles as a result of a heavy swipe are not easily drawn up into the needle. If they are drawn up into the needle they are more likely to stick in the needle. Sperm embedded in the Petri dish are difficult to move. An ideal swipe results in a sperm immediately slowing down and stopping all movement within about 10 seconds. Sperm immobilized like this are easy to pick up because the sperm is not stuck on the dish and the sperm is less likely to be a 'sticky sperm'.

The ease with which a sperm can be immobilized is related to its speed. The slower the sperm the easier the immobilization. Most groups slow down sperm by putting them in a viscous solution of PVP in medium (10%, 360 kDa mol. wt.). In a large number of cases, sperm have slow movement after preparation, and swiping can be performed at a magnification of × 200–× 300, which enables the operator to select sperm on a morphological basis at the same magnification at which they swipe. When dealing with faster sperm it may be necessary to swipe sperm at a lower magnification (× 100–× 150) because at a higher magnification there is not enough time to swipe a fast sperm before it has travelled out of the field of vision. The swiping action is extremely difficult to perform if a sperm is swimming along the 9 o'clock to 3 o'clock position (or vice versa) because it is in the same plane as the needle. However, the swimming direction of the sperm can be altered by tipping the sperm head in the direction the operator wishes it to go. This is only really necessary when there are no, or very few, other sperm to choose from.

## Moving and positioning oocytes during ICSI

During the ICSI procedure the movements of the microtool should be kept to a minimum. In order to move an oocyte from one side of a droplet to the other, one must hold the oocyte and move the microdroplet. Bring the oocyte into focus, lower the holding pipette into the microdroplet until it is in the same optical plane, draw up a small amount on the microinjector and the oocyte will be drawn onto the holding pipette. Move the microdroplet with the stage controls until the oocyte is in the required position and then turn the microinjector screw the opposite way to release the oocyte.

## Picking up sperm

When picking up sperm in the ICSI needle, the in and out movements on the microinjector should be kept to a minimum in order to maintain good control. Move the immobilized sperm to the left of centre of the microscope field by using the stage movement control. Focus on the sperm, then bring the tip of the

ICSI needle into the same optical plane by rotating the joystick. In order to pick up the sperm tail-first, it may be necessary to move the sperm so that the tail is facing the needle tip. This can be performed by gently pushing the sperm with the tip of the ICSI needle in the direction you wish it to move. Sperm can be picked up when the tail is not facing the bevel but the amount of suction required is greater and there will be less control. Place the needle tip slightly behind the end of the tail (about one sperm head in length) and draw up with the syringe slowly. If the sperm does not move, make sure the sperm is not attached to the Petri dish by touching it with the ICSI needle, then draw slowly again.

The sperm may sometimes move downwards towards the needle but fail to go up because it is trying to go up sideways. When this happens, inject out some media until the sperm is released from the needle, and attempt to pick it up again with the needle tip further away from the tail.

If a sperm will not go up the needle because of the shape of the tail, use another one. If there are no other sperm available, then it may be necessary to separate the head from the tail and inject the head only. An immobilized sperm is positioned so that its head is facing 12 o'clock; lower the ICSI needle onto the mid-piece of the sperm, and, as the needle comes into contact with the sperm, move the needle towards the 12 o'clock position. The head will pop off. The parallel part of the needle 50–100 μm from the tip is used to do this. The tailless sperm is very sticky and it readily sticks to the outside of the ICSI needle, or, once picked up, sticks to the inner surface. Speed is therefore speed is required between picking up and the last procedure. During the manipulation move the head up and down the needle frequently to try to prevent sticking.

### Intracytoplasmic sperm injection

When a sperm has been immobilized and picked up, make sure that there is a corresponding movement of the sperm in the ICSI needle when the microinjector is adjusted. This movement should be smooth; if the movement is staggered then it may be better to choose a different sperm. Raise the ICSI needle up out of the plane of the sperm slightly, using the joystick, so that it is just out of focus. Keeping the ICSI needle in the same plane move the oocyte containing the microdroplet into the field of vision using the stage controller (Figure 7). Focus on the oocyte, then lower the ICSI needle into the same optical plane. It will appear on the right of the oocyte. At this point make sure the sperm is not stuck by moving it slightly with the microinjector. Lower the holding pipette into the same optical plane (this will appear on the left of the oocyte). Align the oocyte so that the polar body is at the 12 or 6 o'clock position[15]. This can be done by gently pushing the oocyte with either of the microtools. The oocyte may need to be rotated so that the polar body is in the same optical plane. This is performed by raising the injection needle up and then lowering it on to one end of the oocyte.

Once the oocyte is aligned, move the holding pipette next to the zona and draw up with the coarse microinjector. The oocyte will attach itself to the holding pipette. The oocyte should still be resting on the surface of the Petri dish.

Focus on the portion of the vitelline membrane opposite the holding pipette, bring the ICSI needle into the same optical plane and touch the zona with the tip of the needle. At this time the sperm can be injected towards the tip of the ICSI needle. Push the needle slightly into the oocyte (30–50 μm) so that it penetrates

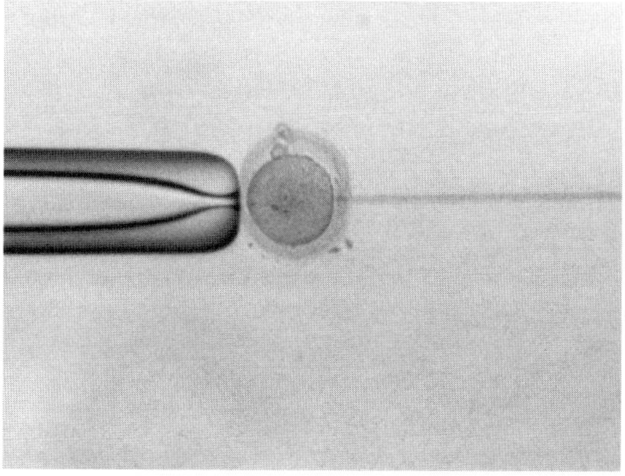

**Figure 7** Intracytoplasmic sperm injection

the zona and makes a <-shaped indent in the vitelline membrane. There may be a need to refocus on the indented vitelline membrane; rotate the joystick to find the maximum definition of the <-shape. Push the needle into the oocyte using the fine right-to-left movement knob (screw), not the joystick. The vitelline membrane will appear to break. Try to inject the sperm. If the sperm enters the cytoplasm then withdraw the needle using the fine left-to-right screw. If the sperm does not enter the cytoplasm draw up on the fine microinjector so there is a pressure in the needle. Do this until the pressure causes the sperm to move to level with the zona. At this point push the needle slightly further into the cytoplasm; the cytoplasm will be disrupted and a small amount will enter the ICSI needle. To keep this to a minimum as the cytoplasm is disrupted, counteract the force by injecting with the fine microinjector, allow the cytoplasm and then the sperm to flow into the oocyte and then withdraw the needle (Figure 8).

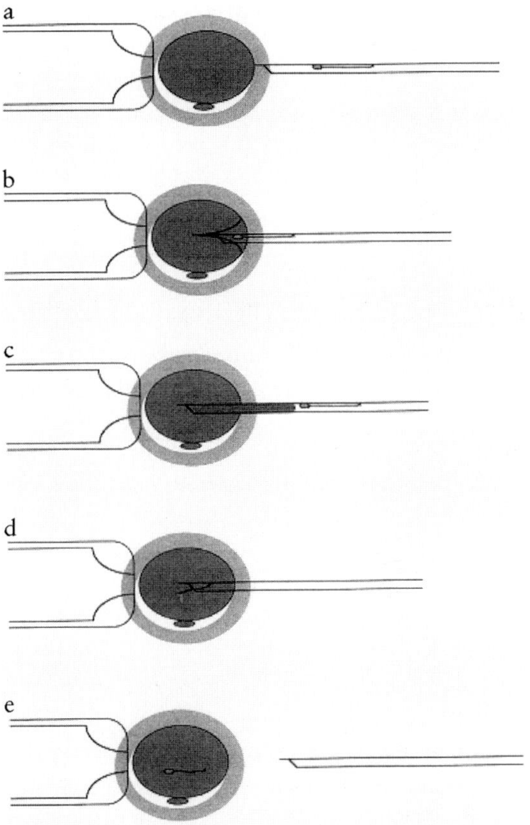


**Figure 8** Sequence of events during the ICSI process: (a) alignment of oocyte holding pipette and injection needle (loaded with one sperm) into the same optical plane; (b) ICSI needle pushed through the zona and indentation of the vitelline membrane; (c) rupture of the vitelline membrane and disruption of the cytoplasm; (d) cytoplasm and sperm re-injected into the cytoplasm; (e) removal of ICSI needle

## Construction of a holding pipette

The holding pipettes are made from borosilicate glass capillary tubes GC100-10 (Clarke Electromedical etc.). Their construction consists of the following steps:

(1) *Pulling:* a reduction of the capillary size to 100 μm using a pipette puller;

(2) *Breaking:* breaking the pipette at the required point;

(3) *Polishing:* a reduction of the internal diameter of the pulled pipette to 20 μm using a microforge; and

(4) *Angling:* the tip of the pipette is bent on the microforge so that it is 30° from the plane of the pipette.

*Pulling*

Place the capillary tube in the micropuller (Research Instruments micropuller) and pull using the following settings: force 7 units, heat 7.5 A, car stop 70 mm.

*Breaking*

Remove the pulled pipette by holding the left-hand portion and pulling the right-hand portion through the coil. The capillary tube will be shaped like an extended hourglass; snap off the right-hand side, leaving the long pulled portion on the left-hand side. The pipette now needs to be broken off at an external diameter of 0.1 mm. This needs to be a straight cut with no jagged edges. It can be performed on the microforge or manually. Take the right-hand portion of the capillary tube; place it across the left-hand portion and use it to stroke along the pulled portion of the pipette; the pipette will snap. Repeat the action with slightly more pressure if it does not break. Aim to make the break between 1 and 1.5 cm from the reduction of the pull.

*Polishing*
Place the pipette vertically in the forge and lower the broken tip next to the ball of glass. Put the heat setting on high. Bring the pipette towards the glass ball. At the right distance and heat setting the pipette's internal diameter should start to close up. The actual settings will differ from one forge to another so some experimenting will be necessary to find the right settings. The internal diameter should be reduced to 20 μm, that is 2 units of the graticule at × 100 magnification using the Narishige forge.

*Creating an angled tip*
Place the polished pipette at an angle to the glass ball. Heat at a high temperature and bring the pipette closer to the ball. At certain settings (again varying with each forge) the pipette will start to bend. Stop the heat when the tip of the pipette reaches a vertical position. In this method the angle of the bend is controlled by the angle of the capillary tube holder. As long as the angle of the tool holder is set at the same angle, and the pipette is bent so that it is vertical, the angle of the bend will be constant.

### Construction of an ICSI injection needle

The ICSI needle is made from a borosilicate glass capillary tube GC100T-10 (Clarke). Its construction consists of the following steps:

(1) *Pulling:* a double pull resulting in 1/100 reduction in size using the pipette puller;

(2) *Breaking:* breaking off the needle at the required point;

(3) *Bevelling:* grinding the needle tip to form a bevel;

(4) *Cleaning:* washing the needle with acid to remove fragments of glass;

(5) *Spiking:* making a fine spike at the tip of the bevel; and

(6) *Angling:* the tip of the needle is bent to form an angle of 30° from the plane of the needle.

*Pulling*
Place the capillary tube in the puller and pull using the following settings: force 6 units, heat 6.4 A, car stop 35 mm. Move the right-hand car to 5 mm and change the settings to force 9 units, heat 7.2 A. Make the second pull. Remove the left-hand portion of the pulled pipette and discard the right.

*Breaking*
Place the pulled pipette horizontally in the view focus, and focus on the tip. This needs to be performed at a high magnification (× 200). Adjust the position of the needle so that the required point of breaking is directly above the mid-point of the glass ball. At × 200 magnification 7 μm is around 1.5 units on the graticule. For a slightly smaller needle, break off the needle so that the internal diameter is 1 unit (5 μm). The ball is heated at a low temperature, so that it is not hot enough to melt the needle, but hot enough for the glass ball to stick to the needle. Attempts may be made with several needles until the right temperature setting is found.

Place the needle above the ball at the required place. Switch on the heat and bring the needle into contact with the ball. Wait 1 or 2 seconds, turn off the heat, and raise up the needle. If the timing and heat setting are correct, the tip of the needle will break off and stay on the glass ball. The tip of the microneedle has an opening at the required position; check the size of the opening and remove.

*Bevelling*
The microneedle is bevelled on the Research Instruments microbeveller MBI. Place the needle in the microbeveller and set to an angle of 30°. Focus on the tip of the needle. Put filtered water in the grinders water bath. Make sure the grinding surface is wet. Bring the grinding

wheel into contact with the needle and grind. Set the grinding speed to the middle position. This may need to be changed but attempt to grind at this speed. Switch off the grinder and move the wheel away from the needle. Remove or repeat grinding.

*Cleaning*
After grinding, the needle is washed in 10% hydrofluoric acid. This is done by using a 20-ml syringe attached to a microtool holder. Put the needle into the tool holder and place the tip in 10% hydrofluoric acid; draw up some acid for 5 s and expel. Repeat and then remove the needle from the acid expelling air at the same time. Place the needle in filtered water and draw up water into the tip and expel. Repeat 10 times. Remove the tool holder/needle from the syringe.

*Spiking*
Place the needle with the tool holder in a vertical position in the microforge. Bring the tip of the needle into view. Use the tool holder to rotate the needle so that the lumen of the bevel is towards the right-hand side. The heat setting in the microforge should be set to make the glass ball sticky, so that when the microtool touches the ball, it will adhere to it. Switch on the heat and then move the needle down to the tip of the bevel. Immediately after touching the ball, raise the needle up and switch off the heat at the same time. This should cause the tip of the bevel to melt and then stretch creating a spike.

*Creating an angled ICSI needle*
After creating a spike rotate the needle 90° clockwise so that the bevel is facing the operator. Place the ICSI needle at 30° to the glass ball. Heat a fairly high temperature and bring the needle closer to the ball. At certain settings (again varying with each forge) the needle will start to bend. Stop the heat when the tip of the needle reaches a vertical position. In this method the angle of the bend is controlled by the angle of the capillary tube holder. As long as the angle of the tool holder is set at the same angle, and the needle is bent so that it is vertical, the angle of the bend will be constant.

## RESULTS

These are the results of 631 ICSI treatment cycles performed at the Lister Hospital, London. Of these 631 cases there were 170 (26.9%) pregnancies. There have been 87 deliveries (25 sets of twins) and there are 48 ongoing pregnancies, making an ongoing/delivery rate of 21.2%. There were 30 (17.6%) miscarriages (18 at less than 8 weeks), three ectopic pregnancies and three patients were lost to follow-up.

Table 7 shows the fertilization rates and pregnancy rates of patients with different indications for ICSI. These are groups 1–5 as discussed earlier. Fertilization is expressed as the total number of 'normal' fertilized oocytes (two pronuclei) from that group divided by the total number of oocytes injected. The pregnancy rate is expressed as the number of pregnant patients within that group over the number of egg collections.

The fertilization rate is approximately 50% for all groups except with testicular sperm (34%) and non-motile sperm (25.7%). It is not uncommon that the testicular fertilization rate is lower than the average[16]. The lower fertilization rate in cases where there are no moving sperm is not surprising as some sperm selected for ICSI will be non-viable and presumably incapable of fertilization even when injected into the cytoplasm. The low pregnancy rate for the non-motile group is a reflection of the fertilization rate. The other groups vary between 18 and 35%.

There are fewer pregnancies in the extreme sperm parameter groups ($< 10^5$, < 1% motility and apparent azoospermia); this may be due to the fact that they involve techniques that are more difficult to perform. When there are so few sperm those found must go into the oocytes even if they are bent or sticky and do not enter the cytoplasm with ease. This situation compares unfavourably to that where there is an excess of sperm and difficult sperm can be discarded. There may be fertilization with a

**Table 7** Fertilization and pregnancy rates of ICSI treatment cycles and indications for treatment

| | *Fertilization rate (no. 2 Pn/no. oocytes injected)* | | *Pregnancy rate per ICSI cycle* | |
|---|---|---|---|---|
| *Indication for ICSI* | *Ratio* | *%* | *Ratio* | *%* |
| *Groups 1 and 2* | | | | |
| Normal sperm but failure or poor fertilization | 212/400 | 52.6 | 12/57 | 21.1 |
| *Group 3* | | | | |
| Epididymal sperm | 370/788 | 47 | 28/79 | 35.4 |
| Testicular sperm | 35/103 | 34 | 4/12 | 33.3 |
| *Group 4: Extreme sperm parameters* | | | | |
| < 100 000 sperm/ml | 173/323 | 53.6 | 7/37 | 18.9 |
| No sperm seen in ejaculate but some found in preparation | 38/78 | 48.7 | 2/8 | 25 |
| Less than 1% motility | 153/327 | 46.8 | 6/33 | 18.2 |
| No motile sperm seen | 36/140 | 25.7 | 2/15 | 13.3 |
| Greater than 95% abnormal sperm | 167/317 | 52.7 | 10/39 | 25.6 |
| *Group 5* | | | | |
| Poor sperm parameters | 1431/2652 | 54 | 98/342 | 28.7 |

no. 2 Pn, number of two-pronuclear zygotes (normal fertilization); ICSI, intracytoplasmic sperm injection

difficult ICSI but subtle damage may have occurred.

There is a lower pregnancy rate in group 1 even though there is good fertilization. It is possible that men with 'normal' sperm parameters that have variable fertilization may occasionally fertilize oocytes and achieve pregnancy naturally, especially if they have fertile partners. This group may have a higher number of partners who contribute to the couples' overall infertility. This is the opposite to group 3 (testicular and epididymal sperm) where the pregnancy rate is high, probably because the fertile partners have not been selected out due to the fact that they have not been exposed to sperm.

There is some variation in pregnancy rates with ICSI but as long as there are some motile sperm, patients have a 50% chance of fertilization and a more than reasonable chance of pregnancy, regardless of the sperm picture. What influences pregnancy rates if the sperm picture is irrelevant? The only parameters which correlate with pregnancies are the age of the woman and the number of embryos available to choose from. Figure 9 shows pregnancy rates in different age groups. The pregnancy rate is much lower in the 40–44 age group, 8/62 (12.9%). There were no pregnancies in the three patients over 44.

Figure 10 compares the pregnancy rates in patients who have different numbers of embryos to choose from for embryo transfer. Out of 631 cycles, 22 cycles did not have any embryos for transfer, and there was a 96.5% ET rate. The pregnancy rate when there was one embryo available was 9.4%. When there were two or three available, the rates were 24.1% and 17.9%, respectively. However, when there was a choice of embryos and three were selected from four or more embryos, the pregnancy rate was 35.9%. This was also true when two were selected from four or more (27.3%) but this is only in a small group of patients.

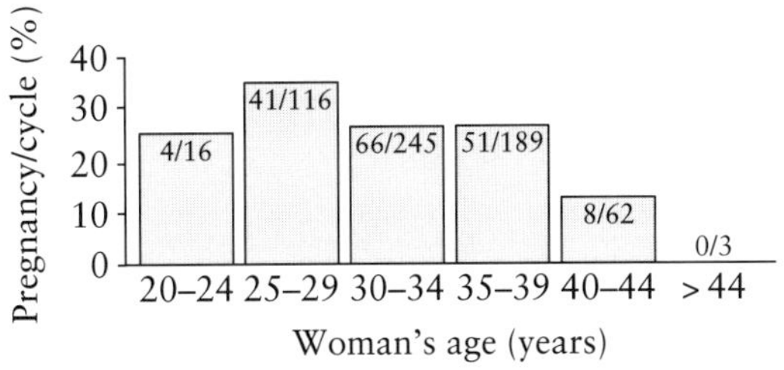


**Figure 9** Pregnancy rates with intracytoplasmic sperm injection (ICSI) in different age groups

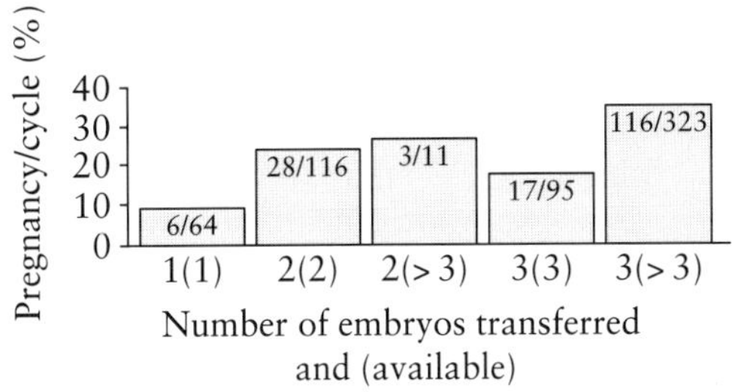


**Figure 10** Pregnancy rates with intracytoplasmic sperm injection (ICSI) according to the number of embryos available for embryo transfer

The factor that most influences the success of ICSI is the number of embryos available to choose from which in turn is related to the number of mature oocytes collected. The author would suggest that if women have a poor response to stimulation (unless there is always a poor response) that they do not proceed with the treatment in that cycle.

## TESTICULAR SPERM EXTRACTION (TESE)

The first reported use of testicular sperm was in 1951 when a pregnancy was achieved by artificially inseminating with macerated testicular tissue. This was regarded with some scepticism as it was thought that it was essential for sperm to pass through the epididymis in order to obtain their fertilizing capability.

In 1993 various workers reported fertilization with testicular sperm using different assisted reproduction techniques; conventional *in vitro* insemination[18] (IVF-ET), subzonal insemination (SUZI)[19] and ICSI[13,20]. In late 1993 Schoysman and colleagues[21] reported pregnancies using testicular sperm. The embryos replaced were a mixture of SUZI and ICSI embryos. A pregnancy was achieved at the Lister Hospital[22] using ICSI and testicular sperm extraction (TESE). Silber and coworkers[23] performed TESE and ICSI on a series of 12 patients with obstructive azoospermia. They achieved a fertilization rate of 46%; nine patients had embryos replaced resulting in five clinical pregnancies.

The combination of TESE and ICSI is now becoming routine throughout the world. It has also been applied to couples where the man has non-obstructive azoospermia. It has been found that small areas of spermatogenesis occur in the testes of men who have severe spermatogenic dysfunction. Devroey and colleagues[24] published the results of 15 patients who were azoospermic and whose histology showed absence or near absence of spermatogenesis. Sperm were found in 13 of these patients. Out of 182 oocytes injected, 57 transferable embryos were obtained. Three pregnancies occurred from 12 embryo transfers. ICSI in combination with TESE can be used to treat couples where the male has non-obstructive azoospermia, small testes and high follicle-stimulating hormone. Only a few years ago this would have been considered as impossible to treat.

## ICSI AND FUTURE DEVELOPMENTS

There have been great advances in the treatment of infertile couples since the introduction of ICSI into clinical practice[5] in 1992. One of the latest developments is the use of spermatids in intracytoplasmic injection. Spermatids are haploid cells and as such have been considered for some time to be an alternative to sperm in cases of spermatogenic arrest.

Vanderzwalmen and colleagues[25] reported fertilization of one oocyte using an elongated spermatid obtained from a testicular biopsy. This patient also had some sperm which were injected into other oocytes. Fishel and coworkers[26] achieved a pregnancy and delivered a normal girl after the intracytoplasmic injection of elongated spermatids and Hannay[27] reported four pregnancies after the injection of spermatid nuclei. These four pregnancies have all spontaneously aborted. Spermatids can be found in the testes. It is not uncommon for seminologists to report the presence of sperm precursors in semen analysis; occasionally they can be seen where there is an absence of sperm.

Tesarik and co-workers[28] published the results of 11 treatment cycles of intracytoplasmic injection with elongated and round spermatids. The mean fertilization rate was 45% but it varied greatly from patient to patient. Ten of these patients had embryos to replace, resulting in two pregnancies. These two pregnancies came to term resulting in two healthy boys.

Tesarik and Mendosa[29] published their laboratory techniques of injecting spermatids. They extracted round spermatids from ejaculates using a five-gradient Percoll technique (100/80/70/60/40% solutions). They found the highest concentration of viable spermatids in the 70% fraction. They also found that those round spermatids, which, when drawn into the ICSI needle, became elongated and then after intracytoplasmic injection returned to their round shape, gave better results. They also noted that after pronuclei formation and nuclear fusion that a single nucleus could be seen in some zygotes 16–18 h after injection. This did not alter the cleavage rate.

## ICSI AND KLINEFELTER'S SYNDROME

There was an interesting paper presented at the annual meeting of the European Society of Human Reproduction and Embryology (ESHRE) in July 1996[30]. Sperm were found in four testicular biopsies from a series of nine apparently non-mosaic Klinefelter men. ICSI was performed with three of these preparations. The resulting embryos were then biopsied and fluorescent *in situ* hybridization (FISH) was performed for the diagnosis of sex chromosomes. Four embryos showed a normal sex chromosome complement and embryo transfer was performed on three patients. One of these patients was reported to have a biochemical pregnancy.

## ICSI AND CONGENITAL MALFORMATIONS

When ICSI was introduced, many workers were worried that oocytes would be fertilized with genetically abnormal sperm because the sperm were not undergoing any natural selection stages. The other concern was that the injection process itself could damage the oocyte and give rise to an abnormal embryo. ICSI is a novel technique with an uncertain risk of fetal abnormality, although there is increasing evidence that the rate of abnormalities in ICSI children is similar to that in the general population.

A follow-up study was presented at the ESHRE meeting in Hamburg in 1995[31] by the Dutch Speaking Brussels Free University group. Out of 1160 pregnancies 479 karyotypes were performed; six were abnormal (1.2%), and five of these had a sex chromosome abnormality. Out of 669 children born, 18 (2.7%) had a major malformation. This group later published a comparative age-matched (female age) study of 130 children born through ICSI and 130 through IVF[32]. They were examined at birth, 2 months and 1 year. In the ICSI group there were four (3%) major abnormalities and 18 minor abnormalities, compared to six (4.6%) major and 21 minor in the control IVF group. They concluded that there was no difference at paediatric follow-up in the age-matched groups.

Wennerholm and colleagues[33] reported lower rates of abnormalities. Out of 273 children born (175 singletons and 98 twins) four had major malformations. There was one abnormal karyotype out of 65 performed.

In a survey of 44 clinics[34] (32 European, five Australian and seven from the Americas) 18 (1.2%) major abnormalities were reported out of 1540 children born after ICSI and 29 (1.9%) minor.

There is some variation in reported rates of major malformations. This could be related to the different definitions of major abnormalities, some clinics treating more older women than others, or some male factor groups may have a higher genetic risk[35].

## REFERENCES


1. Cohen, J., Edwards, R., Fehilly, C., Fishel, S., Hewitt, J., Purdy, J., Rowland, G., Steptoe, P. and Webster, J. (1985). *In vitro* fertilization: a treatment for male infertility. *Fertil. Steril.*, **43**, 422
2. Cohen, J., Malter, H., Fehilly, C., Wright, G., Elsner, C., Kort, H. and Massey, J. (1988). Implantation of embryos after partial opening of oocyte zona pellucida to facilitate sperm penetration (letter). *Lancet*, **2**, 162
3. Ng, S-C., Bongso, A., Ratnam, S. S., Sathananthan, H., Chen, C. L., Wong, P. C., Hagglund, L., Anandakumar, C., Wong, Y. C. and Goh, V. H. H. (1988). Pregnancy after transfer of sperm under zona (letter). *Lancet*, **2**, 790
4. Fishel, S., Antinori, S., Jackson, P., Johnson, J., Lisi, F., Chiarello, F. and Versaci, C. (1990). Twin birth after subzonal insemination (letter). *Lancet*, **355**, 722–3
5. Palermo, G., Joris, H., Devroey, P. and Van Steirteghem, A. C. (1992). Pregnancies after intracytoplasmic injection of single spermatozoon into an oocyte. *Lancet*, **340**, 17–18
6. Van Steirteghem, A. C., Liu, J., Joris, H., Nagy, Z., Janssenswillen, C., Tournaye, H., Derde, M. P., Van Assche, E. and Devroey, P. (1993). Higher success rate by intracytoplasmic sperm injection than by subzonal insemination. Report of a second series of 300 consecutive treatment cycles. *Hum. Reprod.*, **8**, 1055–60
7. Abdalla, H., Leonard, T., Pryor, J. and Everett, D. (1995). Comparison of SUZI and ICSI for severe male factor. *Hum. Reprod.*, **10**, 2941–4
8. Silber, S., Nagy, P., Liu, J., Godoy, H., Devroey, P. and Van Steirteghem, A. C. (1994). Conventional in vitro fertilization versus intracytoplasmic sperm injection for patients requiring microsurgical sperm aspiration. *Hum. Reprod.*, **9**, 1705–9
9. Leonard, T., Abdalla, H., Kirkland, A., Burton, G., Joshi, R., Studd, J. and Pryor, J. (1991). Male factor infertility – which couples do not have a reasonable chance of pregnancy with assisted conception? *Hum. Reprod.*, **6** suppl. 1, 282
10. McClure, R. D., Nunes, L. and Tom, R. (1989). Semen manipulation: improved sperm recovery and function with a two-layer Percoll gradient. *Fertil. Steril.*, **51**, 874–7
11. Ord, T., Patrizio, P., Marello, E., Balmaceda, J. P., and Asch, R. H. (1990). Mini-Percoll: a new method of semen preparation for IVF in severe male factor infertility. *Hum. Reprod.*, **5**, 987–9
12. Nagy, Z., Silber, S., Liu, J., Devroey, P., Cecile, J. and Van Steirteghem, A. (1995). Using ejaculated, fresh, and frozen-thawed epididymal and testicular spermatozoa gives rise to comparable results after intracytoplasmic sperm injection. *Fertil. Steril.*, **63**, 808–15
13. Devroey, P., Tournaye, H., Liu, J., Silber, S. J., Nagy, Z. and Van Steirteghem, A. C. (1994). Normal fertilization of human oocytes after testicular sperm extraction and intracytoplasmic sperm injection. *Fertil. Steril.*, **63**, 639–41
14. Verheyen, G., De Croo, I., Tournaye, H., Pletincx, I., Devroey, P. and Van Steirteghem, A. C. (1995). Comparison of four mechanical methods to retrieve spermatozoa from testicular tissue. *Hum. Reprod.*, **10**, 2956–9
15. Nagy, Z. P., Liu, J., Joris, H., Bocken, G., Desmet, D., Van Ranst, H., Vankelecom, A., Devroey, P. and Van Steirteghem, A. C. (1995). The influence of the site of sperm deposition and mode of oolemma breakage at intracytoplasmic sperm injection on fertilization and embryo development rates. *Hum. Reprod.*, **10**, 3171–7
16. Silber, S. J., Van Steirteghem, A. C., Liu, J., Nagy, Z., Tournaye, H. and Devroey, P. (1995). High fertility rate after intracytoplasmic sperm injection with spermatozoa obtained from testicle biopsy. *Hum. Reprod.*, **10**, 148–52
17. Adler, L. and Macris, A. (1951). Successful artificial insemination with macerated testicular tissue. *Fertil. Steril.*, **2**, 459–61
18. Hirsh, A., Montgomery, J., Mohan, P., Mills, C., Bekir, J. and Tan, S. L. (1993). Fertilisation by testicular sperm with standard IVF techniques (letter). *Lancet*, **2**, 864–5
19. Schoysman, R., Vanerzwalmen, P., Nijs, M., Segal-Bertin, G. and Van de Casseye, M. (1993). Successful fertilization by testicular spermatozoa in an in vitro fertilization programme. *Hum. Reprod.*, **8**, 1339–40
20. Craft, I., Bennet, V. and Nicholson, N. (1993). Fertilising ability of testicular spermatozoa (letter). *Lancet*, **2**, 864

21. Schoysman, R., Vanerzwalmen, P., Nijs, M., Segal, L., Segal-Bertin, G., Geerts, L., Van Roosdaal, E. and Schoysman, D. (1993). Pregnancy after fertilization with human testicular spermatozoa. *Lancet*, **342**, 1237
22. Bettocchi, C., Leonard, T., Abdalla, S. and Pryor, J. P. (1994). Pregnancy following the microinjection (ICSI) of testicular sperm in a man with obstructive azoospermia. Presented at *The Institute of Urology Short Paper Meeting*, March, London
23. Silber, S. J., Van Steirteghem, A. C., Liu, J., Nagy, Z., Tournaye, H. and Devroey, P. (1994). High fertilization and pregnancy rate after intracytoplasmic sperm injection with spermatozoa obtained from testicle biopsy. *Hum. Reprod.*, **10**, 148–52
24. Devroey, P., Liu, J., Goossens, A., Tournaye, H., Camus, M., Van Steirteghem, A. C. and Silber, S. (1995). Pregnancies after testicular sperm extraction and intracytoplasmic sperm injection in non-obstructive azoospermia. *Hum. Reprod.*, **10**, 1457–60
25. Vanderzwalmen, P., Lejeune, B., Nijs, M., Segal-Bertin, G., Vandamme, B. and Schoysman, R. (1995). Fertilization of an oocyte with a spermatid in an *in-vitro* fertilization programme. *Hum. Reprod.*, **10**, 502–3
26. Fishel, S., Green S. and Bishop, M. (1995). Pregnancy after intracytoplasmic injection of spermatid. *Lancet*, **345**, 1641–2
27. Hannay, T. (1995). New Japanese IVF method finally made available in Japan. *Nature Med.*, **1**, 289–90
28. Tesarik, J., Rolet, F., Brami, C., Sedbon, E., Thorel, J., Tibi, C. and Thebault, A. (1996). Spermatid injection into human oocytes. II. Clinical application in the treatment of infertility due to non-obstructive azoospermia. *Hum. Reprod.*, **11**, 780–3
29. Tesarik, J. and Mendoza, C. (1996). Spermatid injection into human oocytes. I. Laboratory techniques and special features of zygote development. *Hum. Reprod.*, **11**, 722–79
30. Tournaye, H., Staessen, C., Liebaers, I., Van Assche, E., Bonduelle, M., Devroey, P. and Van Steirteghem, A. C. (1996). Testicular sperm recovery in 47,XXY Klinefelter patients. *Hum. Reprod.*, **11**, 24
31. Bonduelle, M., Legein, J., Willikens, A., Van Assche, E., Dekoninck, P., Devroey, P., Van Steirteghem, A. and Liebaers, I. (1995). Follow-up study of children born after intracytoplasmic sperm injection. *Hum. Reprod.*, **10**, abstract book 1, 54
32. Bonduelle, M., Legein, J., Derde, M. P., Buysse, A., Schietecatte, J., Wisanto, A., Devroey, P., Van Steirteghem, A. and Liebaers, I. (1995). Comparative follow-up study of 130 children born after intracytoplasmic sperm injection and 130 children born after *in-vitro* fertilization. *Hum. Reprod.*, **10**, 3327–31
33. Wennerholm, U. B., Bergh, C., Hamberger, L., Nilsson, L. and Wikland, M. (1996). Obstetric and perinatal outcome of pregnancies following ICSI. *Hum. Reprod.*, **11**, abstract book 1, 158
34. Vereecken, A. and Keirse, M. J. N. C. (1995). Presented at the *Second International Symposium Andrology in the Nineties*, October, Gent
35. Meschede, D., Lemke, B., De Geyter, C., De Geyter, M., Wittwer, B., Nieschlag, E. and Horst, J. (1996). Genetic risk factors among infertile couples treated with ICSI. *Hum. Reprod.*, **11**, abstract book 1, 158

# Clinical and scientific aspects of human embryo freezing 15

*Peter R. Brinsden and Susan M. Avery*

## INTRODUCTION

The freezing of human embryos is now accepted as being an integral part of most assisted conception treatment units, with frozen/thawed embryo implantation rates as high as or higher than those in many programmes with fresh embryo transfer. Ovarian follicular stimulation is almost universally practised in *in vitro* fertilization (IVF) and other assisted conception treatments in order to maximize a couple's chance of achieving a pregnancy. The number of oocytes collected following stimulation averages 10–12. The maximum number of embryos that may be transferred to the uterus following IVF in the UK is three; in about 50% of women, this will leave some embryos surplus and available for freezing.

The principal advantages of a freezing programme are that no viable normal embryos are wasted and a couple's chances of achieving a pregnancy in any subsequent replacement cycles are enhanced without the need for further ovarian stimulation. However, there are a number of ethical and moral dilemmas thrown up by this relatively new technology that are only just becoming evident – in particular, the fate of stored embryos on the death or divorce of couples, the 'ownership' of the embryos and the accumulation in freezers around the world of large numbers of unclaimed embryos.

## HISTORY OF HUMAN EMBRYO FREEZING

Pregnancies have been achieved with the use of frozen donor semen since 1953[1]. Although the quality of semen is degraded by the freezing process, normal semen generally freezes and thaws well but the same cannot be said for oocytes. Attempts have been made for a number of years to achieve this[2], but, in general, they have met with little success, even though a few pregnancies and births have been reported[3,4].

In the earliest days of IVF, Edwards and Steptoe pointed out the potential benefits of freezing surplus human embryos, but their early attempts were not successful[5]. It was not until 1983 that the first pregnancy[6] was reported following the transfer of frozen/thawed human embryos. Since then, embryo freezing has become an integral part of the majority of programmes practising assisted conception treatment, both in the UK and worldwide. A total of 469 babies were born following the transfer of frozen/thawed embryos in the UK in 1994[7].

## HUMAN EMBRYO FREEZING

### Clinical indications

The modern management of assisted conception treatment cycles generally involves superovulation of the woman, with an average of 10–12 oocytes collected. In normal circumstances, fertilization is achieved in 7–8 of these. By law in the UK, a maximum of three embryos may be transferred to the uterus. Freezing of the remaining good-quality embryos avoids wastage. When the only alternative to freezing these embryos would be their destruction or use in research projects, it is logical to make every effort to conserve all normal embryos for future use by the couple for whom they were originally created.

Another major indication for the freezing of embryos is the occurrence of the ovarian hyperstimulation syndrome (OHSS), which is a relatively rare complication of superovulation. If OHSS occurs, the treatment cycle can be completed, oocytes collected and fertilized and all the embryos frozen, while efforts are made to reduce the clinical effects of OHSS. The embryos may then be thawed and replaced at a later date[8].

Other indications for freezing embryos may arise if, during the stimulation phase of an IVF cycle, a complication occurs such as the appearance of endometrial polyps, or if the endometrium does not develop normally. Sudden ill health or unforeseen domestic circumstances might be reasons for not proceeding with fresh embryo transfer.

Many assisted conception units, both in the UK and elsewhere, have active embryo donation and IVF surrogacy programmes. Embryos are usually donated by couples who have some frozen but who have achieved the children they want for themselves, or by couples who may have decided to discontinue their treatment. Because of the requirement to 'quarantine' embryos in embryo donation and IVF surrogacy programmes in the UK, to protect against the possibility of transmission of the AIDS virus, clinics freeze all embryos for at least 6 months, confirm the negative AIDS status and then proceed to embryo transfer.

An increasing number of young women who are about to receive cancer chemotherapy or radiotherapy are being counselled to have embryos frozen before they undergo their treatment, as it is likely that they will be made infertile by the treatment. If they have partners, then, given time, it is possible in many cases to induce superovulation in the woman, create embryos by IVF with the partner's sperm and store these embryos for their future use. In many cases, however, the younger women do not have partners, and a few centres are now freezing ovarian tissue for possible future use[9].

Frozen embryos may also act as a source of research embryos, since many couples with embryos remaining in storage after completing their families offer to donate the embryos to research projects approved by local ethics committees and, in the UK, by the Human Fertilization and Embryology Authority (HFEA).

### Clinical management of frozen embryo transfer cycles

Frozen/thawed embryos may be transferred to the uterus either in a natural monitored cycle or in a hormone-controlled cycle. The chances of achieving a pregnancy are reported to be the same as for fresh embryo transfer[10,11].

*Treatment in a natural cycle*

Natural cycle replacement is generally recommended when the woman is young and has normal regular menstrual cycles. Women in this group are asked to attend the clinic from day 10 of the menstrual cycle, for the follicular growth and ovulation to be monitored by serial ultrasound scanning and measurement of serial levels of serum oestradiol, luteinizing hormone (LH) and progesterone. When the spontaneous LH surge has been detected, the day of embryo replacement is timed for 3 days later. No luteal phase support is given in these cycles.

*Treatment in a hormone-controlled cycle*

Older women and those with irregular cycles will usually be treated in cycles brought under control by use of a gonadotrophin releasing hormone agonist such as buserelin (Suprefact, Hoechst, UK) or nafarelin (Synarel, Searle, UK). Daily doses of the agonist are usually started on or about day 21 of the cycle preceding the transfer cycle. In amenorrhoeic women, the agonist may be started at any time. Pituitary downregulation is confirmed on the 2nd day of menstruation, or after 10 days of suppression in amenorrhoeic women. If the serum oestradiol level is < 100 pg/ml, the progesterone < 0.5 ng/ml, the LH level is < 5 IU/l and the ovaries quiescent on ultrasound scanning, the dose of agonist is reduced and the hormone replacement therapy (HRT) is started. Oestradiol valerate tablets are given in a dose of 2 mg orally daily, increasing to 4 mg on day 6 and 6 mg on day 10, reducing again to 4 mg from day 14 onwards. Progesterone in the form of Gestone (Paines & Bryne Ltd, UK) 50 mg intramuscularly daily, or Utrogestan (Laboratoires Besins Iscovesco, France) 1 vaginal tablet three times daily, is given on days 15 and 16, and the doses doubled from cycle day 17 (embryo transfer day) onwards[10,12].

**Laboratory techniques**

Embryos may be frozen at the pronucleate, early cleavage, or blastocyst stages. There are advantages and disadvantages to freezing at all three stages. At the pronucleate stage there is no possibility of damage to the meiotic spindle, which is highly susceptible to cooling[13], however this does not allow qualitative selection of embryos on the basis of their morphology. Early cleavage stage embryos can be selected on the basis of morphology, with the proviso that they are at an even-numbered cell stage, since dividing cells are likely to suffer damage to the mitotic spindle and subsequent chromosomal disorganization. This is likely to reduce the number of embryos available for freezing. Cryopreservation of blastocysts represents the ultimate in embryo selection given the small percentage of embryos that reach this stage after culture *in vitro*[14], which means that very few embryos are available for freezing. As there is no significant difference in the survival rates of these different stages after thawing[12], the ideal programme would allow for freezing at all three stages of development, so as to maximize the number of embryos for cryopreservation.

*Cryoprotectants*

Cryopreservation is intended to suspend all chemical reactions within cells. Human embryos are stored under liquid nitrogen at –190 °C, a temperature at which the only deterioration is likely to be due to background ionizing radiation, which would take hundreds of years to do significant damage[15]. If damage does occur it is more likely to be the result of the cooling or thawing process. There are two main causes of possible damage during the cooling process – ice crystal formation and changes in osmotic pressure as a result of water loss from the cell. Both types of damage can be limited by slow cooling, and the use of cryoprotectants such as propanediol, dimethylsulphoxide (DMSO) or glycerol.

Slow cooling slows the rate of water loss from the cell. This water loss occurs as ice crystals form in the surrounding medium. Cryoprotectants also slow the rate of water loss. However, there is a benefit to water loss in that a reduced water content reduces the risk from intracellular ice formation. Cryoprotectants such as propanediol that enter the cell help to reduce the risk of intracellular ice formation.

The current most popular technique for cryopreservation of early cleavage stage embryos and pronucleate oocytes involves the use of propanediol, which penetrates the cells rapidly, in combination with sucrose, which also causes water to leave the cells[16]. This has replaced the earlier freezing method with the use of DMSO, a far more toxic substance that requires a longer, more complicated protocol and which gave disappointing results[17].

*Embryo freezing techniques*

Embryos are equilibrated in phosphate buffered saline, then exposed first to propanediol at 1.5 mol/l and then to medium containing propanediol at 1.5 mol/l and sucrose at 0.1 mol/l. Embryos are subsequently transferred, either to glass ampoules or to plastic straws, and placed in a programmed freezer for cooling. The components of the freezing medium lower the temperature at which ice forms. This is helpful, as it allows more time for water to leave the cell. Ice crystal formation is then induced at a chosen temperature – conventionally –7 °C – by touching the straw or ampoule with a metal object cooled in liquid nitrogen. This prevents further supercooling. Embryos frozen by this technique can be thawed very rapidly by removal of the straw or ampoule from liquid nitrogen, exposure to room temperature for 30 s, and being held in a water bath at 30 °C until thawed; this takes about 30 s. With the use of this procedure, a

75% embryo survival rate can be expected on thawing (see Results, below).

Blastocysts are traditionally frozen with the use of glycerol, which penetrates the cells slowly, and therefore an extended stepwise freezing protocol is necessary. Blastocysts collapse during freezing, but over 80% will survive and re-expand on thawing[12].

*Rapid freezing techniques*

Slow cooling of embryos is time consuming, and the need for a programmable freezer makes it an expensive procedure. Rapid freezing techniques avoid both these problems. The object is to be able to plunge embryos directly into liquid nitrogen after exposure to cryoprotectants. The temperature drop is too rapid to allow water loss from the cells and the use of high concentrations of cryoprotectants leads to the formation of a 'glass' (vitrification) on freezing, which prevents the potential damage caused by the formation of ice crystals. Such high concentrations of cryoprotectant are toxic, but exposure to it is brief before cryopreservation. As some intracellular water may be retained in the form of ice crystals, thawing must also be rapid, to prevent damage. These methods are still under development, but some groups have achieved acceptable success rates[18].

## SAFETY OF EMBRYO FREEZING

Many years of experience of embryo freezing in the animal livestock industry, and with human embryos since 1983, indicate that this is a safe technique. Results published in the UK on the births and short-term follow-up of babies[19,20] have shown no increased incidence of abnormality. However, no long-term studies have yet been carried out, since the oldest child born as a result of frozen embryo transfer is only in the early teens.

Some concern has been expressed about the long-term safety of freezing embryos following the publication of a paper in France which showed that there was an increase in developmental defects in the jaws of a particular strain of mice and that some also developed learning disability in older age[21]. These findings are being followed up and the outcome is awaited with interest. No effect has been observed on the duration of storage of embryos and the outcome of their transfer[22].

## DISADVANTAGES OF EMBRYO FREEZING

The major disadvantage to clinics of freezing embryos is that large numbers of embryos belonging to couples who have lost contact with the clinics are tending to accumulate in freezers. The Human Fertilization and Embryology Act 1990 makes it mandatory in the UK that all such 'orphaned' embryos should be disposed of after 5 years in storage. This destruction of large numbers of embryos has caused concern both in the UK[23] and elsewhere[24,25].

Other ethical dilemmas have arisen following the death of one or both of the partners of couples with embryos in storage, and custody battles for embryos may follow divorce or separation.

Another major disadvantage of freezing embryos is the cost. The equipment required for freezing is expensive, the freezing procedure is labour-intensive and many clinics report poor pregnancy rates following the transfer of frozen/thawed embryos[7]. However, the majority of the larger clinics with active freezing programmes report results at least as good with frozen embryo transfer as with fresh embryos.

## RESULTS OF FROZEN EMBRYO TRANSFER

A number of different factors might be considered to affect the outcome of the replacement of frozen embryos. However, in a recent review of 1009 cycles of frozen embryo replacement carried out at Bourn Hall between 1991 and 1995, the only factors that appeared to have a significant effect were: patient age; the number of embryos replaced; and whether or not the embryos originated from a cycle in which all embryos had been frozen to avoid the effects of ovarian hyperstimulation (FAE cycles).

**Table 1** The effect of patient age on the outcome of frozen embryo replacement

| *Age* (years) | *Number of transfers* | *Mean number of embryos replaced* | *Number pregnant* | |
|---|---|---|---|---|
| | | | *n* | % |
| < 30 | 165 | 2.6 | 43 | 26 |
| 30–34 | 426 | 2.5 | 113 | 27 |
| 35–39 | 331 | 2.5 | 88 | 27 |
| 40+ | 87 | 2.5 | 15 | 17 |

**Table 2** Pregnancy rate in relation to the number of embryos replaced

| *Number of embryos replaced* | *Number of transfers* | *Number pregnant* | |
|---|---|---|---|
| | | *n* | % |
| 1 | 120 | 8 | 7 |
| 2 | 259 | 54 | 21 |
| 3 | 630 | 187 | 29.7 |

**Table 3** Pregnancy rate in relation to the type of replacement cycle

| | *Number of transfers* | *Mean age* (years) | *Mean number of embryos replaced* | *Number pregnant* | |
|---|---|---|---|---|---|
| | | | | *n* | % |
| Natural cycles | 410 | 33.1 | 2.54 | 117 | 28* |
| HRT cycles | 599 | 34.1 | 2.61 | 142 | 24* |

HRT, hormone replacement therapy; *, not significant

The effect of age on the outcome of frozen embryo replacement is shown in Table 1. Pregnancy rates were significantly lower in patients over 40, although there was no significant difference in the number of embryos replaced, and no difference in success between the other age groups. Table 2 shows the relationship between the number of embryos replaced and pregnancy rates, clearly demonstrating the increase in potential for pregnancy with increased numbers of embryos.

The outcome of frozen embryo replacement in relation to the type of replacement cycle, whether natural or hormone controlled, is shown in Table 3. Although it appears that these two treatment methods were equally successful, it should be remembered that patients are assigned to these two groups according to different criteria (already discussed under Clinical management), and it is therefore not surprising that the one method does not demonstrate a significant advantage over the other.

In Table 4, the relationship between the stimulation regime in the originating IVF cycle and the pregnancy rate from the subsequent frozen embryo replacement is shown. These data suggest that the ovarian stimulation regimen used in the originating cycle does not influence the outcome of frozen embryo replacement.

**Table 4** Pregnancy rates in relation to the ovarian stimulation regimen in the originating cycle

| *Stimulation protocol* | *Number of transfers* | *Number pregnant* | |
|---|---|---|---|
| | | *n* | % |
| Long GnRH agonist/ hMG/FSH | 798 | 206 | 26 |
| Short GnRH agonist/ hMG/FSH | 146 | 37 | 25 |
| Clomiphene/hMG/FSH | 65 | 16 | 25 |

Table 5 shows that the cause of infertility does not appear to affect pregnancy rates; neither, in this series, did pregnancy in the originating cycle increase the chance of pregnancy from frozen embryo replacement (Table 6). However, those cases in which the embryos originated from cycles in which all the embryos were frozen, to avoid the potential danger of hyperstimulation, had a significantly higher pregnancy rate.

It appears, therefore, that pregnancy rates following frozen embryo replacement are influenced by the same factors as fresh embryo replacement, i.e. age and number of embryos replaced. The fact that the cause of infertility has no influence may be due to the fact that having sufficient embryos to freeze indicates that these patients are the better responders in each group, having produced sufficient oocytes to have enough to transfer fresh and still having some to freeze. It also excludes all patients with problems related to fertilization, those with a limited response to stimulation and those who have poor-quality oocytes or embryos. The overall clinical pregnancy rate of 26% per cycle compares very favourably with that for fresh embryo transfer over the same period of time (19%).

There has been concern that the length of time embryos have been kept in storage might have a detrimental effect on the outcome of frozen embryo transfer and might also cause an increase in fetal abnormalities. Table 7 shows that there is no apparent effect, although it will be seen that the numbers in some of the groups are small. However, this is the biggest series examined to date, and so far there is no indication that extended storage is detrimental.

**Table 5** The effect of the cause of infertility on the outcome of frozen embryo replacement

| *Diagnosis* | *Number of transfers* | *Number pregnant* *n* | *%* |
|---|---|---|---|
| Tubal damage | 300 | 78 | 26 |
| Unexplained infertility | 162 | 41 | 25.3 |
| Male factor | 172 | 44 | 26 |
| Mixed (male and female) | 202 | 50 | 25 |
| Others | 173 | 46 | 27 |

**Table 6** Pregnancy rates in relation to the outcome of the originating cycle

| *Outcome of originating cycle* | *Number of transfers* | *Number pregnant* *n* | *%* |
|---|---|---|---|
| Pregnant | 96 | 22 | 23 |
| Non-pregnant | 623 | 137 | 22 |
| Freeze all embryos | 290 | 110 | 38 |

## REGULATION OF EMBRYO FREEZING

All infertility treatment involving the use of donor gametes or treatments in which human

**Table 7** The effect of long-term storage on frozen embryos

| *Storage time* (months) | *Number of cycles* | *Number of pregnancies* *n* | *%* | *% survival* | *Number miscarried* *n* | *%* |
|---|---|---|---|---|---|---|
| 3 | 261 | 77 | 29.5 | 81.0 | 16 | 20.8 |
| 6 | 261 | 65 | 24.9 | 80.6 | 9 | 13.8 |
| 9 | 152 | 31 | 20.4 | 77.1 | 6 | 20.7 |
| 12 | 98 | 18 | 18.4 | 79.7 | 1 | 5.5 |
| 18 | 61 | 19 | 31.2 | 80.4 | 5 | 26.3 |
| 24 | 55 | 15 | 27.3 | 86.4 | 4 | 26.6 |
| 36 | 57 | 13 | 22.8 | 73.4 | 3 | 23.1 |
| 48 | 36 | 13 | 36.1 | 78.8 | 1 | 7.7 |
| 60+ | 28 | 8 | 28.6 | 75.4 | 2 | 25 |
| Total | 1009 | 259 | 25.7 | 79.9 | 47 | 18.1 |

embryos are created *in vitro* and all storage of gametes and embryos in the UK are regulated by the HFEA.

The Human Fertilization and Embryology Act (1990), which became effective on 1 August 1991, established a clear rule that embryos could not be frozen for more than 5 years[26]. For all embryos stored before 31 July 1991, the 5-year count-down time started on 1 August 1991. The HFEA made a recommendation to the Secretary of State for Health that the storage period should be extended to a maximum of 10 years[27], except in exceptional cases, such as for young patients with cancer. The Human Fertilization and Embryology Act 1990 was then amended to take account of this recommendation on 1 May 1996. By law, couples may now extend the storage period for a further 5 years, but both partners must specifically sign the consent form to do so. Those couples who had lost contact with their clinics, and whose embryos were stored before 31 July 1991, had all their embryos destroyed on or soon after 1 August 1996.

There has been considerable debate about the fate of these embryos, the genetic parents of which have not been able to be traced. It has been suggested that these so-called 'orphaned' embryos should be donated to other infertile couples or used for ethically approved research projects[25]. Neither of these options is legally possible, since the genetic 'parents' of these embryos will not have given their specific consent.

At present, all couples in this clinic are contacted annually and asked whether they would like their embryos to:

(1) Remain in storage for a further year;

(2) Be allowed to perish;

(3) Be donated to a research project; or

(4) Be donated to infertile couples.

In spite of our best efforts at tracing the genetic 'parents' of many embryos, contact has been lost. Many couples have not been in contact at all with the clinic since their embryos were frozen.

At Bourn Hall Clinic, the embryo freezing programme started in 1984. During the 10-year period to the end of 1994, 3700 couples have had embryos frozen and there are now some 8500 stored. During this same 10-year period, 590 of the 3700 couples have made decisions on the disposal of their embryos. A total of 160 couples have donated their embryos to research programmes and 80 have donated their embryos to other couples in the embryo donation programme; 350 couples have asked to have their remaining embryos destroyed. For those couples who have kept in contact, there has been no problem. The real difficulty has been for those with whom we have lost contact. As a result, in excess of 800 embryos had to be destroyed on 1 August 1996 and hereafter smaller numbers will have to be destroyed each day.

## CONCLUSIONS

The ability to freeze human embryos surplus to IVF/fresh embryo transfer treatment cycles is of great benefit to couples who are fortunate enough to have embryos left over from their IVF stimulation cycle. It allows many couples to have second or third attempts at embryo transfer with, in many clinics, an equal chance of achieving a pregnancy; freezing maximizes the use of these embryos and minimizes wastage.

The Ethics Committee of the American Society for Reproductive Medicine, in a discussion document on the ethics of human embryo cryopreservation[28] states 'The advantages are so compelling that the Committee believes that cryopreservation capacity is an essential component of all programs offering IVF'. They cite the most important reasons for this strong statement as: decreasing cost, decreasing the risk of multiple pregnancies, decreasing the need for controlled ovarian hyperstimulation and decreasing the number of oocyte recovery cycles required for a pregnancy to occur with IVF. They go on to conclude that the procedure 'appears to be safe'. Similarly, the HFEA have encouraged the setting up of cryopreservation programmes in the UK in order to maximize the effectiveness of stimulated IVF cycles and minimize the wastage of human embryos.

However, although there are very real benefits to freezing embryos, a previously unforeseen consequence of this technique is that large numbers of embryos are accumulating in freezers around the world, where the clinics have lost contact with the genetic 'parents' of many of these. The fate of these embryos is causing concern to the clinicians and scientists in assisted conception units everywhere, and has also provoked considerable discussion among the public and in the media about the ethical aspects of this treatment.

## REFERENCES


1. Bunge, R. G. and Sherman, J. K. (1953). Fertilizing capacity of frozen human spermatozoa. *Nature, London*, **172**, 767–8
2. Whittingham, D. G. (1977). Fertilization *in vitro* and development to term of unfertilized mouse oocytes previously stored at –196 °C. *J. Reprod. Fertil.*, **49**, 89–94
3. Chen, C. (1986). Pregnancy after human oocyte cryopreservation. *Lancet*, **1**, 884–6
4. Van Uem, J. F. (1987). Birth after cryopreservation of unfertilised oocytes. *Lancet*, **1**, 752–3
5. Edwards, R. G. and Steptoe, P. C. (1980). *A Matter or Life*, pp. 135–7. (London: Hutchinson)
6. Trounson, A. O. and Mohr, L. (1983). Human pregnancy following cryopreservation, thawing and transfer of an eight-cell embryo. *Nature, London*, **305**, 707–9
7. Human Fertilization and Embryology Authority (1995). *Fourth Annual Report.* (London: Human Fertilization and Embryology Authority)
8. Amso, N. N., Ahuja, K. K., Morris, N. and Shaw, R. W. (1990). The management of predicted ovarian hyperstimulation involving gonadotrophin releasing hormone analog with elective cryopreservation of all pre-embryos. *Fertil. Steril.*, **53**, 1087–90
9. Roy, S. K. and Treacy, B. J. (1993). Isolation and long term culture of human pre-antral follicles. *Fertil. Steril.*, **59**, 783–90
10. Sathanandan, M., Macnamee, M. C., Rainsbury, P., Wick, K., Brinsden, P. and Edwards, R. G. (1991). Replacement of frozen–thawed embryos in artificial and natural cycles: a prospective semi-randomized study. *Hum. Reprod.*, **6**, 685–7
11. Queenan, J. T., Veek, L. L., Seltman, H. J. and Muasher, S. J. (1994). Transfer of cryopreserved–thawed pre-embryos in a natural cycle or a programmed cycle with exogenous hormonal replacement yields similar pregnancy results. *Fertil. Steril.*, **62**, 545–50
12. Sathanandan, M., Macnamee, M., Wick, K. and Matthews, C. (1992). Clinical aspects of human embryo cryopreservation. In Brinsden, P. and Rainsbury, P. (eds.) *A Textbook of In Vitro Fertilisation and Assisted Reproduction*, pp. 251–63. (Carnforth, UK: Parthenon Publishing)
13. Sathanandan, A. H., Trounson, A., Freemann, L. and Brady, T. (1988). The effects of cooling human oocytes. *Hum. Reprod.*, **3**, 968–77
14. Winston, N. J., Braude, P. R., Pickering, S. J., George, M. A., Cant, A., Currie, J. and Johnson, M. A. (1991). The incidence of abnormal morphology and nucleocytoplasmic ratios in 2-, 3- and 5-day human pre-embryos. *Hum. Reprod.*, **6**, 17–24
15. Whittingham, D. G. (1980). Principles of embryo preservation. In Ashwood-Smith, M. J. and Farrant, J. (eds.) *Low Temperature Preservation in Medicine and Biology*, pp. 65–84. (Tunbridge Wells, Kent: Pitman Medical)
16. Lassalle, B., Testart, J. and Renard, J. P. (1985). Human embryo features that influence the success of cryopreservation with the use of 1,2-propanediol. *Fertil. Steril.*, **44**, 645–51
17. Freemann, L., Trounson, A. and Kirby, C. (1986). Cryopreservation of human embryos: progress on the clinical use of the technique in human *in vitro* fertilisation and embryo transfer. *J. In Vitro Fert. Embryo Transfer*, **3**, 53–9
18. Feichtinger, W., Hochfellner, C. and Ferstl, U. (1991). Clinical experience with ultra-rapid freezing of embryos. *Hum. Reprod.*, **6**, 735–6
19. Wada, I., Macnamee, M. C., Wick, K., Bradfield, J. and Brinsden, P. R. (1994). Birth characteristics and perinatal outcome of babies conceived from cryopreserved embryos. *Hum. Reprod.*, **9**, 543–6
20. Sutcliffe, A. G., D'Souza, S. W., Cadman, J., Richards, B., McKinlay, I. A. and Lieberman, B. (1995). Outcome in children from cryopreserved embryos. *Arch. Dis. Child.*, **72**, 290–3

21. Dulioust, E., Toyama, K., Busnel, M. C. *et al.* (1995). Long term effects of embryo freezing in mice. *Proc. Natl. Acad. Sci. USA*, **92**, 589–93
22. Avery, S., Marcus, S., Spillane, S., Macnamee, M. and Brinsden, P. (1995). Does the length of storage time affect the outcome of frozen embryo replacement? *J. Assist. Reprod. Genet.*, **12** (Suppl.), 67S
23. Brinsden, P. R., Avery, S. M., Marcus, S. F. and Macnamee, M. C. (1995). Frozen embryos: decision time in the UK. *Hum. Reprod.*, **10**, 3083–4
24. Saunders, D. M., Bowman, M. C., Grierson, A. and Garner, F. (1995). Frozen embryos: the dilemma ten years on. *Hum. Reprod.*, **10**, 3081–2
25. (1996). *The Times*, London, 31 July
26. Human Fertilization and Embryology Act (1990). (London: Her Majesty's Stationery Office)
27. Human Fertilization and Embryology Authority (1996). *The Human Fertilisation and Embryology (Statutory Storage Period for Embryos) Regulations 1996.* (London: Her Majesty's Stationery Office)
28. The Ethics Committee of the American Fertility Society (1994). Ethical considerations of assisted reproductive technologies. The cryopreservation of pre-embryos. *Fertil. Steril.*, (Suppl. 1), **62**, 56S–59S

# Counselling the infertile couple 16

*Tim Appleton, Margaret Clark and Paul A. Rainsbury*

## THE DISTRESS OF INFERTILITY

Infertility is a major health care problem which has very definite physiological, psychological and sociological implications. The World Health Organization defined infertility as 'a failure to conceive after unprotected intercourse for a period of one year'. A significant number of these will still fail to conceive after 2 years of unprotected intercourse, and it may be several years before a couple realizes that a real problem exists. It has been estimated that between 5 and 9% of couples of child-bearing age in the United Kingdom have a problem in having a baby. Some estimates suggest that this might mean 50–80 million worldwide.

Very often their general practitioner may well have suggested they keep on trying . . . try this . . . try that . . . is the frequent recommendation from the GP and well-meaning friends. What may have seemed 'convenient' in the early days of their relationship now becomes a nightmare. 'When are you two going to have a baby?' is a question they dread and try and avoid, so much so that they will shun social events to protect themselves from distress. The prayers in the wedding service for the 'gift of children' and the injunction to be 'fruitful and multiply' are remembered with bitterness.

Couples suffering from infertility are continually reminded of their situation. When the woman returns to menstruation, there is a sharp reminder that yet another month has gone by – there are only 13 chances of conception in each year assuming a menstrual cycle of 28 days, less if her cycles are longer. The daily measurement of a woman's waking temperature – used as an indicator for the day of ovulation – becomes a sickening chore they dread. Our whole society is based on the family unit. Simple tasks which we take for granted become painful – almost every shop is stocked with goods for the baby or young family; the major stores proudly display their 'back to school' reminders with displays of school uniforms, badges, satchels and useful kits for the classroom; the infertile couple is excluded from this ritual. On one side of the shopping mall is 'Mothercare', on the other an 'Early Learning Centre'. They dodge the prams and push chairs; watch with envy the shopping trolley with the small child sitting at the back; they see the neighbours' washing lines sagging under the weight of nappies, small socks and underwear; they watch their friends fill the car with all the paraphernalia that goes with a visit to the seaside or a day with grandma. The infertile couple are left out – they are on their own.

The stigma of infertility often leads to stress and tensions within the family. They avoid their close friends. It can lead to mental disharmony, to marital and sexual problems, divorce and in some cultures to ostracism from the wider family unit. The suffering is very real.

A couple who have experienced infertility and the eventual relief that successful treatment brings wrote in a letter to the *Daily Telegraph*:

> 'The sorrow of infertility for a happy couple can be compared with the sorrow of bereavement. The 'funeral' starts when a couple first learns the results of the tests which reveal that a problem exists. It continues with surges of hope that a miracle might happen. The sorrow is private, real, and often taboo; failure at any point is always painful.'[1]

The average GP has little time or expertise to provide practical help to the infertile couple. Advice 'to be patient' only prolongs the agony until the time comes when they are too old to consider adoption and the likelihood of successful treatment at specialized clinics is becoming lower. The menopause seems just around the corner and fears that 'she will run out of eggs' or that if a pregnancy does occur the child will be abnormal are only too common. Hopefully, society will become more aware of the scale of infertility and GPs will refer couples for expert help earlier than in the past. It is not uncommon to meet couples who have been 'trying this and that' for 10–15 years, some even longer.

Recently, Child Chat[2], the newsletter of the support group Child, had these comments from couples suffering from infertility:

> 'Although it is mid-October, suddenly everybody is talking of Christmas, the shops are stocking up on and displaying their Christmas goods. For us Christmas is a very painful time and brings with it a feeling of dread. It only seems to heighten your childlessness. Although you enjoy buying and wrapping presents for the children of friends and relatives, a voice inside you is screaming – 'It's not fair . . . we should be doing this for our own children."

Sometimes it is the reaction of society which shows a fundamental misunderstanding of some of the problems. We find it difficult to understand that someone who has had a child can be infertile now.

> 'Infertility is a difficult subject to discuss at any time, but there is a certain understanding for those who never have had children. When I tell people that I am infertile they cannot understand because I already have one child. When I explain the circumstances and that I am desperate to have another child, the usual reply is 'At least you do have a child – you should be thankful for that'. This gives me tremendous feelings of guilt for even wanting another, when some couples have none at all.'[2]

What we cannot tell from that letter is the reason for her 'current' infertility. It is possible that there is now a failure to ovulate or that the condition of the Fallopian tubes has deteriorated. Perhaps she has developed antibodies to sperm or perhaps she was sterilized, now regrets it because her husband has died or she has remarried. Perhaps the problem is not on her side at all but on her partner's side – poor sperm or even none at all. Whatever the reason, it is clear that conception through intercourse appears impossible and her distress very real. However, given limited resources within a state funded health service, someone may have to decide on priorities; that does not mean that we leave her without help – counselling is just as important for those who have reached the 'end. of the road' as for those who do not know who to turn to for help.

Another couple has expressed feelings of guilt for wanting a second child as brother or sister to one born as a result of *in vitro* fertilization (IVF). Their guilt is not because they want a second child but because they feel they would be depriving the existing child by bringing it up as an 'only child'. They had repeatedly tried further attempts at IVF without success. Their guilt, that they have failed the existing child, is in danger of being transferred onto that child. They are concentrating on their weakness rather than on their strengths.

Infertility can dominate the lives of the infertile. One person confessed:

> 'Sometimes, I just long to empty my head of all the feelings of hurt, resentment, shame, anger and bitterness that seem to build up inside me'[3].

Many have found that their relationship with other couples is under strain; their friends have become pregnant when they themselves have failed . . . how can they continue with the friendship with the awkwardness which exists when they meet . . . do they avoid each other, or skirt around the problems . . . often the greater anxiety is with the lucky couple and the unlucky ones cannot understand why they are being avoided, or vice versa. Some couples are able to cope with their infertility, come to terms with it, support each other and remain solidly together. Others have less strength in their relationships and find that they cannot be 'unified' in the absence of a child.

> 'Individuals, who during their younger years have seen their future selves not only as husbands or wives, but as parents, have to make tremendous psychological adjustments to their infertility. They face not only a loss of self as the kind of person they would have become, but loss of image as a family, and with it the kind of life they would have led.'[3]

The new reproductive technologies which have resulted from the work which led to the birth of the first test-tube-baby on July 25th 1978 have raised new hopes for the millions of infertile couples around the world. In this country alone it has been estimated that a million couples of child-bearing age suffer from infertility. It is not just the 'high-tech' methods of treatment, such as IVF and gamete intrafallopian transfer (GIFT) which have benefited from this technology. A better understanding of the processes of human reproduction has meant that many of the simpler methods, such as timing of intercourse, artificial insemination and induction of ovulation using hormones and other drug therapies, have all improved.

Bourn Hall Clinic was founded by Patrick Steptoe and Robert Edwards in 1980. Many countries throughout the world have one or more such clinics, so that the number of babies born from IVF, GIFT and zygote intrafallopian transfer (ZIFT) must be in the tens of thousands. Fifty-three countries with 708 units are now treating patients (Brinsden, private communication).

Justice and equity suggest that all should have equal access to medical care but this would mean stretching limited resources beyond what many might feel is acceptable. Each new announcement in the press or on television brings hope to many but for many others it will also potentiate their distress. The availability of treatment may have come too late for them: they have already reached the menopause; they may not be able to afford it; or they may have doubts about whether such treatment is ethically or morally acceptable – the lobby of religion frequently has a direct or indirect influence on their anxiety. Counselling can help individuals and couples to make adjustments to their life styles, help them maintain the strength in their relationships and equip them to make the choices which are right for them. It can also help them to empty out all those feelings of anxiety, hate, anger and dissatisfaction which can so easily build up in each of us. Sometimes it is enough that there is somebody who has the time and understanding and who is able to listen effectively – to allow the emotions to pour out. At other times counselling in particular areas may need particular counselling skills and we may need the humility to know when we should refer couples to somebody with more experience. A person who knows where to seek that help can be a very valuable member of any team treating those who are infertile. At the same time, if counsellors have managed to develop a good relationship with a couple, it may be more effective for the counsellor to seek advice than to refer the couple onto yet another person.

> 'Counselling is a key element in the provision of any infertility service . . . counselling should be distinct from discussions with a doctor of any treatment he proposes and should be carried out by somebody different, preferably by a qualified counsellor.'[4]

The Warnock Report[5] emphasized the need for counselling when they said that: 'We recommend that counselling should be available to all infertile couples, and third parties, at any stage of the treatment, both as an integral part of the National Health Service provision and in the private sector. We recognize that there may not be sufficient counsellors trained in this field at present, but feel that it is possible for counsellors in other fields to adapt their skills to deal with infertility.' One of the main purposes of this chapter is to help those with experience in counselling methods to understand the clinical and scientific background to the infertility and to help those who do have the working knowledge of infertility to understand the role of counselling in this highly emotive area. The parish priest, teacher, social worker, family doctor and other community welfare workers are in a unique position to assist in the counselling role, particularly when a couple has to come to terms with their childlessness. At the same time, clinicians should not feel that their role is threatened by the involvement of the counsellor. This chapter may help all who are concerned with infertility to understand the problems which infertile couples face and equip them with sufficient insight to join in that counselling role. We will often need to take on the care of those for whom treatment is not possible or for whom treatment has failed – failure is still more likely than success. Support is needed to help them adjust to the realization that they have done everything in their power in exploring all the possibilities and perhaps the time has come for them to concentrate on other aspects of their lives.

Some people have suggested that childless couples should devote more of their energies to considering adoption, service to the community, or caring for the handicapped. There may be times when we, as counsellors, feel we need to help infertile couples come to that realization, that there is more to life than infertility. Treatment, or further treatment, may not always be the right solution. Recently, I was involved in counselling a couple who had asked to review their situation. They had asked for an opportunity to talk over their lack of progress with myself as counsellor and with one of my clinical colleagues. Neither of us made any attempt to influence their decision and we did not know at the time whether our time together had been useful or not, until we received this comment:

> 'I have decided not to go ahead with the treatment offered to me. Since our meetings I have thought long and hard, talking with family and friends – frequently hopelessly muddled. I believe I have reached a resolution with which I can live, my decision is a positive and a life-enhancing one involving a recommitment to my work as a teacher, and a channelling of my energies towards a strength rather than a weakness. Should I become pregnant I would adapt accordingly – meanwhile there is work to be done.'

That decision did not come easily but the outcome for her was one with which she was comfortable and one she could apply with confidence. A successful outcome does not necessarily imply successful clinical treatment. The role in counselling is to help people process their emotions and to arrive at a situation with which they feel comfortable and with which they can live a full life. We need to continually remind ourselves that we are treating 'people who are infertile' rather than just 'treating infertility'. That distinction should underline the point that care goes beyond clinical treatment; that must mean a concern for the whole welfare, with all the stresses and strains that their infertility imposes upon them. Often they will bring with them other concerns which may be a direct result of their infertility or be totally unrelated to it: these too must be our concern if and when they come to the surface. Counselling can be the means which will enable people to uncover those emotions which we all try to hide and which give rise to dissatisfaction and distress and, at the same time, counsellors must be aware that they could unintentionally add to the burdens by imposing on others anxieties which do not already exist.

Counselling must be informed to be effective and can easily become a hindrance and waste of time if it is uninformed or used without thorough experience in counselling skills and an up-to-date knowledge of reproductive medicine.

But what do we mean by counselling? The term counselling is used in many different contexts. It is often taken as meaning 'I asked for their consent' or 'I told them the facts'. Several important areas in infertility counselling have been identified:

(1) Information: whilst this is primarily the task of the clinical team, experience has shown that patients do not always assimilate the information given at a clinical consultation or chat with the nurse coordinator. Tension often erases much of the information which has been given and,

unless written explanations and instructions have been provided, many patients will have not fully digested what has been explained orally. Infertility counsellors will need to be sensitive in detecting where the tension shown by their patients is due to poor understanding of human reproduction.

(2) Implications counselling: this aims to enable people to understand the implications of taking proposed treatments for themselves, their families, and any children which might be born as a result. This will be particularly true of any donor assisted treatments and with surrogacy.

(3) Support counselling: this recognizes the emotional needs and the stress imposed by infertility treatment, drawing upon patients' own resources. It does not seek to provide ready made answers, but draws on the hidden strengths and resources of the patients.

(4) Therapeutic counselling: this seeks to help people cope with the consequences of treatment, helping them understand their expectations and resolve any problems, including the prospect of failure and adjusting to childlessness. It is doubtful whether any childless couple 'comes to terms' with childlessness – many dread the prospect. Counselling can, with time, help people adjust to that situation with a gradual lowering of the stress.

Clinics must take due regard for the future welfare and needs of any resulting child. Several factors have emerged which are common in all donor assisted counselling. Couples should also be aware that the Code of Practice of the UK Licensing Authority requires that information about donors and those treated with those donors is recorded and kept by the authority and that the child has a right to certain non-identifying information on reaching the age of 18 (or on contemplating earlier marriage). This might influence their decision on whether to tell the child/children about the facts of their conception. A child born as a result of egg donation can ask the Licensing Authority whether they are marrying a relative.

These are a vital part of the 'patient's rights', which include education, support and information and which are frequently well catered for by doctors, nurses, nurse counsellors and other health-care professionals who come into contact with the patients. Those roles, while being important, are, I believe, quite different from the role of counselling. Yet it is highly probable that the counsellors will need to ensure that these particular needs have been adequately covered since a considerable amount of distress is grounded in an inadequate understanding of the facts. Counsellors also need to have an independence which may sometimes mean that they must pursue the 'cause of the patients', take, if you like, their side in the pursuit of their 'peace of mind'.

> 'Counselling does not ignore the obvious, but seeks to reach behind it. It requires the giving of sufficient time to help a person in distress to uncover and reach behind some of the less obvious and less acceptable feelings and thoughts which contribute to unhappiness and dissatisfaction. It is an approach which has isolated certain factors in caring relationships and stressed them, while at the same time playing down other factors such as giving answers, expressing sympathy, or actively trying to change the circumstances which appear to contribute towards that distress . . . it is above all an approach which tries to understand what goes on inside people, and how internal difficulties can stand in the way of change, rather than looking at external factors or external solutions.'[6]

We all have to learn to listen more carefully so that we can help others more effectively. Counselling can only be really effective when we have heard the needs of each individual cry . . . there is no rigid formula to follow . . . each cry will be different . . . each approach will be individual, and a careful watch for body language may provide a valuable clue to the direction, or change of direction, which must be adopted. Counsellors within a clinical situation must be a part of the team so that they can listen to both patients and staff; they should be respected by that team so that they can play their part in formulating new protocols as new advances are made. At the same time, it is vital that the counsellor keeps him/herself informed and up to date. It is only by informed counselling that we shall be able to 'seek behind the obvious'.

At one time there was little that a childless couple could do to seek effective help – the new technologies have changed that. In the past, the cause of infertility was always assumed to be the fault of the woman. That too has changed. We now know that male factor infertility is the biggest single cause of infertility, but that does not imply impotence. Injecting the sperm directly into the egg (intracytoplasmic sperm injection; ICSI) has certainly revolutionized the treatment of male factor infertility, but we should not lose sight of the simpler and often more accessible forms of treatment such as donor insemination. The additional 'interference factor' which micromanipulation imposes has led many couples to fight for what they feel is more realistic for them. *In vitro* fertilization plus ICSI is expensive and beyond the resources of many couples and many men have expressed feelings of guilt that, where the problem lies with them, the suggested treatment imposes superovulation on their partner for ICSI to be contemplated. They have often reached a difficult point in coming to terms with the use of donor sperm, only to have that acceptance dashed by an understandable enthusiasm on behalf of the clinician to suggest a new 'solution' such as ICSI.

Childless women often share their problems with other women but few men want to share their problems with other men – infertility has been associated with impotence, particularly in some parts of the United Kingdom. In some cultures childlessness is considered to be grounds for divorce. In many cultures it is the woman who is blamed, even when tests have clearly shown that there is a male 'factor' present.

Progress in the treatment of infertility has meant that we can tackle problems which seemed insurmountable just a decade ago. It has raised alarm bells in our society! Is technology moving ahead too fast? The introduction of cryopreservation of embryos in the early 1980s seemed to provide a solution to the creation of 'spare' embryos in IVF. Those who pioneered the new techniques predicted that the ability to freeze embryos would solve many problems: many couples would need all the embryos they could get; others might want to try for a sibling and 'space their family'. However, the number of embryos going into the freezers exceeds the number being used after thawing. The embryo bank gets bigger and bigger and many couples have been faced with having to make desperate decisions about what to do with the embryos they no longer need. The law imposes a limit on the time embryos can be frozen and the first time that the law insisted on decisions was on July 31st 1996. Couples had to choose between:

(1) Using the embryos for themselves;
(2) Donating the embryos to another couple;
(3) Donating the embryos for research;
(4) Allowing the embryos to die; and
(5) Continuing the storage for another 5 years (only possible with the consent of all parties and when the embryos were to be used for themselves).

In the absence of any of those choices the embryos had to be destroyed after the storage interval of 5 years. For many, the choices were too difficult and many couples admitted to not being able to make a decision and hence left the decision 'to the law'.

Many sections of society have expressed their concern about such issues. We cannot ignore the concerns shown by different groups in our society and we must be careful not to dismiss lightly those concerns which differ from our own – their concerns are often transferred onto the couples who are seeking our help and we may need to help them uncover those concerns. We will need to use a pragmatic approach which puts the modern technology into perspective without forgetting the dream which infertile couples experience. For some that dream will be realized but for many the dream will not come true. Our care must be for them all, not forgetting those for whom the treatment has been successful but who may still need support and counselling.

## FERTILITY COUNSELLING: A PERSONAL VIEW

### The feelings of the childless

Working at the fertility unit has made me aware of the deep emotional suffering that infertile couples experience. In the past, childless couples had two choices – either to accept the childless state or to adopt someone else's child. Readily available abortion has reduced the numbers of such children.

In the past 10 years, great strides have been made to assist couples to conceive and create life. However, these techniques have brought their own problems. First, because there is still a comparatively low success rate, couples often have to face disappointment. Second, the procedures can often be uncomfortable, mechanical and time-consuming. This is a particular difficulty for the woman who is also trying to hold down a full-time job. She faces the difficulty of juggling her working hours to make frequent visits to the hospital, which is fine if she has an understanding boss but difficult if she does not. She also has the problem of how much to tell people. The tension, anxiety and fear can sometimes rise to intolerable levels.

The comparatively low success rate can make it very difficult for the couple to hold on to hope that the treatment will work. They long to conceive and create a baby of their own, just as their parents, siblings and friends have done and are doing. Often, as anxiety and despair begin to build, each will try to protect the other from their feelings for fear of upsetting them. This pressure of feelings will frequently show itself by the expression of anger which only adds to hidden feelings of shame and guilt. It is often at the time when the couple need each other most that they pull back and withdraw into themselves. This withdrawal leaves each of them isolated and the very mention of babies often causes distress. Family and friends often pick up this distress and have great difficulty in knowing how to respond. In this way a distance builds. No-one dares to speak so that as the treatment continues and failures occur, the couple, and indeed each partner, can feel very alone.

In order to deal with this awful feeling of being alone, the woman will often create a fantasy world where she will visit baby shops and buy clothes to store in a bottom drawer in preparation for the longed-for baby. This will often distress the man who is excluded from the fantasy. Usually no-one speaks about it and the man withdraws, feeling helpless.

### Facing the loss

The experience of Margaret Clark confirms that of others that the loss of a potential baby is equivalent to a death and bereavement. The couple go through the same processes of shock, confusion, fear, anger, despair, shattered dreams, depression, feelings of failure, blaming and withdrawal, which are typical of mourning.

In more global terms, childless couples feel in a dead end and excluded from playing their part in the biological future of the human race. They find this hard to accept and to discuss.

The infertile couple's problems have, of course, started some time, perhaps even a long time, before they seek help. When they are told that something is wrong, the first reaction is shock that what seems to be so natural for so many is not going to be for them. Alarm and anxiety usually follow: who best to turn to for help; who to trust, how long to wait? When they finally reach the hospital, there is often a seemingly endless wait for tests. When the tests confirm infertility and need for treatment, there is often more delay because waiting lists are full. There is a feeling of confusion: 'why us'?

Very little of this distress seems to be communicated to doctors. Perhaps our faith in their omnipotence and their tendency to reassurance makes it difficult for patients to disappoint or anger the doctor by showing anxiety and uncertainty.

The role of the counsellor, in being available to help the couple to express these hidden feelings and to do the work of grieving, is therefore very important.

### How to cope with facing the loss

The options that may be offered include individual, couple or group counselling. All these options offer both support and therapeutic counselling.

*Individual counselling*
Because of the overwhelming nature of the feelings between the partners it is not always possible for the infertile couple to come together in the first instance. One, usually the woman, will ask to see me alone. Coming to see me can take the pressure off the relationship and therefore help make the situation more manageable.

Ideally the person (or couple) needs to experience a non-directive approach in the quiet, containing atmosphere of the consulting room, which allows the person to reach the deep hidden feelings which I have described. The awful sadness and despair which, in my experience, they feel when they are told that IVF treatment has failed, is particularly poignant and painful. At that moment they are usually devastated and they lose all hope. It is important for the therapist to be still at this time. There is often no word that can bring comfort at such a time. A silent sharing and understanding is very important.

When the woman has developed more confidence in expressing feelings, I will suggest that, since they have a common problem, they should come as a couple or come to a group.

*Couple counselling*
My experience is that the attitude of many men to their infertility is different from most women and very defensive; 'the stiff upper lip'. They often say, 'I am doing this for her'. The common childhood indoctrination of boys to be brave and not cry, makes it difficult for the man to express sadness and disappointment. He dare not acknowledge that he feels the same as his partner. He deals with this by denial and by projecting these feelings onto his partner. This explains why it is the woman who first seeks help.

Working together with his partner, he can begin to acknowledge these feelings so that they can share them and confront them together.

*Group counselling*
Couples come to the group with the disquieting thought that they are unique in their wretchedness, that they alone have thoughts and feelings which are unacceptable. Very quickly they discover that this is not so and soon begin to exchange their experiences and feelings and obtain mutual support.

They have often been given useless advice by well-meaning family and friends. Common examples are: 'Stop worrying and it will just happen'; 'Have a bottle of wine'; 'Relax'; 'Who wants to be up in the middle of the night to see to a screaming baby anyway'. They complain that they are too often called upon to be godparents, 'a poor substitute', they say.

Christmas and other occasions associated with family are painful times for childless couples. One couple said that last Christmas they had tried to cope by having 'all the family', including several children. They spent all day in the kitchen which kept them busy. After the family had left they were exhausted and felt empty. They vowed that next Christmas they would go away.

The group is a mixed group. It includes couples who have just begun treatment, couples who have experienced one or more failures and couples who have been successful. The latter are very important, as hope is essential. The group is open and non-directive. The therapist is there to facilitate, not direct.

Groups have an interesting effect on men. At first they are shy; 'the stiff upper lip' again! The company of other men, often with the same problems, e.g. male infertility, seems to give them confidence to open up and share their feelings.

Aggression and anger are more often expressed by men. It seems easier for them to be in touch with these emotions than the sadness and pain which so often underlies the anger.

The childhood exhortation to the boy to be strong prevents him from showing the 'weak' emotions for fear of being seen to be a weakling and different from his brothers and friends. The therapist's task here is to facilitate the emergence of these feelings; give him permission to express the rage which is often directed towards the professionals, doctors, health services and society in general.

One man in a group said that he and his wife had agreed that they would go only so far. They could not bear the thought of their whole life being taken over by their wish to have a baby. They had spent so much money on treatment that they had had to go without clothes, holidays and a better home. 'There would have to be an end'.

Another man, whose wife also felt that there was a limit for her, said that he could not imagine a future life without children. 'We will keep going until we have achieved our goal'.

### Conclusion

Support and therapeutic counselling is a vital part of the services provided by a fertility unit. The distress of the infertile state, the fear and discomfort associated with the treatment programmes, the uncertainty of success and the possibility of having to accept failure, are all situations for which few can ever be equipped by their past experience. They can be made bearable by expert counselling.

## EGG DONATION: SOME COUNSELLING THOUGHTS

### Introduction

Somebody once said that the single most important cell in human reproduction is the egg. A good egg stands a good chance of fertilizing easily, results in a strong embryo which implants with vigour and energy and results in a pregnancy. In IVF the likelihood of a pregnancy decreases with a woman's age and by about 38 is declining steadily. With egg donation (where the eggs are donated from a young woman) the pregnancy rate per embryo transfer remains steady and the statement that 'there is no biological reason why eggs from a young woman cannot be successfully transferred to a woman of any age' is borne out by the Italian experience where a 59-year-old woman gave birth to twins and a 63-year-old to a singleton. How far we should go in trying to do the best for our patients is a subject of debate. In my role as a fertility counsellor I would want to take several factors into consideration when exploring the complex mixture of the desire for a child with the feelings and concerns which all parties must face.

This contribution arises out of over 10 years of implications counselling in donor assisted treatments – sperm donation and more recently egg donation and surrogacy – as an independent fertility counsellor working with three clinics in the United Kingdom (Bourn Hall Clinic, Cambridge; The Hallam Medical Centre, Harley Street, London; BUPA Roding, Ilford; and others for surrogacy). In all these clinics, counselling has been an integral part of donor assisted treatment for some years and arose out of an experience some 10 years ago when a couple who had been through IVF with donor sperm regretted their decision – twins had been born but because of complications during pregnancy had suffered severe brain damage. The father, on hearing the prognosis, had walked out on his wife with the exclamation 'well they certainly aren't mine'. A careful examination of the patient's notes showed concern over the use of donor gametes and yet full consent had been given. Similar, though less dramatic, reservations have been expressed by some undergoing egg donation (recipients and donors). Patients had then not been given adequate opportunity to consider all the issues and implications. For some years all patients, after clinical consultation (donors and recipients), have been asked to make contact with the counsellors and over 90% have responded gratefully; counselling is, nevertheless, voluntary and patients have a perfect right to decline. Even those who already have children by donor assisted methods welcome the chance to explore their attitudes further.

**Shortage of donors – what are the alternatives?**

Few clinics are able to recruit sufficient egg donors to meet demands. Waiting lists invariably cause distress and can be from a few weeks to 18 months or longer. Recipients are understandably concerned that:

(1) Their chances might be slipping away?

(2) The age difference between parent and child is getting too large?

(3) They want to enjoy their children while they are young enough and not to be looking after their own ageing parents as well; and

(4) That, because donor eggs are in short supply and therefore 'precious', there will be some selection process as to who is deemed acceptable as recipients!

Sharing eggs has been suggested as one way of overcoming the shortage. Couples undergoing IVF or GIFT are asked to share their eggs (anonymously?) with recipients who need donor eggs. What difficulties does this raise for donors and recipients? Have any inducements or payment been offered or asked for?

Does the use of known donors, i.e. egg donation between friends and relatives, put additional pressures on donors and recipients? Some patients prefer a known donor because they know something about the genetic pool. Is there a danger of a 'possessive' attitude from the donor as opposed to the possibility of reciprocity from the recipient's side, i.e. a feeling that they must be continually saying 'thank-you' to their friend/sister? In some cases the pressure between friends and sisters has been too intense and the counsellor has had to act as 'referee' and help them to resolve those anxieties.

**Counselling**

In the United Kingdom, all clinics treating patients with IVF (but not GIFT) or with donor gametes must be licensed by the Human Fertilisation and Embryology Authority, and must provide proper implications counselling. Counselling should be an integral part of any donor assisted treatment so that patients are automatically 'routed' through independent counselling; this applies to donors and recipients. Counselling cannot be compulsory but most patients appreciate the counselling 'route' and the take-up rate exceeds 95% when the cost of counselling is included with their treatment. Good information booklets which can be given to the patients at clinical consultation, provide the means for patients to explore their feelings together in the privacy of their own homes. Counselling in donor assisted treatments is even more effective if it too can take place in the home rather than in the fertility clinic. The agenda then becomes that of the patients rather than the counsellor and patients will have had the opportunity to think through the issues for themselves and make the maximum use of counselling.

Several important principles have evolved in counselling for donor assisted treatments.

*For recipients*

There must be sufficient time and space for recipient patients to get over the shock of hearing that their gametes are not suitable or likely to achieve a pregnancy. We need to recognize that they often need or seek permission to grieve for what is, for many, a major loss. Something which was alive is either useless or dead and the depth of that loss becomes greater as they progress along the lines of failure – from failure in fertilization, to implantation, blighted ovum, miscarriage, stillbirth, etc.

The best place for them to take stock of their feelings is in the privacy of their own homes and so there needs to be a time interval between first hearing the news about their gametes and meeting the counsellor. The length of this interval varies from person to person and may be just a few days to weeks, months or even years. Given such a gap, the agenda for counselling often (but not always) becomes theirs rather than the counsellor's.

Once they feel that they can contemplate the idea of donor eggs the concerns become more practical but are still intertwined with their emotions, religious backgrounds, cultural and domestic factors, etc. and frequently include the following:

*Why do women donate eggs?* Ninety-five per cent of donors have experienced infertility at some level amongst their friends, colleagues at work or relatives, and when they see articles, advertisements, TV programmes, etc. they are reminded of the joy they have experienced in having children. The majority are altruistic but I am sure that some may have other and very different motives.

*What sort of woman donates?* In the last year I have been counselling all patients from BUPA Roding's Donor Egg programme in their homes. Donors come from all spectra of society, from the unemployed, full-time housewives, through shop and factory workers, domestic cleaners to sophisticated business women.

*What sort of screening is done?* Screening for human immunodeficiency virus (HIV), karyotype (chromosomal abnormalities), VDRL, hepatitis B and C, etc. is carried out and donors are asked many questions about their medical history and that of their family (physical, mental, psychological). During counselling they need to understand the importance of being honest because the law in the UK makes it clear that if a donor wilfully withholds information and the child does inherit a genetic abnormality then the child may sue the donor. Sometimes, during counselling, donors will suggest reasons why they should not be a donor which were not revealed during clinical consultation. Sometimes other members of their families will raise such questions.

*Are there any risks?* Can fresh eggs be safely used? This is an important question for many people. What is best for them? The register of information about donors from the Licensing Authority makes provision for tracing the donor in the unlikely event of abnormalities which might be felt to be genetic in origin.

*Who is the mother?* What is the legal situation? In the UK and within many cultures, the mother is defined as the woman who gives birth to the child, and her husband/partner is the father. Who we think of as our mother is the woman who gave birth to us. Telling the child may be easier in egg donation when compared with sperm donation.

*Should they tell the child? When and how?* Many people might be tempted to draw a comparison with adoption where an open policy is advocated. Others feel that the parallel is not a useful one and that much will have to depend on the child, that no-one has the right to tell a couple that they must tell the child or that they should not tell the child. The decision must be theirs, but it is the duty of counsellors to help them to understand the different options and arguments, bearing in mind that what is said cannot be unsaid.

Does keeping secrets impose strains on the family? Some recent research[7] compared the quality of parenting on donor assisted treatment (DI), IVF, adoption and a control group of naturally conceived children. Preliminary findings suggest that 'the quality of parenting in families with a child conceived as a result of assisted conception is superior to that shown by families with a naturally conceived child'. In another study by Bolton and colleagues (personal communication), parents demonstrated uncertainty on the issue of giving information to children . . . but held positive attitudes towards counselling of both donors and recipients.'

Patients do appreciate being provided with booklets and leaflets prior to counselling. This does not replace the opportunity to explore their feelings during the counselling but sets their agenda.

### *For donors*

Many of the concerns expressed by the recipients are shared by the donors and donors frequently want assurances that the recipients have also been counselled (personal communications). There is often a high drop-out rate, which can occur after clinical consultation, after counselling, or as a result of changing circumstances within their lives. In addition, counselling needs to take into account the following factors:

(1) What are their motives?

(2) The procedures involved? Many donors are unaware of what treatment will be necessary for them to donate eggs. They need to understand the nature of their commitment in terms of time, inconvenience, pain, etc.

(3) Risks? Although the risks are small, many potential donors are concerned about ovarian hyperstimulation syndrome (OHSS) and although many clinicians will have covered this adequately the donors appreciate the opportunity to talk this through with an independent counsellor. The risks which donors take in travelling to a clinic are probably greater than any medical risks from OHSS.

(4) What sort of couples either need or are seeking donor eggs?

(5) Will their eggs be used to treat women significantly past the normal age for the menopause (i.e. about 50)? Many potential donors are alarmed at the use of their eggs beyond nature's normal cut-off point.

(6) Embarrassment? Some donors have expressed embarrassment that they are to be 'subject to the indignities' of a gynaecological examination and egg recovery.

(7) They revoke all rights to their donated eggs.

(8) They have no obligations towards any future children.

(9) Knowing whether treatment is successful or not?

(10) Help in understanding that they should not blame themselves if treatment fails.

Above all, counselling must establish that they are comfortable with their own decisions, that they have the support of their families, that they are under no pressures to donate and that there is an avenue of support available to them all.

## SURROGACY

At BUPA Roding Hospital, we carry out about four surrogacy cases per year, which compared, for example, to Bourn Hall is a small programme. The indications for surrogacy are presented in Chapter 10 and will not be repeated here.

Each case is presented in detail (and anonymously) to the Roding Ethics Committee and is considered on its own merits. We are sensitive to the fact that this procedure is potentially an ethical minefield, so an independent unbiased overview is essential.

One of the more interesting cases is still under consideration by the Committee. A 29-year-old patient was undergoing IVF at another hospital, the indication being blocked Fallopian tubes. At the time of oocyte retrieval, an unusual ovarian mass was detected. Subsequent investigation unfortunately showed this to be a malignant growth. Bilateral oophorectomy was carried out followed by chemotherapy. The patient presented to one of the authors (P.R.) requesting that her frozen embryos (which had been cryopreserved following discovery of the tumour) be transferred to the Roding Hospital for replacement into a friend who was prepared to act as a surrogate host for her.

The case has now been muted by the Ethics Committee and embryo transfer will probably have taken place in a buserelin/hormone replacement cycle upon publication of this textbook.

## FURTHER READING

*All these publications are available from The IFC Resource Centre, 44 Eversden Road, Harlton, Cambridge, CB3 7ET, UK.*

Appleton, T. (1994). *The Pain of Childlessness; an Illustrated Guide to the Treatment of Infertility*

Appleton, T. (1995). *Male Factor*

Appleton, T. (1995). *Egg Donation*

Appleton, T. (1996). *My Beginnings – A Very Special Story*

Appleton, T. (1996). *I'm a Little Frostie*

## REFERENCES


1. Henderson, H. (1985). Adapted from a letter to the *Daily Telegraph* June 6th 1985
2. *Child Chat*, **42** (the magazine of Charter House, 43 St. Leonards Rd., Bexhill on Sea, UK)
3. Brebner, C. (1986). Psychiatrist quoted by Thomas Prentice, Science Correspondent of *The Times*, April 8 1986
4. Secretary of State for Social Services (1987). Government White Paper *Human Fertilization and Embryology; a framework for legislation*, Cm259. (London: HM Stationery Office)
5. Secretary of State for Social Services (1984). *Report of the Committee of Enquiry into Human Fertilization and Embryology*, Chairman, Dame Mary Warnock, Cmnd.9314. (HM Stationery Office)
6. After Michael Jacobs in *Still Small Voice*, (London: SPCK)
7. Golombok, S., Cook, R., Bish, A. and Murray, C. (1995). Families created by the new reproductive technologies: quality of parenting and social and emotional development of children. *Child. Dev.*, **66**, 285–98

# Infertility and the nurse's role 17

*Frances Plowman*

## INTRODUCTION

This chapter will give an overview of infertility, the developing role of the clinical nurse specialist working within the field and the specific role of the clinical nurse in the treatment programmes.

In the United Kingdom infertility tends to affect one in six couples[1] and up to 25% of these will require the services of an Assisted Conception Unit (ACU) in the hope that medical treatment may achieve a pregnancy. For many couples who long for a child but cannot achieve a pregnancy, efforts to conceive may replace all other considerations and the sense of despair and failure can be overwhelming, ultimately placing a great strain on their relationships. Causes of infertility are broadly considered in four categories: failure of ovulation, male factor, tubal disease and those that are undiagnosed (Table 1). Each of these accounts for approximately 25%, the remainder are due to less common causes mainly accounted for by endometriosis and cervical factors. Many couples have more than one cause.

Patients are classified as being infertile if pregnancy has not occurred after one year of regular unprotected intercourse. On average, a normal fertile couple aged about 25 years who are having regular sexual intercourse (three to four times a week) have a 1 in 4 chance of conceiving each month. Most couples will have achieved conception within a year. As women get older they become less fertile, for example, a woman in her mid-20s takes on average 2–3 months to conceive compared with 6 months or more for a woman in her mid-30s. There are several reasons that can account for this. All women are born with all their eggs already *in situ* in their ovaries. An ovum released each month therefore, is as old as the woman herself, as it has resided in her body virtually unchanged for the whole of her life to date.

A woman of 40 is therefore ovulating eggs that are 40 years old. Eggs ovulated from older women may be of relatively poor quality; older women ovulate less regularly and their eggs may have poor fertilizing ability. In contrast, sperm are produced all the time from puberty onwards and they take about 3 months to mature. Men tend to remain fertile when they are older with little decline until after they have reached their 60s.

The emphasis in today's society on controlling fertility through contraception and on choosing whether to have children, has reinforced the assumption that, once the decision has been made to have a child, conception and pregnancy will soon follow[2]. The inability to reproduce can represent a failure to meet cultural norms and affects both men and women.

Infertility can occur in anyone, regardless of class, race or social background. It is generally thought by society to be a female problem, which seems to be more socially acceptable. The pressure of infertility on a couple can cause

**Table 1** Causes of infertility

| | |
|---|---|
| Male factors | 32% |
| Hormonal abnormalities | 28% |
| Tubal factors | 22% |
| Uterine abnormalities | 11% |
| Unknown causes | 4% |
| Cervical | 3% |

Data from 'Infertility' Postgraduate Update Series, 1995 edn. Reed Health Care Communications sexual problems. Sexual problems could be attributed to the couple not making love due to pressure of work and hospital visits or anxieties about failing to conceive. When sex becomes an exercise whose only function is to achieve a pregnancy, the basis is laid for a great deal of tension within the couple's relationship. It is very common for couples to find that they are suddenly unable to have sexual intercourse at a specified time – making love on demand can be very different to making love for fun. Quite often, by the time the couple talk to the nurse in the clinic, their sex life will be suffering.

Patients may bring up their concerns about their fertility at any time: sometimes to their practice nurse; in the family planning clinic; they may have been 'trying' for months or maybe even years. The nurse must remember that it has taken a lot of courage to mention something that the patient feels deeply embarrassed or upset about.

## THE CLINICAL NURSE SPECIALIST

The nurse's role within this specialty has advanced with increasing technology and innovation. The range of skills and responsibilities undertaken can be impressive, although the nurse's role varies enormously from clinic to clinic.

The Royal College of Nursing Fertility Nurses Group (RCN FNG), in their professional survey report[3], showed that the roles of nurses in the United Kingdom working within this field varied enormously, usually dictated by the needs of the doctor and the type of clinic.

It has been widely accepted that, in many clinics throughout the UK, nurses working in this specialty have extended their roles to perform tasks such as venepuncture, chaperoning doctors, giving information to patients and many other tasks. Their skills have developed to undertake specialized procedures including patient consultations, vaginal ultrasonography, postcoital testing, semenology and semen preparation, performing intrauterine insemination (IUI) and embryo transfers (ET). It must be stressed, however, that nurses who are multiskilled need to have clearly defined guidelines for practice and limits of responsibility, as well as appropriately supervised training.

The Human Fertilisation and Embryology Act 1990 states that people having licensed treatments must be given 'a suitable opportunity to receive proper counselling about the implications of taking the proposed steps' (schedule 3, para. 3(1)(a)). The Code of Practice[4] gives guidance to clinics on how to fulfil this statutory obligation and describes the types of counselling that should be available in licensed clinics. In many clinics this has become part of the nurse's role. Nurses should seek recognized training courses to acquire the knowledge and expertise to effectively manage the degree of stress, anxiety and complexity of feelings encountered by couples attending infertility units.

In many clinics it is compulsory for human immunodeficiency virus (HIV) antibody blood tests to be performed prior to licensed treatments. The responsibility to carry out the pretest counselling is usually a function of the nurse. It is vital that the nurse performing this counselling has attended a study day on the topic and attends regular updates.

Corrigan[5] states: 'in general infertility nurses are keen to extend their boundaries. It therefore follows that pioneering and developing the role is essential and should run in parallel to medical and scientific progress'.

Recently the term 'named nurse' has become widespread following the introduction of the Patient's Charter (1991)[6]. The Charter gave governmental approval for 'high quality patient focused care' as advocated by the nursing profession. The concept of the named nurse would provide the delivery of continuous co-ordinated care for couples attending the assisted conception unit. The role of the nurse is to assess, plan, implement and evaluate the care given. This is achieved by applying knowledge and skills acquired through education, training and research. Nelson[7] has pointed out that increasing one's range of technical skills does not necessarily lead to a well-being of the patient. Keywood[8] maintains that all patients, whatever their state and condition, need tender loving care, which is the first and oldest principle of nursing.

The United Kingdom Centre and Council (UKCC) recommendations regarding exercising accountability, the Code of Professional Conduct[9] and more recently *Scope of Practice*[10] have created channels of role development within clinical specialties. Postregistration education and practice (PREPP) within the UKCC aims to achieve, through perceptorship and clinical supervision, a continuum in nursing practice, leading to clinical and advanced nurse practitioners.

The RCN FNG was established in 1987 with the aim of providing a professional focus for nurses working within the specialty, to consider education, support, guidance and quality of patient care. The FNG Committee recognizes that nurses working within this specialty require that their training and skills should be constantly reviewed to ensure that appropriate care is provided for couples as scientific and clinical management progresses. The group aims to:

(1) Promote the development and recognition of the nurse's role in the treatment of infertility;

(2) Advocate and promote the education and training of nurses to fulfil this role;

(3) Define and promote higher standards of care for the infertile;

(4) Provide a source of expertise for nurses facing clinical and managerial challenges in the field of infertility treatments;

(5) Increase public and professional awareness of the requirements for the provision of infertility services;

(6) Promote and support research into all aspects of infertility treatments, particularly those of interest and concern to nurses and to patient care; and

(7) Provide a forum for the dissemination of developments and knowledge in the field of infertility treatments.

The FNG has also produced Standards of Care for Fertility Nurses[11] which cover:

(1) Professional development and responsibilities;

(2) Safety;

(3) Patient care;

(4) Counselling; and

(5) Ethical matters.

The RCN FNG has also produced guidelines for practice for infertility nurses to perform IUI and ET. The following guidelines should only be used as a guide to emphasize the key points when units are writing their own protocols.

**Intrauterine insemination, the nurse's role: training protocol**

(1) The nurse must have a thorough knowledge of infertility treatments and the indications for performing IUI.

(2) The nurse must be aware of the need to ensure that patients are fully informed about all aspects of the procedure including the side-effects and the risk of multiple pregnancy if ovarian stimulation is used. Patients must be offered the opportunity for professional counselling. Licensed centres using donor gametes must adhere to the Human Fertilisation and Embryology Authority (HFEA) Code of Practice[4].

(3) The nurse must ensure that patients are aware of the risk of ovarian hyperstimulation syndrome (see later).

(4) If ovulation stimulation is used, the nurse must understand the action of the drugs and their side-effects.

(5) The nurse must understand how the cycles are monitored using both ultrasound scans and hormone assessments.

(6) The nurse must have a thorough knowledge of the anatomy of the pelvis.

(7) The importance of the preparation of the semen sample and the guidelines used must be understood.

*Clinical training*
The nurse must observe an experienced practitioner performing a minimum of three IUIs. The trainee then has to perform a minimum of three procedures under supervision and assessment should continue until the trainee is competent and confident.

*Practice protocol*
This should be developed within individual units as part of the nursing procedures. The protocol must be written out and the following key points should be considered:

(1) Although nurses are indemnified to carry out IUIs by the RCN, they must always adhere to the UKCC Code of Practice in all professional activities.

(2) Each unit must have a routine procedure for the technician preparing the sample and the nurse to currently identify the patient and ensure the correct semen sample is used.

(3) There must be an experienced doctor available to take over from the nurse in the event of any technical difficulties arising with the IUI and in case of an emergency, for example, if the patient goes into shock.

(4) The nurse must ensure that all patients have been offered counselling and that all appropriate consent forms are signed.

(5) The nurse must decline to perform IUI if she is concerned about any aspect of the procedure.

### Embryo transfer, the role of the nurse: training protocol

The following key points should be incorporated into the training programmes for nurses performing ETs:

(1) The nurse must have a thorough knowledge of the UKCC Code of Professional Conduct[10] and Scope of Professional Practice[11] and the HFEA Code of Practice[4].

(2) The nurse must have a thorough knowledge of all aspects of treatment relating to *in vitro* fertilization (IVF) procedures.

(3) The nurse must have thorough knowledge of the pelvic anatomy.

(4) The nurse must be aware of the need to ensure that patients are fully informed about all aspects of IVF, including the risk of multiple pregnancy, depending upon how many embryos are transferred.

(5) The nurse must ensure that all patients have been offered counselling and all appropriate consent forms have been signed.

(6) The nurse must ensure that patients are aware of the risk of ovarian hyperstimulation (OHSS) and that they have written information about it and who to contact in an emergency (Chapter 10).

*Clinical training*
This will follow the same principles as for IUI, the only difference being that the trainee will observe and perform a minimum of ten supervised embryo transfers.

*Practice protocol*
This should be developed within individual units as part of the nursing procedures. According to the RCN FNG guidelines of professional practice 1994[12], the protocol must take into consideration and include the following points:

(1) There must be a routine procedure for the embryologist and the nurse to correctly identify the patient and ensure that the correct embryos are transferred.

(2) It is essential that the number of embryos to be transferred is discussed with the patient. There must be a routine procedure for making this decision and it must be

clearly documented in the patient's record what this decision is and who made it. The nurse must document the details of the ET clearly in the patient's notes in line with the routine practice of the centre. At oocyte retrieval, a trial transcervical catheterization should be performed to identify any technical difficulties in passing the catheter (known as a 'dummy run').

(3) The nurse must decline to perform the embryo transfer if she is concerned about any aspect of the procedure.

More recently the FNG has published guidelines on transport IVF (TIVF)[13] to assist nurses involved in setting up and developing a transport programme. It is only now with the recent development of TIVF that high-tech treatments are becoming more widely available. This treatment describes exactly what is involved in transporting the oocytes collected from the local unit to a specialist licensed centre, where fertilization takes place using the sperm of the partner or a donor.

Using a central laboratory has many attractions. It avoids the expense of setting up and staffing an additional laboratory. The HFEA does not require transport clinics to be licensed, however, they should follow the guidelines of the HFEA[4] and should be regarded as an integral part of the treatment services provided by the central licensed unit. The Authority may also inspect the satellite unit.

Efficient channels of communication are required if a high standard of care is to be maintained. The central unit must have a named co-ordinator in post, as contact for the transport unit and clear and concise protocols need to be agreed between units to ensure that everyone is aware of their particular responsibilities for the treatment cycle.

## The nurse's role within the assisted conception unit

Many of the couples who attend an assisted conception unit have been fully investigated and have been given a diagnosis as to the cause of their infertility. Prior to the initial consultation with the doctor, the couple should have received written information about the treatments offered at the clinic and the unit's success rates. The first consultation provides the opportunity for the couple to ask questions relating to the information supplied in order that they may come to an informed decision about the treatment most appropriate for them. The nurse then reinforces the details of the treatment. The timing and logistics of a treatment cycle need to be discussed with the couple, and a decision is made on which menstrual cycle the couple wish to commence treatment.

It is important that any couple seeking treatment are given advice about preconceptual care, the risk of miscarriage and the health of the future child[14]. Kiddy and colleagues further suggest that a woman trying to conceive should have a healthy well-balanced diet and that she should restrict alcohol consumption and smoking[14]. It is well recognized that infertility investigations, treatments and the time spent at the clinic waiting for results can be extremely stressful. Many couples choose not to share their infertility problems with anyone outside the clinic, thus increasing the stress they are experiencing. Cant[15] highlighted the need for couples to be able to control part of their treatment and suggested alternative therapies such as massage and relaxation techniques within the privacy of their own homes to help minimize stress.

The nurse should familiarize the couple with the unit's consent forms, the HFEA consent forms if licensed treatments are required and the significance of the Consent to Disclosure of Identifying Information about their infertility treatment to people not covered by a HFEA licence. The HFEA Act requires clinics to take into account the 'welfare of the child who may be born as a result of treatment'. It is the clinic's responsibility to carry out a non-clinical assessment of the couple before treatment is commenced.

Details of an independent counsellor and how to make an appointment should be given to the couple at their initial consultation with the doctor.

## OVULATION INDUCTION

To increase the chance of success, the doctor will prescribe gonadotrophin releasing hormone (GnRH) analogues which act by 'switching off' the pituitary (down-regulation). Whilst this is happening the woman may experience hot flushes and may feel depressed and have headaches. Once down-regulation has been achieved, human menopausal gonadotrophin (hMG) is used to stimulate follicular development within the ovary. Follicles are sacs of fluid, each with a single egg. Human chorionic gonadotrophin (hCG) is a hormone identical in its action to luteinizing hormone (LH). It is administered intramuscularly and mimics the LH surge. Progesterone is given to support the endometrial lining following insemination or embryo transfer and this can be administered intramuscularly, orally or by the use of pessaries. It is essential for the nurse to know the effects and side-effects of each of these drugs so that they can be explained to the couple.

The nurse's role is to co-ordinate the treatment schedule. She will arrange scheduling of appointments for monitoring of follicular growth both by ultrasound scanning and taking blood for hormone assays (oestradiol levels). The nurse will discuss the administration of the drugs with the couple. It is important that the couple understands that the treatment can be quite stressful, with several hospital visits being required. If the woman, her partner or a friend agrees to administer the drugs they will find it an easy technique to learn, under tuition by the nurse who will be happy to teach them following the clinic's guidelines. It is important that the couple understands the need for the correct dose, timing and administration of the drugs to avoid complications. Any woman undergoing ovulation induction is at risk of OHSS; she must be aware of the early warning signs and symptoms such as nausea, reduced urinary output, and abdominal distension and pain. A protocol should be in place within the unit for the management of OHSS, as without appropriate treatment the patient's condition can deteriorate rapidly (Chapter 10). There should be ongoing support for patients and contact numbers should be available for out-of-hours calls.

Ovulation stimulation protocols will vary from clinic to clinic according to individual clinician's preferences. It will be the nurse's responsibility to give couples clear instructions about the timing of their treatment. The following protocols have been successfully introduced in the author's clinic.

### Ovulation induction and intrauterine insemination using partner/donor sperm

Clomiphene citrate or tamoxifen can be used to stimulate the ovaries and should be given orally on days 2–6 of the cycle or sometimes gonadotrophins may be indicated.

*Alternate day hMG therapy*

For a woman aged up to 35 years, the stimulation protocol is as follows: hMG two ampoules (150 IU) intramuscularly on alternate days, starting on day 3 of the cycle.

For a woman aged over 35 years, the stimulation protocol is hMG three ampoules (225 IU) intramuscularly on alternate days, starting on day 3 of the cycle.

For subsequent cycles, the dose of hMG should be calculated according to the patient's previous response.

*Daily hMG therapy*

This is similar to the alternate day schedules referred to above, except that the starting dose is lower, i.e. 75–150 IU (one to two ampoules) per day.

Daily administration of follicle stimulating hormone (FSH) may be prescribed for women diagnosed with polycystic ovaries as these women are known to be particularly sensitive to gonadotrophins and they tend to have high LH concentrations.

*Induction of ovulation*

Human chorionic gonadotrophin, 10 000 IU, should be injected intramuscularly 36 h prior to insemination, when the leading follicle is greater than 18 mm in diameter with no more than two further follicles of > 14 mm.

The ovarian follicular response is regularly monitored by vaginal ultrasonography. The treatment cycle should be abandoned if more than three preovulatory follicles are present over the sizes mentioned above. The insemination is usually carried out by the nurse who has had appropriate training and follows the unit's protocols. This involves the preparation of sperm, either from the partner or donor, being deposited into the uterine cavity via the cervix using a small catheter (the preparation of the sample is described in Chapter 13).

## TREATMENT PROTOCOL FOR *IN VITRO* FERTILIZATION

A long buserelin or Syneral® protocol is used and patients commence on either day 1 or 21 of their menstrual cycle (Figure 1):

(1) Buserelin 500 μg subcutaneously daily;

(2) Syneral nasal spray – two sniffs, one into each nostril, twice daily.

Couples who intend to administer their own injections are given written instructions on how to do this, together with a practical demonstration by the fertility nurse. After 14 days, an oestradiol blood test is performed to see whether the pituitary has been down-regulated. Then hMG is commenced and administered at a previously determined dosage and the buserelin is reduced to 200 μg daily. Ultrasound monitoring of follicular growth is performed regularly and when the follicles are large enough an hCG injection is administered 34.5 h prior to oocyte retrieval. Once the hCG has been administered, buserelin/syneral and hMG treatment is stopped. Progesterone support will commence the day before egg collection and will continue. The partner should ejaculate 3–4 days prior to oocyte retrieval and abstain until

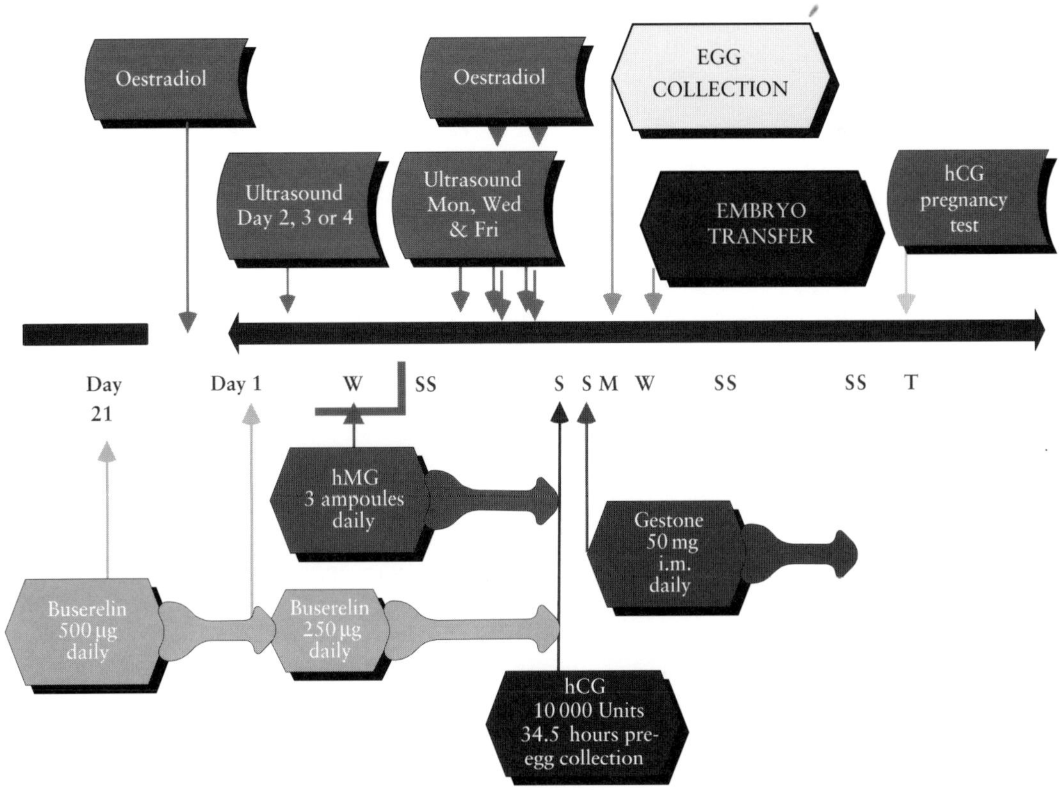


**Figure 1** BUPA Roding Hospital IVF unit

he produces a sample of semen on the day of oocyte retrieval.

The patient will be admitted as a day case for the egg collection. The procedure is carried out in the theatre using transvaginal ultrasound-directed follicular aspiration. The procedure is usually carried out under sedation and takes approximately 40 min. Follicles are aspirated into falcon tubes and given to the embryologist to identify eggs for fertilization (Chapter 13). If fertilization has occurred, a maximum of three embryos are transferred into the uterine cavity 48 h later. By using a small catheter, the procedure usually takes approximately 10 min. A maximum of three embryos can be transferred under HFEA regulations; this is to minimize the risk of multiple pregnancies. Any remaining embryos can be cryopreserved for use in a subsequent cycle. If the woman has not bled after 14 days a β-hCG blood test is performed. If the result is positive, the couple is given an appointment for a transvaginal ultrasound scan to assess the viability of the fetus.

## CONCLUSION

Infertility nursing can vary from clinic to clinic, however, nurses who come into this specialty need to have the correct knowledge and training to effectively meet both the physical and psychological needs of their client group. Due to rapid changes within assisted conception, there is a potential risk for nurses to lose sight of their caring and supportive role, which is essential to this specialty.

## REFERENCES


1. Hull, M. G. R., Glazener, C. M. A., Kelly, N. J. *et al.* (1985). Population study of the causes, treatment and outcome of infertility. *Br. Med. J.*, **291**, 1693–7
2. Pearson, L. H. (1992). The stigma of infertility. *Nursing Times*, **88**, 36–8
3. The Royal College of Nursing Fertility Nurses Group (1990). Report of a professional survey. (London: Royal College of Nursing)
4. HFEA (1993). Code of Practice. (London: Human Fertilisation and Embryology Authority)
5. Corrigan, E. (1996). Rules and expectations of infertility nurses. *J. Br. Fertil. Soc.*, **1**, 61–4
6. Patients' Charter (1991). (London: Her Majesty's Stationery Office)
7. Nelson, P. (1987). The issues to be considered when developing an outline curriculum for an advanced nurse course in fertility control nursing. Reprinted from *Br. J. Fam. Plann.*, 1987, **13**(1). *National Association of Family Planning Nurses Newsletter*, **13**, 32–4
8. Keywood, O. (1986). *Personal and Community Health*. (Oxford: Blackwell Scientific)
9. United Kingdom Centre and Council (1992). *The Scope of Professional Practice*. (London: United Kingdom Centre and Council for Nursing, Midwifery and Health Visiting)
10. United Kingdom Centre and Council (1992). *The Code of Professional Conduct*. (London: United Kingdom Centre and Council for Nursing, Midwifery and Health Visiting)
11. RCN FNG (1993). *Standards of Care for Fertility Nurses*. (London: Royal College of Nursing Fertility Nurses Group)
12. RCN FNG (1994). *Guidelines of Professional Practice*. (London: Royal College of Nursing Fertility Nurses Group)
13. RCN FNG (1996). *Transport IVF: Guidelines for Nurses Working in Units Offering Transport* In Vitro *Fertilization*. (London: Royal College of Nursing Fertility Nurses Group)
14. Kiddy, O., Cant, S. and Corrigan, E. (1995). The nurse's role in specific treatments. In Meerabeau, L. and Denlan, J. (eds.) *Infertility: Nursing and Caring*. (London: Scutari)
15. Cant, S. (1996). Complementary therapies – stress management strategies. *Fertility Nurses Newsletter*, Spring, issue 17

# Subfertility services in the National Health Service

# 18

*Satha M. Sathanandan and Parameswaran Kishore*

## INTRODUCTION

The provision of services for subfertility (infertility) in the National Health Service (NHS) has always been controversial; this is because of the lack of clarity as to whether subfertility is a disease or not. Infertility has always emerged low in surveys of community health need priorities[1]. The controversy is even greater when it comes to assisted reproductive treatments (ART). Even international organizations such as the World Health Organization (WHO) have pronounced that governments are under no obligation to ensure the availability of *in vitro* fertilization (IVF) treatments to any person who may desire to have a child[2].

The purpose of this chapter is to provide a review of the current provision of infertility services in the NHS, to explore the problems and identify a way forward. As the issue of whether or not to provide assisted conception techniques in the NHS is an important one, we have attempted to provide a brief review of the process of priority setting or rationing. We conclude the chapter by exploring the possible future trends in the incidence of the condition and provide options for consideration.

## PROVISION OF SERVICES

Traditionally the provision of fertility services in the NHS can be divided into three levels of care[3].

### Level 1

At this level, a detailed history is obtained from both partners followed by physical examination and simple investigations to test the three major factors contributing to subfertility. These are semen analysis, tests of tubal patency in the form of hysterosalpingogram (HSG), or laparoscopy and dye test, and evidence of ovulation in the form of mid-luteal phase serum progesterone. This service is provided by some general practitioners (GP) or by hospital gynaecologists.

### Level 2

This level is provided by a gynaecologist with special interest in infertility. Usually, there is a separate clinic in which the couple are seen together. Some of these clinics could offer donor insemination and ovulation induction with gonadotrophins. A proportion would offer tubal microsurgery if the consultant has received appropriate training.

### Level 3

Usually, this is provided in the regional centres where there is a subspecialist in reproductive medicine. The centre also has infertility nurses and has access to trained infertility counselling. Most of these centres provide all types of assisted conception including IVF, gamete intrafallopian tubal transfer (GIFT) and intrauterine insemination (IUI). Some can provide micromanipulation treatments such as intracytoplasmic sperm injection or embryo biopsy for diagnosis of genetic diseases. Even though these centres are available in most regions, the majority are established by university departments in NHS hospitals. NHS funding for these centres is patchy.

The Scottish Office Home and Health Department appointed a committee to recommend how the infertility services in Scotland should be provided. The committee's recommendations, which were published in 1993, include the following[4].

(1) Every infertile couple is entitled to receive a proper and well-ordered investigation leading to a diagnosis wherever possible and treatment under the general provision of the NHS.

(2) At level 1, a well-defined initial plan of investigation should be agreed between the GP and the local gynaecology department. The GP should be encouraged to arrange basic investigations provided the following conditions are observed[3].

  (a) The regionally agreed protocol for investigation and management is in place and is complied with.
  (b) The semen analysis should be carried out in the laboratory, which serves the secondary or tertiary care clinics, to which couples might eventually be referred or in a laboratory with a recognized quality control.
  (c) That all patients should be seen as couples with sufficient time set aside for the initial assessment.

(3) At level 2, the investigations should be limited to those which are most likely to lead to a realistic prospect of treatment. The plan of investigation should contain a specific end-point so that both the nature and the extent of the treatment are fully comprehended by the couple. At secondary care level, there should be a separate session for the infertility clinic and at least one consultant with special interest in infertility.

(4) The use of protocols should be mandatory and applicable to all levels of care with some element of flexibility for individual patients. These protocols should be subject to review and updated on a regular basis.

(5) Treatment of infertility should be made available through the NHS for women with ovulatory problems, damaged tubes and for selected cases of endometriosis and oligospermia, and women with unexplained infertility of more than 4 years' duration.

(6) IVF should be offered by the NHS to women up to and including 40 years of age. Except in exceptional circumstances, unexplained infertility should be of at least 4 years' duration. Unless exceptional circumstances dictate to the contrary, women who have had failed reversal of sterilization and/or women with responsibility for at least two children within their present relationship should not be eligible for infertility treatment within the NHS. Patient selection criteria should be subject to regular review. Whether to provide IVF or tubal surgery should be selected by a centre which performs both and is funded for both. We would also like to add that regular audit reports should be provided by all centres providing ART.

### Laboratory services

The Scottish report also commented on the possibility of rationalizing the existing laboratory resources. Highly specialized tests should be restricted to specialist centres employing subspecialists in reproductive medicine or clinicians with a special interest or expertise in reproductive medicine.

The important feature of the Scottish recommendations, is that the committee was formed by medical and lay people who did not have any special interest in reproductive medicine or infertility. However, experts were consulted whenever needed. Although a similar committee has not been appointed in England and Wales, the Scottish recommendations should be equally applicable throughout the UK.

## OUTCOMES OF TREATMENT

### Positive outcomes

Outcome as measured by number of maternities is reasonably good. One in six women need some form of help to achieve a pregnancy during their life. One in eight will need help in their first pregnancy. However, only 4% remain involuntarily childless at their menopause. This means 75–80% of couples seeking help succeed in eventually having a child. Of the patients referred for subfertility treatment 16–25% would need assisted conception in the form of IVF or GIFT.

Outcome in terms of pregnancies is best in anovulatory subfertility, especially where the specific problem is in the hypothalamic–pituitary–ovarian axis. Success is low when the age of the woman is more than 40 or if a significant male factor problem exists. These factors need to be taken into account when cost-effective purchasing is contemplated. However, when assessing outcome, reproductive outcome should not be the only factor considered. The degree to which the treatment has been successful in reducing the stress, distress or social handicap due to subfertility also needs to be evaluated. This could involve for example, measures of the extent to which treatment helps couples come to terms with their childlessness. However, this is difficult and there is a need for the development of valid and standardized measures of quality of life.

A brief discussion on the outcome measures available in the UK is given in a subsequent section.

### Negative outcomes

Although subfertility treatment results in about 75% success as regards achievement of pregnancy, it is important to realize its potential complications[5]. The complications are maximal with ART.

The important complications are:

(1) Ovarian hyperstimulation;

(2) Multiple pregnancies;

(3) Obstetric/neonatal risks;

(4) Possible ovarian cancer risk;

(5) Psychosexual problems.

## OVARIAN HYPERSTIMULATION SYNDROME

Ovarian hyperstimulation syndrome (OHSS) results from a combination of ovarian enlargement and increased capillary permeability which causes a loss of protein rich fluid from the intravascular compartment. Based on the clinical presentations and laboratory findings, the syndrome is divided into mild, moderate and severe OHSS. The overall incidence of OHSS with exogenous gonadotrophins is estimated at 4% with the severe form between 0.5 and 1%[6,7]. The severe forms need hospitalization for management. The factors favouring OHSS are young age (less than 35 years), polycystic ovarian syndrome, luteal phase supplementation with human chorionic gonadotrophins (hCG) as well as the use of gondotrophic releasing hormone analogues (GnRHa) in the stimulation protocols. The severe OHSS is also more common in women who had more than 30 eggs retrieved (23%) and those with serum oestradiol levels more than 6000 pg/ml (20 000 pmol/l) on the day of hCG administration (38%); patients having both these factors had an 80% chance of developing severe OHSS. The use of prophylactic albumin and withholding gonadotrophins and allowing serum oestradiol to fall below 6000 pg/ml before administering hCG are measures known to minimize the development of severe OHSS[8].

Hospitalization and intravenous therapy are mandatory should haemoconcentration (haematocrit greater than 45%) and massive ascites occur. Human albumin is the volume expander of choice at doses of 50–100 g repeated every 2–12 h, after which haematocrit is returned to normal and diuresis resumed. In the presence of tense ascitis, paracentesis may be needed. Thromboprophylaxis is also needed in severe forms. Therapeutic termination of pregnancy may be life saving in those who are pregnant, when all other measures have failed, but with immense psychological consequence to the patient.

## MULTIPLE PREGNANCIES

The incidence of twins from ART is around 25% (compared to 1 in 80 in the general population). While spontaneous occurrence of triplets and higher order gestations is rare (1 in 7925 and 1 in 600 000 deliveries) following ART, they are considerably increased[9].

## OBSTETRIC/NEONATAL RISKS

There is an increased risk of obstetric and neonatal complications in pregnancies resulting from ART, not only in multiple but also in singleton pregnancies[10]. While spontaneous abortion, perinatal mortality and congenital malformations and chromosomal defects are similar in singleton pregnancies resulting from ART and spontaneous pregnancies, ectopic pregnancies (five-fold increase), Caesarean section rate (46% versus 18%), preterm deliveries (15% versus 8%) and low birth weight babies (13% versus 8%) are increased after ART.

## POSSIBLE ASSOCIATION BETWEEN CONTROLLED OVARIAN HYPERSTIMULATION AND OVARIAN CANCER

Joly and associates, in their analysis of 399 women with ovarian cancer, found that these patients had an increased incidence of nulliparity, a lower mean number of pregnancies and a higher incidence of miscarriage[11]. It is also well established that the use of oral contraceptives is associated with a lower frequency of ovarian cancer. Other factors reducing the number of ovulations (late menarche, early menopause and prolonged lactation) are also associated with a decreased risk of ovarian cancer[12]. Based on this, any factor increasing the rate of ovulation could augment the risk as well.

Recently a series of articles published by Whittemore and colleagues focused attention on this association, suggesting that some increased risk of ovarian cancer associated with infertility may be due to the use of fertility drugs[13]. Although this study has a number of limitations (small numbers, no information on the dosage and type of drug used, aetiology of infertility, outcome of treatments etc.) and by no means provides evidence of a cause and effect, it has created a great deal of concern among patients and physicians. On the other hand, a previous long-term follow-up study[14] did not detect an increased risk of ovarian cancer among infertile women treated with fertility drugs, although it did find an increased risk of endometrial cancer. In view of the controversy, this subject needs appropriately designed studies to be performed before reaching final conclusions.

## PSYCHOLOGICAL AND PSYCHOSEXUAL IMPACT OF ART

Infertility diagnosis and treatment represent a stressful experience for many patients (daily appointments, ultrasounds, blood tests, scheduled intercourse, postcoital tests, periods of abstinence, invasive procedures etc.) and are associated with a feeling of loss of control over the situation. A period of impotence is reported in 60% of male partners once they find out they are azoospermic[15]. Sexual dysfunction occurs in 50% of women in primary infertility – the commonest dysfunction is loss of libido[16,17].

## ORGANIZATION AND MANAGEMENT OF INFERTILITY SERVICE

In order to avoid unnecessary duplication of diagnostic testing and treatment and to reduce the stress experienced by patients it is important that all providers of services to a given population agree on and adhere to a common management philosophy and framework. This is likely to optimize the continuity of care for individuals as they move between primary, secondary and tertiary levels of care.

Protocols for the management of subfertility for a Health Authority population should be agreed with the tertiary centres with which contracts are placed. These protocols should address the roles of primary and secondary care in early management depending on the expertise available locally.

To treat couples too early leads to inefficient use of resources as there is a high spontaneous pregnancy rate. Therefore clear guidelines should be written for referral by primary care.

## MODELS OF CARE

### Comprehensive subfertility service

These are centres which provide all three levels of infertility investigations and treatment. At present they are mainly situated in the large teaching hospitals and in a few major district hospitals where the expertise is available. The latter act as subregional centres for the neighbouring smaller district hospitals. The patients are referred to these centres by their GP. The patients could progress from simple investigations and treatment to the most complex micromanipulation techniques in the same centre. As all options are available in the same centre, the decision to institute a specific treatment should be entirely based on clinical needs. These centres are desirable for the local residents as the couple is looked after by the same team and investigations are not duplicated. These tertiary centres may also receive referral from primary or secondary centres for a higher level of care. Unfortunately there are very few of these centres in the UK that are fully funded by the NHS at present.

### Limited subfertility service

Most district hospitals in this country and some of the teaching hospitals only provide specific levels of services. This could be level 1 or level 1 and 2 or level 1 and 2 together with part of level 3. This is either because they do not have a consultant with special interest in infertility and/or the local purchasers only purchase limited service for their population. Once the patient has completed the level of care available without success, she could be referred to the regional or subregional centre with facilities for tertiary care provided the local purchasers are prepared to fund the service. Otherwise, the patient has to go to a private centre for further treatment as is often the case at present. Limited subfertility centres are sometimes forced to offer inappropriate treatments particularly due to pressure by the couple. The classical example is a woman with significant distal tubal disease where IVF is more successful than tubal surgery. If IVF is not funded by the NHS, tubal surgery may be performed leading to poor results.

The ideal cost-effective situation is for the whole range of service to be funded by the NHS. In this case, depending on the local expertise available, either level 1 and/or level 2 can be carried out at the local hospital and the patient can be referred for level 3 care to the regional or subregional centre. It is important that the primary centres work in close collaboration with tertiary centres to an agreed protocol of investigation and treatment so that none of the tests performed locally have to be repeated by the tertiary centre.

There are also some secondary centres where all the clinical expertise is available but the laboratory facilities for ART treatments are not. In this situation, the level 3 care, and particularly IVF, could be shared between the secondary and tertiary care centres. This could take one of two forms.

*Transport IVF*

Here patients have all the counselling, ovulation induction and egg collection done in their local hospital. The eggs are transported to the tertiary centres, usually by the husband, who also provides a specimen of semen on the same day to the tertiary centre. The *in vitro* fertilization of the eggs occurs in the tertiary centre laboratory and the embryos are replaced at the tertiary centre. The rest of the patient care is done locally in the secondary centre. Excess embryos resulting from this treatment are frozen for future use in the tertiary centre. The advantage of this model of treatment is that the patient visits the tertiary centre only once during her whole treatment cycle. The balance of treatment is done locally in a hospital close and convenient to her where she is cared for by staff known to her. The success of this treatment is comparable to one centre treatment with significantly more patient satisfaction. The embryos cannot be transferred back to the local hospital for replacement due to an HFEA regulation which stipulates that the centres handling the embryos have to be licensed.

*Satellite centre IVF*

The treatment is similar to that of transport IVF except the patient has the egg collection and embryo replacement done at the tertiary centre. This type of treatment needs significantly more co-ordination and co-operation between the secondary and tertiary centres as the tertiary centre relies on the judgement of the secondary centre gynaecologist to decide on the timing of hCG for egg collection. Satellite centre IVF is not as common as transport IVF due to reluctance of the tertiary centres. However, one of the authors has been carrying out this treatment with success rates similar to that of the parent centre but with great satisfaction to the patients.

As IVF success rates are higher in centres carrying out more than 200 (medium) to 400 (large) cycles per year, both transport IVF and satellite IVF treatments should be encouraged as a cost-effective and satisfying treatment both to the doctors and their patients. This enables the laboratory scientists in the tertiary centres to maintain their skills at their optimum which is a crucial factor for success in IVF as well as micromanipulation treatments. In this way the NHS resources could be spent in the most cost-effective way without compromising patient satisfaction and reproductive outcomes.

## RATIONING AND PRIORITY SETTING – IS AN INFERTILITY SERVICE A LUXURY?

Health care rationing and priority setting in health care are two sides of the same coin. The inevitability of rationing health care arises from the fact that, while the needs for health care are infinite, the resources available to meet those needs are finite. Hence, there is a necessity to make choices and this means that not all needs can be satisfied and somewhere someone has to be denied access to health care.

Rationing is not a new phenomenon. It has always existed. What has recently changed is that rationing has been made more explicit with each organization trying to identify explicit criteria to demystify the rationing process, often with increasing involvement of the public.

The method used to ration health care depends on the type of health-care system. In a privately funded, often insurance-based health-care system such as exists in the USA, the ability to pay acts as a rationing factor. However, even in such a system there is a need to provide health care for those who cannot afford to pay an insurance contribution; Medicaid is a scheme which provides all 'medically necessary' services to certain categories of poor people. The question of what is 'medically necessary' is an open one and in the USA, different states use different definitions. One well-known approach to define what is medically necessary was pioneered in the state of Oregon[18,19]. This involved asking members of the public to rank, in order of priority, a list of 709 items and Oregon legislature agreed to fund the first 587 items. The Dutch health-care system had to tackle the same issues, and the Government set up the Dunning Committee. This committee came up with a 'basic' package to which all citizens should be entitled. The treatments and service in the basic package should satisfy four criteria: community approach, effectiveness, cost-effectiveness and individual responsibility[20].

In the NHS, rationing had always existed but was implicit. With the introduction of the NHS reforms and the separation of the roles of the purchasers and providers, the need for explicit rationing became inevitable.

The role of the Health Authorities (formerly District Health Authorities) is to assess the health needs of their residents and to purchase services to meet those needs. As mentioned previously, it is never possible to meet infinite needs with finite resources and hence choices have to be made. This has meant that Health Authorities have had to make explicit decisions regarding what type of treatment to purchase, and for whom. Different Health Authorities have used a variety of approaches[21].

Most approaches have involved consulting the public regarding priorities. In public consultation exercises regarding priorities, infertility services have been ranked low. This is especially the case with IVF so that many Health Authorities could sacrifice it entirely[1]. The reason for this may include the public perception of infertility as a social rather than a medical problem; that resources are limited and should be directed at 'saving lives' and above all, the ignorance regarding the condition. In view of this, there is a tendency to regard the treatment of infertility, especially IVF, as a 'luxury' that is completely excluded by many Health Authorities. A detailed discussion of the provision of infertility services in the NHS is given in the next section.

## AVAILABILITY OF INFERTILITY SERVICES IN THE NHS ACROSS ENGLAND AND WALES

There is tremendous variation across England and Wales in the availability of infertility services within the NHS. It is fair to comment that almost all the variation is confined to the NHS funding of assisted conception; in line with the purchaser/provider split, it is the Health Authorities who decide on the funding of assisted conception as well as the criteria for the same. Different Health Authorities use various approaches – while some Health Authorities do not fund assisted conception at all, most do but place restrictions such as age limits.

### National surveys of NHS funding of infertility services

The College of Health, on behalf of the National Infertility Awareness Campaign, has undertaken three nationwide surveys regarding NHS funding of infertility services. The surveys were conducted in 1993, 1994 and 1995. The reports provide the most comprehensive account of the availability of NHS-funded infertility services across England and Wales and include details of the criteria used by each Health Authority[22–24]. The following account represents a summary of these reports.

*Changes in NHS funding*

The NHS funding of infertility services remained static or increased between 1994/5 and 1995/6 in most Health Authorities although in a small proportion it had been reduced.

*Policy on infertility services*

There has been a rise in the proportion of Health Authorities which have a formal policy on the purchase of infertility services; it increased from 21% in 1993 to 57% in 1995.

*Number of IVF treatments purchased*

There were 27 Health Authorities reporting that they purchased no IVF treatments in 1994/5; this includes some authorities who completely exclude IVF from their purchasing programme, while a few others do not formally have an exclusion policy for IVF, but have not funded any. Compared to figures in the 1994 survey, there was an increase in the proportion of authorities who do not purchase IVF treatment, from 22 to 28%.

One method of comparing the IVF policies is to calculate the IVF rate as the number of IVF cycles funded per 100 000 population. The optimal figure for this, as estimated in the *Effective Health Care* bulletin on subfertility services[25] is 40 IVF treatments per 100 000 population. There was enormous variation between District Health Authorities in rates of IVF purchased – from 0 to over 30 per 100 000 population. The rates can also be examined at Regional level by aggregating the rates in Districts: this varies from 0 (in Northern Ireland) to 14.5 (in Scotland) (for purpose of aggregation, Scotland, Northern Ireland and Wales are considered as NHS 'Regions').

*Eligibility criteria*

Over half the authorities use formal eligibility criteria for IVF treatment; of these, the majority specified limits on the woman's age, 14% on the man's age, 90% on the number of previous children, 31% on the length of the couple's relationship and 71% on the number of previous cycles of assisted conception.

Three authorities specified a minimum period of residence within the authority's boundary. Regarding maximum age for the woman, it varied from 34 to 40 in all districts except one in Scotland, where the cut-off age was 42.

With regard to the number of children, some authorities specified absence of children in current relationship as a criterion while others were more restrictive and excluded anyone with any children in either current or previous relationships. There were other criteria used by different Health Authorities, such as the woman must be a non-smoker. Some authorities specified a minimum period of stable relationship (2 years, 3 years, 5 years, etc.) for the couple, while a few mentioned that the couple must have been married for a minimum number of years. All authorities specified a maximum number of IVF cycles, varying from one to three[25], some included private sector treatment in the calculation of the number of cycles.

*Cost of drugs for assisted conception*

There were again differences in the policy on meeting the cost of drugs for assisted conception. Of the authorities purchasing IVF, 59% met the cost of drugs, 27% did not, and the remainder did not give a definite answer.

## EFFECTIVENESS AND COST-EFFECTIVENESS OF INTERVENTIONS

There is an increase in the emphasis on effectiveness and cost-effectiveness in health-care systems all over the western world; the NHS is no exception. This arises from the fact that limited resources available for health care must be deployed to yield maximum benefit; this would mean that interventions, before they become widespread, have to be shown to be effective.

### Outcome measures for subfertility services

A special feature of assisted conception treatment in the UK is that valid outcome measures are available. The Human Fertilization and Embryology Authority (HFEA) obtains detailed information from every clinic performing assisted conception procedures and analyses the data to provide comparative information on outcomes. The following are the outcome measures used by the HFEA.

*Adjusted live birth rate*

Crude live birth rate (number of live births per 100 IVF cycles) is not an appropriate outcome measure as it does not take into consideration the case mix and hence is of limited use for comparative purposes. The adjusted live birth rate adjusts for factors such as the age profile of the patients, the duration of infertility, the causes of infertility etc., so that the effect of these factors is excluded. The HFEA undertakes this analysis and provides information on adjusted live birth rate for each clinic. Since this rate is derived by statistical adjustment, there is an error factor and hence the 95% confidence interval is also provided.

*Multiple birth rate/triplet birth rate*

This is the percentage of births in which more than one child (or a triplet) was born.

### 'Soft' outcome measures

One of the criticisms regarding the use of measurable outcomes such as live birth rate is that it ignores other benefits of treatment. It is known that a certain proportion of couples derive satisfaction knowing that 'everything possible was done' even though there was no live birth. It is difficult to assess this, but it is an important issue which needs consideration.

### Sources of information on effectiveness

In addition to the peer-reviewed journals, there are other sources of information on effectiveness such as the *Effective Health Care* bulletin and the *Cochrane Database of Systematic Reviews* (CDSR).

The *Effective Health Care Bulletin: No. 3* deals with the management of subfertility. *Effective Health Care* is based upon a systematic literature review and is compiled and published by a consortium of the School of Public Health, University of Leeds, the Centre for Health Economics, University of York and the Research Unit of the Royal College of

Physicians. The CDSR has been developed by the Cochrane collaboration. A section entitled *Subfertility Group* is available and included under this are systematic reviews on specific topics such as clomiphene citrate versus placebo for ovulation induction in oligo-amenorrhoeic women, and the medical treatment of idiopathic oligo/asthenospermia: androgens versus placebo or no treatment. The CDSR deals exclusively with specific medical interventions and does not provide any information on models of health-care delivery, or issues such as organization of service. However, the database is an invaluable source of information on effectiveness, especially in a rapidly advancing field such as subfertility.

A detailed discussion of effectiveness of individual interventions is beyond the scope of this chapter.

**Cost-effectiveness of interventions**

This is another important consideration in health-care provision. Cost, measured in monetary terms, on its own is not a useful indicator to judge whether a particular treatment or intervention is to be provided in a health-care system. The cost has to be related to the chances of success or otherwise and this is the basis of economic analysis. For a full discussion on the various types of economic analyses, the reader is referred to a standard text book on health economics[26,27].

The cost of assisted conception consists of the following:

(1) The cost of investigations, drugs, monitoring and surgery employed whilst trying to achieve conception;

(2) The extra costs associated with high-risk obstetric care particularly because of the high incidence of multiple pregnancies following treatment for infertility;

(3) The extra costs associated with increased need for neonatal intensive care as the incidence of multiple pregnancy and low birth weight is increased following infertility treatment; and

(4) The costs falling on the couple and their family.

Of these, (4) is difficult to quantify while (1), (2) and (3) can be estimated. In most published studies (4) has been omitted.

A recent UK study[28] estimated the costs of (1), (2) and (3) and related them to the average success rate to obtain the average cost per maternity. The most cost-effective form of treatment was found to be drug treatment of amenorrhoea where the average cost per maternity was estimated to be £3430. In the case of IVF, the average cost per maternity, assuming a success rate of 13%, was estimated to be £22 491. However, because the success rate of IVF is closely related to the indication, it is misleading to provide a single estimate. A study undertaken in the USA (since the USA has a totally different health-care system, the costs are not directly comparable) provided figures based on the indication, age of the women, etc.[29]. The cost per maternity increases from \$66 667 for the first cycle of IVF to \$114 286 by the sixth cycle; for those with tubal disease, the cost ranges from \$50 000 for the first cycle to \$72 727 for the sixth. For couples in which the woman is older and there is a diagnosis of male factor infertility, the cost rises from \$160 000 for the first cycle to \$800 000 for the sixth.

It is also worth pointing out that in most economic analyses, the emphasis has been on cost per maternity; as noted previously, there are other benefits such as the psychological comfort from knowing that all possibilities have been exhausted which helps couples to come to terms with infertility. A study in Australia attempted to estimate this using the 'willingness to pay' approach[30]. The study estimated the average willingness to pay to be Au \$ 2506; it was found that individuals who agreed with the statement 'even if I leave the service childless, I will be glad I tried it' were willing to pay more than the average. This study clearly provides testimony to the fallacy of evaluations, both epidemiological and economic, which concentrate solely on 'hard outcomes' (such as maternity rate) and shows that women do derive benefit from IVF over and above the production of a successful pregnancy.

## TRENDS IN INFERTILITY AND ITS TREATMENT

It is likely that the need for infertility treatment will increase; the following factors are contributory:

(1) A possible reduction in sperm quality;

(2) Social changes such as women planning to start a pregnancy at a relatively late age; and

(3) Medical advances increasing public expectations.

### Reduction in sperm quality

The question of whether there has been a significant reduction in the quality of seminal fluid over the past 20–50 years is a much debated issue. Carlsen and colleagues[31], based on a meta-analysis of 61 papers, concluded that there has been a significant decline in mean sperm density from $113 \times 10^6$/ml in 1940 to $66 \times 10^6$/ml in 1990, and in mean seminal volume from 3.40 ml to 2.75 ml over the same time. The authors hypothesized that this is probably due to environmental factors. There is also evidence of deteriorating sperm quality among semen donors over the past 20 years[32–34]. While the issue of deteriorating sperm quality is not proven, the evidence seems to favour this, although the decrease could have been a cohort effect. It is difficult to predict whether this is likely to continue.

### Social changes

Two social changes are worth considering.

*Postponement of pregnancy*

Increasingly women are postponing their first pregnancy to enable them to pursue their careers. In 1992, for the first time in recorded history, the number of births for every thousand British women in their early 30s, exceeded that in women in their early 20s; the rate in older women is also on the increase[35]. The tendency to postpone child-bearing is most noticeable in women with higher educational qualifications. In addition, some women who have had children in a previous relationship wish to have another child with a new partner. The problem with delaying child-bearing is that there is an age-related reduction in fertility. The reduction, and eventual disappearance, of oocytes is the main factor responsible for this age-related reduction in fertility[36,37] and higher pregnancy rates can be achieved by transferring donated eggs from younger women to older women[38].

*Increasing public expectation*

There is evidence to suggest that public expectation of health care has increased. A study in Somerset, England, showed that while the prevalence of infertility had not increased, greater use was made of services[39].

### Medical advances

Treatment of fertility problems is a very rapidly advancing field; this makes it possible to provide effective interventions in conditions for which no treatment was previously available. Using techniques such as microepididymal sperm aspiration (MESA) and intracytoplasmic sperm injection it is possible to obtain sperm for IVF from men who are azoospermic. Similarly, oocyte donation and surrogacy further extend the available options.

## INFERTILITY TREATMENT IN THE FUTURE

As a consequence of the factors discussed above, the need for infertility treatment will increase and with the availability of sophisticated techniques the cost will soar. Even at present in the UK, about a quarter of Health Authorities do not fund IVF and most do not fund oocyte donation. Furthermore, increase in demand would mean tighter rationing as it is unlikely that the resources devoted to infertility services will increase in tandem. Faced with this dilemma, alternative ways of financing such services need consideration. Some are briefly discussed below.

### Private sector treatment

At present in the UK, there is a varying proportion of ART carried out in the private sector because Health Authorities either do not fund the treatment, or place restrictions. However, this undermines the basic principle of the NHS and assumes that 'the willingness and ability to pay' should be the main criterion. It is clearly inequitable; however, such inequalities are known to exist in other countries; the real issue is whether society as a whole considers having children as a right (and hence everyone can expect the health service to respond to their need, irrespective of their ability to pay). Unfortunately, there is often a tendency for many Health Authorities to make decisions without exploring all the ramifications.

### Public/private mix

This would mean that the NHS and private sector collaborate; the 'private sector' could include private hospitals, private facilities in NHS premises, private sector purchasers such as insurance agencies and the pharmaceutical industry. The basis of this is that it will be advantageous to both sectors and would ensure that treatment is available free at the point of consumption.

### NHS-assisted, patient-financed schemes

In these, the patient bears part of the cost (for example, for IVF, the NHS bears the cost of drugs, the patient pays for the rest). Already, some NHS hospitals are operating such a scheme where each patient has to pay a fixed sum or the patient is asked to 'top up' the NHS contribution (e.g. when the Health Authority funds IVF, but not intracytoplasmic sperm injection, and the patient is asked to pay the difference). However, even this is inequitable and undermines the fundamental principle of the NHS, as the ability to pay becomes a criterion. It would be more equitable if a means-tested co-payment scheme were introduced (in which the patient is asked to make a contribution, depending on the income of the couple).

## REFERENCES


1. Redmayne, S. and Klein, R. (1993). Rationing in practice, the case of *in vitro* fertilisation. *Br. Med. J.*, **306**, 1457–8
2. World Health Organization (1990). Consultation on the place of *in vitro* fertilization in infertility care. Report. EUR/ICP/MCH 122(s) (WHO: Geneva)
3. Fertility Committee of the Royal College of Obstetricians and Gynaecologists (1992). *Infertility Guidelines for Practice.* (London: RCOG Press)
4. Scottish Health Service Advisory Council (1993). *Infertility Services in Scotland.* (Edinburgh: The Scottish Office, Home and Health Dept.)
5. Goldsman, M. P. and Asch, R. H. (1995). Negative aspects of assisted reproductive technology. In Asch, R. and Studd, J. (eds.) *Progress in Reproductive Medicine,* Vol. 2, pp. 67–81. (Carnforth, UK: Parthenon Publishing)
6. Golan, A., Ron El, R., Herman, A., Weinraub, Z., Soffer, Y. and Caspi, E. (1988). Ovarian hyperstimulation syndrome following D-Trp-6 luteinizing hormone microcapsules and menotropin for *in vitro* fertilization. *Fertil. Steril.*, **50**, 912–16
7. Royal College of Obstetricians and Gynaecologists (1995). *Management and Prevention of Ovarian Hyperstimulation Syndrome (OHSS) – RCOG Guidelines.* (London: RCOG Press)
8. Asch, R. H., Li, H. P., Balmaceda, J. P., Weckstein, I. N. and Stone, S. C. (1991). Severe ovarian hyperstimulation syndrome in assisted reproductive technology: definition of high risk groups. *Hum. Reprod.*, **6**, 1395–9
9. Kerin, J. F., Warnes, G. M., Quinn, P. J., Jeffrey, R. and Kirby, C. (1983). Incidence of multiple pregnancy after *in vitro* fertilization and embryo transfer. *Lancet,* **2**, 537–40
10. Mahoul, S., Manzur, A. and Asch, R. H. (1995). The obstetric outcome of assisted reproductive techniques. In Asch, R. H. and Studd, J. (eds.) *Progress in Reproductive Medicine,* Vol. 2, pp. 23–34. (Carnforth, UK: Parthenon Publishing)
11. Joly, D. J., Lilenfield, A. M. and Diamond, E. L. (1974). An epidemiologic study of the rela-

tionship of reproductive experience to cancer of the ovary. *Am. J. Epidemiol.*, **99**, 190
12. Daly, M. B. (1992). The epidemiology of ovarian cancer. *Hematol. Oncol. Clin. N. Am.*, **6**, 729
13. Whittemore, A., Harris, P. and Itnyre, J. (1992). The collaborative ovarian cancer group: collaborative analysis of 12 US case control studies II. Invasive ovarian cancer in women. *Am. J. Epidemiol.*, **136**, 1184–203
14. Ron, E., Lunenfeld, B., Menczer, J., Blumstein, T., Katz, L., Oelsner, G. and Serr, D. (1987). Cancer incidence in a cohort of infertile women. *Am. J. Epidemiol.*, **125**, 780–90
15. Berger, D. (1980). Impotence following discovery of azoospermia. *Fertil. Steril.*, **34**, 154–6
16. Wylie, K. (1994). Psychosexual aspect of infertility. *Br. J. Sex. Med.*, May/June, 6–8
17. Wright, S., Bromham, D. and Cottle, C. (1990). Infertility and psychological well being: effect of treatment stage, childlessness, aetiology and sex. *Health Psychol. Update*, **5**, 15–19
18. Strosberg, M. A., Weiner, J. M., Baker, R., Fein, I. A. (eds.) (1992). *Rationing America's Medical Care: The Oregon Plan and Beyond.* (Washington DC: The Brookings Institute)
19. Oregon Health Services Commission (1991). *Prioritisation of Health Services.* (Portland: Oregon Health Services Commission)
20. Dunning, A. J. (Chairman) (1992). *Choices in Healthcare: A Report by the Government Committee on Choices in Healthcare.* (Rijswijk, Netherlands: Ministry of Health, Welfare and Cultural Affairs)
21. Ham, C. (1993). Priority setting on the NHS: reports from six districts. *Br. Med. J.*, **307**, 435–8
22. College of Health (1993). *Report of the National Survey of the Funding and Provision of Infertility Services.* (London: College of Health)
23. College of Health (1994). *Report of the Second National Survey of the Funding and Provision of Infertility Services.* (London: College of Health)
24. College of Health (1995). *Report of the Third National Survey of the Funding and Provision of Infertility Services.* (London: College of Health)
25. *Effective Healthcare: The Management of Subfertility.* (Leeds: School of Public Health, University of Leeds) 1992
26. Mooney, G. (1992). *Ecomonics, Medicine and Health Care* (Harvester Wheatsheaf)
27. Drummond, M. F., Stoddart, G. L. and Torrance, G. W. (1987). *Methods for the Ecomonic Evaluation of Health Care Programmes.* (Oxford: Oxford University Press)
28. Ryan, M. and Donaldson, C. (1996). Assessing the costs of assisted reproductive techniques. *Br. J. Obstet. Gynaecol.*, **103**, 198–201
29. Neumann, P. J., Gharib, S. D. and Weinstein, M. C. (1994). The cost of a successful delivery with *in vitro* fertilisation. *N. Engl. J. Med.*, **331**(4), 239–43
30. Ryan, M. (1994). *Evaluating Assisted Reproductive Technology Programmes: An Australian Pilot Study Using Willingness to Pay.* (Sydney: Sydney Centre of Health Economics Research and Evaluation, University of Sydney)
31. Carlsen, E., Giwercmann, A., Keiding, N. and Skakkeback, N. E. (1992). Evidence for decreasing quality of semen during past 50 years. *Br. Med. J.*, **305**, 609–13
32. Auger, J. Czyglik, F., Kunstmann, J. M. and Jouannet, P. (1994). Significant decrease of semen characteristics of fertile men from Paris area during the last 20 years. *Hum. Reprod.*, **9** (Suppl. 4), 72
33. van Waeleghem, K., De Clercq, N., Vermeulen, L. *et al.* (1994). Deterioration of sperm quality in young Belgian men during recent decades. *Hum. Reprod.*, **9** (Suppl. 4), 73
34. Irvine, D. S. (1994). Falling sperm quality. *Br. Med. J.*, **309**, 476
35. Office of Population Censuses and Surveys (1994). *Birth Statistics 1992.* Series FM1, No. 21. (London: HMSO)
36. Gosden, R. and Rutherford, A. (1995). Delayed childbearing. *Br. Med. J.*, **311**, 1585
37. Navot, D., Bergh, P. A., Williams, M. A. *et al.* (1991). Poor oocyte quality rather than implantation failure as a cause of age-related decline in female infertility. *Lancet*, **337**, 1375–7
38. Sauer, M. V., Paulson, R. J. and Lobo, R. A. (1995). Pregnancy in women 50 or more years of age: outcome of 22 consecutively established pregnancies from oocyte donation. *Fertil. Steril.*, **64**, 111–25
39. Gunndl, D. J. and Ewings, P. (1994). Infertility prevalence needs assessment and purchasing. *J. Public Health Med.*, **16**(1), 29–35

# The outcome of infertility treatment

# 19

*David A. Viniker, Terry Matthews, Henry Okuson and Paul A. Rainsbury*

## INTRODUCTION

The fundamental objective of infertility treatment is for the couple to bring a healthy child into a family environment. The desire to have children is one of the most natural of instincts. For those who continue to have difficulties achieving parenthood there remains a feeling of lost happiness and reduced well-being. Several studies have suggested that mothers in particular are more prone to disturbances of psychological well-being after long-term infertility. Depression, anxiety[1], health complaints and lack of self-esteem are more prevalent for the woman; support counselling and supportive psychotherapy are often required[2–5]. Problems with excessive anxiety may be even more acute in women with a traditional feminine sex-role type[6]. Men do not escape psychological consequences, however: they have been shown to have a tendency towards repressed anxiety, leading to a greater risk of psychosomatic illness[3].

In this chapter, we aim to summarize the outcomes of infertility treatments, and also the emotional effects on the families involved. When comparing the outcomes of pregnancies achieved by the various infertility treatment modalities with each other and also against spontaneous pregnancies, allowance must be made for a number of confounding factors. Couples seeking infertility treatment are likely to be slightly older, which confers a negative bias. However, those staying the course and achieving pregnancy by high-tech regimens are more likely to be educated and of higher socioeconomic status, which confer more positive influence. Treatments using ovulation induction, and in particular gonadotrophin therapy, are more likely to result in multiple pregnancy and this is associated with higher obstetric risk.

The rate of spontaneous abortion was found to be significantly greater in women with endometriosis than in a fertile non-endometriosis affected group[7]. Treatment of severe endometriosis before *in vitro* fertilization (IVF) can improve success rates[8,9] and reduce the incidence of associated early pregnancy loss[9]. When there are hydrosalpinges, salpingectomy before IVF may improve success rates (Chapter 8).

Results reported from individual departments are more likely to be from the pioneers or those achieving excellent results. Meta-analyses and national statistics provide a better reflection of the overall situation. Technological advances are occurring so frequently that trends and audit are difficult to interpret: intracytoplasmic sperm injection (ICSI) has resulted in fertilization success where there has been recurrent failure with IVF previously and, furthermore, it has been associated with a fall in the number of donor insemination (DI) treatment cycles.

The first description of *in vitro* fertilization and embryo transfer (IVF–ET) startled the world. Within two decades, however, this revolutionary treatment, for couples with previously insurmountable infertility, has become socially accepted. There are a large amount of data bearing testimony to its success[10–17]. The number of treatment cycles per annum is increasing (Figure 1) and many thousands of healthy babies have been delivered.

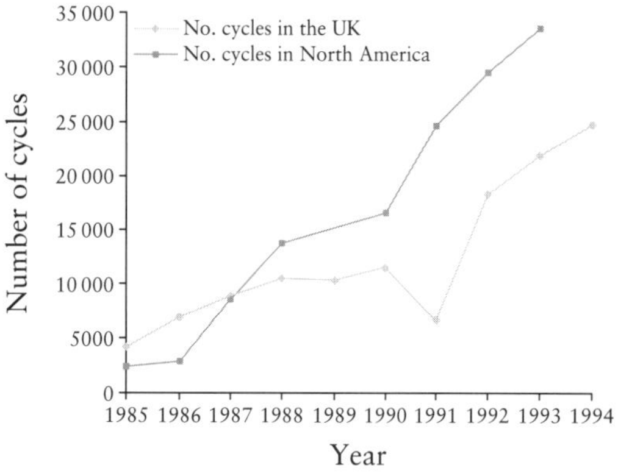


**Figure 1** Annual number of *in vitro* fertilization cycles in the United Kingdom and in North America[10–18]

It is now appropriate to determine how successful infertility treatments have become and we must also consider the risks. Remarkable developments are occurring at ever shorter intervals. Ovulation induction techniques have been with us for 35 years (Chapter 8), IVF (Chapter 10) for 20 years and ICSI (Chapter 14) for 5 years. Cryopreservation (Chapter 15), multifetal embryo reduction and embryo biopsy for inherited disorders are examples of additional technical developments requiring consideration. Each requires not only scientific analysis of statistical data but also consideration of more difficult ethical and counselling questions.

Comparison of success rates, between different treatments and between fertility departments, is extremely difficult (Chapter 8). A variety of confounding factors need to be taken into account, the most important being the duration of infertility, female partner's age, previous therapy, obstetric history, semen quality and pelvic pathology, particularly Fallopian tube pathology (Chapters 7 and 9) and severe endometriosis (Chapters 7 and 23). The Human Fertilisation and Embryology Authority (HFEA) has tried to allow for adverse factors that could affect results between the different British fertility units by providing 'adjusted' live birth rates in their guide for patients[18].

## PREGNANCY

All parents-to-be have natural anxieties about the outcome of pregnancy. Will the baby be healthy? How will they cope with parenting? How will the new arrival change their lives? For couples who have experienced delays in achieving pregnancy, these anxieties may be understandably magnified. A comparative study of adaptation to pregnancy, however, found no increased latent effects of stress in subfertile women in the first trimester[19].

Every pregnancy and baby is precious to the professionals caring for pregnancy and childbirth. Obstetricians and midwives must tread a delicate tight-rope between allowing nature to take its course and intervention when this is to the benefit of mother and baby. A woman who has required infertility treatment, particularly assisted conception, is likely to accept, and probably expect, increased vigilance and intervention during her pregnancy. We believe that there is self-evident advantage, both for patients and doctors, when the team involved in successful infertility treatment can continue care through the pregnancy. Some of the details of the 48 pregnancies (58 babies) achieved at the BUPA Roding Hospital and managed at Whipps Cross Hospital over the last year are presented in this chapter.

## EARLY PREGNANCY COMPLICATIONS

There are many common symptoms reported by patients during pregnancy. Research suggests that there is no notable difference in these symptoms between fertile women and those who have previously experienced infertility[20].

### Early pregnancy loss

Miscarriage is defined as the spontaneous termination of a clinical pregnancy before 24 weeks gestation or with a fetal weight of less than 500 g. An early study of IVF pregnancies reported the spontaneous abortion rate rose from 24.1% for women aged 30–34 years to 41.9% for women over 40 years[21]. This may be a reflection of oocyte quality as miscarriage rates with donor eggs and women aged more than 40 are lower. Our own miscarriage rates have been consistently less than 5% although we have not been able to explain this low figure. The incidence of miscarriage with spontaneous pregnancies is estimated to be between 10 and 20%[22,23]. A meta-analysis of assisted conception has shown a spontaneous abortion rate of 22%[24].

In a study of 161 patients with positive serum human chorionic gonadotropin (β-hCG) following infertility treatment, serial vaginal ultrasound examinations were performed from the 5th to the 12th week. One hundred and fourteen (71%) had fetal heart movements, of whom 106 (93%) had continuing pregnancy and eight patients (7%) had a first trimester miscarriage. Less than 2% miscarried when there had been fetal heart movement after 9 weeks. There were no differences whether conception cycles had been unstimulated or associated with clomiphene, gonadotrophins or gonadotrophin releasing hormone (GnRH)[25].

Harrison and his colleagues[26] have compared the outcome of pregnancies achieved from IVF with those of patients conceiving spontaneously whilst awaiting IVF in the Republic of Ireland. There were 16.5% spontaneous abortions in the IVF group compared with 5% in the spontaneous pregnancy group.

The psychological effects on couples following miscarriage should not be underestimated and when this occurs following infertility treatment, considerable clinical and counselling skills are often required. There is evidence that 50% of male partners suffer significant psychological disturbance[27].

### Ectopic pregnancy

The ectopic pregnancy rate for spontaneous conception is about one in 200 pregnancies. As tubal pathology is relatively common in the infertile population, it is not surprising that ectopic pregnancy is more common when previously infertile women conceive either spontaneously or following treatment[28]. Unfortunately, even when the embryos are transferred to the uterine cavity in IVF there is still an average ectopic rate averaging 4.5%[24]. To date, we have had just one ectopic pregnancy from the BUPA Roding Hospital Fertility Unit.

### Heterotopic pregnancy

Natural heterotopic pregnancy (simultaneous intrauterine and extrauterine gestation) is a relatively rare condition occurring once in 30 000 pregnancies. Infertility is associated with an increased risk of ectopic pregnancy and ovulation induction increases the chance of multiple pregnancy. The incidence of heterotopic pregnancy has increased in recent years as a result of assisted reproductive technology. Ultrasound has improved early diagnosis; with skillful treatment, the outcome of the intrauterine pregnancy has improved. In a study of the English literature, Tal and his colleagues[29] found 139 case reports. The incidence of heterotopic pregnancy with assisted reproductive technology was about 1 : 100. The ectopic pregnancy was in a Fallopian tube in 89% of cases and the ectopic was in the cornua in six cases. Two-thirds of the intrauterine pregnancies resulted in livebirths; 76 deliveries were singleton, 13 were twins and three were triplets.

## MULTIPLE PREGNANCY

Infertility treatments involving ovulation induction are associated with a higher incidence of multiple pregnancy[24,30]. Attention has largely focused on assisted conception, which in the UK requires documentation of outcome. An Australian epidemiological study of twin confinements delivered in 1991 found that there were nearly twice as many twin confinements associated with ovarian stimulation given alone as with IVF and gamete intrafallopian transfer (GIFT) combined[31]. Table 1 summarizes our latest year's experience with pregnancies achieved at the BUPA Roding Hospital and managed at Whipps Cross Hospital.

The incidence of twin pregnancy in a meta-analysis of 26 498 deliveries achieved by assisted reproductive technology (ART)

**Table 1** Numbers of pregnancies achieved at the BUPA Roding Hospital and managed at Whipps Cross Hospital in 1995

| *Order* | *Number* |
|---|---|
| Singleton | 40 |
| Twins | 5 |
| Triplets | 3 |
| Total | 48 |

showed a 25-fold increased incidence of twins (23.3%) and a 350-fold increase in the incidence of triplets (4.4%)[24]. A study from France compared the perinatal outcome of twin pregnancies in three groups of patients[32]. The first group had IVF–ET ($n$ = 72), the second had ovarian stimulation only ($n$ = 82) and the third group were spontaneous ($n$ = 164). The patients in the IVF–ET group were older and of higher socioeconomic class. The Caesarean section rate for the IVF–ET twins was significantly higher (54.2% compared to 41.5% and 43.3% in the other groups, respectively). There were no significant differences in the rates for prematurity, growth retardation or perinatal mortality.

Multiple pregnancy constitutes a 'high-risk' in obstetrics as there is an increased risk for most important complications. Maternal problems include anaemia, urinary tract infection, hypertension and haemorrhage (antepartum and postpartum). Rates for miscarriage, low birth weight from prematurity and growth retardation, and increased perinatal mortality are more common for twins; higher order multiple pregnancy rates are associated with an even greater incidence of complications.

## Higher order pregnancies

The higher order (triplet and quadruplet) birth rates rose from 3.5 per 10 000 in 1982 to 10.9 per 10 000 in 1990 in the State of Victoria, Australia. Of these, 42% were attributable to ART in 1990[33]. In the other Australian states, the birth rates for higher order pregnancy increased nearly twice as much during this period[33]. Friedler and associates[34] analyzed the data on 151 triplets. Fifty-six had been conceived with ART, 55 after gonadotrophin therapy, 27 following clomiphene citrate and 13 were spontaneous. The mean gestational age following ART was 33.2 weeks and was not different from those conceived following gonadotrophins (33.4 weeks) or clomiphene citrate (34.2 weeks) but these were significantly less than in spontaneous conception (35.3 weeks). The mean birth weight following ART (1743 g) did not significantly differ from those after gonadotrophin therapy or clomiphene but was significantly less than after spontaneous conception (1963 g). There was no significant difference in perinatal mortality between the groups.

## Selective termination

The majority of pregnancies with three early gestation sacs reduce spontaneously. In a study of 38 pregnancies in which there were three gestation sacs between 21 and 28 days following ART, 18.4% delivered singletons, 31.6% twins and 47.4% triplets and only one patient spontaneously miscarried all three embryos. Even when all three embryos showed fetal heart beats, only 69.2% delivered triplets[35].

Selective termination is usually associated with the termination of one fetus that has an abnormality in a multiple pregnancy. The objective is to allow the pregnancy to continue with the expectation that the remaining healthy infant(s) will be delivered. Multifetal pregnancy reduction is the termination of one or more apparently healthy fetuses with the objective of reducing the risks of extreme premature delivery associated with higher order multiple pregnancies. From our own data in The North Thames Regional Health Authority, the neonatal death rate for a singleton pregnancy is 3.4, for twins is 25.4 and for higher order it is 93.8 (Hilder, personal communication). Multifetal pregnancy reduction has improved the perinatal outcome for pregnancy with four or more fetuses[36], although the procedure carries a risk of losing the entire pregnancy (9%). For the remaining 91%, the evidence is generally reassuring[37].

We have had six triplet pregnancies from the BUPA Roding Hospital Fertility Unit and we have felt it appropriate to discuss the question of selective embryo reduction with the parents. The first two couples elected to undergo the procedure. They were referred to different appropriate specialist units in London; sadly, following selective termination, both pregnancies miscarried completely. The last four couples decided against selective termination. One developed pre-eclampsia and was delivered by Caesarean section at 32 weeks' gestation. Two pregnancies were uneventful and were delivered by elective Caesarean section at 36 weeks gestation. All nine babies are healthy. The sixth has reached 29 weeks' gestation at the time of writing. It is our policy to offer admission for rest at 26 weeks' gestation and to commence steroid administration[38].

The ethical issues relating to selective termination of an anomalous fetus are identical to those pertaining to pregnancy termination of a singleton fetus with significant abnormality. The ethics of multifetal pregnancy reduction is a more difficult area as it involves the sacrifice of one or more normal fetuses in the belief that this will improve the chances of healthy survival of the remainder. Long-term paediatric and psychological follow-up of surviving offspring and their parents subsequent to multifetal pregnancy reduction has been carried out in Holland[39]. There were no apparent adverse effects on either the infants or their families subject to adequate counselling before and after the procedure.

Selective embryo transfer is becoming an option for couples at risk of transmitting inherited disorders. The embryos are produced by standard IVF techniques. Three days after insemination one or two cells are removed from the 6–10 cell embryos. Up to 25% of the embryo is removed during the procedure. In one recent series of 16 pregnancies following IVF–ET of embryos biopsied, including four sets of twins, 15 healthy infants were delivered[40].

## MODE OF DELIVERY

The decision to undertake a Caesarean delivery is usually reached by taking into acount a combination of factors. A history of infertility, particularly when pregnancy has been achieved after many years and perhaps following high-tech treatment, is generally considered to be one factor in favour of operative delivery. For these women, nature has needed assistance and 'natural childbirth' may not sound quite so appealing. Maternal age tends to be higher than average and hypertension and placental insufficiency are more likely. There is a reduced chance of further pregnancy so that the small risks associated with Caesarean section scars in future pregnancy do not constitute a significant clinical problem. Multiple pregnancy is more common when ovulation induction has been required and would be an additional factor in favour of elective Caesarean section.

During the last 20 years there has been a rise of Caesarean section rates in industrialized countries[41–44] but this may be stabilizing at about 23% in the United States[44]. The increased rate of Caesarean section has probably not resulted in a rise in maternal complications and there may have been a favourable influence on infant morbidity[41].

The debate on whether obstetricians undertake too many or too few Caesarean sections can never be resolved because it is impossible to state what the 'ideal' operative delivery rates should be. There are those who believe that many Caesarean sections are performed unnecessarily[45,46], although individual auditors frequently give inconsistent assessment when faced with identical information at different times[45]. Some of the increase in Caesarean section rates can be attributed to patient request[43]. Ultimately, it should be for the individual informed patient to decide with her obstetrician how they plan delivery. Safety and patient satisfaction are the quality measures that should be audited.

In the Dublin study, the Caesarean section rate for women conceiving with IVF was 55.7% compared to 10.9% in the group conceiving spontaneously whilst awaiting IVF[26]. In a meta-analysis of five studies totalling 1343 deliveries, the Caesarean section rate for singletons was 46.4% compared to 18.2% of the controls and for twins the Caesarean section rate was 64.1% compared to 52.4% of the controls[24]. In our series of 48 deliveries, 18 (37.5%) were spontaneous vaginal deliveries, six (12.5%) were instrumental and 24 (50%) were by Caesarean section.

A comparative study in Michigan, using a specially designed questionnaire completed at the postnatal assessment, demonstrated no apparent latent effects of the stress of infertility[19].

## THE BABIES

### Take-home-baby rate

Ultimately successful treatment of infertility results in a couple taking home a healthy baby. For the couple to achieve this ultimate goal, a number of hurdles must be successfully overcome. If we consider IVF, these hurdles are as follows:

(1) Adequate follicular development;

(2) Egg collection;

(3) Fertilization;

(4) Embryo transfer;

(5) Implantation (positive pregnancy test);

(6) Clinical pregnancy (fetal heart movement seen on ultrasound examination);

(7) The pregnancy must not miscarry;

(8) Negative antenatal screening tests (e.g. screening for Down's syndrome and spina bifida);

(9) Pregnancy complications (e.g. hypertension, placental insufficiency);

(10) Livebirth (preferably not premature); and

(11) Neonatal complications (including neonatal death).

For fertile couples, the conception rate in early cycles is at best 30%. It would be optimistic to believe that for couples with infertility, treatment even with ART would prove to have greater success. There is, therefore, likely to be merit in quoting success rates over a given number of treatment cycles[47]. Cumulative pregnancy rates have been quoted for oral ovulation induction[48,49], intrauterine insemination[50], IVF and ICSI[51].

### Live birth rate

The live birth rate is the most widely accepted measure of success in fertility treatment. The overall pregnancy rate for IVF seems to be settling at about 18% per treatment cycle and the live birth rate at 14% (Figure 2). There are many confounding factors that influence the birth rate, maternal age being the most important (Figure 3). For older women, donated eggs appear to provide significantly better success (Figure 3). *In vitro* fertilization is associated with a relatively high incidence of multiple pregnancy (Figure 4) and perinatal loss is increased with multiple pregnancy (Figure 5). In the latest HFEA annual report of British centres[18], there were 19 983 IVF treatment cycles with a live birth rate of 14.9% (Figure 6) (range 5–23%; the BUPA Roding Hospital is centre number 3).

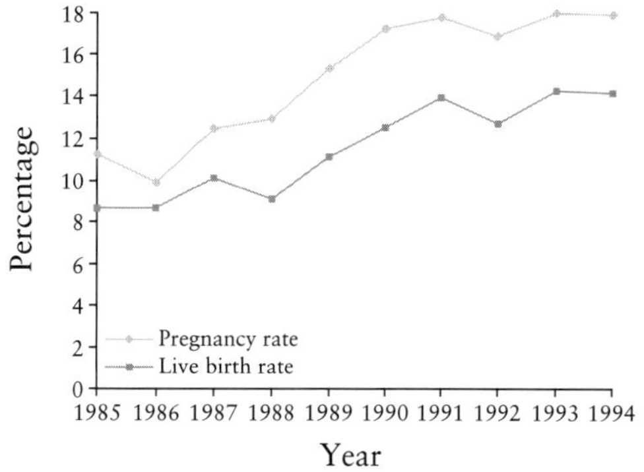


**Figure 2** *In vitro* fertilization pregnancy rate (%) and live birth rate (%) per treatment cycle in the United Kingdom[18]

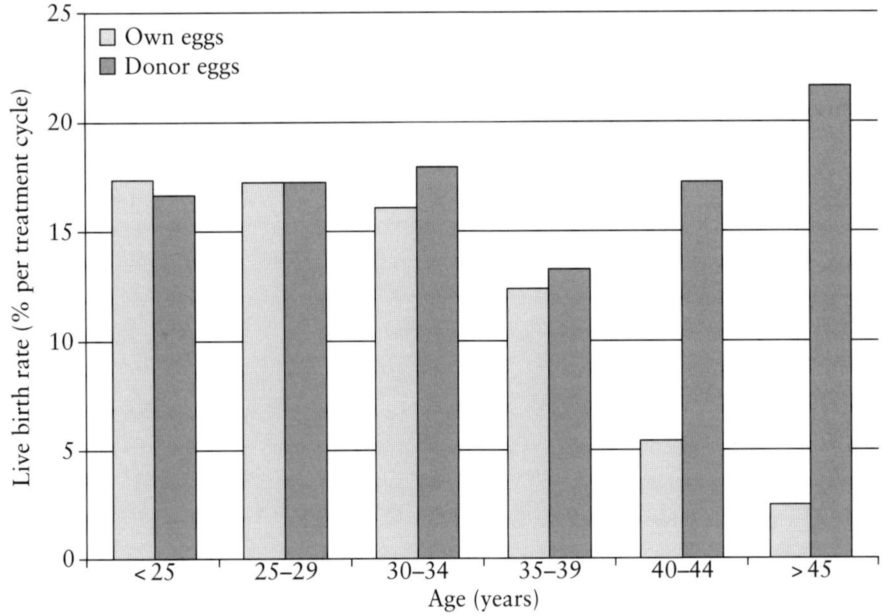


**Figure 3** Live birth rate from *in vitro* fertilization by woman's age (% per treatment cycle; United Kingdom, 1994–95)[18]

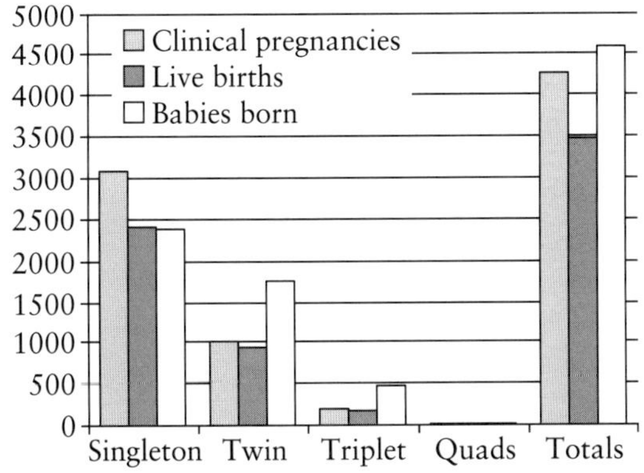


**Figure 4** Single and multiple clinical pregnancy outcomes after *in vitro* fertilization (United Kingdom, 1994–95)[18]

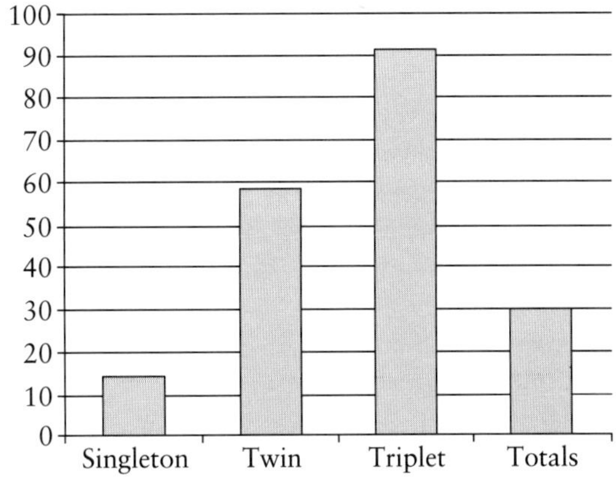


**Figure 5** Perinatal deaths (per 1000 births) in pregnancies achieved through *in vitro* fertilization (United Kingdom, 1994–95)[18]

## LOW BIRTH WEIGHT

A birth weight of less than 2500 g occurs in 7% of deliveries. The three factors associated with low birth weight are prematurity, intrauterine growth retardation and multiple pregnancy. There is evidence that there is a relatively high incidence of preterm labour and low birth weight babies following IVF[52]. Small-for-gestational-age remains more prevalent even for singleton IVF babies. Analysis by multiple regression demonstrated that hypertension and antepartum haemorrhage were independent

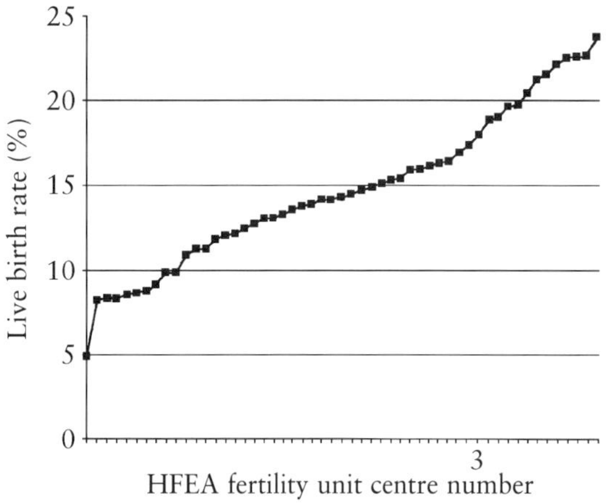


**Figure 6** Live birth rate per *in vitro* fertilization treatment cycle (United Kingdom; BUPA Roding Hospital is centre number 3)[18]

factors[52]. In our own recent series of 58 babies, none had a birth weight of less than 2000 g, 12 had birth weights between 2000 and 2500 g and four had birth weights greater than 4000 g. All were delivered beyond 32 weeks' gestation.

### Premature delivery

Delivery before 37 weeks gestation occurs in 8% of spontaneous singleton pregnancies and in 15% following ART[24]. Premature delivery occurs in 51% of twins in spontaneous and also ART pregnancies[24]. Premature delivery is associated with an increased risk of perinatal mortality and morbidity and all ART pregnancies should therefore be clinically managed as high-risk.

### Neonatal care

In a retrospective study of neonatal intensive care unit admissions in a hospital with a large IVF programme, the IVF livebirths accounted for only 5.1% of total ventilator bed days[53]. The IVF babies were more likely to require ventilation when compared to non-IVF booked livebirths, mainly as a result of multiple pregnancy and prematurity. Singleton IVF babies, however, were still at increased risk of requiring ventilatory support.

### Congenital abnormality rate

Children conceived after donor insemination are at similar risk for congenital anomalies as normally conceived children and there is evidence that they experience a significantly lower rate of family dissolution[54]. There is no apparent increased risk of congenital abnormality with clomiphene citrate or gonadotrophin therapy[55].

*In vitro* conception and additional technological advances, including ICSI and cryopreservation of embryos, circumvent natural selection. In IVF the dominant follicle is in competition with an average of ten follicles, and sperm that would never have reached an ovum, are placed in direct contact with the female gametes. There has been understandable concern that the children of ART will be at greater risk of problems than those conceived naturally. The mean maternal age of mothers following ART is greater than for spontaneous conception mothers and fetal chromosome abnormalities, notably Down's syndrome, is more common with increasing maternal age.

So far, the universal evidence has been reassuring, with the prevalence of congenital abnormality following IVF being no higher than the general population. This has been reported from France[30], Canada[56], England[57], Sweden[58], and Israel[59], with reported rates at about 1.8%[24]. Intracytoplasmic sperm injection (Chapter 14) and cryopreservation of embryos[60] (Chapter 15) do not appear to increase the incidence of congenital abnormality.

### Perinatal mortality rate

There are a variety of terms used to define fetal demise around the time of delivery. Different countries may use different definitions and may change their definitions over time so that comparisons need to be made with caution. Perinatal mortality rate is the number of fetal deaths after 24 weeks' gestation and neonatal deaths during the first 7 days after delivery per 1000 deliveries. The stillbirth rate is the number of fetal deaths per 1000 deliveries beyond 24 weeks' gestation and the neonatal mortality rate is the number of deaths of liveborn infants occurring in the first 28 days of life per 1000 live births. Although the overall perinatal mortality rate of ART is at least double the rate for spontaneous pregnancy, this seems to be related to the relatively high incidence of multiple pregnancy associated with ART. The perinatal mortality rates for singleton pregnancy in ART conceptions is similar to the rate for spontaneous conception[24].

## THE CHILD AND LATE SEQUELAE OF INFERTILITY TREATMENT

For those who sadly do not achieve parenthood even with ART, there is at least the knowledge that all avenues have been explored.

Should management of infertile couples by specialists cease at the point of conception, establishment of pregnancy, delivery, or are there sufficient problems common to parents who have had assisted conception to suggest that the service to them would be improved by providing dedicated advice on child care?

In addition to the psychological profiles of the individual parents there is a social dimension which may also be important for the development of the children. In Australia, IVF parents have been reported by Munro and colleagues[61] to have deficient social relationships compared to non-IVF parents, both in the size and the quality of the relationships. The matched comparison of 157 parents of preschool twins conceived spontaneously, after ovulation induction therapy or IVF showed that the IVF parents were not as well integrated when compared to the other families. Socialization skills become increasingly important for successful integration into society as it becomes ever more complex: to have parents who may be less able to instil these skills may introduce a significant handicap to a child who is anyway less likely to have siblings. This would suggest that ongoing support and counselling may be appropriate for these families.

Whether these problems significantly affect the children born to couples after long-term infertility is less clear. There is a degree of secrecy inherent in the families involved after a successful result that makes studying the well-being of the offspring difficult[62]. Many social and developmental problems are difficult to measure and may require long-term follow-up with current assessment techniques to demonstrate significant differences. Until long-term longitudinal studies on a large number of children are reported from many centres, it will not be possible to categorically state that the parents need no dedicated management after birth, or that the children are totally unaffected.

In the meantime, there is cause for optimism. Studies from Australia suggest that donor insemination produces children with the same psychosocial achievements as matched adopted and naturally conceived children[63]; that donor insemination, ovum donation, IVF and GIFT children show no adverse physical or psychosocial effects[64]; and that there was no independent IVF effect on growth and physical outcome in children at 2 years when matched for plurality and gestation[65]. In the UK, the development of children who were conceived from cryopreserved embryos showed no significant differences compared to matched controls, although the formal testing had highlighted small differences[66]. One study has even suggested that the quality of the parenting in families with a child conceived following assisted conception is superior to that of a naturally conceived child[67], following standardized interviews and questionnaires.

In Sweden, 99 IVF children have been studied up to 85 months of age[68]. Profiles of 50 different behaviours and mental development were assessed and all the children were examined by a paediatric neurologist. Their cognitive development was described as excellent and their behaviour proved to be no different from other children. It was concluded that development, behaviour and social adaptation of these IVF children was 'very satisfactory'. Gonadotrophin releasing hormone agonists do not have any apparent adverse effects on perception, motor or memory indices in the children conceived when these agents have been administered[69].

Comparisons with experience gained from the outcome of adopted children suggest that it will be some time before it is known whether the children of infertile couples are more prone to certain physical or psychological difficulties[2] just because of their parents' experiences and, furthermore, whether any intervention would improve the outcome for families.

Children born into a family which has been successfully treated for infertility have some obvious advantages. They are clearly much wanted even if the motives for wanting children can be very mixed. The parents are more likely to be affluent, conferring the advantages of a higher socioeconomic group on the developing child, although as treatment for infertility becomes more widely available this advantage is likely to disappear. The 'emotional investment' in such children can be a mixed blessing but the basic attitude of wanting the very best for the child at all times, which is so commonly observed after infertility, nearly always works to the advantage of the child.

However, there are couples who translate their yearning for a child and the associated emotional (and often financial) investment into excessive anxiety about all issues related to the child's health and well-being after birth. It is understandable that against the background of assisted conception, extra concern by parents about the safety of immunizations, the side-effects of essential drugs such as anti-asthma medication, or the risks of disasters such as cot death, may be found by paediatricians. It is therefore suggested that all those involved in the monitoring and treatment of children born after assisted conception specifically seek evidence of any inappropriate concerns so that they may be helped by suitable reassurance (Table 2).

Careful questioning and authoritative reassurance will ensure that the parents feel more comfortable with their much wanted children, especially in the early worrying stages and that the benefits of assisted conception will be as complete as possible.

## CONCLUDING REMARKS

In 1959, Lord Jacobovits[70] wrote that 'It is estimated that man doubles his scientific knowledge every eight years. In other words, within the span of eight years we accumulate as much new understanding about the universe in which we live as the knowledge mankind amassed in all the preceding millennia of observation, enquiry and research'. By such calculation, in the intervening 38 years, the scientific database should have increased approximately 32-fold. There can be little doubt that our knowledge about infertility and its treatment has increased at least as much as would have been predicted. Computers can assist the clinician and medical researchers to access the enormous amount of data and to analyse it (Chapter 30). We must also ensure that patients are adequately informed of their options (Chapter 2), the potential problems and the likelihood of successful outcome.

Modern treatment of infertility is remarkably successful. If we leave out economic arguments, the majority of couples presenting with infertility should become parents. There are a number of counter-arguments to providing an infertility service.

(1) 'Infertility treatment has poor success rates'. This statement can only be made by those who have not kept themselves abreast of developments. The vast majority of couples attending fertility clinics can achieve parenthood when they are in a position to receive the full range of available treatments.

(2) 'Infertility is not a healthcare issue'. The British government and the majority of socially conscious people recognize that infertility (Chapter 16) is amongst the most important of health needs and is more than worthy of treatment. There is a large body of literature relating to the negative effects on women's and men's well-being as a result of infertility. The overall effects of parenthood have been assessed in a group of 174 infertile couples achieving parenthood. The positive effects

**Table 2** Examples of questions to be considered when interviewing parents of children born after assisted conception

| *Information* | *Questions* |
|---|---|
| Details of assisted conception | Are you worried that the method of conception will influence the health or development of your baby? |
| Perinatal history | Do you have any worries about anything happening around the time of birth that could affect your baby? |
| Neonatal period | Are you experiencing difficulties with feeding or basic care and would you like some extra help? |
| Immunizations | What worries do you have about your child receiving immunizations? |
| Early growth record and developmental progress | Do you think anything related to your infertility or assisted conception could affect your child's growth or development? |
| Non-specific symptoms (e.g. fever, irregular breathing, diarrhoea) | Do you think your child is ill whenever these symptoms occur? |
| Health problems | Do you think your child has a serious disease? Are you worried about the drugs recommended? |
| Family background | Are you worried that any health problem in your (or donor's) family may be associated with health problems in your child? |
| Other concerns | Do you worry about cot death, meningitis epidemics, environmental pollution? |

on well-being were more obvious in the mothers than the fathers, although there were some negative effects on the marital relationship[71].

(3) 'The world is over populated and couples who cannot achieve pregnancy by natural means should accept nature's decision'. It is a fundamental medical principle that we should strive to offer the best treatment available to the individual. For those who have difficulty in understanding this concept, let them consider whether they would wish doctors to withhold treatment for themselves, or those close to them, when they are experiencing 'natural' but remedial medical problems.

## REFERENCES


1. Achmon, Y., Tadir, Y., Fisch, B. and Ovadia, J. (1989). Emotional characteristics and attitudes of couples during *in vitro* fertilization treatment. *Harefuah*, **116**, 189–92
2. Golombok, S. (1992). Psychological functioning in infertility patients. *Hum. Reprod.*, **7**, 208–12
3. Tarlatzis, I., Tarlatzis, B. C., Diakogiannis, I., Bontis, J., Lagos, S., Gavriilidou, D. and Mantalenakis, S. (1993). Psychosocial impacts of infertility on Greek couples. *Hum. Reprod.*, **8**, 396–401
4. van Balen, F. and Trimbos-Kemper, T. C. (1995). Involuntarily childless couples: their desire to have children and their motives. *J. Psychosom. Obstet. Gynecol.*, **16**, 137–44
5. Halman, L. J., Andrews, F. M. and Abbey, A. (1994). Gender differences and perceptions about childbearing among infertile couples. *J. Obstet. Gynecol. Neonat. Nurs.*, **27**, 593–600
6. Cook, R. (1993). The relationship between sex role and emotional functioning in patients undergoing assisted conception. *J. Psychosom. Obstet. Gynecol.*, **14**, 31–40
7. Pittaway, D. E., Vernon, C. and Fayez, J. A. (1988). Spontaneous abortions in women with endometriosis. *Fertil. Steril.*, **50**, 711–15
8. Dlugi, A. M., Loy, R. A., Dieterle, S., Bayer, S. R. and Siebel, M. M. (1989). The effect of

endometriomas on *in vitro* fertilization outcome. *J. In Vitro Fertil. Embryo Transf.*, **6**, 338–41
9. Dicker, D., Goldman, J. A., Levy, T., Feldberg, D. and Ashkenazi, J. (1992). The impact of long-term gonadotropin-releasing hormone analogue treatment on preclinical abortions in patients with severe endometriosis undergoing *in vitro* fertilization-embryo transfer. *Fertil. Steril.*, **57**, 597–600
10. Anonymous (1988). *In vitro* fertilization/embryo transfer in the United States: 1985 and 1986 results from the National IVF/ET Registry. Medical Research International. The American Fertility Society Special Interest Group. *Fertil. Steril.*, **49**, 212–15
11. Anonymous (1989). *In vitro* fertilization/embryo transfer in the United States: 1987 results from the National IVF/ET Registry. *Fertil. Steril.*, **51**, 13–19
12. Anonymous (1990). *In vitro* fertilization-embryo transfer in the United States: 1988 results from the IVF/ET Registry. Medical Research International, Society for Assisted Reproductive Technology, American Fertility Society. *Fertil. Steril.*, **53**, 13–20
13. Anonymous (1991). *In vitro* fertilization-embryo transfer (IVF-ET) in the United States: 1989 results from the IVF/ET Registry. Medical Research International, Society for Assisted Reproductive Technology, American Fertility Society. *Fertil. Steril.*, **55**, 14–22
14. Anonymous (1992). *In vitro* fertilization-embryo transfer (IVF-ET) in the United States: 1990 results from the IVF/ET Registry. Medical Research International, Society for Assisted Reproductive Technology (SART), The American Fertility Society. *Fertil. Steril.*, **57**, 15–24
15. Anonymous (1993). Assisted reproductive technology in the United States and Canada: 1991 results from the Society for Assisted Reproductive Technology generated from The American Fertility Society Registry. *Fertil. Steril.*, **59**, 956–62
16. Anonymous (1994). Assisted reproductive technology in the United States and Canada: 1992 results generated from the American Fertility Society/Society for Assisted Reproductive Technology Registry. *Fertil. Steril.*, **62**, 1121–8
17. Anonymous (1995). Assisted reproductive technology in the United States and Canada: 1993 results generated from the American Fertility Society for Reproductive Medicine/Society for Assisted Reproductive Technology Registry. *Fertil. Steril.*, **64**, 13–21
18. Anonymous (1996). *The Patients' Guide to DI and IVF Clinics*. (London: Human Fertilisation and Embryology Authority)
19. Halman, L. J., Oakley, D. and Lederman, R. (1995). Adaptation to pregnancy among subfecund and fecund primiparous women. *Matern. Child Nurs. J.*, **23**, 90–100
20. Black, B. P., Holditch-Davis, D., Sandelowski, M. and Harris, B. G. (1995). Comparison of pregnancy symptoms of infertile and fertile couples. *J. Perinat. Neonat. Nurs.*, **9**, 1–9
21. Steptoe, P. C., Edwards, R. G. and Walters, D. E. (1986). Observations on 767 clinical pregnancies and 500 births after human *in vitro* fertilization. *Hum. Reprod.*, **1**, 89–94
22. Whittaker, P. G., Taylor, A. and Lind, T. (1983). Unsuspected pregnancy loss in healthy women. *Lancet*, **1**, 1126–7
23. Sweeney, A. M., Meyer, M. R., Aarons, J. H., Mills, J. L. and LaPorte, R. E. (1988). Evaluation of methods for prospective identification of early fetal losses in environmental epidemiology studies. *Am. J. Epidemiol.*, **127**, 843–50
24. Maloul, S., Manzur, A. and Asch, R. H. (1995). The obstetric outcome of assisted reproductive techniques. In Asch, R. and Studd, J. (eds.) *Progress in Reproductive Medicine*, vol II, pp. 23–34. (Carnforth, UK: Parthenon Publishing)
25. Molo, M. W., Kelly, M., Balos, R., Mullaney, K. and Radwanska, E. (1993). Incidence of fetal loss in infertility patients after detection of fetal heart activity with early transvaginal ultrasound. *J. Reprod. Med.*, **38**, 804–6
26. Harrison, R. F., Hennelly, B., Woods, T., Lowry, K., Kondaveeti, U., Barry-Kinsella, C. and Nargund, G. (1995). Course and outcome of IVF pregnancies and spontaneous conceptions within an IVF setting. *Eur. J. Obstet. Gynecol. Reprod. Biol.*, **59**, 175–82
27. Daly, S. F., Harte, L., O'Beirne, E., McGee, H. and Turner, M. J. (1996). Does miscarriage affect the father? *J. Obstet. Gynaecol.*, **16**, 260–1
28. Tuomivaara, L. and Ronnberg, L. (1991). Ectopic pregnancy and infertility following treatment of infertile couples: a follow-up of 929 cases. *Eur. J. Obstet. Gynecol. Reprod. Biol.*, **42**, 33–8

29. Tal, J., Haddad, S., Gordon, N. and Timor-Tritsch, I. (1996). Heterotopic pregnancy after ovulation induction and assisted reproductive technologies: a literature review from 1971 to 1993. *Fertil. Steril.*, **66**, 1–12
30. Anonymous (1995). Pregnancies and births resulting from *in vitro* fertilization: French national registry, analysis of data 1986 to 1990. *Fertil. Steril.*, **64**, 746–56
31. Kurinczuk, J. J., Pemberton, R. J., Binns, S. C., Parsons, D. E. and Stanley, F. J. (1995). Singleton and twin confinements associated with infertility treatments. *Aust. NZ J. Obstet. Gynaecol.*, **35**, 27–31
32. Olivennes, F., Kadhel, P., Rufat, P., Fanchin, R., Fernandez, H. and Frydman, R. (1996). Perinatal outcome of twin pregnancies obtained after *in vitro* fertilization: comparison with twin pregnancies obtained spontaneously or after ovarian stimulation. *Fertil. Steril.*, **66**, 105–9
33. Jonas, H. and Lumley, J. (1993). Triplets and quadruplets born in Victoria between 1982 and 1990. The impact of IVF and GIFT on rising birthrates. *Med. J. Aust.*, **158**, 659–63
34. Friedler, S., Mordel, N., Lipitz, S., Mashiach, S., Glezerman, M. and Laufer, N. (1994). Perinatal outcome of triplet pregnancies following assisted reproduction. *J. Assist. Reprod. Genet.*, **11**, 459–62
35. Manzur, A., Goldsman, M. P., Stone, S. C., Frederick, J. L., Balmaceda, J. P. and Asch, R. H. (1995). Outcome of triplet pregnancies after assisted reproductive techniques: how frequent are the vanishing embryos? *Fertil. Steril.*, **63**, 252–7
36. Berkowitz, R. L., Lynch, L., Stone, J. and Alvarez, M. (1996). The current status of multifetal pregnancy reduction. *Am. J. Obstet. Gynecol.*, **174**, 1265–72
37. Berkowitz, R. L. (1996). From twin to singleton. *Br. Med. J.*, **313**, 373–4
38. Robson, S. C. (1995). Antenatal management of higher order pregnancies and embryo reduction. In Ward, R. H. and Whittle, M. (eds.) *Multiple Pregnancy*, pp. 203–17. (London: RCOG Press)
39. Kanhai, H. H., de Haan, M., van Zanten, L. A., Geerinck-Vercammen, C., van der Ploeg, H. M. and Gravenhurst, J. B. (1996). Follow-up of pregnancies, infants, and families after multifetal pregnancy reduction. *Fertil. Steril.*, **62**, 955–9
40. Soussis, I., Harper, J. C., Handyside, A. H. and Winston, R. M. L. (1996). Obstetric outcome of pregnancies resulting from the embryos biopsied for pre-implantation diagnosis of inherited disease. *Br. J. Obstet. Gynaecol.*, **103**, 784–8
41. Baille, M. F., Grandjean, H., Arnaud, C., Lesourd, F., Fournie, A., Reme, J. M. and Pontonnier, G. (1995). Caesarean section trends at the Toulouse University Hospital, from 1983 to 1993. Determinants and consequences. *J. Gynecol. Obstet. Biol. Reprod. (Paris)*, **24**, 763–71
42. Elferink-Stinkens, P. M., Brand, R. and Van Hemel, O. J. (1995). Trends in Caesarean section rates among high- and medium-risk pregnancies in The Netherlands 1983–1992. *Eur. J. Obstet. Gynecol. Reprod. Biol.*, **59**, 159–67
43. Signorelli, C., Cattaruzza, M. S. and Osborn, J. F. (1995). Risk factors for Caesarean section in Italy: results of a multicentre study. *Public Health*, **109**, 191–9
44. Clarke, S. C. and Taffel, S. (1995). Changes in Cesarean delivery in the United States, 1988 and 1993. *Birth*, **22**, 63–7
45. Barrett, J. F. R., Jarvis, G. J., MacDonald, H. N., Buchan, P. C., Tyrell, S. N. and Lilford, R. J. (1990). Inconsistencies in clinical decisions in obstetrics. *Lancet*, **336**, 549–51
46. Francome, C., Savage, W., Churchill, H. and Lewison, H. (1993). *Caesarean Birth in Britain*, p. 1. (London: Middlesex University Press)
47. Rainsbury, P. A. and Rizk, B. (1992). The outcome of IVF. In Brinsden, P. R. and Rainsbury, P. A. (eds.) *A Textbook of* In Vitro *Fertilization and Assisted Reproduction*, pp. 325–43. (Carnforth, UK: Parthenon Publishing)
48. Fukaya, T., Tsuiki, A., Mansfield, C. and Yajima, A. (1994). Is treatment of long-term and consecutive use of clomiphene citrate effective in anovulatory patients? Results of multicentric retrospective studies. *Tohoku J. Exp. Med.*, **172**, 205–8
49. Viniker, D. A. (1996). Late luteal phase dydrogesterone in combination with clomiphene or tamoxifen in the treatment of infertility associated with irregular and infrequent menstruation: enhancing patient compliance. *Hum. Reprod.*, **11**, 1435–7
50. Robinson, J. N., Forman, R. G., Nicholson, S. C., Maciocia, L. R. and Barlow, D. H. (1995). A comparison of intrauterine insemina-

tion in superovulated cycles to intercourse in couples where the male is receiving steroids for the treatment of autoimmune infertility. *Fertil. Steril.*, **63**, 1260–6

51. Comhaire, F., Milingos, S., Liapi, A., Gordts, S., Campo, R., Depypere, H., Dhont, M. and Schoonjans, F. (1995). The effective cumulative pregnancy rate of different modes of treatment of male infertility. *Andrologia*, **27**, 217–21
52. Doyle, P., Beral, V. and Macnochie, N. (1992). Preterm delivery, low birthweight and small-for-gestational-age in liveborn singleton babies resulting from *in vitro* fertilization. *Hum. Reprod.*, **7**, 425–8
53. Leslie, G. I., Bowen, J. R., Arnold, J. D. and Saunders, D. M. (1992). *In vitro* fertilisation and neonatal ventilator use in a tertiary perinatal centre. *Med. J. Aust.*, **157**, 165–7
54. Amuzu, B., Laxova, R. and Shapiro, S. S. (1990). Pregnancy outcome, health of children, and family adjustment after donor insemination. *Obstet. Gynecol.*, **75**, 899–905
55. Shoham, Z., Zosmer, A. and Insler, V. (1991). Early miscarriage and fetal malformations after induction of ovulation (by clomiphene citrate and/or human menotropins), *in vitro* fertilization, and gamete intrafallopian transfer. *Fertil. Steril.*, **55**, 1–11
56. Alsalili, M., Yuzpe, A., Tummon, I., Parker, J., Martin, J., Daniel, S., Rebel, M. and Nisker, J. (1995). Cumulative pregnancy rates and pregnancy outcome after *in vitro* fertilization: > 5000 cycles at one centre. *Hum. Reprod.*, **10**, 470–4
57. Rizk, B., Doyle, P., Tan, S. L., Rainsbury, P., Betts, J., Brinsden, P. and Edwards, R. (1991). Perinatal outcome and congenital malformations in *in vitro* fertilization babies from the Bourn-Hallum groups. *Hum. Reprod.*, **6**, 1259–64
58. Wennerholm, U. B., Janson, P. O., Wennergren, M. and Kjellmer, I. (1991). Pregnancy complications and short-term follow-up of infants born after *in vitro* fertilization and embryo transfer (IVF/ET). *Acta Obstet. Gynecol. Scand.*, **70**, 565–73
59. Friedler, S., Mashiach, S. and Laufer, N. (1992). Births in Israel resulting from *in vitro* fertilization/embryo transfer, 1982–1989: National Registry of the Israeli Association of Fertility Research. *Hum. Reprod.*, **7**, 1159–63
60. Wada, I., Macnamee, M. C., Wick, K., Bradfield, J. M. and Brinsden, P. R. (1994). Birth characteristics and perinatal outcome of babies conceived from cryopreserved embryos. *Hum. Reprod.*, **9**, 543–6
61. Munro, J. M., Ironside, W. and Smith, G. C. (1992). Successful parents of *in vitro* fertilization (IVF): the social repercussions. *J. Assist. Reprod. Genet.*, **9**, 170–6
62. Sokoloff, B. Z. (1987). Alternative methods of reproduction. Effects on the child. *Clin. Pediatr. (Philadelphia)*, **26**, 11–17
63. Kovacs, G. T., Mushin, D., Kane, H. and Baker, H. W. (1993). A controlled study of the psycho-social development of children conceived following insemination with donor semen. *Hum. Reprod.*, **8**, 788–90
64. Kovacs, G. T. (1996). Assisted reproduction: a reassuring picture. *Med. J. Aust.*, **164**, 628–30
65. Saunders, K., Spensley, J., Munro, J. and Halasz, G. (1996). Growth and physical outcome of children conceived by *in vitro* fertilization. *Pediatrics*, **97**, 688–92
66. Sutcliffe, A. G., D'Souza, S. W., Cadman, J., Richards, B., McKinlay, I. A. and Lieberman, B. (1995). Outcome in children from cryopreserved embryos. *Arch. Dis. Child.*, **72**, 290–3
67. Golombok, S., Cook, R., Bish, A. and Murray, C. (1995). Families created by the new reproductive technologies: quality of parenting and social and emotional development of the children. *Child. Dev.*, **66**, 285–98
68. Cederblad, M., Friberg, B., Ploman, F., Sjoberg, N. O., Stjernqvist, K. and Zackrisson, E. (1996). Intelligence and behaviour in children born after *in vitro* fertilization treatment. *Hum. Reprod.*, **11**, 2052–7
69. Ron-El, R., Lahat, E., Golan, A., Lerman, M., Bukovsky, I. and Herman, A. (1994). Development of children born after ovarian superovulation induced by long-acting gonadotropin-releasing hormone agonist and menotropins, and by *in vitro* fertilization. *J. Pediatr.*, **125**, 734–7
70. Jacobovits, I. (1959). *Jewish Medical Ethics*, p. 251. (New York: Bloch Publishing Company)
71. Abbey, A., Andrews, F. M. and Halman, L. J. (1994). Infertility and parenthood: does becoming a parent increase well-being? *J. Consult. Clin. Psychol.*, **62**, 398–403

# The Human Fertilisation and Embryology Authority and the law

# 20

*Ruth Deech*

## INTRODUCTION

The Human Fertilisation and Embryology Act (HFE Act) was passed by Parliament in 1990. Its introduction broke new ground in the relationship between medicine, law and ethics. For the first time, an area of medicine, assisted reproduction, was to be controlled by an independent statutory body rather than by voluntary or self-regulation.

The HFE Act provided for this statutory body to be set up and the Human Fertilisation and Embryology Authority (HFEA) was formally established in November 1990. Its principal role is to regulate specified fertility treatments in the UK. It must also keep the whole area of fertility treatment under review for the Secretary of State for Health.

In this chapter, three main areas will be covered regarding regulation of fertility treatment in the UK. Initially, the background to the legislation will be described, as well as the framework of the HFE Act. Second, the powers of the HFEA and its means of regulation, particularly its Code of Practice, will be outlined. Finally, some legal developments since 1990 will be summarized.

## THE LEGISLATION

### Background to legislation

It was in July 1978 that the public became widely aware of scientific developments in the field of infertility treatment with the first report of the successful birth of a baby through the technique of *in vitro* fertilization (IVF).

The birth of what the media dubbed the first 'test-tube' baby created a great deal of excitement, and a certain amount of anxiety. People recognized the benefits which new techniques of assisted reproduction could bring. However, as they began to understand what IVF involved, some grew increasingly concerned about the scientific possibilities which might ensue and how they would be controlled. Where would science and technology lead us next?

As a result of the public concern, the Government set up a Committee of Enquiry in 1982. This Committee was chaired by Mary Warnock, now Baroness Warnock. The prime function of the Warnock Committee was to consider what policies and safeguards should be adopted for infertility treatments and embryo research. The Committee published its findings 2 years later in 1984. The Warnock Report, as it became known, was debated extensively in Parliament and there was much public consultation. One of the main recommendations of the Report was that a statutory body should be set up to license and monitor research on embryos and infertility treatment, particularly IVF and any treatment involving the use of donated sperm, eggs or embryos.

While the Government began preparing and framing its proposals for legislation, the Royal College of Obstetricians and Gynaecologists and the Medical Research Council established the Voluntary Licensing Authority (later renamed the Interim Licensing Authority) which, as the name suggests, operated a voluntary system of regulation of clinics providing IVF treatment, and embryo research.

The Government's White paper, its proposals for legislation, appeared in 1987. Its content was remarkably similar to the recommendations of the Warnock Report. Debates on the White Paper were held in both Houses of Parliament in 1988. The Human Embryology Bill was introduced in 1989 and became an Act of Parliament in November 1990.

### Provisions of the HFE Act 1990

The HFE Act states that certain activities must only be carried out under licence from the Authority. These include:

(1) The creation of an embryo outside the body, whether for treatment or research;

(2) The use, in treatment, of donated human sperm or eggs;

(3) The storage of human eggs, sperm or embryos; and

(4) Research involving the creation or use of human embryos.

It was clear that these needed to be monitored and regulated, and thus the Act brought into being the HFEA to replace the Interim Licensing Authority.

For the doctors, nurses, embryologists and other professionals working in the field, this prompted fears about bureaucracy and, more significantly, the role of the new Authority whose approval they needed in order to carry out the activities in which they were already involved. The remit of the HFEA is wider than that of the voluntary authority – for example, donor insemination is now regulated for the first time and the Act imposed new responsibilities on all clinics. It has been the responsibility of the HFEA to ensure that clinics have complied with these demands.

The HFE Act distinguishes clearly between what is allowed under licence and what is wholly prohibited by law. Such activities, if carried out, are punishable by criminal prosecution, and include[1]:

(1) Keeping or using an embryo after the appearance of the primitive streak (this usually appears at 14 days);

(2) Placing an embryo in any animal;

(3) Keeping or using an embryo in any circumstances in which regulations prohibit its keeping or use; and

(4) Replacing a nucleus of a cell of an embryo with a nucleus taken from a cell of any person, embryo or subsequent development of an embryo.

As well as inspections and licensing of clinics, the Act sets out other general functions of the Authority. It must also:

(1) Keep under review information about embryos and any subsequent development of embryos and about the provision of treatment services and activities governed by (the) Act, and advise the Secretary of State, if he asks it to do so, about those matters;

(2) Publicise the services provided to the public by the Authority or provided in pursuance of licences;

(3) Provide, to such extent as it considers appropriate, advice and information for persons to whom licences apply or who are receiving treatment services or providing gametes or embryos for use for the purposes of activities governed by this Act, or may wish to do so; and

(4) Perform such other functions as may be specified in regulations[2].

One of its main statutory obligations is the keeping of a register of information. All licensed treatment cycles carried out in the UK must be recorded on the HFEA register, as well as the subsequent outcomes[3]. The purposes of this information and the register will be described below.

The HFE Act also introduced a number of new and unique statutory duties for licensed clinics. Compliance with these duties is monitored by the Authority through its inspection system.

*The welfare of the child*
An interesting aspect of the HFE Act is that it requires certain non-clinical assessment of people seeking treatment. The Act requires clinics, before deciding whether or not to offer treatment, to take account of 'the welfare of any child who may be born as a result of the treatment (including the need of that child for a father), and of any other child who may be affected by the birth'[4]. Detailed guidance on what factors should be considered when assessing the welfare of the child are given in the Authority's Code of Practice, which is described later.

*Consent*
Consent is paramount to the HFE Act and to all work in licensed clinics. Consent to the use and storage of gametes and embryos is comprehensively covered in Schedule 3 to the Act. Patients and donors must give their written consent before treatment or a programme of donation can begin. The HFEA provides consent forms for both patients and donors to complete which the clinics must keep on file.

Embryos and gametes cannot be used in any circumstances except in accordance with the specific terms of that consent. For a couple to use an embryo produced from their own gametes, each of their consents must be compatible. Therefore, in the event of a divorce, one cannot use the embryo without the other's consent. Anyone can vary or withdraw their consent at any time.

*Counselling*
It is a requirement of the Act that counselling be offered to all patients and donors. The Code of Practice gives thorough guidance of how it expects clinics to fulfil their statutory obligation in this respect and describes the various types of counselling that should be made available.

*Information*
A further requirement of the Act is that all potential patients and donors must be given 'such relevant information as is proper'[5]. The Authority believes that it is highly important that all patients and donors be given as much information as is needed for them to make fully informed decisions, and they should be encouraged to ask for further information.

## HFEA Directions and the Code of Practice

The Act allows the Authority to make Directions about certain aspects of its own and clinics' activities[6]. Some matters covered by directions are purely procedural, while others raise ethical and social issues. Directions enable the Authority in effect to impose additional conditions on licensed activities. These directions cover areas where primary legislation would be inappropriate because of the need for flexibility. Directions can be applied to an individual clinic or generally.

Directions provided for under the HFE Act cover some of the following areas:

(1) The form in which licensees' records are to be maintained;

(2) Payment or benefits given to donors for supply of gametes or embryos; and

(3) Export and import of gametes and embryos.

The Act also states that the Authority is required to 'maintain a code of practice giving guidance about the proper conduct of activities carried on in pursuance of a licence under this Act and the proper discharge of the functions of the person responsible and other persons to whom a licence applies'[7]. This Code of Practice, which will be described in more detail below, provides the basis for much of the Authority's monitoring work.

## Regulations

Most Acts of Parliament contain regulation-making powers. Usually they confer on the relevant Government Minister powers to determine detailed subordinate legislation. Regulations are sometimes also known as 'secondary legislation' or 'statutory instruments'.

In relation to the HFE Act, the Secretary of State for Health has the power to make regulations. This allows the law to be changed to keep in tune with advances in technology and science or changes in public opinion. The power to make regulations is exercisable by statutory instruments which means that Parliament must agree to them.

Certain sections of the HFE Act have a regulation-making power attached. These pertain to surrogacy, storage of gametes and licensing. Regulations are further discussed below.

## FUNCTIONS OF THE HFEA

As discussed above, the Authority has a number of statutory obligations. The Authority must operate a licensing system and collect information and maintain an information register of all licensed treatments. The Authority is also required to produce a Code of Practice.

### Membership of the HFEA

The HFEA is a non-departmental public body, consisting of 21 members appointed by the Secretary of State. It employs a staff of 25 to implement its policy. It is a requirement of the Act that both the chairman and the deputy chairman, as well as at least half of the membership, are not involved in medical or scientific practice. Members come from fairly diverse walks of life.

It is also a requirement of the Act that the Authority should consist of both men and women, and currently the ratio is 10 women to 11 men. Appointments are for terms of up to 3 years, which may be renewed, and the members are chosen because of their personal experience and abilities and not as representatives of any particular group or organization.

### Code of Practice

The Code represents the translation of legal and ethical issues into practical applications. It provides guidance to licensed clinics as to their duties, responsibilities and practice. It remains under constant review and has been amended twice since it was first published in July 1991.

First, there are sections on staff and facilities. These give guidelines on what is expected of the different personnel working in a treatment or research centre, and on the standards expected in the premises and equipment they use.

Detailed guidance is given also in the Code of Practice on what factors should be considered when assessing the welfare of the child. In deciding whether or not to offer treatment, clinics should take account of both the wishes and needs of the people seeking treatment and of the needs of any children who may be involved.

There is a section on assessing donors and potential patients. Amongst its many detailed provisions, age limits for donors are set (35 for women and 55 for men); and it stipulates that clinics should carry out tests, including tests for human immunodeficiency virus (HIV), on donors.

There is a section on the information which must be given to potential patients and donors, including the physical effects of treatment, the risks and costs, as well as the written consents that must be obtained from them, making it clear who the legal father will be. This is almost always the husband or partner of the patient.

Counselling is covered very comprehensively and forms a pivotal part of the service the HFEA expects clinics to provide. The Act requires that counselling must be offered to anyone wanting treatment, anyone wishing to be a donor, and anyone wishing to store sperm or embryos. The aim is threefold: to help people understand the implications of treatment, donation or storage; to give emotional support; and to offer therapeutic counselling where needed.

In short, the Code seeks to protect the interests of infertile people, the donors and the resulting children. It also seeks to guarantee to the general public that research on human embryos will only be carried out when absolutely essential without hindering potential benefits and that human life will be respected at all stages of development. It promotes the best possible professional practice.

The Code of Practice is regularly reviewed and updated. The second revision of the Code

(December 1995) incorporates policy decisions which the HFEA has made and notified to licensed clinics. These include policy on sex selection of children by means of assisted conception (only permitted in licensed clinics for medical reasons), and policy on cloning by making identical twins artificially (not permitted).

The new edition also explains the requirements of the law on Access to Health Records and the Parental Orders Regulations which provide a procedure in surrogacy cases for transferring legal responsibility for a child from its birth parents to its commissioning parents.

There is also clarification on a number of issues, including:

(1) Taking account of the welfare of the child before offering treatment (clinics must now have clear written procedures for this; the Code stresses the need for a stable and supportive environment);

(2) The consent required for use and storage of gametes and embryos (reminds clinics that consent from sperm donors pre-August 1991 is not needed to continue storage but is needed if using gametes and embryos in treatment);

(3) Responsibility for controlling the number of offspring from a donor (responsibility is clearly put on suppliers and users of donor sperm); and

(4) The relevance of the guidelines in cases where material is stored for cancer patients (a new section).

**Breaches of the HFE Act, Directions or Code of Practice**

In the case of an alleged breach of the HFE Act or of the Code of Practice, the HFEA will make preliminary enquiries to establish whether there is *prima facie* evidence of a breach. If this is found to be the case, the HFEA will investigate the facts and circumstances and take specialist advice, including legal advice, where necessary.

Evidence will then be referred to a licence committee which will decide what further action, if any, needs to be taken. Where there is the possibility that a criminal offence may have been committed, a decision will be taken as to whether the matter should be referred to the Director of Public Prosecutions and whether the police should also be involved in any investigation.

The HFEA insists on the maintenance of the highest standards and any breach of the HFE Act or the Code of Practice could result in a licence being revoked or suspended. Since its establishment, licence committees have revoked one licence and refused to renew two others. One of these is currently the subject of an appeal. Committees have also refused to grant several applications for new licences and to vary existing ones.

Where an appeal is made by a clinic against a licence committee decision, it will be heard by the HFEA, excluding the members of the licence committee which made the decision under appeal. An appeal takes the form of a rehearing and both the appellant and the licence committee are entitled to be represented. If the HFEA decides, following the appeal, to refuse a licence, to refuse to vary a licence or to vary or revoke a licence, there is the right of appeal to the High Court on a point of law.

**Licensing function**

The Authority's licensing function absorbs a lot of time and effort by members and staff. As described above, a licence is required for certain specific activities:

(1) IVF treatment and any fertility treatment involving donated human eggs or sperm;

(2) Storage of human eggs, sperm or embryos for treatment or for research; and

(3) Embryo research.

When the HFEA receives an application for a licence, an inspection of the clinic is arranged. The inspection team usually consists of four people with relevant expertise, at least one of whom will be a member or employee of the Authority. The report of the inspection team goes to a licence committee which is made up of members of the Authority. This licence committee will decide whether or not to grant a licence, and with what specific conditions, if any. These conditions will normally relate to breaches of the Code of Practice, where aspects of a clinic's practice must be improved within a certain time scale – certainly before the next inspection.

The role of the inspectors is crucial – they form the direct link between the Authority and the clinics; they report back to the Authority any breaches of the Act and Code of Practice as well as new developments and good practice.

**Information function**

Under the Act, the Authority must provide information to the patients and the public. It is also obliged to keep a detailed register of:

(1) The treatment of individual patients;

(2) The use made of all sperm or eggs provided by donors; and

(3) All outcomes of licensed treatments.

Information gathering is complex but required by the Act. The HFEA receives over 200 treatment and outcome forms each day. These need to be input into the HFEA register. It is important that these are completed and that procedures are in place to obtain the outcomes. Procedure notes on how to fill in the forms are included with the Manual for Centres, of which each licensed clinic has a copy.

The register has a three-fold purpose. First, it is obviously a potential method of monitoring the work of treatment centres. Second, it provides statistics, such as national pregnancy and live-birth rates. The third use is possibly the most controversial. The Act permits anyone over the age of 18 to have access to information about their genetic background. For instance, they would be able to determine if they were genetically related to someone they want to marry.

The Act goes further than this, however. It allows for future regulations to be made (in Parliament, as Parliament is needed to introduce or change regulations) to allow not only the physical characteristics of the donor to be released, but also the donor's name. Such regulations have *not yet been formulated*, and are unlikely to be so until public opinion has been consulted nearer the time when people born as a result of treatments that have been registered are reaching the age of maturity. In any event, if they were made to reveal the donor's identity, the Act expressly forbids them from being retrospective.

The Government may decide that there should be a period of time for further consultation before such far-reaching changes are implemented. Some think that the child should indeed have full rights to information about its genetic history, while others think the wishes of the parents should be paramount. It has been argued that the disclosure of the donor's identity will greatly inhibit people's willingness to donate.

*The patient's guide to donor insemination and in vitro fertilization clinics*

As the HFEA's register of information holds comprehensive and validated data for about 40 000 IVF and donor insemination treatment cycles each year, the Authority is therefore in a unique position to publish a patient's guide containing information about the results of individual clinics. Each year the HFEA receives thousands of requests for information. By far the majority of these concern information on choosing a clinic and many people ask for the results of individual clinics.

The patient's guide, titled *The Patient's Guide to IVF and DI Clinics*, is published annually. It offers a consistency in the presentation of data within the context of a range of other relevant information. It is freely available to prospective patients and the public.

In publishing the Guide, the Authority felt that it would be wrong to withhold information unless it would be unfair to clinics and unhelpful to patients. Raw treatment data would have presented such problems, but the Authority has been able, using its database, to produce statistically adjusted figures which compensate for the main factors, such as the woman's age, which affect IVF and donor insemination outcomes.

**Policy function**

The policy making of the Authority is divided between its committees and its working groups. These working groups and committees consider policy matters in detail before bringing their recommendations to the full Authority. The Authority recognizes that there is a wide range of views on most of the matters with which it deals.

The Authority decided early on that it should continue to debate the ethical aspects of research and treatment in fairly broad terms. Ethical debate is very important to the Authority. The members provide a balance of views but by no means a full range of views. In reaching its conclusions, the Authority has two overriding priorities. These are that the interests of all those involved, including the public interest, are recognized by properly informed analysis of the issues, and that people seeking treatment and donors should receive the highest possible standards of service.

The Authority recognizes that the field that it is regulating is dynamic and contains few absolutes. It is therefore important that it consults, by public debate if appropriate, and listens to as wide a range of views as possible. This is not least because it should anticipate future possibilities which raise important social and ethical issues and encourage informed debate. The Authority has consulted the wider public on issues of major importance, such as sex selection and the use of donated ovarian tissue in treatment and research.

## SOME LEGAL DEVELOPMENTS SINCE 1990

As with any piece of legislation, the passage of time brings to light possible improvements that could be made to make the legislation work more effectively. Though the HFE Act gives powers to the Authority which allow it to make certain Directions, Parliament must be relied upon to make changes to the primary legislation or, where allowed by the Act, to enforce regulations (also known as statutory instruments).

Since 1990, no changes have been made to the primary legislation. However, in the last 5 years, certain parts of the HFE Act have come into force, some regulations have been made, and a new Act has been passed by Parliament concerning aspects of the HFE Act.

Given below are brief descriptions of some of the most important legal developments in the area of reproductive technologies in the UK.

**Disclosure of Information Act 1992**

Section 33(5) of the Act prevents any person to whom a licence applies from giving identifying information about a patient or donor to any other person who is not covered by a licence, except in a few clearly defined circumstances. The penalty under the Act for an unlawful disclosure of such information is up to 2 years' imprisonment. While it is recognized that this restriction quite reasonably gives the patient an extra degree of control over information relating to their own treatment, it soon became evident that the extent of the restriction had consequences which were previously unforeseen and potentially dangerous.

The confidentiality provisions of the Act were identified early on as a matter of concern. The provisions were in some cases too restrictive and it was feared that patient care was being jeopardised. The Authority collected information from clinics about the practical difficulties encountered due to the restrictions and concluded that an amendment to the Act was required.

In November 1991, the Authority sought the help of the Minister for Health in obtaining an amendment to the Act. On 16 July 1992, the Human Fertilisation and Embryology (Disclosure of Information) Act became law. This Act relaxed some of the restriction on liaison between different doctors involved in patient care (particularly in an emergency situation) and between lawyers and their clients. At the same time it maintained the safeguards which gave patients control over who had access to their personal information. The Code of Practice section on confidentiality was revised to reflect the changes in the law.

**Parental Orders 1994**

Section 30 of the HFE Act was the last remaining major section of the Act to be given effect. This happened in November 1994. It brought into being new legal instruments called parental orders. In the case of the birth of a child to a surrogate mother, parental orders allow the transfer of legal parental responsibility to the commissioning parents from the surrogate parents without the need for full adoption procedures. The Code of Practice gives clear guidance about the role of licensed clinics and clinicians in applications for parental orders. It explains what needs to be stated on the birth certificate when a birth to surrogate parents is registered, a matter which has caused some confusion in the past.

**Statutory storage period for embryos**

Since 1991, the law has required that, before people agree to the storage of embryos, they must be informed of the statutory storage period and be offered counselling about the implications before they consent to the procedures. They must give specific consent to the use and storage of their embryos, including what should be done with them in the event of their death or some event which would prevent them making decisions for themselves. Though people need to consent to the storage and use of their embryos, they do not own their embryos. In law, embryos are not to be seen as property.

When the Human Fertilisation and Embryology Bill was going through Parliament, it was decided that embryos should be stored for only 5 years. This limit of 5 years was chosen for reasons of caution given that state of knowledge at the time when the Bill was drafted, though there was no evidence that 5 years was the maximum period of viability of embryos.

Parliament decided that the maximum storage period for gametes should be 10 years and for embryos it should be 5 years. Patients can, of course, have their embryos stored for a shorter period of time if they so wish, and clinics can operate policies offering embryo storage for a shorter period of time. This took effect on 1 August 1991 and for all embryos in storage on that date, the 5-year period ended on 31 July 1996. However, Section 14 (5) of the HFE Act provides that the maximum storage period may be lengthened by regulations.

In 1994, the Secretary of State for Health asked for the Authority's recommendations concerning the statutory storage period. In making its recommendations, the Authority had found that there were advantages to increasing the storage period, such as:

(1) Patients would have more time to decide whether to continue treatment or decide what to do with the embryos;

(2) Patients would have more time to save money for what is often expensive treatment;

(3) Female cancer patients in particular might benefit from an increase in the storage period for embryos, as freezing oocytes is not yet a viable option (regulations allow extended storage of sperm for medical reasons until the man concerned is 55 years old); and

(4) Research into the effects of longer storage periods would be possible.

Parliament decided to accept the recommendations of the Authority which stated that the storage period should be extended. On 1 May 1996 the regulations came into force. Most patients may now opt for a further extension of 5 years for their embryos. Some women, in exceptional circumstances, will be able to store their embryos until they are 55. Such women will have to have two doctors confirm that they are completely infertile, such as from chemotherapy or if they were born without a womb.

## CONCLUSION

Britain has responded to the ethical and social concerns about artificial reproductive technology by means of statutory control. No other country in the world has a national regulatory system similar to the legislation and regulation in Britain.

In response to the Human Fertilisation and Embryology Act, the statutory body has turned ethical issues into practical applications. The legislation and the Authority's Code of Practice have gone some considerable way to address society's concerns. Undoubtedly, there will be new concerns with future developments in treatment and research. The Authority will continue to monitor the field and be ready to offer information and guidance to clinics, patients, donors and the public.

## REFERENCES


1. Human Fertilisation and Embryology Act 1990, s. 3(3)
2. Human Fertilisation and Embryology Act 1990, s. 8
3. Human Fertilisation and Embryology Act 1990, s. 31
4. Human Fertilisation and Embryology Act 1990, s. 13(5)
5. Human Fertilisation and Embryology Act 1990, s. 13(6)
6. Human Fertilisation and Embryology Act 1990, s. 23,24
7. Human Fertilisation and Embryology Act 1990, s. 25(1)

# Investigation and treatment for recurrent pregnancy loss

# 21

*Howard J. A. Carp*

## INTRODUCTION

Pregnancy loss is a common occurrence. Approximately 15% of pregnancies terminate in clinical abortions, and 0.5–1% of couples may experience recurrent pregnancy losses[1] (usually defined as three or more consecutive pregnancy losses). Pregnancy loss, whether sporadic or habitual, is psychologically distressing for the couple, requiring the patient to come to terms with having lost the 'baby' that was expected. When the anger and the mourning period are over, the patient seeks diagnosis, requires to know her prognosis, and usually requests the best that medical science can offer, in order to prevent a recurrence. However, the reality is often different. Clinical investigation seldom reveals the cause, and the literature is vague as to the chance of a recurrence. The chance of a fourth miscarriage after three previous miscarriages is usually quoted to be 40–50%. In other forms of recurrent pregnancy loss, the recurrence rate is unknown, e.g. recurrent biochemical pregnancies, after *in vitro* fertilization, antiphospholipid syndrome, or in the older woman. Most physicians believe that the majority of abortions are due to a chromosomal anomaly incompatible with life. Hence, treatment is usually empiric, rather than being based on an accurate diagnosis and specific treatment.

In this chapter, we shall attempt to clarify some of the causes of recurrent pregnancy losses and discuss some of the pitfalls which may be encountered in interpreting this condition, and advising patients.

## NOMENCLATURE AND POPULATION CHARACTERISTICS

The World Health Organization (WHO), in 1977, defined an abortion as the expulsion of an embryo weighing less than 500 g[2]. However, while this definition defines the end point for abortion, it does not define the starting point. At present, there is no agreement as to whether early chemical pregnancies should be counted as abortions. Missed abortions are outside the WHO definition as they are often not expelled from the uterus. Similarly, recurrent fetal deaths may occur after the weight of 500 g has been reached. Hence, the term 'recurrent pregnancy loss' is replacing terms such as habitual abortion or recurrent miscarriage. The term recurrent pregnancy loss may itself soon become passé and the type of loss will need to be defined. Table 1 lists a proposed method of classifying pregnancy losses according to their clinical presentation.

Primary aborters are defined as those who abort all their pregnancies, whereas secondary aborters have had one or more pregnancies develop beyond 20 weeks. We have recently

**Table 1** Types of pregnancy loss

| |
|---|
| Chemical pregnancy |
| Blighted ova |
| Missed abortion |
| Abortion of live embryo |
| Mid- or third-trimester fetal death |
| Premature labour in mid- or third trimesters |
| Mixed pattern of pregnancy loss |

described another pattern of abortion, in patients whom we have called tertiary aborters. These are patients with abortions, followed by a live birth, then a further string of abortions. In the author's series of 489 patients with recurrent pregnancy loss, 58% were primary aborters, 32% secondary aborters and 10% tertiary aborters.

The author distinguishes between three types of abortion: abortion of a live fetus, a missed abortion in which a fetal heart was previously present, and blighted ova. Missed abortions may be expelled quickly or retained in the uterus for a relatively long period. We term a pregnancy a blighted ovum when no fetal echo can be detected on ultrasound and no embryonic tissue is detected on histological examination.

In the first 186 patients to present to us with 899 previous abortions, 800 (89%) were in the first trimester and 99 (11%) in the second trimester[3]. Abortions of live fetuses occurred in only 31 (4%) of 800 first-trimester abortions, but in 30 (37%) of 81 second-trimester abortions. In a subsequent prospective follow-up study of 83 miscarriages[3], 77% were blighted ova. An international register has been compiled by the Recurrent Miscarriage Immunotherapy Trialists Group (RMITG), under the auspices of the American Society for Reproductive Immunology[4]. In consists of 1753 patients with 6625 miscarriages, drawn from 16 centres. As a contributing centre, we have analyzed the results. Of the 6625 abortions, only 1543 were defined. In this series, 71% of the 1543 were blighted ova.

In a population with recurrent pregnancy loss, there are many more patients with three losses than ten losses. Figure 1 shows the number of previous pregnancy losses in the author's series.

Therefore in any study that assesses recurrent pregnancy loss by the standard definition of three or more losses, it should be ascertained that the population consists of approximately two-thirds primary aborters and one-third secondary aborters, with approximately 90% of losses in the first trimester, approximately

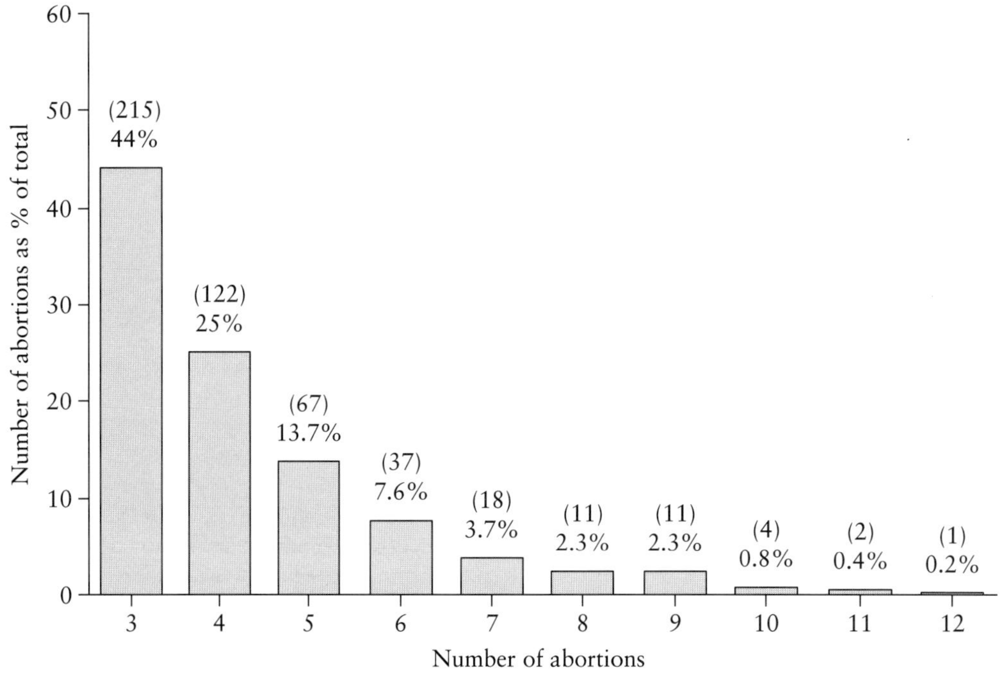


**Figure 1** Number of pregnancy losses in 489 recurrently aborting women (author's series). The number of patients with 3, 4, 5 abortions, etc. is shown in brackets

75% blighted ova, and no more than 30% of patients with five or more abortions. Any significant deviation from this distribution may produce different conclusions as to the subsequent spontaneous live birth rate and the efficacy of treatment.

## PITFALLS IN INTERPRETING THERAPY

The first potential pitfall is that miscarriages cannot yet be classified satisfactorily on a laboratory basis, but in many cases the cause of abortion can be related to a clinical picture, for example, cervical incompetence presents as second-trimester abortion of a live fetus, starting with painless dilatation, etc.; chromosome 16 trisomy presents as missed abortion of a 2 mm embryo[5]; triploidy as a blighted ovum[5]; antiphospholipid-related fetal loss as growth retardation probably leading to fetal death in the second or third trimesters[6]. The classification shown in Table 1 may help us to reach a more accurate diagnosis and prognosis. However, most patients do not know the character of the miscarriage, nor are these details available from hospital records. Most miscarriages are classified as inevitable or incomplete. Over 70% of recurrent miscarriages are blighted ova[3]. No trial of treatment has assessed blighted ova as a separate group from other abortions.

The second point is that a diagnosis is rarely reached. We have published the results of the first 186 patients who presented to us[3]. We reached a diagnosis in 42 (22%). Even when a presumptive cause of abortion is found, it is not certain that the specific cause of this patient's abortion has been diagnosed, e.g. Figure 2 is the hysterosalpingogram of a patient with five previous blighted ova. Although we advised further investigation to diagnose whether the uterus was septate or bicornuate, and then appropriate surgery, the patient refused, and was immunized with paternal leukocytes. Her sixth pregnancy terminated in a normal delivery at 38 weeks. Therefore, the uterus was probably not the cause of her first-trimster miscarriages.

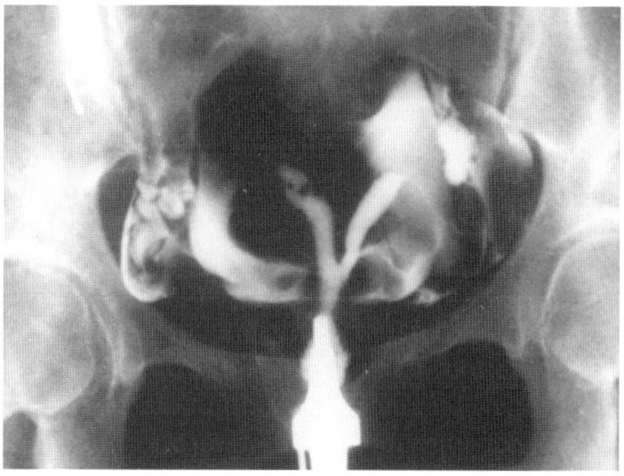

**Figure 2** Hysterosalpingogram of septate or bicornuate uterus. This patient had five previous missed abortions or blighted ova in the first trimester. She had no treatment for the uterus and delivered two subsequent live births at 38 weeks after paternal leukocyte immunization

It is usual practice to take the outcome of the first subsequent pregnancy as a measure of the efficacy of treatment. However, even after the next pregnancy, the effect of treatment is uncertain if abortions are not classified. A patient presented to us with three miscarriages of live fetuses at 12–16 weeks, all starting with contractions and bleeding. A fetal heart was present after the start of bleeding and persisted until the fetus was expelled. A uterine septum was found and resected hysteroscopically. The fourth pregnancy was a missed abortion at 8 weeks. However, this was not a failure of treatment as the fifth and sixth pregnancies terminated in the deliveries of infants of 3800 g and 3900 g at 42 weeks, after induced labours. The fourth abortion was almost certainly due to a different cause, possibly genetic.

The third point concerns the chance of the subsequent pregnancy developing to term. Although the figure of 50–60% is often quoted, the subsequent live birth rate is different in different patients, and dependent on certain predictive factors. These are summarized in Table 2.

The most important predictive factor is the number of previous miscarriages. The higher the number of previous miscarriages, the lower

**Table 2** Factors influencing a subsequent live birth (from references 4, 132 and 133)

| |
|---|
| Number of previous abortions |
| Presence of live birth (primary or secondary aborter) |
| Karyotype of previous miscarriage |
| Concurrent infertility |
| Maternal age |
| Antipaternal complement dependent antibodies (APCA) |
| Luteinizing hormone levels |

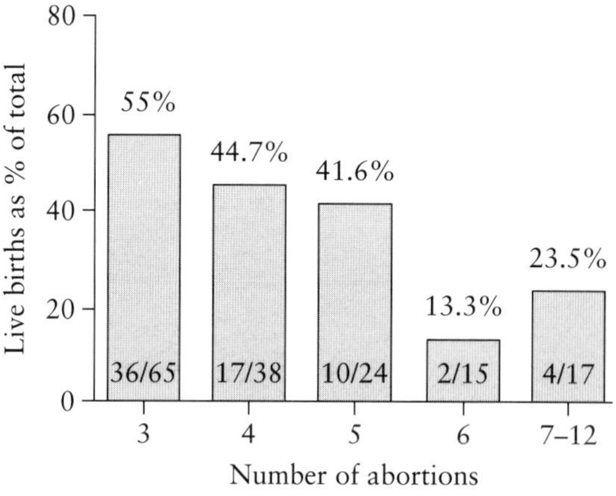


**Figure 3** Effect of number of previous abortions on outcome of subsequent pregnancy in untreated patients (author's series)

the live birth rate. Each subsequent miscarriage lowers the live birth rate by 23%[4]. This causes error in assessing results. If the chance of a live birth is 80% after two miscarriages, any treatment can only affect 20% of patients. Any trial using historical controls will show an excellent live birth rate, but any comparative trial (whether double-blind or not) will show treatment to be futile. After three miscarriages, the live birth rate is approximately 50–60%. This means that treatment can affect 40–50% of patients, and just allows for showing a treatment effect. Most treatment effects will be small if patients with three or more miscarriages of any kind are assessed, and whether the treatment effect is statistically significant will depend, to a large extent, on the sample size. After five or more miscarriages, the chance of a subsequent live birth is 25–30%, and it might be easier to show a treatment effect. However, the number of patients with five or more abortions is relatively small. Hence, there are very few such trials. Figure 3 shows the chance of a live birth in untreated patients with three or more pregnancy losses, in the author's series.

In order to interpret published figures, the number of previous abortions must be taken into account. However, no trial of treatment stratifies the results according to the number of abortions, whether primary or secondary, live or missed abortions, nor has any trial corrected for the cause of a subsequent pregnancy loss. So even if treatment is highly effective, the results are skewed, creating an illusion of futility. If we are ever going to assess treatment effectively, we must stop assuming that all abortions are identical and that there is one treatment which is a panacea. Second-trimester premature labour of a live fetus is not identical to a blighted ovum; the patient with three pregnancy losses is not identical to the patient with ten pregnancy losses.

## Theoretical considerations

The development of pregnancy, from conception to delivery, is dependent on numerous events which can encourage development or lead to pregnancy loss. The pregnancy loss may be diagnosed by its direct effect or may trigger a vicious circle as in Figure 4, leading to some overlap in clinical presentation. For pregnancy to develop normally, there must be a normal embryo which is capable of further development, and a receptive maternal environment. Whether the embryo is normal may be intrinsic or dependent on extrinsic factors occurring in the mother. The most obvious type of abnormal embryo is one with chromosomal rearrangements, e.g. monosomy X, trisomy 16, triploidy, etc. If chromosomal anomalies are due to chance, no treatment affecting maternal factors will affect the chromosome anomaly rate. However, abnormal embryos may also be due to extrinsic maternal factors which cause lethal anomalies. The serum of women with

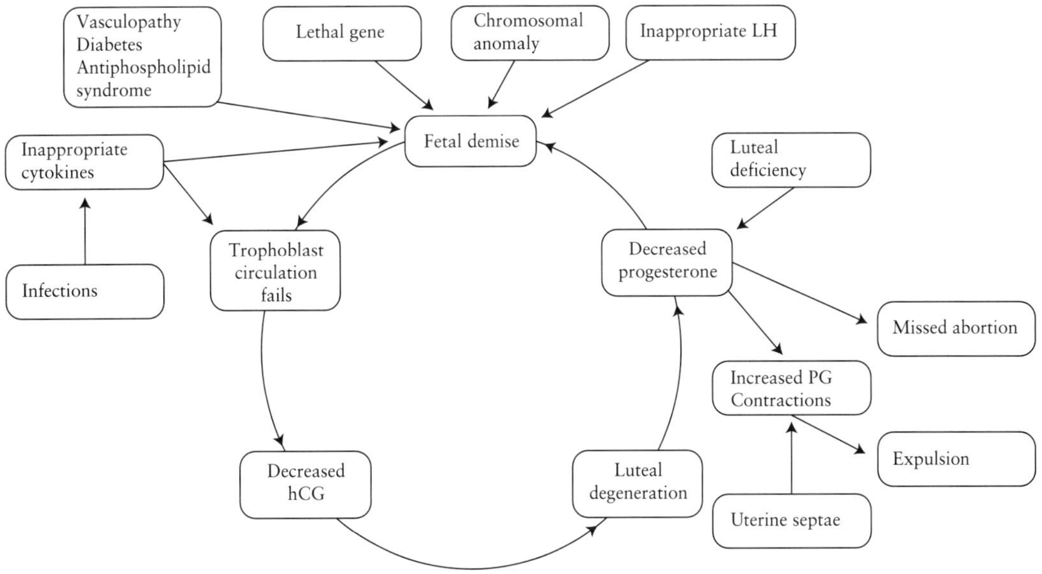


**Figure 4** Inter-relationship of various causes of pregnancy loss. LH = luteinizing hormone; PG = prostaglandin; hCG = human chorionic gonadotrophin

pregnancy loss is toxic to preimplantation embryos and blastocysts[7,8]. Abir and co-workers[9] have shown that this toxicity causes a higher incidence of malformations in 10-day mouse embryos, including exencephaly, microcephaly, anophthalmia, cardiac defects and yolk sac anomalies, and hence a high subsequent pregnancy loss rate. In a subsequent paper[10], she showed that in some cases the incidence of anomalies could be reduced in these embryos if immunoglobin G (IgG) interchange was first performed on the habitually aborting women's serum. She therefore defined two groups of embryos, those whose anomalies could be reduced and those whose anomalies could not be reduced by immunomanipulation. It is conceivable that chromosome segregation and non-disjunction at meiosis and mitosis may also be affected by maternal factors. The manipulation of anomalies has not been studied in humans, but it is possible that women with intractable infertility or that some women with recurrent miscarriage are forming abnormal embryos, and that some of them may be amenable to therapy for maternal factors.

The maternal prerequisites for a successful pregnancy are largely unknown, but certainly include a normal hormonal milieu and possibly appropriate immunological responses. The normal development of pregnancy is probably dependent on communication between embryo and trophoblast. Early pregnancy factors have been defined, e.g. preimplantation factor, pregnancy-associated plasma protein 1 and SP-1. Cytokines have been defined which are produced by the maternal immune system and encourage trophoblastic proliferation, e.g. granulocyte/macrophage colony stimulating factor (GM-CSF), epidermal growth factor (EGF-1), etc. There are also cytokines which cause natural killer (NK) cells to attack the trophoblast (e.g. interleukin-2 (IL-2), interferon-γ (IFNγ)). Although no factors have been defined which are produced by, or act on, the embryo, co-culture of embryonic explants with trophoblast has shown profound effects on trophoblast function, such as human chorionic gonadotrophin (hCG) secretion[11], and may well affect cytokine production too. Some embryos are inherently abnormal and are not amenable to any form of therapy. Others have been made abnormal by maternal factors. They may cause their trophoblasts to fail or may be aborted by maternal factors and they may be amenable to treatment. Other embryos may be normal but lost due to maternal factors. They may be influenced by treatment.

## CLINICAL FEATURES OF RECURRENT PREGNANCY LOSS

The incidence of various obstetric complications is higher in patients after recurrent pregnancy loss[12–15]. The most common obstetric complication is vaginal bleeding, occurring in 31%[13] to 50%[15] of patients. As over 70% of habitual abortions are blighted ova[3], the reason for bleeding when there is a live embryo within the uterus remains unclear. Beard[12] has quoted a perinatal mortality incidence of 12.3% (21 perinatal deaths in 171 patients), whereas we[15] have found an incidence of 3.8% (six of 157 patients). However, perinatal mortality is a measure of obstetric care as well as of underlying pathology. The cause of the perinatal mortality was mainly due to preterm labour and placental insufficiency. Even when perinatal mortality was not involved, the incidence of preterm labour was increased; it was found in 21% of the patients in Reginald and colleagues' series[13], in 14.3% of patients in Seidman and co-workers' series[14] and 18% of the patients in our series[15]. In 62% of the infants with perinatal deaths, the weight was below the 10th percentile, thus implicating placental insufficiency as the most likely cause of perinatal death. Intrauterine growth retardation without mortality has been reported to occur in between 7.6%[15] and 28.5%[12] of patients.

In Beard's series[12], 2.6% of infants had anomalies (seven of 267). In our series the incidence has been slightly higher, 6.0% (nine anomalies in 150 infants). Although this incidence is higher than in the general population, it is probably less than expected if most abortions had an underlying chromosomal basis.

## SPECIFIC CAUSES OF ABORTION

Numerous factors have been claimed to cause recurrent miscarriage. These include abnormal fetal karyotypes; anatomical causes including Müllerian duct malformations, cervical incompetence, fibroids and intrauterine adhesions; endocrine disorders such as luteal phase deficiency and inappropriate luteinizing hormone (LH) secretion; infections; autoimmune (antiphospholipid antibody syndrome) and alloimmune factors; general maternal disease such as thyroid disorders and diabetes; environmental toxins and psychological causes. Only certain factors which seem topical will be discussed. We apologise for not discussing the other causative factors which are considered to be outside the scope of this chapter.

### Genetic anomalies causing abortion

Until recently, the investigation of genetic causes of pregnancy loss was limited to chromosomal rearrangements. Only recently, with the development of molecular and DNA techniques, is it becoming feasible to diagnose other genetic causes of pregnancy loss. When a patient has a single spontaneous miscarriage, chromosomal anomalies have been reported in as many as 50–60%. However, there are problems involved in karyotyping the abortus; curetted placental tissue may be contaminated by maternal tissue, missed abortion usually produces necrotic tissue which does not grow in culture. In the series of Ornoy and colleagues[16] only 65 of 360 abortuses could be karyotyped (18%). Table 3 shows that, even today in a university unit with highly devoted staff, only 59% of abortuses could be karyotyped.

When anomalies are found, over 49% are autosomal trisomies, almost 20% are sex chromosome monosomies, over 19% polyploidies, 3.8% structural anomalies and 3.2% mixoploidy[5]. Chromosomal anomalies do have typical clinical presentations. Autosomal trisomies, except trisomies 13, 18, 21, 22 and X, allow very little embryonic development. Trisomy 16, which is relatively frequent, does not allow the embryo to develop to more than 2 mm in length. Triploid abortuses show variable morphology, from empty sacs to embryos with anomalies. With the increased use of early

**Table 3** Karyotypes of 37 abortuses from recurrently miscarrying women (author's series). Mean maternal age was 29.8 years (range 25–39) and mean number of abortions 4.36 (range 3–9)

| | *Number of abortuses* | *Percentage* |
|---|---|---|
| *No growth* | 15 | 41 |
| *Normal karyotype* | 13 | 35 |
| *Abnormal karyotype** | 9 | 24 |
| Trisomy (total) | 6 | 66 |
| trisomy 16 | 3 | 33 |
| trisomy 21 | 2 | 22 |
| trisomy 7 | 1 | 11 |
| Translocation | 2 | 22 |
| Triploidy | 1 | 11 |

*Abnormal karyotypes occurred in 9 out of 22 (41%) of abortuses that could be karyotyped

ultrasound, it may be possible accurately to describe the patient's type of miscarriage, allowing a more accurate classification than is presently available.

It is questionable whether recurrent miscarriage may be due to recurring chromosomal aberrations. The only study on the karyotype of recurrent abortions is that of Stern and associates[17]. They reported that, when 94 abortuses of recurrently miscarrying women were karyotyped, 57% were found to have aneuploidy. This was a similar incidence to that found in the abortuses of 130 women without recurrent abortion. However, recurrent spontaneous abortion was not defined in that study, as to the character or even the number of abortions. In our study on 37 abortuses from recurrently aborting women, the incidence of chromosomal anomalies was 41% of those that could be karyotyped (Table 3). Although the risk of a subsequent trisomic abortion is approximately 1% after a previous trisomy[18], most series agree that the risk of a further abortion is more common after euploidic abortions than aneuploidic abortions[19,20], indicating that a different factor must operate in a significant proportion of cases.

It is logical to assume that a carrier state should exist in one of the parents in a high proportion of cases. However, chromosome anomalies are only found in 4–8% of parents[21,22]. These are usually structural abnormalities such as translocations and inversions. Theoretically, the risk of a structural anomaly passing on to the gametes is 50% but in fact the risk is much lower. Parents with chromosomal disorders usually pass normal chromosomes to their offspring[22]. There have been seven patients with major chromosomal anomalies diagnosed at the Sheba Medical Center. Six of these subsequently delivered healthy babies[23]. In this group of parents, one had 47,XXX, five had translocations and one had a pericentric inversion of chromosome 2.

*De novo* aneuploidy or structural anomalies could arise in spermatogenesis, oogenesis or cleavage. Rosenbusch and Sterzik[24] have studied the chromosome complement of sperm of men whose partners had recurrent miscarriages. There was no increased incidence of aneuploidy or structural anomalies above the level seen in normally fertile men. Examination of oogenesis or cleavage is much more difficult as neither eggs nor embryos are readily available. However, it does seem that a maternally derived factor is mainly responsible. In the case of Down's syndrome, the recurrence risk is 10–15% if the mother is the carrier, but only 2% if the father is the carrier[22].

The effects of imprinting of either parental genome have hardly been investigated. When the entire paternal genome is imprinted, a hydatidiform mole ensues which is eventually aborted[25]. It appears that a maternal component is essential for the development of an embryo.

Point genetic mutations could be responsible for abortion by causing a gene to become lethal. Mutation could cause severe abnormalities incompatible with life, or may code for an antigen to which the mother's immune response is aberrant. An example of the former is the T complex in the mouse. This complex of genes occurs on chromosome 17. A complete T haplotype carries two non-overlapping inversions in the proximal segment of chromosome 17 with a small segment of normal chromatin separating them[26]. These two inversions are associated with segregation distorters, causing a high degree of transmission of T chromosomes via the male germ cells. Homozygous T/T embryos die *in utero* at 10.5 days due to irregularities of the neural tube and notochord. Heterozygotes show shortening of the tail but no other abnormalities. A similar lethal gene could conceivably exist in humans[27].

### Infections

Rushton[28] has investigated the pathology of 1426 pregnancy losses. He classified these losses as blighted ova, macerated or fresh fetuses. The inflammatory changes of chorioamnionitis were present in 8.5% of macerated fetuses (29 of 339) and 30.1% of fresh fetuses (125 of 415). Villitis of probable viral origin was seen in 1% of cases.

Many organisms have been implicated as causative agents of abortion: *Chlamydia, Brucella,* Cytomegalovirus, *Toxoplasma*, Herpes, *Mycoplasma* and *Listeria monocytogenes*. However, it is unclear whether these organisms cause abortion or merely infect an abortion which is already taking place. The only organism which has been shown to cause abortion is *Toxoplasma gondii.* However, toxoplasmosis may cause sporadic abortion while in the acute stage but probably not repeated abortion. Until specific organisms can be isolated and shown to be associated with abortion, no real clinical presentation can be described.

Septic abortion is relatively rare in recurrent miscarriage. In the cases which we have seen, there has been a mixed pattern of abortions, with one sporadic septic abortion, e.g. in one patient there was a blighted ovum, followed by a septic abortion at 14 weeks, followed by a missed abortion at 12 weeks, in whom there was a fetal heart beat 2 weeks previously. We felt that each miscarriage was probably due to a different agent.

In view of Rushton's work[28] showing that most cases of chorioamnionitis occur in cases of fresh pregnancy loss, we assume that most bacterial agents probably cause contractions in the second or third trimesters, leading to the abortion of a live or freshly dead fetus. This is usually the case in septic abortion or in chorioamnionitis after ruptured membranes in the third trimester. We have seen patients with this type of history, and no anatomical or other abnormalities. We have treated them with antibiotics, with good results, but the cases are anecdotal. No scientific study has been performed. The role of infectious agents in the first trimester, if any, remains to be elucidated.

### Uterine anomalies

The incidence of uterine anomalies is unknown in the general population, as many patients with anomalies may deliver successfully and are not diagnosed. The conditions determining which anomalies cause pregnancy loss and which allow term delivery are unknown. Table 4 shows the incidence of uterine anomalies and interuterine adhesions in the author's series.

The patient with a septate uterus is said to have the worst prognosis with a higher incidence of abortion[29] and live birth rates as low as 15–28%[30,31]. However, it has been reported that only one in five patients with a bicornuate uterus has reproductive difficulties[29,32]. Both have a high rate of premature deliveries (approximately 20%). Until recently, the diagnosis of these conditions was made at hysterosalpingography (HSG). However, the hysterosalpingogram does not distinguish between the bicornuate or septate uterus. Ultrasound can be used to distinguish between

**Table 4** Uterine factor in abortion (author's series)

| | |
|---|---|
| Number of patients assessed | 476 |
| Intrauterine adhesions | 64 |
| Bicornuate and septate uterus | 17 |
| Arcuate | 9 |
| Polyp | 3 |
| T-shaped | 9 |
| Diethylstilboestrol exposure | 9 |
| Cervical incompetence | 5 |

the two, if ultrasound of a sufficient standard is available. Otherwise, laparoscopy may be necessary. This distinction is important as the septate uterus can be operated upon hysteroscopically. The ratio of septate to bicornuate uteri is 2 : 1[33].

A typical history has been described by Rock and Jones[29], with expulsion of a fully formed fetus early in the second trimester, following uterine contractions after a 'mini-labour'. In our experience too, uterine anomalies probably cause mid-trimester abortions of live fetuses, rather than first-trimester missed abortions.

The mechanism of abortion is unknown. The endometrium of the septum appears normal histologically, but pregnancy loss may possibly be due to the septum having a poorer blood supply than the rest of the uterus[34]. In the case of unicornuate uterus, it is possible that the reduced capacity of the uterine cavity is responsible for pregnancy loss.

Muasher and colleagues[35] have fully described the management of such patients and the place of metroplasty. When uterine anomalies are taken as a whole, it is doubtful if metroplasty improves the outcome of subsequent pregnancies. In the case of bicornuate uterus, surgical correction is possible by Strassman, Jones or Tomkin's operation (after determining the external configuration of the uterus). However, there are no controlled studies, and none limited to patients with the clinical presentation described by Rock and Jones[29].

In the septate uterus, hysteroscopic resection has become the treatment of choice as the operation is relatively simple and safe, requiring minimal hospitalization. Success rates have been quoted to be high[36,37]. However, reports of successful outcomes have included patients with just two abortions, and most reports refer to anatomical correction, rather than live births compared to control patients matched for the size of septum. In our experience, the best results are probably obtained from septal resection in patients with abortions of live fetuses. Hence, we tend to resect septae in cases of mid-trimester missed abortions, but are doubtful about its necessity in patients with first-trimester missed abortions, blighted ova or secondary abortions. In the patient with recurrent first-trimester missed abortions or blighted ova, uterine anomalies, if found, may be an incidental finding.

A higher incidence of cervical incompetence (38%) has been reported in the bicornuate uterus[38]. It has therefore been suggested that a prophylactic cervical cerclage may be helpful[38–40]. Heionen and associates[40] have claimed that cervical cerclage increased the fetal survival rate from 53% to 100%, and decreased the prematurity rate from 53% to 31%. However, this is controversial, as many of these pregnancy losses may start with contractions rather than silent dilatation of the cervix, and it is impossible to determine accurately which are the patients requiring cerclage. The author tends not to perform cerclage prophylactically, but performs regular ultrasonic assessment of the internal os, as suggested by Michaels and co-workers[41], and only stitches the cervix if there is funneling of the internal os. Although the incidence of cervical incompetence may be raised with a bicornuate uterus, cerclage has not been shown to improve the live birth rate in other forms of Müllerian duct anomalies.

We have recently recognized a factor responsible for late second-trimester abortions which we call luminal incompetence. Figure 5 shows the hysterosalpingogram of a patient exposed to diethystilboestrol (DES) *in utero*. She aborted four times, at 23 weeks. Each time she presented with ruptured membranes, but the cervix was tightly closed. On each occasion, she needed a large quantity of either synthetic oxytocin or prostaglandin to induce contractions. This is not cervical incompetence, but a different entity with a very high risk for further pregnancy losses in the second and third trimesters. Exposure to DES is one cause of this presentation and the high rate of pregnancy loss after DES exposure has been well documented[42]. However, there are numerous patients with T-shaped and other deformed uterine cavities in whom no history of DES exposure can be elicited. Luminal enlargement by hysteroscopic diathermy, as suggested by Nagel and Malo[43], may improve the outcome.

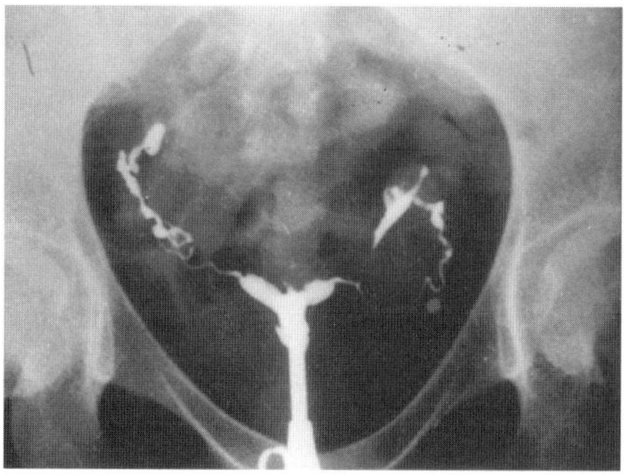

**Figure 5** Hysterosalpingogram of diethylstilboestrol exposure. This patient had four abortions of live fetuses at 23 weeks, after ruptured membranes with a closed cervix. Note the constriction rings at each horn

Intrauterine adhesions, as seen in Asherman's syndrome, have been described as a cause of abortion[44]. However, only 40% of patients in Schenker and Margalioth's series[45] of 292 women with intrauterine adhesions had miscarriages, and only 14% had recurrent miscarriage. It is questionable whether the adhesions are a cause of pregnancy loss or a result of previous abortions. If the adhesions are mild, they probably cause no problem. If severe, they probably cause hypomenorrhoea, amenorrhoea or infertility. Until the introduction of hysteroscopic surgery, dilatation and curettage was often used to divide the adhesions. Today, hysteroscopic adhesiolysis is more often used. This procedure has been reported to produce live birth rates of 90%[44,46]. However, these reports refer to all patients with adhesions, including those with infertility, and are not confined to patients with pregnancy losses. There is as yet no controlled trial matched for the severity of adhesions, nor matched for the number of pregnancy losses. In order to evaluate the role of intrauterine adhesions, such trials will need to show a subsequent live birth rate significantly greater than 60% in the case of three abortions and greater than 30% in the case of five abortions. We have seen patients with complete occlusion of the uterine cavity by adhesions have subsequent live births, once the problem of infertility had been overcome[47].

### Luteal phase deficiency

Luteal insufficiency has long been suspected to be a cause of miscarriage[48]. The corpus luteum and its hormones are essential to support early pregnancy. Lutectomy before 7 weeks causes abortion[49]. It is therefore conceivable that a defective corpus luteum may produce low levels of progesterone which are insufficient to allow adequate ripening of the endometrium, implantation and placentation.

Various methods have been used to diagnose the condition, including a short luteal phase of less than 10 days, plasma progesterone levels and endometrial biopsy. The most reliable diagnostic method has always been thought to be the endometrial biopsy which is taken 2 days prior to menstruation and histologically dated according to the criteria of Noyes and colleagues[50]. Luteal deficiency is said to occur if the dating lags more than 2 days behind the chronological age. This technique has produced a positive diagnosis in 26–35% of cases[51,52]. However, if the dating is more accurately determined by ultrasonic monitoring of follicle rupture, and biopsy timed to 12 days later, the incidence falls to 4%[53]. Horta and coworkers[48] found lower progesterone levels than normal in ten of 15 women with recurrent miscarriages. These patients aborted subsequently between 7 and 12 weeks. However, other reports such as that of Portuondo and associates[54] have shown a lack of correlation between plasma progesterone levels and endometrial histology, thus casting doubt on the whole concept of luteal deficiency. It must be remembered, however, that progesterone is secreted in a pulsatile fashion, and blood may be drawn at a pulse peak or nadir. These may vary tenfold[55], and therefore serial progesterone estimations may be more reliable[56]. Normal hormone levels in the presence of abnormal histology may also be due to progesterone receptor deficiency, rather than absolute hormone levels.

As with other presumptive causes of abortion, low hormone levels may be a result of abortion rather than its cause. In the blighted ovum or after embryonic death, villous circulation fails[28], leading to trophoblast failure. Trophoblast failure after villous circulatory failure may cause progesterone levels to fall, partly explaining the mechanism of expulsion, but not necessarily that of embryonic death. Another objection to the concept of luteal deficiency is that the corpus luteum is a transitory organ which functions for one cycle only. It is nearly always assessed in a non-conception cycle, and the results are assumed to apply in a cycle which uses a different corpus luteum.

Both progesterone and hCG have been administered to prevent abortion in cases of luteal deficiency. Wentz and co-workers[57] showed that 21 out of 26 patients corrected their luteal phase detect when progesterone was administered. However, the effect on the live birth rate has been more difficult to assess. Balasch and colleagues[58] have reported on a double-blind trial of progesterone vaginal tablets. This trial showed progesterone to have a distinct advantage over no treatment, but other comparative studies of progesterone have shown it to have no advantage[57,59]. However, these trials, while randomized, are not matched for the predictive factors listed above, and no correction has been made for chromosomally abnormal pregnancies. There has also been a tendency to administer progesterone in threatened abortion whether habitual or not. Hence, the results are almost impossible to analyse. In our opinion, a trial needs to be carried out which is matched for the number of abortions, patient's age, etc. It must then correct the results for patients aborting chromosomally abnormal fetuses. The progesterone should also be administered early, prior to fetal demise in missed abortions or blighted ova. After a fetal heart is detected, there is a 98% chance of a live birth[60]. Therefore, no drug which is administered late will improve the live birth rate.

Exogenous administration of hCG has been used to stimulate hormone production in a live pregnancy. In a placebo-controlled trial[61] of 20 women, there were no abortions in the hCG group, but seven of ten aborted in the placebo group. It is possible that the effect is due to the hCG being contaminated by early pregnancy factor, anti-idiotypic antibodies, growth factors, etc. All of these could conceivably allow the pregnancy to develop. Quenby and Farquarson[62] have reported that hCG supplementation increased the live birth rate in women who were oligomenorrhoeic, but not in women with normal menstrual cycles. Although this study included women with only two miscarriages, where a live birth rate of 80% would be expected, it is possible that hCG has a place in women with associated infertility, but little place in women with miscarriages but no infertility.

### Inappropriate luteinizing hormone as a cause of abortion

Increased follicular phase serum LH levels (above 10 mIU/ml) have been reported to lead to pregnancy loss in addition to infertility[63,64]. It has even been claimed that, if follicular LH levels are high in the conception cycle, it may predict abortion. However, others have disputed whether raised LH levels are associated with an adverse pregnancy outcome[65,66]. Kovacs and co-workers[65] have even reported that fertile women undergoing donor insemination had a higher incidence of abortion when LH levels were low. Thomas and associates[66] showed that raised serum LH levels did not predict the outcome of 331 conceptions following *in vitro* fertilization (IVF).

Based on the assumption that LH can predict the likelihood of abortion, it has been suggested that suppression of LH secretion by gonadotrophin releasing hormone (GnRH) analogues can lower the abortion rate[64]. However, these reports also assessed all patients with three or more abortions, and have not matched them for any of the predictive factors above. Additionally, there is confusion about the exact criteria. Polycystic ovaries, when diagnosed ultrasonically, are relatively common in recurrent miscarriage: 82% of the patients in Sagle and colleagues' series[68], and 56% in the series of Clifford and co-workers[67]. However, the incidence of raised LH is low in recurrently aborting women, whether LH is assessed in serum (0 of 82 patients in Sagle and colleagues' series[68], 36% of the patients in our series[69]) or assessed in urine (32% of the patients in Clifford and associates' series[67]). Furthermore, follicular phase LH levels might vary from cycle to cycle.

In order to clear the confusion, we assessed serum LH levels in 153 women (aged 20–44) with three to eight prior miscarriages[69]. LH levels were not suppressed. During the study period, 103 of the 153 couples conceived. The patients with normal or raised LH levels were of similar maternal age and had a similar number of previous abortions. Of those 103 pregnancies that were followed prospectively, 65 (63.1%) resulted in the birth of a live infant. The pregnancy outcome was slightly better in women with a low LH level; 67% of pregnancies terminated in live births compared to 56% in women with an increased LH level. This difference was not statistically significant. There was no significant difference between primary or secondary aborters. There was no difference in the mean LH level in women with a live birth (12.43 mIU/ml) and those that subsequently aborted (12.68 mIU/ml). Hence, we concluded that inappropriate LH is not a major cause of recurrent miscarriage, but may be associated with miscarriage in a certain proportion of patients. Treatment by LH suppression is probably not indicated in most cases. Inappropriate LH may be associated with pregnancy loss in patients with concurrent infertility and possibly less in patients who conceive without difficulty.

## Antiphospholipid antibodies and pregnancy

Injection of serum from mice with a high titre of antiphospholipid antibodies (APLA) to naive mice induces resorption of pregnancies in the recipient[70], indicating that APLAs have a direct action on pregnancy loss and are not just epiphenomena. There are three relevant antibody assays: lupus anticoagulant (LA), anticardiolipin antibody (ACA) and the antibody responsible for false-positive syphilis serology. Other antiphospholipid antibodies are still experimental and their association with the APLA syndrome remains to be confirmed. Phosphatidyl inositol, phosphatidylserine and phosphatidylethanolamine are three such examples.

The most commonly used diagnostic assay is the enzyme-linked immunoabsorption assay (ELISA) for anticardiolipin antibodies. However, this test has a number of drawbacks. There is wide interlaboratory variation requiring the clinician to use skill and experience in interpreting the results. Peaceman and associates[71] have reported that, when they sent 20 serum samples, reported to be ACA-positive, to five laboratories, the results only concurred for five samples. Additionally, although the test is highly sensitive, it has a relatively low specificity. Therefore, the presence of anticardiolipin antibody alone does not mean that the fetal loss is related to antiphospholipid antibody[72], but that additional features such as a high level of antibody (above 40 IgG phospholipid units), concurrent thromboses and additional antibodies such as antinuclear factor or lupus antiocoagulant should be present before it is assumed that the fetal loss is due to APLA.

The prevalence of pregnancy loss is high in the presence of APLA syndrome. Rote and co-workers[73] have claimed it to be 80%, Branch and colleagues[74] have reported an 89% fetal loss rate in 43 women with antiphospholipid antibodies and a perinatal survival of only 14%. In our series of 19 patients with lupus anticoagulant, there were 66 previous fetal losses[75].

The incidence of APLA is low in women with normal pregnancies (0.2% for LA and 2% for ACA)[6,76]. In an unselected population with recurrent miscarriage, we have found the incidence of LA to be approximately 5% (19 of 360 patients)[77]. Tincani and associates[78] found anticardiolipin antibodies or lupus anticoagulant in eight of 103 women with three or more fetal losses. Lockwood and co-workers[79] found anticardiolipin antibodies in 27% of 55 women with a poor obstetric outcome, but lupus anticoagulant in four. As transiently raised levels of ACA, which soon return to normal, may be found after viral infections[80], persistently raised levels are necessary to be meaningful[81].

Although much has been elucidated with regard to the APLA syndrome, the nature of the phospholipid antigen is unknown, as are the mechanisms involved in the binding of APLA to phospholipid (it may be dependent on a 50 kDa cofactor called apolipoprotein H[82]). The unknown antigen is thought to reside in thrombocyte and small vessel membranes. Antiphospholipid antibodies may cause binding of platelet membrane phospholipid to antiphospholipid antibodies and hence aggregation and thrombosis[83]. Thrombi have been described to be widespread, involving almost any arteries or veins. Thrombosis has been reported as due to an inhibitory effect on prekallikrein, a prolonged *N*-globulin lysis time due to the low activity of plasminogen activators, a low level of antithrombin III, or low activity of protein C. This may also explain the increased incidence of thrombocytopenia in patients with APLA antibodies.

Antiphospholipid antibodies have also been reported to react with phospholipids of endothelial cells, inhibiting arachidonic acid release[84] which is essential for prostacycline production, thus altering the thromboxane/prostacyclin balance[85]. However, recent studies have suggested that APLAs may not act on the thromboxane/prostacyclin balance at all, but may affect the adhesion molecules between the elements of syncytiotrophoblast[86]. Cytotrophoblast cells express phospholipid on their surface. Phospholipids function as adhesion molecules[87]. Hence APLAs may damage the trophoblast unrelated to thrombosis. Women with APLA have been found to have decreased vasculosyncytial membranes, increased syncytial knots, substantially more fibrosis, hypovascular villi and infarcts than women without APLA[88]. Therefore APLAs have even been reported to cause preclinical pregnancy loss, presenting as infertility. Rote and co-workers[73] and ourselves[89] have summarized other series in the literature. Approximately 50–60% of fetal losses occurred in the first trimester, 30% in the second trimester and 10–20% in the third trimester. These figures show a higher incidence of second- and third-trimester losses than is usual in an unselected group of habitual aborters (in our series of 899 fetal losses in an unselected group of 186 habitual aborting patients, 800 abortions were in the first trimester and 99 in the second trimester).

There have been few attempts to define the character of the pregnancy loss. Lockshin[6] has described a typical clinical picture. The first trimester is normal. Fetal growth slows in mid-pregnancy and oligohydramnios becomes apparent. Tests of fetal well-being will show signs of fetal compromise. Either fetal death ensues or delivery of a live but growth-retarded fetus. The placenta is small, and usually has a vasculopathy.

We attempted to determine the effect of treatment on recurrent first-trimester abortions. We compared 15 patients with APLA and five or more first-trimester abortions to 19 patients with recurrent first-trimester miscarriages without APLAs[89]. The 15 APLA patients had 24 subsequent pregnancies. They were treated by prednisone 30 mg and aspirin 100 mg daily. The 19 control patients had 22 subsequent pregnancies. The rate of first-trimester abortions was similar in both groups. The number of subsequent mid- or third-trimester fetal deaths was higher in the APLA patients, five of 12 pregnancies reaching the second trimester, compared to none of the eight pregnancies reaching the second trimester in the control patients. Although the live birth rate was similar in both groups of patients, there was a higher incidence of growth retardation in APLA syndrome patients (six of 12 pregnancies in the presence of APLA compared to one of eight pregnancies in control patients). This difference was statistically significant. We concluded that treatment of APLA may not be necessary in patients with first-trimester recurrent abortions, but may be necessary to prevent the effects of APLA in the second and third trimesters. Due to the high incidence of growth retardation and the necessity for preterm induction of labour, the author monitors these patients intensively throughout pregnancy. All forms of fetal monitoring should be used, including Doppler flow studies, serial growth on ultrasound and electronic monitoring to detect changes in the non-stressed cardiotocograph, etc.

Most patients have a mild form of the condition with the presence of antibodies only. The next stage may be the presence of APLA and fetal death, with or without previous thromboses. These patients may have an early form of the condition and the general widespread clinical effects may develop later. It is rare to find a patient with generalized disease present in pregnancy. The Sheba Medical Center is a referral centre for patients with APLA syndrome. Of 100 patients with APLA, only nine had the severe form of the disease.

The first regimen to be used as treatment was to lower antibody levels with steroids and aspirin to prevent platelet aggregation[90]. Although many workers, including the author[75], have found this regimen to improve the live birth rate, Lockshin and co-workers[91] have cast doubt on the efficacy of steroids. This, coupled with the toxicity of steroids (Cushing's syndrome, acne, osteoporosis, etc.), has led various workers to seek less toxic regimens. Aspirin has been used alone[92,93] with a good success rate. An alternative treatment regimen has been heparin which has been used in a low dose or in the full dose[94]. The rationale is as an anticoagulant and immunoadsorbent. Recently, low molecular weight heparins have been used[95,96]. Dulitzky and colleagues[97] have used enoxaparin subcutaneously by a once-daily injection. The advantages of low molecular weight heparin over classical heparin include a higher antithrombotic/anticoagulant ratio; hence, there is less bleeding, a better antithrombotic effect, and a longer half-life requiring only one injection per day. Hence, there is little need for laboratory monitoring as with unfractionated heparin. There may also be less heparin-induced thrombocytopenia or osteoporosis[98]. A few authors have reported good results using prednisone and azathioprine[99] or intravenous immunoglobulin[100,101]. However, these series are small, usually involving individual patients who were refractory to other forms of treatment.

Every regimen of treatment has been claimed to produce a higher live birth rate than no treatment. Many and associates[102] have published a meta-analysis on all the regimens, and reported that successful pregnancies have been reported in as many as 70% of patients following suppression of the antibody's activity by any treatment (whether prednisone, antiaggregants or anticoagulants). However, it is difficult to compare these results. Information does not always exist concerning the number of prior pregnancy losses in each patient, level of APLA, basic primary disease, or previous thromboembolic phenomena. There are only two comparative studies. One compares prednisone and aspirin to heparin and aspirin[103]. It showed a similar result in both groups. This paper is one of the significant works resulting in the decreased use of steroids. The other study[93] compares aspirin to heparin with aspirin, showing a higher live birth rate when heparin is included in the regimen. The authors have compared steroids and aspirin to enoxaparin and aspirin. Enoxaparin and aspirin seem to be associated with a higher birth rate (82% as opposed to 50% with steroids and aspirin). However, this was not a controlled trial. We used steroids up to 1991 and enoxaparin thereafter.

In the absence of an optimal therapeutic schedule, only guidelines can be suggested regarding treatment. Low-dose aspirin is recommended in patients with pregnancy losses and APLA. Anticoagulants should be added if they have suffered previous thromboembolism or have had further pregnancy losses when treated with aspirin alone. The use of corticosteroids should be based on the presence of other autoimmune phenomena such as vasculitis or a relapse of the original autoimmune condition in the previous or present pregnancy. We tend to base treatment on the features of the patient rather than using a standard regimen. Figure 6 shows our treatment protocol.

Unfortunately, changes in the antibody levels do not correlate with fetal death. In our series, only one patient showed a correlation. Anticardiolipin antibodies do not change under the influence of treatment. Although steroids return the LA activity (as diagnosed by clotting tests) to normal, there is no test to measure cofactors; hence treatment is empirical and tests

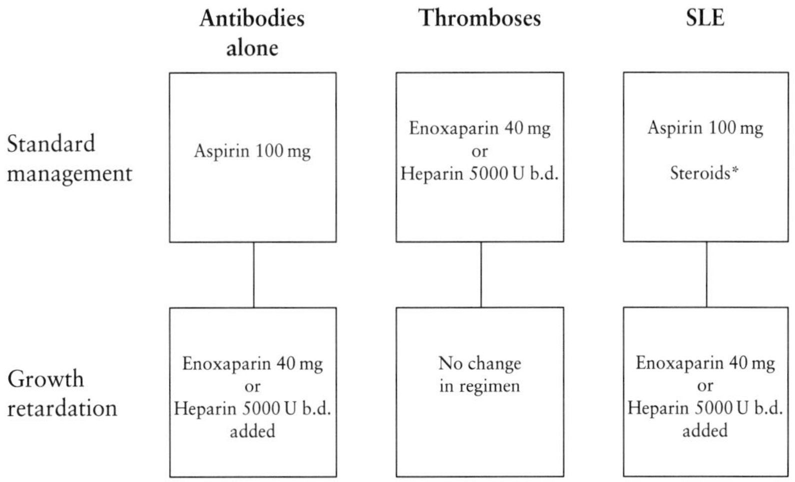


**Figure 6** Algorithm for treatment of antiphospholipid antibody (APLA) syndrome. SLE = systemic lupus erythematosus; *steroids are used only when medically indicated

of fetal well-being are presently more reliable than antibody levels.

## Alloimmune pregnancy loss

In the 1980s, there was a concept that the pregnant woman needs to mount an active immune response to trophoblast or fetal antigens in order to protect the fetoplacental unit, and that these responses are either not initiated or aberrant in women with habitual miscarriage. Based on this concept, immunopotentiation was used in order to boost the immune response. It was originally attempted as a means of preventing abortion by Beer and coworkers[104] and Taylor and Page Faulk[105] independently in 1981. Since then, two forms of immunization have been used, active, involving immunization of the mother with either paternal or donor leukocytes, or passive immunization with immunoglobulin. Both forms of immunization have been used to prevent further miscarriage in recurrently miscarrying women, or to improve the implantation rate after repeated failure of implantation and *in vitro* fertilization (IVF) and embryo transfer (ET).

Active immunization has been used since 1981. Donor immunization is not often used today due to the risk of transmission of acquired immune deficiency syndrome (AIDS). Paternal leukocyte immunization, however, has been widely used. Its use became much more popular after the double-blind trial of Mowbray and associates[106] showed immunopotentiation to have a distinct advantage in preventing further abortions. However, this therapy has been controversial since its inception. Controversy has been based on four main contentions: whether treatment is effective, that the mode of action is unknown, which patients should be selected for treatment, and the possible side-effects.

Even today (after 15 years of use), it is still debatable whether this treatment improves the live birth rate. Since the trial of Mowbray and associates[106], numerous other trials have been performed. Most show a slight benefit from immunization[107–109] but the benefit failed to reach statistical significance. They therefore generally concluded that immunotherapy was not helpful. Only Cauchi and colleagues[110] have claimed that immunized patients did less well than non-immunized patients. As most of the trials were too small to allow the benefit to reach statistical significance, it was decided to carry out a large world-wide collaborative meta-analysis on the results of immunization. This meta-analysis was performed on the results of an international register of 1753 patients with recurrent miscarriage. The method of data collection for the international register has been fully described[4]. Briefly, centres practising paternal leukocyte or other forms of immunopotentiation for recurrent miscarriage submitted data forms with 140 variables for each patient, including history, details of investigation and treatment. Data were collected from nine centres which had carried out randomized studies and seven centres which had performed non-randomized studies. The analysis was performed by two independent teams on over 400 patients from the randomized trials alone. The overall benefit was 8–10%, which was statistically significant. However, the result is confusing, as it allows physicians who do not believe in immunization to contend that a 10% benefit is not worthwhile, and it allows those who believe that immunization is beneficial to continue using it. However, this analysis also included all patients with three or more abortions of any type. The other results obtained from the meta-analysis are probably more important, even though they are not often quoted. They are summarized in Table 5. When the results were corrected for predictive factors, there was a 24% benefit.

**Table 5** Conclusions of the world-wide observational study and meta-analysis on allogeneic leukocyte immunotherapy for recurrent spontaneous abortion

| |
|---|
| Overall benefit from immunization is 8–10% |
| The number of patients needed to achieve one extra live birth is 10–13 |
| The benefit when corrected for predictive factors is 24% |
| The benefit was statistically significant |
| Immunotherapy improved the live birth rate in the primary aborters |
| There was no beneficial effect in the secondary aborter |
| The live birth rate was 70% in control patients with pretreatment evidence of antipaternal complement dependent antibody (APCA) |
| The live birth rate was 37% higher in immunized patients who seroconverted to APCA positive |

These results led to the conclusions that immunotherapy may be an effective treatment, but for a relatively small number of patients; in other words, that a more effective diagnosis is necessary, or that this treatment may only be partially effective. The second approach has led to wider use of immunoglobulin to prevent further miscarriages.

In 1990, we published our results[111] which showed that immunopotentiation improved the live birth rate in the primary but not secondary aborter. We also showed that the patient with pretreatment evidence of antipaternal complement dependent antibody (APCA) has a live birth rate of 70%, and suggested that she does not require immunization. We also showed that it was not enough to immunize a patient. It was necessary to show that something in the immune response had changed. We took seroconversion to APCA positive as such a marker. These antibodies are detected clinically in a cross-match between maternal serum and paternal lymphocytes[112]. Antipaternal complement dependent antibody is not a specific marker and not an essential prerequisite for pregnancy to develop. The presence of this antibody merely indicates that an immune response has occurred to paternal antigens. This antibody is present in maternal and fetal circulations[113]. It is not harmful to the trophoblast or fetus and seems to be absorbed by the placenta[114]. Its value is controversial as it is only present in approximately 20% of normal parous women's serum and only produced at or near term in successful pregnancies[115]. Absence of this antibody in habitual aborters could be normal, as suggested by Regan and Braude[116], or could be a reflection of maternal immune hyporesponsiveness.

In order to take such considerations into account, Daya and Gunby[117] carried out a subsequent meta-analysis on the same register of patients from the double-blind randomized studies in the RMITG register, but only included the primary aborters who were APCA negative at initial testing. This analysis consisted of 285 patients. They found immunization to be effective and increased the live birth rate by 46%. This figure was highly statistically significant. In other words, six patients needed treatment to achieve one extra live birth.

As our unit acts as a tertiary referral unit for patients with recurrent miscarriage, we see a large number of patients with a higher number of pregnancy losses. We therefore asked about the patient with five or more abortions. We originally published an analysis of our results in 1993[15]. In this report, we showed that the patient with five or more abortions derives a greater benefit from immunization than the patient with three or more abortions. Daya and Gunby[117] have also shown that, as the number of abortions increases, the number of patients needed to be treated in order to obtain one extra live birth decreases. We have analysed our figures and those of the RMITG register for patients with five or more abortions who were APCA negative, and seroconverted after immunization. Immunization was effective in primary and tertiary aborters but not in secondary aborters. The number of patients needed to be treated for an extra live birth is three primary or two tertiary aborters.

There is an anomalous situation; immunization is generally thought to be of only marginal benefit, as the patient with three abortions has a relatively good chance of a live birth. Therefore, the patient with ten abortions may be inappropriately advised against immunotherapy on the basis that the patient with three abortions does relatively well in her fourth pregnancy.

Immunization has also been used in IVF failure. The rationale has been that these patients have numerous embryos in the uterus, but failure to implant could be a form of early abortion. Hasegawa and colleagues[118] claimed that one patient of the three that they immunized had a subsequent pregnancy. We have not found immunization to increase the conception rate in IVF failure[119].

There has been much concern over the possible side-effects of immunization, as it carries the same risk as with any transfer of blood products. Menge and Beer[120] have suggested that immunization may cause intrauterine growth retardation. However, as quoted above, these patients are prone to growth retardation even if not immunized. Beard[12] has shown growth retardation in the 30% of habitual aborters whose pregnancies succeed without immunization, but in only three of 92 (3.26%) habitual aborters immunized by paternal leukocytes. In fact, all side-effects were reported to the RMITG register and have been fully described in the 1753 patients in that register[121]. The conclusion reached in the RMITG meta-analysis[4] was that side-effects seemed to be minimal.

If immunotherapy has any place, it is necessary to ask what its action may be. Unfortunately, very little is known of the functioning of the immune system in pregnancy. It has been assumed that the success of the 'fetal allograft' must depend on preventing a potentially harmful maternal immune response. Current thoughts on the functioning of the immune system include altered suppressor cells, involvement of non-specific immunostimulators and activation of certain cytokines. A full review of the functioning of the immune system has been provided elsewhere[122]. However, no immunological mechanism has been proven to cause abortion. Immunomodulation could act on other systems. As mentioned above, serum from habitually aborting women inhibits the ability of rat blastocysts to spread, attach and implant[8]. This effect is reversed by immunization. Serum from habitually aborting women causes exencephaly, microcephaly, anophthalmia, cardiac defects and yolk sac anomalies in 10-day mouse embryos[9]. Exchanging the IgG fraction of the serum reversed this effect in a large proportion of cases[10]. Hence, malformed fetuses may die *in utero* and be reabsorbed or aborted. Modulation of the immune response may prevent some of these malformations and subsequent pregnancy loss. It is known that progesterone is essential for pregnancy and that early pregnancy can be terminated by blocking the progesterone receptors, e.g. with RU 486. Szekeres-Bartho and co-workers[123] have reported that an immune stimulator may induce the progesterone receptors necessary to support pregnancy.

In view of the American Society for Reproductive Immunology meta-analysis showing that immunotherapy has a treatment effect, the need to explain the mechanism and develop accurate diagnostic tests to identify the patient who can benefit, is greater than ever. Until that is done, immunization will be offered to all habitual aborters, including many who will not benefit from treatment.

As the overall benefit from immunization appears marginal when all patients with three or more miscarriages are treated, various workers have sought other forms of treatment which might be more effective. Intravenous infusion of immunoglobulin (IVIG) is a passive form of immunization, as it contains a normal complement of antibodies from a pool of many donors. The exact mode of action has not been fully elucidated. The initial reports on the use of this drug for recurrent miscarriage have been encouraging[124–126]. Due to these results, two randomized studies have been carried out but their results are conflicting. The German Recurrent Spontaneous Abortion/IVIG group[127] has claimed that IVIG is ineffective and have ceased using it, whereas Coulam[128] claims IVIG is effective in preventing abortion. Therefore, the same situation may occur with IVIG as with paternal leukocyte immunization, i.e. after 14 years of use, there is still no consensus as to its efficacy.

We have used immunoglobulin in a small series of patients[129] considered to have such a poor prognosis that they have little chance of ever sustaining a pregnancy to viability, i.e. patients with five or more abortions and miscarriages after paternal leukocyte immunization or continued miscarriages despite the presence of APCA at initial testing, or a contraindication to paternal leukocyte immunization, e.g. if the husband is hepatitis B antigen positive, etc. In these cases, immunoglobulin was administered in the follicular cycle in which a pregnancy was planned and again at the beginning of pregnancy. Ten patients out of 15 have conceived and five had live births. This is an encouraging result, which requires a larger series of patients. The only side-effect was an allergic reaction in one patient.

Immunoglobulin has also been used in implantation failure at IVF. There are presently two series with conflicting results. Coulam and associates[130] have claimed a 56% pregnancy rate in women in whom over 50% of their eggs were fertilized. However, Balasch and colleagues[131] obtained no implantations in a similar group of patients, and therefore abandoned the use of immunoglobulin in IVF–ET failure.

The prohibitive cost of immunoglobulin probably precludes its use in large numbers of patients, but it has a place in patients who are refractory to other forms of treatment. Figure 7 shows our current protocol for immunization in women with recurrent pregnancy loss.

## INVESTIGATION OF RECURRENT PREGNANCY LOSS

Ideally, it should be possible to make a specific diagnosis and offer the patient specific treatment based on that diagnosis. However, as research in reproductive immunology, genetics, endocrinology, etc. has not yet provided sufficiently clear answers as to the mechanisms involved, this is rarely possible. The best that can be offered is to achieve a rough idea of the cause of pregnancy loss and then offer empirical treatment. The literature contains many suggested schemes for managing these patients. Tables 6 and 7 show how we investigate and treat our patients. As there is no accurate laboratory test to diagnose the cause of the pregnancy losses, the importance of an accurate history cannot be overstated. Some patients have a mixed pattern of pregnancy losses. In these patients, the losses are most likely due to chance or possibly due to chromosomal disorders in the fetus. There is no treatment for this at present. The secondary aborter is a problem. If she has three miscarriages, she has a relatively good chance of a live birth, but after ten abortions, her chance of a live birth is as poor as that of a primary aborter. She does not have a high incidence of raised LH, nor does she respond to paternal leukocyte immunization. Immunoglobulin has still to be evaluated in these patients. If the patient has had a high number of pregnancy losses, surrogacy may be her only choice. The patient who is APCA positive similarly has a good chance of a live birth

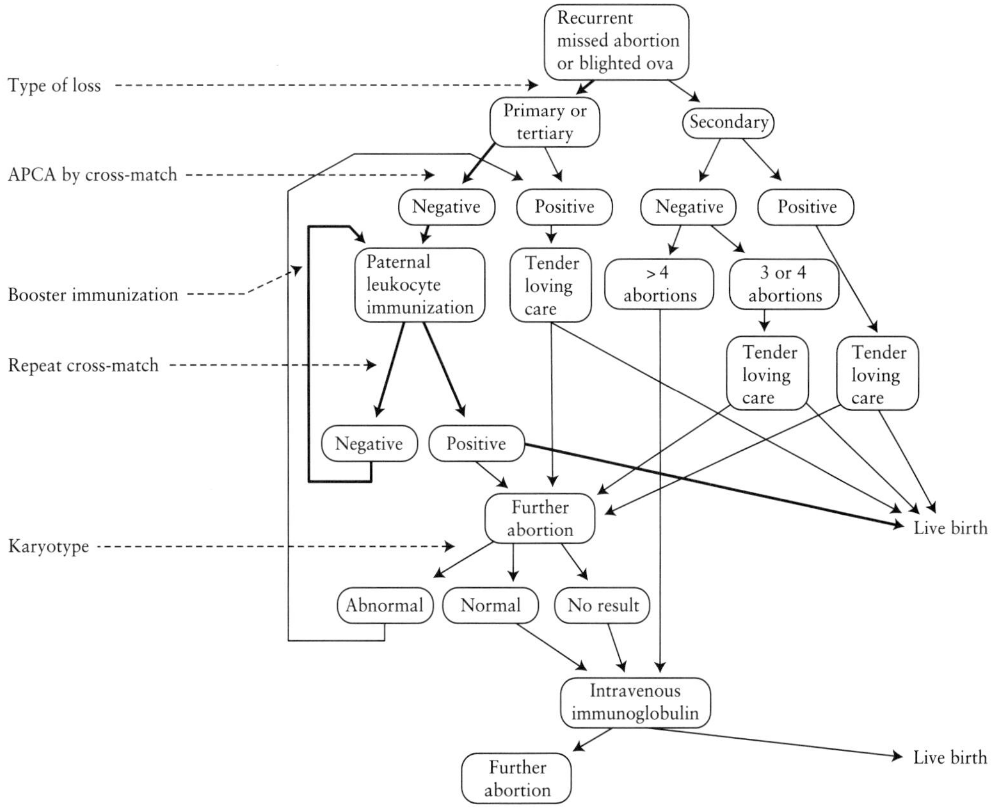


**Figure 7** Author's suggested scheme of immunopotentiation. Booster immunizations are used by the author. It is not standard management. 70% of patients follow the path in bold type. APCA = antipaternal complement dependent antibody

if she has three abortions. However, if she continues aborting, this chance significantly decreases since she also does not seem to respond to paternal leukocyte immunization. We have tried immunoglobulin in these patients but with only a few successes. Paternal leukocyte immunization remains controversial. We find it beneficial in primary or tertiary aborters who are APCA negative. Immunization is then most effective when the patient seroconverts. In patients in whom immunization is followed by a further pregnancy loss, immunoglobulin looks a promising form of treatment. Hysteroscopic surgery of a septate uterus is also effective treatment, but in our opinion only effective in patients with an appropriate history.

In conclusion, even today very little is known about the pathology leading to pregnancy loss. Therefore, patients are usually not

**Table 6** Investigation of recurrent pregnancy loss

| |
|---|
| Accurate history of past losses, missed abortions, blighted ova, abortions of live embryos, mixed pattern of losses, primary or secondary aborters |
| Treatment given in past pregnancies |
| Cycle length |
| History of associated conditions, diabetes, thyroid disease, infertility or autoimmune disease |
| Karyotype of previous abortions (if available) |
| Karyotype of both parents |
| Luteal progesterone level and endometrial biopsy |
| Hysterosalpingogram or hysteroscopy |
| Autoantibody screen for antinuclear antibody, anticardiolipin antibody, recalcification time and kaolin clotting time |
| Cross-match for antipaternal complement dependent antibody |
| Follicular phase follicle stimulating hormone, luteinizing hormone and ultrasound of ovaries to exclude polycystic ovaries |

**Table 7** Suggested treatment of recurrent pregnancy loss

| *Presumed cause* | *Clinical features* | *Management* |
|---|---|---|
| Septate uterus | abortion of live fetus in second or third trimesters | hysteroscopic resection |
| Bicornuate uterus | as above | ultrasound assessment of cervix if open, cerclage if another pregnancy loss, metroplasty |
| Luteal deficiency | abnormal biopsy in two cycles | progesterone or hCG supplements |
| Chromosomal disorders in parents | dependent on disorder | genetic counselling and amniocentesis in next pregnancy |
| Chromosomal disorder in abortus | as above | no treatment necessary, good prognosis |
| APLA syndrome | second- or third-trimester fetal death after IUGR | if APLA antibodies alone, aspirin; if APLA and thrombosis, aspirin and heparin and enoxaparin (see Figure 6) |
| Alloimmune | first-trimester blighted ova or missed abortions, APCA negative | paternal leukocyte immunization; if another abortion, immunoglobulin (see Figure 7) |

hCG = human chorionic gonadotrophin; APLA = antiphospholipid antibodies; IUGR = intrauterine growth retardation; APCA = antipaternal complement dependent antibody

diagnosed and treatment is empirical. Many modes of treatment have been examined as to efficacy in patients with three or more pregnancy losses. However, no treatment has been found to be a panacea for all pregnancy losses. In our opinion, research should attempt to define patients with a specific diagnosis. Treatment can then become rational and specific.

## REFERENCES


1. Salat-Baroux, J. (1988). Recurrent spontaneous abortions. *Reprod. Nutr. Dev.*, **28**, 1555–68
2. World Health Organization (1977). WHO recommended definitions, terminology and format for statistical tables related to the perinatal period. *Acta Obstet. Gynecol. Scand.*, **56**, 247–53
3. Carp, H. J. A., Toder, V., Gazit, E., Orgad, S., Mashiach, S., Serr, D. M. and Nebel, L. (1988). Paternal leucocyte immunization and habitual abortion. *Contemp. Rev. Obstet. Gynecol.*, **1**, 49–59
4. Recurrent Miscarriage Immunotherapy Trialists Group (1994). Worldwide collaborative observational study and meta-analysis on allogenic leucocyte for recurrent spontaneous abortion. *Am. J. Reprod. Immunol.*, **32**, 55–72
5. Creasy, R. (1988). The cytogenetics of spontaneous abortion in humans. In Beard, R. W. and Sharp, F. (eds.) *Early Pregnancy Loss: Mechanisms and Treatment*, pp. 293–304. (London: Royal College of Obstetricians and Gynaecologists)
6. Lockshin, M. D. (1992). Antiphospholipid antibody syndrome. *J. Am. Med. Assoc.*, **268**, 1451–3
7. Chavez, D. J. and McIntyre, J. A. (1984). Sera from women with histories of repeated pregnancy losses cause abnormalities in mouse preimplantation blastocysts. *J. Reprod. Immunol.*, 6, 273–81
8. Zigril, M., Fein, A., Carp, H. J. A. and Toder, V. (1991). Immunopotentiation reverses the embryotoxic effect of serum from women with pregnancy loss. *Fertil. Steril.*, **56**, 653–9
9. Abir, R., Ornoy, A., Ben Hur, H., Jaffe, P. and Pinus, H. (1994). The effects of sera from

women with spontaneous abortions on the *in vitro* development of early somite stage rat embryos. *Am. J. Reprod. Immunol.*, **32**, 73–81
10. Abir, R., Ornoy, A., Ben Hur, H., Jaffe, P. and Pinus, H. (1993). IgG exchange as a means of partial correction of anomalies in rat embryos *in vitro*, induced by sera from women with recurrent abortions. *Toxicol. In Vitro*, **7**, 816–26
11. Barnea, E. R. and Barnea, J. D. (1995). Embryonic signals (Abstract). *Am. J. Reprod. Immunol.*, **33**, 429
12. Beard, R. W. (1988). Clinical associations of recurrent miscarriage. In Beard, R. W. and Sharp, F. (eds.) *Early Pregnancy Loss: Mechanisms and Treatment*, pp. 3–8. (London: Royal College of Obstetricians and Gynaecologists)
13. Reginald, P. W., Beard, R. W., Chapple, J., Forbes, P. B., Liddell, H. S., Mowbray, J. F. and Underwood, J. L. (1987). Outcome of pregnancies pregressing beyond 28 weeks gestation in women with a history of recurrent miscarriage. *Br. J. Obstet. Gynaecol.*, **94**, 643–8
14. Seidman, D. S., Gale, R., Ever-Hadani, P., Slater, P. E. and Stevenson, D. K. (1990). Reproductive complications after previous spontaneous abortions. *Pediatr. Rev. Commun.*, **5**, 1–10
15. Carp, H. J. A., Toder V. and Mashiach, S. (1993). Immunotherapy of habitual abortion. *Am. J. Reprod. Immunol.*, **28**, 281–4
16. Ornoy, A., Salomon, J., Ben Zur, Z. and Kohn, G. (1981). Placental findings in spontaneous abortions and stillbirths. *Teratology*, **21**, 243–52
17. Stern, J. J., Dorfman, A. D., Gutierez-Najar, M. D., Cerillo, M. and Coulam, C. B. (1996). Frequency of abnormal karyotypes among abortuses from women with and without a history of recurrent spontaneous abortion. *Fertil. Steril.*, 65, 250–3
18. Stene, J., Stene, E. and Mikkelsen, M. (1984). Risk for chromosome abnormality at amniocentesis following a child with non-inherited chromosome aberration. *Prenat. Diagn.*, **4**, 81–95
19. Morton, N. E., Chiu, D., Holland, C., Jacobs, P. A. and Pettay, D. (1987). Chromosome anomalies as predictors of recurrence risk of spontaneous abortion. *Am. J. Med. Genet.*, **28**, 353–60
20. Warburton, D., Kline, J., Stein, Z., Hutzler, M., Chin, A. and Hassold, T. (1987). Does the karyotype of a spontaneous abotion predict the karytope of a subsequent abortion? Evidence from 273 women with two karyotyped spontaneous abortions. *Am. J. Hum. Genet.*, **41**, 465–83
21. Simpson, J. L., Meyers, C. M. and Martin, A. O. (1989). Tranlocations are infrequent among couples having repeated spontaneous abortion but no other abnormal pregnancies. *Fertil. Steril.*, **51**, 811–14
22. Boue, A. and Gallano, P. (1984). A collaborative study of the segregation of inherited chromosome structural arrangements in 1356 prenatal diagnoses. *Prenat. Diag.*, **4**, 45–67
23. Carp, H. J. A., Ben Shlomo, I., Toder, V., Nebel, L. and Mashiach, S. (1993). Congenital malformations after immunotherapy for habitual abortion: is there an increase? *Gynecol. Obstet. Invest.*, **36**, 198–201
24. Rosenbusch, B. and Sterzik, K. (1991). Sperm chromosomes and habitual abortion. *Fertil. Steril.*, **56**, 370–2
25. Lawler, S. D., Porey, S., Fisher, R. A. and Pickthall, V. J. (1982). Genetic studies on hydatidiform moles. *Ann. Hum. Genet.*, **46**, 209–22
26. Shin, H. S., Flaherty, L., Artzt, K., Bennett, D. and Ravetch, J. (1983). Inversion in the H-2 complex of t-haplotype in mice. *Nature (London)*, **306**, 380–3
27. Gill, T. J. (1983). Immunogenetics of spontaneous abortion in humans. *Transplantation*, **35**, 1–6
28. Rushton, D. I. (1984). The classification and mechanisms of spontaneous abortion. *Perspect. Pediatr. Pathol.*, **8**, 269–87
29. Rock, J. A. and Jones, H. W. (1977). The clinical management of the double uterus. *Fertil. Steril.*, **28**, 798–806
30. Buttram, V. C. (1983). Muellerian anomalies and their management. *Fertil. Steril.*, **40**, 159–63
31. Musich, J. R. and Behrman, S. J. (1978). Obstetric outcome before and after metroplasty in women with uterine anomalies. *Obstet. Gynecol.*, **52**, 63–8
32. Steinberg, W. (1955). Strassmann's metroplasty with management of bipartite uterus causing sterility or habitual abortion. *Obstet. Gynecol. Surv.*, **10**, 400–30
33. Capararo, V. J., Chaung, J. T. and Randall, C. L. (1968). Improved fetal salvage after

etroplasty. *Obstet. Gynecol.*, **31**, 97–103

34. Candiani, G. B. and Fedele, L. (1987). Recurrent spontaneous abortion: state of the art and new horizons. *Acta Eur. Fertil.*, **18**, 91–104
35. Muasher, S. J., Acosta, A. A., Garcia, J. E., Rosenwaks, Z. and Jones, H. W. (1984). Wedge metroplasty for the septate uterus: an update. *Fertil. Steril.*, **42**, 515–19
36. DeCherney, A. and Polan, M. L. (1993). Hysteroscopic management of intrauterine lesions and intractable uterine bleeding. *Obstet. Gynecol.*, **61**, 392–7
37. Israel, R. and March, C. M. (1984). Hysteroscopic incision of the septate uterus. *Am. J. Obstet. Gynecol.*, **149**, 66–73
38. Golan, A., Langer, R., Wexler, S., Seveg, E., Niv, D. and Menachem, P. D. (1990). Cervical cerclage – its role in the pregnant anomalous uterus. *Int. J. Fertil.*, **35**, 164–70
39. Keetle, W. C. (1963). Comment on Barter *et al.* Further experience with the Shirodkar operation. *Am. J. Obstet. Gynecol.*, **85**, 801–5
40. Heinonen, P. K., Saarikoski, S. and Pystyne, P. (1982). Reproductive performance of women with uterine anomalies. *Acta Obstet. Gynecol. Scand.*, **61**, 157–62
41. Michaels, W. H., Montgomery, C., Karo, J., Temple, J., Ager, J. and Olson, J. (1986). Ultrasound differentiation of the competent from the incompetent cervix: prevention of preterm delivery *Am. J. Obstet. Gynecol.*, **154**, 537–46
42. Berger, M. J. and Goldstein, D. P. (1980). Impaired reproductive performance in DES-exposed women. *Obstet. Gynecol.*, **55**, 25–7
43. Nagel, T. C. and Malo, J. W. (1993). Hysteroscopic metroplasty in the diethyl stilbestrol-exposed uterus and similar non-fusion anomalies: effects on subsequent reproductive performance; a preliminary report. *Fertil. Steril.*, **59**, 502–6
44. March, C. M. and Israel, R. (1981). Gestational outcome following hysteroscopic lysis of adhesions. *Fertil. Steril.*, **36**, 455–9
45. Schenker, J. G. and Margalioth, E. J. (1982). Intrauterine adhesions: an updated appraisal. *Fertil. Steril.*, **37**, 593–610
46. Valle, R. F. and Sciarra, J. J. (1988). Intrauterine adhesions: hysteroscopic diagnosis, classification, treatment and reproductive outcome. *Am. J. Obstet. Gynecol.*, **158**, 1459–70
47. Carp, H. J. A., Ben Shlomo, I., Mashiach, S. and Nebel, L. (1992). Complete Asherman's syndrome as a cause of infertility and embryo loss. *Fertil. Steril.*, **58**, 419–21
48. Horta, J. L. H., Fernandez, J. G. and DeSoto, L. B. (1977). Direct evidence of luteal insufficiency in women with habitual abortion. *Obstet. Gynecol.*, **49**, 705–8
49. Csapo, A. I. and Pulkkinen, M. O. (1978). Indispensability of the human corpus luteum in the maintenance of early pregnancy: lutectomy evidence. *Obstet. Gynecol. Surv.*, **3**, 69–81
50. Noyes, R. W., Hertig, A. T. and Rock, J. (1950). Dating the endometrial biopsy. *Fertil. Steril.*, **1**, 3–10
51. McNeely, M. J. and Soules, M. R. (1989). The diagnosis of luteal phase deficiency: a critical review. *Fertil. Steril.*, **51**, 582–7
52. Noyes, R. W. and Haman, J. O. (1953). Accuracy of endometrial dating: correlation of endometrial dating with basal body temperature and menses. *Fertil. Steril.*, **4**, 504–9
53. Peters, A. J., Lloyd, R. P. and Coulam, C. B. (1992). Prevalence of out-of-phase endometrial biopsy specimens. *Am. J. Obstet. Gynecol.*, **166**, 1738–41
54. Portuondo, J. A., Agustin, A., Herran, C. and Echanojauregui, A. D. (1981). The corpus luteum in infertile patients found during laparoscopy. *Fertil. Steril.*, **36**, 37–40
55. Abraham, G. E., Maroulis, G. B. and Marshall, J. R. (1974). Evaluation of ovulation and corpus luteum function using measurements of plasma progesterone. *Obstet. Gynecol.*, **44**, 522–7
56. Olive, D. L., Thomford, P. J., Torres, S. E., Lambert, T. S. and Rosen, G. F. (1989). Twenty-four hour progesterone and luteinizing hormone profiles in the midluteal phase of the infertile patient: correlation with other indicators of luteal phase insufficiency. *Fertil. Steril.*, **51**, 587–91
57. Wentz, A., Herbert, C., Maxson, W. and Garner, C. (1984). Outcome of progesterone treatment of luteal phase inadequacy. *Fertil. Steril.*, **41**, 856–62
58. Balasch, J., Vanrell, J., Marquez, M., Burzac, I. and Gonzalez-Merlo, J. (1982). Dehydrogestone versus vaginal progesterone in the treatment of the endometrial luteal phase deficiency. *Fertil. Steril.*, **37**, 751–4
59. Huang, E. (1986). The primary treatment of luteal phase inadequacy: progesterone versus

clomiphene citrate. *Am. J. Obstet. Gynecol.*, **155**, 824–8
60. Achiron, R., Tadmor, R. and Mashiach, S. (1991). Heart rate as a predictor of first trimester spontaneous abortion after ultrasound proven viability. *Obstet. Gynecol.*, **78**, 330–4
61. Harrison, R. (1988). Early recurrent pregnancy failure: treatment with human chorionic gonadotrophin. In Beard, R. W. and Sharp, F. (eds.) *Early Pregnancy Loss: Mechanisms and Treatment*, pp. 421–8 (London: Royal College of Obstetricians and Gynaecologists)
62. Quenby, S. and Farquarson, R. G. (1994). Human chorionic gonadotrophin supplementation in recurring pregnancy loss: a controlled trial. *Fertil. Steril.*, **62**, 708–15
63. Homburg, R., Armer, N. A., Eshel, A., Adams, J. and Jacobs, H. S. (1988). Influence of serum luteinising hormone concentrations on ovulation, conception, and early pregnancy loss in polycystic ovary syndrome. *Br. Med. J.*, **297**, 1024–6
64. Regan, L., Owen, E. J. and Jacobs, H. S. (1990). Hypersecretion of luteinizing hormone, infertility, and miscarriage. *Lancet*, **336**, 1141–4
65. Kovacs, G. T., Baker, H. W., Burger, H. G., Lee, J. and Summerbell, D. (1990). Prognosis of pregnancies conceived by donor insemination with respect to the late follicular phase luteinizing hormone levels. *Br. J. Obstet. Gynaecol.*, **97**, 654–6
66. Thomas, A., Okamoto, S., O'Shea, F. O., MacLauchlan, V., Besanko, M. and Healy, D. (1989). Do raised serum luteinising hormone levels during stimulation for *in vitro* fertilisation predict outcome? *Br. J. Obstet. Gynaecol.*, **96**, 1328–32
67. Clifford, K., Rai, R. and Regan, L. (1984). An informative protocol for the investigation of recurrent miscarriage: preliminary experience of 500 consecutive cases. *Hum. Reprod.*, **9**, 1328–32
68. Sagle, M., Bishop, K., Ridley, N., Alexander, F. M., Michel, M. and Bonney, R. C. (1988). Recurrent early miscarriage and polycystic ovaries. *Br. Med. J.*, **297**, 1027–8
69. Carp, H. J. A., Perla, Y., Rabinovici, J. and Mashiach, S. (1995). The effect of serum follicular phase LH levels in habitual abortion: correlation with paternal leucocyte immunization. *Hum. Reprod.*, **10**, 1702–5
70. Blank, M., Cohen, J., Toder, V. and Shoenfeld, Y. (1991). Induction of anti-phospholipid syndrome in naive mice with mouse lupus monoclonal and human polyclonal anti-cardiolipin antibodies. *Proc. Natl. Acad. Sci. USA*, **88**, 3069–73
71. Peaceman, A. M., Silver, R. K., MacGregor, S. N. and Socol, M. L. (1992). Interlaboratory variation in antiphospholipid antibody testing. *Am. J. Obstet. Gynecol.*, **166**, 1780–6
72. Harris, E. N. (1988). Clinical and immunological significance of antiphospholipid antibodies. In Beard, R. W. and Sharp, F. (eds.) *Early Pregnancy Loss: Mechanisms and Treatment*, pp. 43–60. (London: Royal College of Obstetricians and Gynaecologists)
73. Rote, N. S., Walter, A. and Lyden, T. W. (1992). Antiphospholipid antibodies – lobsters or red herrings. *Am. J. Reprod. Immunol.*, **28**, 31–7
74. Branch, D. W., Scott, J. R., Kochenour, N. K. and Hershgold, E. (1985). Obstetric complications associated with the lupus anticoagulant. *N. Engl. J. Med.*, **313**, 1322–6
75. Carp, H. J. A., Frenkel, Y., Many, A., Menashe, Y., Mashiach, S., Serr, D. M., Toder, V. and Nebel, L. (1989). Fetal demise associated with lupus anticoagulant: clinical features and results of treatment. *J. Gynaecol. Obstet. Invest.*, **28**, 178–84
76. Lockwood, C. J., Romero, R., Feinberg, R. F., Clyne, L. P., Coster, B. and Hobbins, J. C. (1989). The prevalence and biologic significance of lupus anticoagulant and anticardiolipin antibodies in a general obstetric population. *Am. J. Obstet. Gynecol.*, **161**, 369–73
77. Carp, H. J. A., Toder, V., Mashiach, S., Nebel, L. and Serr, D. M. (1990). Recurrent miscarriage: a review of current concepts, immune mechanisms, and results of treatment. *Obstet. Gynecol. Surv.*, **45**, 657–69
78. Tincani, A., Cattenco, M. and Martinelli, D. (1987). Anti-phospholipid antibodies in recurrent fetal loss: only one side of the coin? *Clin. Exp. Rhematol.*, **5**, 390–1
79. Lookwood, C. J., Reece, E. A., Romero, R. and Hobbins, J. C. (1986). Antiphospholipid antibody and pregnancy wastage. *Lancet*, **2**, 742–3
80. Vaarala, O., Palosuo, T., Kleemola, M. and Abo, K. (1986). Anticardiolipin response in acute infections. *Clin. Immunol. Immunopathol.*, **41**, 8–15
81. Ishii, Y., Nagasawa, K., Mayumi, T. and Nibo,

Y. (1990). Clinical importance of persistence of anticardiolipin antibodies in systemic lupus erythematosus. *Ann. Rheum. Dis.*, **49**, 387–90
82. Galli, M., Comfurius, P., Maassen, C., Hemker, H. C., De Baets, M. H., Van Breda-Vriesman, P. J. C., Barburi, T., Zwaal, R. F. A. and Bevers, E. M. (1990). Anti-cardiolipin antibodies (ACA) directed not to cardiolipin but to a plasma protein cofactor. *Lancet*, **335**, 1544–7
83. Khamashta, M. A., Harris, E. N. and Gharavi, A. E. (1988). Immune mediated mechanism for thrombosis: antiphospholipid antibody binding to platelet membranes. *Ann. Rheum. Dis.*, **47**, 849–54
84. Carreras, L. O., Defreyen, G. and Machin, S. J. (1981). Arterial thrombosis, intra-uterine death and 'lupus' anticoagulant: detection of immunoglobulin interfering with prostacycline formation. *Lancet*, 1, 244–6
85. Peaceman, A. M. and Rehnberg, K. A. (1993). The effect of immunoglobulin G fractions from patients with lupus anticoagulant on placental prostacycline and thromboxane production. *Am J. Obstet. Gynecol.*, **169**, 1403–6
86. Lyden, T., Vogt, E., Ng, A. K., Johnson, P. M. and Rote, N. S. (1992). Monoclonal antiphospholipid antibody reactivity against human placental trophoblast. *J. Reprod. Immunol.*, **22**, 1–14
87. Sessions, A. and Horowitz, A. F. (1983). Differentiation related differences in the plasma membrane phospholipid asymmetry of myogenic and fibrogenic cells. *Biochem. Biophys. Acta*, **728**, 103–11
88. Out, H. J., Kooijman, C. D., Bruinse, H. W. and Derksen, R. H. W. M. (1991). Histopathological findings from patients with intrauterine fetal death and antiphospholipid antibodies. *Eur. J. Obstet. Gynaecol.*, **41**, 179–86
89. Carp, H. J. A., Menashe, Y., Frenkel, Y., Many, A., Nebel, L., Toder, V., Serr, D. M. and Mashiach, S. (1993). Lupus anticoagulant: significance in first trimester habitual abortion. *J. Reprod. Med.*, **38**, 549–52
90. Lubbe, W. F., Butler, W. S., Palmer, S. J. and Liggins, G. G. (1983). Fetal survival after prednisone suppression of maternal lupus anticoagulant. *Lancet*, **1**, 1361–3
91. Lockshin, M. D., Druzin, M. L. and Qamar, T. (1989). Prednisone does not prevent recurrent fetal death in women with antiphospholipid antibody. *Am. J. Obstet. Gynecol.*, **160**, 439–43
92. Cowchock, S. (1991). The role of antiphospholipid antibodies in obstetric medicine. *Curr. Obstet. Med.*, 1, 229–47
93. Kutteh, W. H. and Webster, R. M. (1993). A prospective controlled trial of aspirin for the treatment of recurrent pregnancy loss associated with antiphospholipid antibodies. *Fertil. Steril.*, **60** (Suppl.), S68–9
94. Rosove, M. N., Tabsh, K., Wasserstrum, N., Howard, P., Hahn, B. H. and Kalunian, K. C. (1990). Heparin therapy for pregnant women with lupus anticoagulant or anticardiolipin antibodies. *Obstet. Gynecol.*, **75**, 630–4
95. Lorber, M. and Blumenfeld, Z. (1992). Low molecular weight heparin (Clexane): a promising treatment in women with recurrent abortions in SLE and antiphospholipid antibody syndrome. *Lupus*, **1** (Suppl.), 162–4
96. Salzman, E. W. (1992). Subcutaneous low molecular weight heparin and other new antithrombotic drugs. *N. Engl. J. Med.*, **326**, 1017–19
97. Dulitzki, M., Pauzner, R., Langevitz, P., Livneh, A., Many, A. and Schiff, E. (1996). Low molecular weight heparin during pregnancy and delivery: preliminary experience with 41 pregnancies. *Obstet. Gynecol.*, **87**, 380–3
98. Babcock, R. B., Dumper, C. W. and Scharfman, W. B. (1976). Heparin-induced immunothrombocytopenia. *N. Engl. J. Med.*, **295**, 237–41
99. Reece, E. A., Gabrielli, S., Cullen, M. T., Zheng, X. Z., Hobbins, J. C. and Harris, E. N. (1990). Recurrent adverse pregnancy outcome and antiphospholipid antibodies. *Am. J. Obstet. Gynecol.*, **163**, 162–9
100. Scott, J. R., Branch, W., Kochenour, N. K. and Ward, K. (1988). Intravenous immunoglobulin treatment of pregnant patients with recurrent pregnancy loss caused by antiphospholipid antibodies and Rh immunization. *Am. J. Obstet. Gynecol.*, **159**, 1055–6
101. McVerry, B., Spearing, R. and Smith, A. (1985). SLE anticoagulant: transient inhibition by high does immunoglobulin infusions. *Br. J. Haematol.*, **61**, 579–80
102. Many, A., Pauzner, R., Carp, H. J. A., Langevitz, P. and Martinowitz, U. (1993). Treatment of patients with antiphospholipid antibodies during pregnancy. *Am. J. Reprod. Immunol.*, **28**, 216–18
103. Cowchock, F. S., Reece, E. A., Balaban, D., Branch, D. W. and Plouffe, L. (1992). Repeated fetal losses associated with antiphospholipid

antibodies: a collaborative randomized trial comparing prednisone to low dose heparin treatment. *Am. J. Obstet. Gynecol.*, **166**, 1318–27

104. Beer, A. E., Quebbman, J. F., Ayres, J. W. T. and Harines, R. F. (1981). Major histocompatibility complex antigens. Maternal and paternal immune responses and chronic habitual abortions. *Am. J. Obstet. Gynecol.*, **141**, 987–99
105. Taylor, C. and Page Faulk, W. (1981). Prevention of recurrent abortion with leucocyte transfusions. *Lancet*, **2**, 68–9
106. Mowbray, J. F., Gibbings, C. R., Lidell, H., Reginald, P. W., Underwood, J. and Beard, R. W. (1985). Controlled trial of treatment of recurrent spontaneous abortions by immunisation with paternal cells. *Lancet*, **1**, 941–3
107. Ho, H. N., Gill, T. J., Hsieh, H., Jiang, J., Lee, T. and Hsieh, C. (1991). Immunotherapy for recurrent spontaneous abortions in a Chinese population. *Am. J. Reprod. Immunol.*, **25**, 10–15
108. Gatenby, P. A., Cameron, K., Simes, R. J., Aldstein, S., Bennet, M. J., Jansen, R. P. S., Shearman, R. P., Stewart, G. J., Whittle, M. and Doran, T. J. (1993). Treatment of recurrent spontaneous abortion by immunization by paternal lymphocytes: results of a controlled trial. *Am. J. Reprod. Immunol.*, **29**, 88–94
109. Chrisatiansen, O. B., Mathiesen, O., Husth, M., Lauritzen, J. G. and Grunne, N. (1994). Placebo controlled trial of active immunization with third party leucocytes in recurrent miscarriage. *Acta Obstet. Gynecol. Scand.*, **73**, 261–8
110. Cauchi, M. N., Lim, D., Young, D. E., Kloss, M. and Pepperell, R. J. (1991). Treatment of recurrent aborters by immunization with paternal cells – controlled trial. *Am. J. Reprod. Immunol.*, **25**, 16–17
111. Carp, H. J. A., Toder, V., Gazit, E., Orgad, S., Mashiach, S., Serr, D. M. and Nebel, L. (1990). Selection of patients with habitual abortion for paternal leucocyte immunization. *Arch. Gynaecol. Obstet.*, **248**, 93–101
112. Mittal, K. K., Mickey, T. R., Singall, D. P. and Terasaki, P. I. (1968). Serotyping for transplantation XVIII. Refinement of microdroplet cytotoxicity test. *Transplantation*, **6**, 913–27
113. Gazit, E., Efter, T., Mizrachi, Y., Mashiach, I., Mashiach, S. and Serr, D. M. (1977). Acquisition of typing serum from postpartum blood clots. *Tiss. Antigens*, **9**, 66–8
114. Wegmann, T., Singh, B. and Carlson, G. (1979). Allogenic placenta is a paternal strain immunoabsorbent. *J. Immunol.*, **122**, 270–4
115. Regan, L. (1988). A prospective study of habitual abortion. In Beard, R. W. and Sharp, F. (eds.) *Early Pregnancy Loss: Mechanisms and Treatment*, pp. 23–37. (London: Royal College of Obstetricians and Gynaecologists)
116. Regan, L. and Braude, P. B. (1987). Is antipaternal cytotoxic antibody a valid marker in the management of recurrent abortion? (Letter) *Lancet*, **2**, 1280
117. Daya, S. and Gunby, J. (1994). The effectiveness of allogeneic leucocyte immunization in unexplained primary recurrent spontaneous abortion. *Am. J. Reprod. Immunol.*, **32**, 294–302
118. Hasegawa, I., Tani, H., Takakuwa, K., Yamada, K., Kanazawa, K. and Tanaka, K. (1992). Immunotherapy with paternal lymphocytes preceeding *in vitro* fertilization embryo transfer for patients with repeated failure of embryo transfer. *Fertil. Steril.*, **57**, 445–7
119. Carp, H. J. A., Toder, V., Mashiach, S. and Rabinovici, J. (1994). The effect of paternal leucocyte immunization on implantation after recurrent biochemical pregnancies and repeated failure of embryo transfer. *Am. J. Reprod. Immunol.*, **31**, 112–15
120. Menge, A. C. and Beer, A. E. (1985). The significance of human leucocyte antigen profiles in human infertility, recurrent abortion and pregnancy disorders. *Fertil. Steril.*, **43**, 693–5
121. Mowbray, J. F. and Underwood, J. L. (1994). Abstracts of contributors' individual data submitted to the worldwide prospective observational study on immunotherapy for treatment of recurrent spontaneous abortion. *Am. J. Reprod. Immunol.*, **32**, 261–74
122. Toder, V. and Carp H. J. A. (1994). Maternal immune recognition of pregnancy. *Israel J. Med. Sci.*, **30**, 787–91
123. Szekeres-Bartho, J., Varga, P., Kinsky, R. and Chaouat, G. (1990). Progesterone mediated immunosuppression and the maintenance of pregnancy. *Res. Immunol.*, **141**, 175–84
124. Coulam, C. B. and Coulam, C. H. (1992). Update on immunotherapy for recurrent pregnancy loss. *Am. J. Reprod. Immunol.*, **27**, 124–7
125. Mueller-Eckhardt, G., Heine, O. and Polten, B. (1991). IVIG to prevent recurrent spontaneous abortion. *Lancet*, **1**, 337

126. Maruyama, T., Makino, T., Sugi, T., Iwasaki, K., Umeuchi, M., Saito, S. and Nozawa, S. (1991). Alternative treatment for unexplained recurrent spontaneous abortion. *Acta Obstet. Gynecol. Jpn.*, **43**, 1581–2
127. German RSA/IVIG group (1994). Intravenous immunoglobulin in the prevention of recurrent miscarriage. *Br. J. Obstet. Gynaecol.*, **101**, 1072–7
128. Coulam, C. B. (1995). Immunotherapy for recurrent spontaneous abortion. *Early Pregnancy*, **1**, 13–26
129. Carp, H. J. A., Ahiron, R., Mashiach, S., Schonfeld, Y., Gazit, E. and Toder, V. (1996). Intravenous immunoglobulin in women with five or more abortions. *Am. J. Reprod. Immunol.*, **35**, 360–2
130. Coulam, C. B., Krysa, L. W. and Bustillo, M. (1994). Intravenous immunoglobulin for *in vitro* fertilization failure. *Hum. Reprod.*, **9**, 2265–9
131. Balasch, J., Font, J., Creus, M., Martorell, J., Fabregues, F. and Vanrell, J. A. (1996). Intravenous immunoglobulin preceding *in vitro* fertilization-embryo transfer for patients with repeated failure of embryo transfer. *Fertil. Steril.*, **65**, 655–8
132. Cauchi, M. N., Pepperell, R., Kloss, M. and Lim, D. (1991). Predictors of pregnancy success in repeated miscarriages. *Am. J. Reprod. Immunol.*, **26**, 72–5
133. Cowchock, F. S., Smith, J. B., David, S., Scher, J., Batzu, F. and Corson, S. (1990). Paternal mononuclear cell immunization. Therapy for repeated miscarriage: predictive values for pregnancy success. *Am. J. Reprod. Immunol.*, **22**, 12–17

# Hormonal contraception 22

*James O. Drife*

## INTRODUCTION

Part of the fascination of reproductive medicine is the interaction between scientific advances and cultural attitudes in society. This is particularly important in relation to hormonal contraception. The science of contraception has advanced dramatically over the last 30 years and our knowledge continues to increase. Science, however, is only part of the story. As with other aspects of reproductive medicine, our willingness to apply scientific knowledge is influenced by deeply held beliefs about sex and reproduction. Indeed, in the case of hormonal contraception, cultural attitudes may affect our interpretation of the scientific data.

### The risks of excessive fertility

Much of reproductive medicine is concerned with treating infertility, but the greatest challenge facing our species is population growth. 'The past century has been characterized by unnaturally high fertility, first in the West during Victorian times and more recently in the developing world'[1]. The causes have included a decline in mortality rates, a fall in the age at puberty and a change from breastfeeding on demand to scheduled or artificial feeding.

There is now a strong desire for contraception in the developing world, but, unfortunately, access to contraception is often difficult. The problems include restrictive medical practices. For example, in parts of Africa access to hormonal contraception is contingent on expensive tests or on a prolonged physical examination[1]; these are regarded as unnecessary in the UK[2].

In the developed world, hormonal contraception is available and relatively cheap, but there are still large numbers of unwanted pregnancies. In Britain around 25% of women will have at least one abortion by the age of 25 and around 20% of all pregnancies are terminated. Many Western countries have rates of abortion that are higher than those in Britain. For example, in the USA the abortion rate (28/1000 women aged 15–44) is double that in Britain; about half of American women have an abortion at some time in their life. Some countries, such as the Netherlands and Germany, have lower rates than those in Britain, and there is a correlation between low abortion rates and contraceptive use.

The reasons that there are still so many unplanned pregnancies lie in attitudes to contraception[3]. The British media often feature sex in a lurid or facetious way, but play a small role in the health education of teenagers. Over the years, much more publicity has been given to the possible adverse effects of hormonal contraception than to its benefits. This has resulted in women having a biased and inaccurate view of its risks.

Another factor that influences people's perceptions of hormonal contraception is the fact that marketing is directed towards doctors and not to the public. Direct marketing to consumers would emphasize its positive aspects. Advertising to doctors has, at least in the past, concentrated on side-effects, reinforcing a perception that hormonal contraception carries important risks.

### Non-contraceptive benefits

Hormonal contraception is highly effective in preventing unwanted pregnancy, but may also have other benefits for health. The greatest benefits are conferred by methods that suppress the natural ovarian cycle. Ovarian activity involves the production of relatively high levels of oestradiol (in the preovulatory phase) and progesterone (in the postovulatory phase), and these hormone levels, rising and falling month after month, may have adverse effects ranging from psychological effects (premenstrual syndrome) to malignant disease. Incessant ovulation has been linked with risks of subsequent ovarian cancer; suppressing ovulation with the combined pill has been shown to reduce this risk. This is discussed further below.

## PHYSIOLOGY AND PHARMACOLOGY

Steroid contraceptives have three antifertility actions: suppression of ovulation, thickening of cervical mucus and effects on the endometrium. The relative importance of each depends on the type of preparation. With the combined oral contraceptive pill, for example, the most important action is the suppression of ovulation[4]. Both the oestrogen and the progestogen components of the combined oral contraceptive act on the hypothalamus, affecting the physiological negative feedback mechanism to suppress the production of follicle stimulating hormone (FSH) and luteinizing hormone (LH).

During the normal menstrual cycle, the cervical mucus becomes penetrable to spermatozoa at the time of the preovulatory oestrogen surge, when the mucus is thin and stretchy and has spinnbarkheit. By preventing the oestrogen surge, the combined oral contraceptive prevents this change. The progestogen component keeps the mucus scanty and viscous, with low spinnbarkeit. This type of mucus impairs sperm transport.

The endometrium during the normal cycle undergoes a synchronized series of changes in preparation for implantation[5]. Their significance is still not fully understood, but it is clear that hormonal contraception disrupts endometrial development and leads to the formation of a thin endometrium with poorly developed secretory ability.

## ORAL CONTRACEPTION

### Combined oral contraceptives

In spite of the years of adverse publicity, by 1991 nearly 50% of 20-year-old women in the UK were taking combined oral contraceptives[6]. The following sections summarize some salient points about the pharmacology of these compounds and discuss recent concerns about cardiovascular disease and breast cancer.

*Pharmacology*

The first combined oral contraceptive introduced on the market, Enovid®, was approved in the USA in 1959 and in the UK in 1961. It contained 150 μg of mestranol and 10 mg of norethynodrel. These are very high doses. Over the next 20 years, there was a steady trend towards the use of lower-dose formulations. In the UK by 1980, well over 50% of combined oral contraceptive prescriptions were for formulations containing less than 50 μg of oestrogen[7]. As much of the original data on risks came from studies carried out before 1980, this change may be important in interpreting epidemiological studies.

One aspect of combined oral contraceptive use that has not changed is that the pill is almost always taken in a monthly cycle of 3 weeks 'on' and 1 week 'off'. Follicular development occurs during the 'pill-free' week, increasing the chance of accidental ovulation if a pill is forgotten towards the beginning or the end of a packet. If the pill were taken in a cycle of perhaps 9 weeks on and 1 week off, there would be much less chance of conception if a pill were missed. Such regimens are safe[8] but have not become popular, because the pattern of monthly bleeds seems 'normal' to both women and doctors. An alternative strategy for reducing the number of pill failures would be to shorten the pill-free week to 5 or 6 days[9].

*Metabolic effects*
Both components of the combined oral contraceptive affect other organs in addition to the hypothalamus and genital tract. For example, oestrogens affect bone, connective tissue and pelvic blood flow, while progesterone elevates body temperature and has mild diuretic effects. Oestrogens and progestogens both affect the breast. The potency of a progestogen is assessed by its ability to induce secretory change in the endometrium, but this may not reflect the relative potencies of progestogens on other organs.

Oestrogens and progestogens are metabolized in the liver, and the resultant slight alteration in liver function underlies most of the metabolic changes produced by the pill. Combined oral contraceptives increase serum levels of triglyceride and low-density lipoprotein cholesterol, and decrease high-density lipoprotein cholesterol. They reduce glucose tolerance and increase insulin levels. These metabolic changes are similar to those associated with an increased risk of coronary heart disease. Modern formulations containing low doses of oestrogen and progestogens reduce these adverse metabolic effects.

Combined oral contraceptives affect blood clotting by increasing plasma fibrinogen and the activity of coagulation factors, especially factors VII and X. There is also a reduction in the coagulation inhibitor, antithrombin III. These changes tend to create a hypercoagulable state, although this is largely counterbalanced by increased fibrinolytic activity. The coagulation effects depend on the dosage of oestrogen and the type of progestogen, and new low-dose formulations should therefore reduce the risk of thromboembolic complications.

The third-generation progestogens (desogestrel, norgestimate and gestodene) appear to have a balanced effect on coagulation factors and may improve the ratio of low-density lipoprotein to high-density lipoprotein[10]. Thus they may carry lower risks of cardiovascular disease than the older progestogens. Never-the-less, the metabolic basis of cardiovascular disease is still incompletely understood, and it is important to remember that low-dose combined oral contraceptives containing second-generation progestogens have not resulted in a high incidence of adverse side-effects[11].

*Cardiovascular disease*
*Venous thromboembolism* Studies from the USA and the UK, and a collaborative study by the World Health Organization (WHO) have indicated that the combined oral contraceptive causes a three- to six-fold increase in venous thromboembolism. The risk is unrelated to duration of use[12,13]. Some studies have suggested that the reduction in oestrogen dosage to 20–35 μg of oestradiol has brought about a reduction in risk[14].

In 1995, this trend towards lower risk was confirmed, with the WHO international study giving a relative risk of 4.1 in Europe and 3.2 in developing countries[15]. The increased risk appeared within 4 months of starting the combined oral contraceptive and disappeared within 3 months of stopping it. The study also confirmed that increased body mass index is an independent risk factor for venous thromboembolism.

An unexpected finding in the WHO study was that the progestogen component of the combined oral contraceptive may affect the risk of venous thromboembolism. When low-oestrogen preparations containing second- and third-generation progestogens were examined separately, the risk appeared to be 2–3 times greater for preparations containing desogestrel and gestodene than for those containing levonorgestrel[16].

This finding was checked in two other studies. One, based on the UK General Practice Research Database, also concluded that combined oral contraceptives containing third-generation progestogens had approximately double the risk of those containing levonorgestrel. The other, a case–control study based on the Leiden Thrombophilia Study, concluded that combined oral contraceptives containing desogestrel carried a higher risk than did other combined oral contraceptives[17]: it also pointed out that some women (e.g. those carrying the factor V Leiden mutation) are already at increased risk of thromboembolism, but the higher risk of third-generation combined oral contraceptives was not confined to this subgroup.

When UK cases in the WHO study were analysed, the risk estimates were 2.6, 5.3 and 5.7 for levonorgestrel, desogestrel and gestodene, respectively. These are within the range that has been widely known for several years. The UK media, however, gave the public the impression that the new studies had revealed an unexpectedly high risk of venous thromboembolism[18]. In reality, the 1995 studies show, if anything, an unexpectedly low risk for combined oral contraceptives containing levonorgestrel. In all these 1995 studies, bias or confounding factors cannot be ruled out – for example, there may have been a tendency for doctors to prescribe third-generation progestogens to women whom they believed to be at higher risk of venous thromboembolism.

The mortality from venous thromboembolism is low (estimated at 1% of cases) and the risk of death from thromboembolism among combined oral contraceptive users is no higher than 2–3 per million users[19]. Therefore, the difference in fatality rates between second- and third-generation progestogens is about 1 in a million[20]. This should be weighed against the known benefits of third-generation progestogens, in terms of improved cycle control[11], and the possibility that they may carry a lower risk of other types of cardiovascular disease[21].

*Myocardial infarction* Early studies, based on high-dose combined oral contraceptives, indicated that the overall risk of myocardial infarction is increased about 3–5 times[22,23]. This increase was related to smoking and age. Among smokers using the combined oral contraceptive, the risk of death from circulatory causes is 1 in 10 000 until the age of 35. Between the ages of 35 and 44, the risk increases among smokers to 1 in 2000, but for non-smokers the risk remains less than 1 in 6000. Above age 45, the respective figures are 1 in 550 and 1 in 2500. Therefore, combined oral contraceptives are contraindicated over the age of 35 in smokers, although not necessarily in non-smokers.

After the changes in combined oral contraceptive formulation in the UK, a new case–control study was started in 1986[24,25]. All women in England and Wales between 16 and 39 years, who died of myocardial infarction, subarachnoid haemorrhage, other stroke and pulmonary embolism and/or deep vein thrombosis, were included in the study and preliminary data suggested that the risk of myocardial infarction associated with combined oral contraceptives was indeed lower than it had been in the past. The authors commented, 'It may be that any increase in risk is associated solely with the older combined preparations containing 50 μg of oestrogen'[25].

The most recent studies, in the USA of non-fatal disease[22] and in the UK of fatal myocardial infarction[26], found an unadjusted relative risk of 1.1 for combined oral contraceptive use, i.e. no increased risk of coronary artery disease in pill users. However, the relative risk rose to a two-fold increase in risk after adjustment for other risk factors. In the UK study, the relative risk associated with older combined oral contraceptives containing 50 μg of ethinylestradiol was 4.2. The increase in risk applied only to current users: among women who had stopped using the pill, the risk was not significantly raised[23].

*Stroke* In young women, haemorrhagic stroke is more common than occlusive stroke. A case–control study of women suffering a stroke at age less than 40 concluded that the relative risk of occlusive stroke was 4.4 among ever-users: for the commoner type, subarachnoid haemorrhage, the relative risk was 1.1 for current users and 1.3 for ever-users[27].

Recently, a hospital-based case–control study was conducted in 21 centres in 17 countries[28]. Each centre recruited cases and controls from collaborating hospitals. The cases were women aged 20–44 years admitted with a stroke between February 1989 and January 1993.

The study found that, in Europe, the overall odds ratio of ischaemic stroke was 2.99, but lower in younger women and those who did not smoke, and less than 2 in women who did not have hypertension and whose blood pressure had been checked before combined oral contraceptive use. The odds ratio associated with low-dose combined oral contraceptives (less than 50 µg of oestrogen) was 1.53. The study concluded 'The incidence of ischaemic stroke is low in women of reproductive age and any risk attributable to oral contraceptive use is small. The risk can be further reduced if users are younger than 35 years, do not smoke, do not have a history of hypertension and have blood pressure measured before the start of oral contraceptive use. In such women, oral contraceptive preparations with low oestrogen doses may be associated with even lower risk.'

The study also examined haemorrhagic stroke. There was a slightly increased overall risk which was not significant in Europe but was significant in developing countries. In women under 35, however, combined oral contraceptive use did not affect the risk of haemorrhagic stroke in either group of countries. The risk was greatly increased, however, by a history of hypertension and was also increased by smoking[29].

*Hypertension* The combined oral contraceptive causes a rise in blood pressure in most women[30]. A recent study of users of combined oral contraceptives containing 35 µg of ethinyloestradiol showed a rise of about 1.0 mmHg in diastolic pressure, which, as the authors remarked, is 'statistically significant but clinically unimportant'[31].

*Age and smoking* Much attention has been paid to the effect of combined oral contraceptives on myocardial infarction[32], but in young women the effect of smoking is much more important. Recent studies show a seven-fold increase in relative risk of myocardial infarction in women under 50 who smoke 35 or more cigarettes a day. The apparent link between combined oral contraceptive use and myocardial infarction may have been due to the association between combined oral contraceptive use and smoking: there is no excess risk of heart attacks in combined oral contraceptive users who are non-smokers[33].

It is clear that women over 35 who smoke should not take the combined oral contraceptive. It is not clear how soon the risk returns to normal in ex-smokers, but it seems prudent to advise that an older woman who has recently given up heavy smoking should be advised not to start the combined oral contraceptive. Women who have never smoked, however, may continue to use combined oral contraceptives after the age of 35, provided other risk factors – particularly hypertension and a previous history of cardiovascular disease – are not present[34].

*Cancer*

*Ovary* The combined oral contraceptive has a well-established protective effect against ovarian cancer. At least a dozen case–control studies have shown that former users of combined oral contraceptives have a diminished risk compared to women who have not used the pill[35]. The relative risk in former combined oral contraceptive users is about 0.6 that of controls[36]. A recent study in the USA concluded that a protective effect is not detected among women who have used the combined oral contraceptive for less than 3 years and does not become greater if the combined oral contraceptive is used for more than 4 years. The effect, however, is apparent for as long as 15–19 years after cessation of combined oral contraceptive use. Data on newer types of combined oral contraceptive were limited in this study, but the investigators concluded that protection is not confined to any particular type of formulation[37].

The Oxford–FPA cohort study suggested an even greater protective effect, with an overall relative risk among combined oral contraceptive users of 0.4. No protective effect was seen in up to 2 years of combined oral contraceptive use, but this study indicated that prolonged use might give greater protection, as the relative risk for users of 97 months' duration or more was only 0.3[38]. Vessey and Painter[38] pointed out that, in several countries, a decline in the mortality from ovarian cancer in women aged under 55 years has been noted since the early

1970s, and suggested that this may well reflect an effect of combined oral contraceptive use.

Although the protective effect against ovarian cancer is clear, the biological mechanism underlying it is not fully understood. Suppression of ovulation abolishes the dramatic monthly growth in ovarian follicular size (and, incidentally, in endometrial thickness) and it is not surprising, therefore, that inhibiting this process causes a reduction in the disordered growth that could lead on to cancer. The persistence of the effect is more puzzling, however. It may possibly be explained by lack of hormonal support for transformed cells, which then differentiate and die.

*Uterus* Unopposed oestrogen stimulation is a risk factor for endometrial cancer and, in combined oral contraceptive-controlled cycles, oestrogen is opposed by a progestogen throughout the 21 days of pill-taking. It is therefore not surprising that the combined oral contraceptive reduces the risk of endometrial malignancy. This protective effect, like that against ovarian cancer, has been well established by numerous studies[39], and again a relative risk of 0.6 for these cancers can be detected after only 12 months or less of combined oral contraceptive use, and persists for at least 15 years after the combined oral contraceptive is stopped.

Again, the protective effect shown by case–control studies has been confirmed in cohort studies. Both the RCGP study and the Oxford–FPA study have shown a very marked protective effect, with relative risks of 0.2 and 0.1, respectively[38].

*Breast* Breast cancer is one of the most common fatal malignancies among women, and the effect of combined oral contraceptives on breast cancer incidence is therefore a very important question. After many case–control studies, it was concluded that, in the middle of reproductive life (between the ages of 25 and 39), the combined oral contraceptive has no effect on cancer risk[40]. A review and meta-analysis of the epidemiological studies concluded that there was no increase in the risk of breast cancer for women who had ever used combined oral contraceptives, even after a long duration of use[41].

Attention has, however, focused on young women – those under 25, or women who have not yet had their first full-term pregnancy[42]. There have been suggestions of an increased risk in these groups but the results remain inconclusive[43]. At least ten studies have addressed the question of breast cancer risk related to duration of combined oral contraceptive use before the age of 25. Three showed no increase in risk and six suggested a positive relation. The excess risk for long duration of use before age 25 was estimated at 1.5. Four studies have shown an increased risk for early age at first combined oral contraceptive use and four others have reported no such association[44].

A recent case–control study of breast cancer among Dutch women aged 20–54 at diagnosis found that long-term combined oral contraceptive use (more than 12 years) had a relative risk of 1.3. This positive trend was found in women aged under 36 and over 46, but not in women aged 36–45. The relative risk of developing breast cancer before age 36 was 2.1 for 4 or more years of use, and the risk increased for longer use before age 20 (1.44 per year). Recent use was associated with an increased risk among women of 46–54 (relative risk 1.9). The authors concluded that 4 or more years of use, especially before age 20, are associated with increased risk of breast cancer at an early age, but there is limited evidence that this increased risk disappears with age[45].

The UK National Case–Control Study published evidence that the risk of breast cancer under age 36, which is already known to be related to duration of use (relative risk 1.07 per year: 2.57 for > 8 years of use) is not modified by interrupting pill use either by pregnancy or for any other reason[46].

Why does this question remain so controversial? One difficulty is the long latent period between combined oral contraceptive use and clinical cancer. Not only does this make it difficult to ascertain the duration of combined oral contraceptive use in cases or controls, but also, and more importantly, current studies often relate to dosages no longer used. Discrepancies between studies may arise because they may relate to different dosages of combined oral contraceptive or possibly to studies being carried out before the end of the latent period[47].

There is no evidence at present that combined oral contraceptive use early in reproductive life increases the risk of breast cancer after the menopause[48]. A collaborative re-analysis has recently been published[49] of data from 54 studies involving 53 297 with, and 100 239 women without, breast cancer. The results indicate that during combined oral contraceptive use, there is a small increase in the relative risk of breast cancer and this increase persists for 10 years after use, falling steadily during this time. Ten years after stopping combined oral contraceptives, there is no increased risk. These data provide reassurance that combined oral contraceptive use early in reproductive life will not affect the risk of breast cancer in later life when the disease becomes common.

There is an increase in the activity of the normal breast in the luteal phase of the normal menstrual cycle[50,51]. The combined oral contraceptive mimics the effect of the normal cycle on mammary glands: low-dose combined oral contraceptives produced a level of stimulation similar to that in the normal cycle, but higher levels of stimulation were seen with combined oral contraceptives with higher oestrogen contents[52]. These laboratory studies explain why no protective effect of the combined oral contraceptive against breast cancer has been detected, and suggest that the reduction of dosage may have reduced the risk to the breast. Because of the long latency of breast cancer, further studies are needed to establish the effects of current low-dose combined oral contraceptives.

*Cervix* The incidence of cervical carcinoma is heavily influenced by sexual behaviour, but, in the 1980s, case–control studies which controlled for the number of sexual partners concluded that there is a modest increase in risk in long-term combined oral contraceptive users. Cohort studies came to similar conclusions. The Oxford-FPA study showed a trend in the incidence of all forms of cervical neoplasia with duration of combined oral contraceptive use, rising from 0.9 per 1000 women-years with up to 2 years' use, to 2.2 per 1000 women-years after eight years' use. It is impossible, however, to be certain that the apparent effects of the combined oral contraceptive were not due to incompletely controlled confounding by sexual factors[53].

In a recent study in New Zealand, over 6000 women were followed up for over 5 years. They consisted of three cohorts using combined oral contraceptives, intrauterine devices or depot medroxyprogesterone acetate (MPA). Over 300 cases of cervical dysplasia were detected during the 5 years, and no differences in risk were found among the three cohorts[54].

One review concluded: 'after differences in sexual activity and the use of barrier methods of contraception (which have a protective effect) have been accounted for, there appears to be no increase in the risk of cervical cancer among women who take combined oral contraceptives'[55].

Nevertheless, there is no change in the advice that has been standard for many years, that it is important for combined oral contraceptive users to have regular screening by cervical cytology[56].

*Other cancers* Hepatocellular carcinoma is a very rare disease, but is probably increased at least three-fold among combined oral contraceptive users. Recent studies have shown that the combined oral contraceptive does not increase the risk of choriocarcinoma or malignant melanoma[57].

*Gynaecological disease*

Rates of carriage of *Candida albicans* are similar in women taking the pill, those using an intrauterine device (IUD) and those using no contraception[58].

The combined oral contraceptive does not confer protection against herpes, the human immunodeficiency virus (HIV) or *Chlamydia*[59,60], but it does protect against sexually transmitted bacterial infection, presumably by thickening the cervical mucus, and reduces the risk of pelvic inflammatory disease by about 50%.

The risk of uterine fibroids (leiomyomata) is also reduced by the combined oral contraceptive, with a reduction of 17% for every 5 years of combined oral contraceptive use[61]. This may seem surprising, as fibroids are oestrogen-dependent tumors, but suggests that the total amount of oestrogenic stimulation provided by the combined oral contraceptive is in fact less than the total amount during the normal menstrual cycle.

Ovarian suppression by the combined oral contraceptive reduces the risk of functional ovarian cysts. In the Oxford–FPA study, corpus luteum cysts were reduced by 78% and follicular cysts by 49%[62]. The progestogen-only pill does not confer this protection.

Combined oral contraceptive use suppresses endometrial proliferation and produces a 50% reduction in the incidence of menorrhagia and iron deficiency anaemia. The combined oral contraceptive also reduces the incidence of dysmenorrhoea by about 50%.

*Summary*

The combined oral contraceptive pill confers significant health benefits by suppressing ovulation. Its risks have been reduced by the steady reduction in dosage of both components to a total daily dosage only slightly higher than that of hormone replacement therapy. Further reduction in dosage is not possible without losing contraceptive efficacy, as hormone replacement therapy itself does not fully suppress ovulation[63].

## Emergency contraception

The chance of conception after unprotected intercourse has been calculated as around 28%[64]. Sperm can survive for at least 4 days in the female reproductive tract and the fertile period is usually regarded as 3 days before and 1 day after the estimated day of ovulation. However, because of the difficulty in pinpointing the day of ovulation in most women, the 'fertile period' is difficult to define in practice.

The standard method of emergency postcoital contraception is the so-called 'Yuzpe' regimen, in which a woman is given two doses of a combination of 100 μg ethinyloestradiol and 500 μg levonorgestrel, the second dose being given 12 h after the first. This is available as the proprietary preparation PC4®, or in the form of two tablets of Ovran® for each of the doses. Some women have the impression that emergency contraception involves very large doses of hormones, and this misapprehension may be one of the reasons that so many women do not use it[65].

The exact mode of action of hormonal postcoital contraception is not known, but there is some evidence that it inhibits ovulation (if given before release of the oocyte), interferes with corpus luteum function, and inhibits or disrupts implantation by a direct action on the endometrium. The suggestion that it may increase the chance of ectopic pregnancy by inhibiting tubal motility has not been confirmed.

Hormonal postcoital contraception is effective up to 72 h after intercourse. (It should therefore not be called 'morning after' contraception, as this may mislead some women into thinking that there is a very tight time limit to its effectiveness.) The incidence of vomiting is around 16% and some clinics give extra tablets or antiemetics in case this occurs. The failure rate is difficult to calculate, but is around 1%[64]. As this refers to a single cycle, it is much higher than that of the combined oral contraceptive (around 1% per year), and women should be strongly advised not to rely on postcoital contraception routinely.

If the method fails, the woman is likely to be concerned about the possibility of fetal abnormality. Although there are few data about this, it seems that there is at most a minimal increase, if any, in the risk of fetal abnormality.

When a woman presents more than 72 h after intercourse, postcoital contraception can be offered by the insertion of an intrauterine device. This works by disrupting implantation and is highly effective up to 5 days after intercourse.

Surveys of UK women show that only a minority have accurate information about the appropriate timing of postcoital contraception[64,66]. Getting this information to sexually active women, particularly teenagers[67], would be an effective way of lowering the rates of unwanted pregnancy[68], but, once again, cultural attitudes inhibit widespread advertising of this effective method of preventing unwanted pregnancy and abortion.

An associated problem is the availability of postcoital contraception 'out of hours', particularly at weekends[69]. Making it available through pharmacies could reduce this problem, and would be preferred by many women[70]. Nevertheless, some doctors are unhappy about this suggestion, despite there being few, if any, contraindications to its use in an emergency[71]. An alternative is to make it available through trained family planning nurses in community clinics[72].

### Progestogen-only pills

Progestogen-only pills were introduced to avoid the side-effects of oestrogen, but with modern low-dose combined oral contraceptives this has become less of an issue[73]. The concept of progestogen-only contraception, however, stimulated the development of long-acting hormonal contraception, discussed below.

The main mode of action of low-dose progestogens is through interference with cervical mucus and endometrial function, although there may be some effect on follicular and luteal function. This is why careful pill-taking is essential, as the effect on the cervical mucus may wear off in just over 24 h.

In the UK six brands of progestogen-only pill are available: three contain levonorgestrel (at a dose of 30 or 37.5 μg), two contain 350 μg of norethisterone and one contains 500 μg of ethynodiol diacetate. The choice depends on the woman's or the doctor's preference.

The main indications for use of the progestogen-only pill are during breastfeeding (as oestrogen may diminish the milk supply in some women) and when there are other contraindications to the combined oral contraceptive, e.g. in smokers over the age of 35, or just before major surgery.

The major disadvantage is the possibility of menstrual disturbance and the persistence in some women of ovarian follicles, which usually regress spontaneously after a month or two. The health benefits of the combined oral contraceptive are not necessarily conferred by the progestogen-only pill, as it does not reliably suppress ovulation.

## LONG-ACTING METHODS

Most long-acting methods of hormonal contraception involve progestogen only, delivered by depot injection, implant or vaginal rings (see Table 1). Combined hormonal contraception can also be delivered by vaginal rings. With all the progestogen methods, the main mode of action is by thickening the cervical mucus and affecting the endometrium, although there is often an effect on ovulation as well. The main side-effect limiting the acceptability of these methods is menstrual disturbance.

### Injectables

Intramuscular injections are the most commonly used long-acting delivery system, and the most frequently used is Depo-Provera®, depot medroxyprogesterone acetate: one injection lasts for 3 months, during which time the failure rate is below 0.5 in 100 woman-years. An alternative is norethisterone enanthate, given every 2 months. Over time, the woman may develop amenorrhoea, which some women like and others find unacceptable. The effects may take several months to wear off and users should be warned that the timing of the return of fertility is unpredictable[73].

When Depo-Provera was first introduced in the UK, there was opposition from some feminist and consumer groups, who claimed that some women, particularly those whose first language was not English, had been given the injection without adequate counselling. Opposition to the method, in the form of

**Table 1** Long-acting methods of contraception (modified from reference 75)

| |
|---|
| *Injectable preparations* |
| Progestogen only |
| medroxyprogesterone acetate 150 mg every 12 weeks |
| norethisterone enanthate 200 mg every 8–10 weeks |
| Combined injectables |
| oestradiol valerate 5 mg plus medroxyprogesterone acetate 25 mg (Cyclofem) |
| oestradiol cypioniate 5 mg plus norethisterone enanthate 25 mg (Mesigna) |
| *Vaginal rings* |
| Progestogen only systems |
| levonorgestrel 20 μg/day (Femring) |
| 3-ketodesogestrel 25 μg/day |
| progesterone 15 mg/day |
| Combined ring systems |
| ethinyloestradiol 12 μg/day plus 3-ketodesogestrel 120 μg/day |
| norethisterone acetate plus ethinyloestradiol |
| *Implants* |
| Norplant-6 (six capsules of levonorgestrel) |
| Norplant-2 (two covered rods of levonorgestrel) |
| Implanon (one rod of 3-ketodesogestrel) |
| *Hormone-releasing intrauterine devices* |
| Mirena (20 μg/day levonorgestrel) |

'ban-the-jab' campaigns, led to debates about its safety. Animal studies showed increased rates of mammary cancer in beagles given high doses on a long-term basis, and endometrial cancers were reported in rhesus monkeys on long-term treatment. It is now clear that Depo-Provera, as would be expected, provides a major degree of protection against endometrial carcinoma, and that there is no overall increase in the risk of breast cancer, although there may be a very small risk in long-term users. In spite of the negative views expressed by some consumer activists, many women are keen to use Depo-Provera, because of its high effectiveness and the relative infrequency of the injections. Marketing approval for it was finally given in the USA in 1992.

*Combined oestrogen–progestogen preparations*
Combinations of oestradiol valerate and a progestogen given by injection are used by around 2 million women worldwide[74]. 'Chinese injectable no. 1' is used mainly in China and nearby countries, and other combined preparations have recently been approved. Failure rates as low as 0.6% are reported.

## Rings

The search for an ideal delivery system has produced two types of vaginal ring: progestogen-only rings and combination rings containing ethinyloestradiol and desogestrel. The former is left in the vagina for 3 months and the latter for 21 days, with a 7-day break. The purpose is to maintain steady levels of steroid in the circulation rather than the daily fluctuations which result from oral administration of pills[75].

With the progestogen-only ring, pregnancy rates are around 3% per year and initial studies showed discontinuation rates of almost 50% at 1 year, the main single reason for discontinuation being menstrual problems.

### Implants

Four types of implant are being evaluated and one (Norplant®) is in widespread use in more than 50 countries. The principle underlying them is that steroids can be released at a steady rate through silicone, which is tissue compatible. Various progestogens were tried and the lowest pregnancy rates were found with levonorgestrel. Norplant consists of six rods implanted under the skin and can be left in place for 5 years. The pregnancy rate during the first year of use is less than 0.3% and the effect is rapidly reversible when the implants are removed.

Like other progestogen-only methods, however, Norplant can cause irregular vaginal bleeding. The method quickly became popular in Britain when it was introduced in 1994, but this side-effect, coupled with media reports of difficult removals, rapidly reduced demand. There have also been difficulties over the question of remuneration for doctors inserting these implants. In spite of this, studies are showing that many users find Norplant an acceptable method and are happy with the prospect of a 5-year lifespan for these implants[76].

Other implants are Norplant II®, which consists of two rods rather than six, and has a similar clinical performance to Norplant; Implanon®, which contains a metabolite of desogestrel and consists of a single rod that can be inserted without an incision; and new implants under development which use new progestogens[77].

### Intrauterine devices

An intrauterine device releasing progesterone (Progestasert®) was marketed in the UK, but its use was discontinued because of concern about an increased risk of ectopic pregnancy. It is still available in the USA.

Mirena® is an intrauterine device that contains levonorgestrel. It was developed in Finland and consists of a Nova-T frame carrying a silastic sheath impregnated with levonorgestrel, which is released at the rate of 20 μg/day. It can be left in place up for up to 5 years[78].

The device functions by exerting a strong progestational effect on the cervical mucus and on the endometrium. Ovulation is not normally inhibited, but there may be some effects on ovulation. Attempts to recover fertilized eggs from the Fallopian tubes have not succeeded, suggesting that this device acts mainly by preventing conception[79].

Pregnancy rates as low as 0.2% per year have been reported, with no increase in the rate of ectopic pregnancy. Fertility returns immediately after the device is removed.

The device markedly reduces menstrual flow and is an effective treatment for menorrhagia. It also reduces the risk of pelvic infection because of its effect on cervical mucus. However, some women become worried because it can cause amenorrhoea; careful counselling is necessary because of this.

## NEW HORMONAL METHODS

### GnRH analogues

It has been suggested on theoretical grounds that the safest hormonal contraception could be provided by suppressing gonadal function with gonadotrophin releasing hormone (GnRH) analogues, and providing replacement therapy with low doses of steroid hormones. This would reduce to a minimum the risk of subsequent hormone-dependent cancer, particularly breast cancer.

GnRH analogues are peptides similar to GnRH itself, but with modifications to make them resistant to enzymic breakdown and increase their affinity for receptors. They can be administered by nasal spray, injection or subcutaneous implant.

Women with severe menstrual problems may be treated with GnRH analogues along with low-dose oestrogen replacement therapy, and intermittent progestogen therapy to induce withdrawal bleeding and protect the endometrium. This provides effective contraception, but the regimen is very expensive and is not approved solely as a method of family planning.

In men, initial trials showed that prolonged treatment with GnRH agonists produced oligospermia, but inhibition of FSH secretion was apparently incomplete and consistent suppression of spermatogenesis was not achieved. Testosterone secretion was suppressed, however, leading to loss of libido and impotence, and confirming that testosterone replacement therapy was necessary. Further trials showed that a combination of GnRH and testosterone enanthate could maintain libido and potency: azoospermia was achieved in 6–12 weeks in most of the subjects[80]. This combination, however, seems at present to be less effective than steroids alone, which are discussed in the next section.

### Hormonal contraception for men

Normal spermatogenesis depends on a high concentration of testosterone within the testis (about 50–100 times higher than in peripheral blood) and the synergistic action of FSH[81]. Therefore, spermatogenesis can be abolished by inhibiting FSH and is not restored by adding exogenous testosterone. Other possible modes of action for male contraception would be to target the epididymis, where the spermatozoa acquire motility and fertilizing potential. Unfortunately, not enough is yet known about epididymal function to allow the development of male contraceptives of this type[81].

Hormonal suppression of spermatogenesis was first attempted by testosterone enanthate injections, on the principle that they would inhibit FSH production by negative feedback, like the female combined oral contraceptive. This produced azoospermia in most men, but oligospermia in some. It seems likely that pregnancy will not occur if the sperm density is less than 5 million/ml, possibly because the residual sperm are functionally impaired.

Further trials conducted by the World Health Organization between 1990 and 1994 accumulated 283.5 years of exposure. Nine pregnancies occurred and analysis of the data indicated a threshold sperm density of 3 million/ml, above which pregnancy rates were unacceptably high. For men with densities below that level, the failure rate was 1.4 per 100 person-years – similar to that of the female combined oral contraceptive.

Current developments with testosterone-only contraception include improved delivery systems for testosterone, such as implants, depot injections or transdermal patches. However, it seems likely that, in order to achieve maximal suppression of spermatogenesis, supraphysiological levels of testosterone are required. Research is therefore being carried out on other regimens in which testosterone is combined with progestogens, anti-androgens or oestrogen. The last combination has been the most effective in animal studies.

For many years, it was widely assumed that men would be reluctant to use hormonal contraception and that women would not trust men to use it correctly. Now, however, with the realistic prospect of effective male hormonal methods, these assumptions are being questioned[82]. There may be some substance to the criticism that research on male hormonal methods has been slow for cultural rather than technical reasons. If hormonal contraception is going to become available to men, there will have to be a change in attitude among family planning doctors as well as the public.

### Antigestogens

Mifepristone (RU486®) is now familiar to gynaecologists because of its use in medical abortion. It is a competitive inhibitor of progesterone and when used for therapeutic abortion it is given in association with prostaglandin. It may, in the future, be used to induce labour and promote lactation[83].

When given in the follicular phase of the menstrual cycle, RU486 can inhibit ovulation. Given in the luteal phase of the cycle, it can be used as a postcoital contraceptive. When it was used for postcoital contraception and administered within 72 h of a single act of unprotected intercourse, it seemed to be more effective than the Yuzpe regimen (see above) and causes less vomiting, although it causes more menstrual disturbance[83].

If RU486 is given at the time of the expected menses (as a so-called 'once a month' contraceptive) there appears to be an unacceptably high incidence of continuing pregnancy (around 15%), although bleeding occurs in almost all women. If RU486 is to be developed as a late postcoital method of contraception, it will probably have to be combined with prostaglandin. The legal and ethical boundary between late postcoital contraception and early abortion is unclear, and this method is unlikely to be acceptable to the majority of women[84].

## THE FUTURE

Looking further into the future, Lincoln[85] has suggested that attention in contraceptive research will turn from the use of steroids to more direct manipulation of molecular mechanisms. He suggested three possible targets. First, there could be selective inhibition of FSH in the male, leaving LH action (and androgen secretion) intact. This might be achieved by altering the structure of FSH to produce an antagonist. There could be problems in ensuring that such an antagonist were resistant to enzymic degradation and in administering it in sufficient quantities to antagonize FSH *in vivo*.

A second target is the neutralization of human chorionic gonadotrophin (hCG). If this were achieved early enough after fertilization, the menstrual cycle need not be affected. Vaccines against the carboxy-terminal of the hCG molecule (the region of greatest specificity) have been developed and are being tested in clinical trials.

The third possible target is blocking of the interaction between the sperm and the oocyte. Vaccines based on peptides of the zona pellucida or the sperm are being developed, and a particularly attractive aim is to target the proteins involved in binding the sperm to the plasma membrane of the oocyte. This would leave the rest of the reproductive system, including the normal menstrual cycle, intact.

Lincoln concluded his look into the future by suggesting that even if some of these new contraceptive techniques come to fruition, there will still be a place for steroids 'for purposes of positive health care, with respect to cancer, osteoporosis and well-being'.

## CONCLUSION

Although further advances in the design of the combined oral contraceptive pill seem unlikely, a number of developments are taking place with other types of delivery system, which will increase the range of options available to women (and men) who wish to use hormonal contraception. The biggest challenge remains public education, to ensure that the risks of modern low-dose contraceptives are not exaggerated in people's minds, and that the health benefits are known.

## ACKNOWLEDGEMENT

Parts of this chapter were adapted from: Drife, J. (1996). *The Risks and Benefits of Oral Contraceptives Today*. (Carnforth, UK: Parthenon Publishing)

## REFERENCES

1. Potts, D. M. and Crane, S. F. (1993). Contraceptive delivery in the developing world. *Br. Med. Bull.*, **49**, 27–39
2. Owen-Smith, V., Hannaford, P. and Webb, A. (1996). What do family planning providers do before prescribing combined oral contraceptives? *Br. J. Fam. Plann.*, **22**, 103–4
3. Drife, J. O. (1993). Contraceptive problems in the developed world. *Br. Med. Bull.*, **49**, 17–36
4. Guillebaud, J. (1995). Combined hormonal contraception. In Loudon, N., Glasier, A. and Gebbie, A. (eds.) *Handbook of Family Planning and Reproductive Health Care*, 3rd edn., pp. 19–36. (Edinburgh: Churchill Livingstone)
5. Bell, S. C. and Drife, J. O. (1989). Secretory proteins of the endometrium – potential markers for endometrial dysfunction. *Baillière's Clin. Obstet. Gynaecol.*, **3**, 271–91
6. Hepburn, M. (1995). Factors influencing contraceptive choice. In Loudon, N., Glasier, A.

and Gebbie, A. (eds.) *Handbook of Family Planning and Reproductive Health Care*, 3rd edn., pp. 19–36. (Edinburgh: Churchill Livingstone)

7. Thorogood, M. and Vessey, N. P. (1990). Trends in use of oral contraceptives in Britain. *Br. J. Fam. Plann.*, **16**, 41–53
8. Cachrimanidou, A.-C., Hellberg, D., Nilsson, S., von Schoulz, B., Crona, N. and Siegbahn, A. (1994). Hemostasis profile and lipid metabolism with long-interval use of a desogestrel-containing oral contraceptive. *Contraception*, **50**, 153–65
9. Korver, T., Goorisen, E. and Guillebaud, J. (1995). The combined oral contraceptive pill: what advice should we give when tablets are missed? *Br. J. Obstet. Gynaecol.*, **102**, 601–7
10. Gillmer, M. D. G., Walling, M. R. and Povey, S. J. (1996). The effect on serum lipids and lipoproteins of three combined oral contraceptives containing norgestimate, gestodene and desogestrel. *Br. J. Fam. Plann.*, **22**, 67–71
11. Fotherby, K. and Caldwell, A. D. S. (1994). New progestogens in oral contraception. *Contraception*, **49**, 1–32
12. Drife, J. (1989). Complications of oral contraception. In Filshie, M. and Guillebaud, J. (eds.) *Contraception: Science and Practice*, pp. 39–51. (London: Butterworths)
13. WHO Collaborative Study (1989). Cardiovascular disease and use of oral contraceptives. *Bull. W.H.O.*, **67**, 417–23
14. Gerstman, B. B., Piper, J. M., Tomita, D. K., Ferguson, W. J., Stadel, B. V. and Lundin, F. E. (1991). Oral contraceptive estrogen dose and the risk of deep venous thromboembolic disease. *Am. J. Epidemiol.*, **133**, 32–7
15. World Health Organisation Collaborative Study of Cardiovascular Disease and Steroid Hormone Contraception (1995). Venous thromboembolic disease and combined oral contraceptives: results of international multicentre case–control study. *Lancet*, **346**, 1575–82
16. World Health Organisation Collaborative Study of Cardiovascular Disease and Steroid Hormone Contraception (1995). Effect of different progestagens in low oestrogen oral contraceptives on venous thromboembolic disease. *Lancet*, **346**, 1582–8
17. Bloemenkamp, K. W. M., Rosendaal, F. R., Helmerhorst, F. M., Buller, H. R. and Vandenbroucke, J. P. (1995). Enhancement by factor V Leiden mutation of risk of deep-vein thrombosis associated with oral contraceptives containing a third-generation progestagen. *Lancet*, **346**, 1593–6
18. Editorial (1995). Sensible alerts. *Lancet*, **346**, 1569
19. Gillebaud, J. (1995). Advising women on which pill to take. *Br. Med. J.*, **311**, 1111–12
20. Weiss, N. (1995). Third-generation oral contraceptives: how risky? *Lancet*, **346**, 1570
21. Jick, H., Jick, S. S., Gurewich, V., Myers, M. W. and Vasilakis, C. (1995). Risk of idiopathic cardiovascular death and non-fatal venous thromboembolism in women using oral contraceptives with differing progestagen components. *Lancet*, **346**, 1589–93
22. Rosenberg, L., Palmer, J. R., Lesko, S. M. and Shapiro, S. (1990). Oral contraceptive use and the risk of myocardial infarction. *Am. J. Epidemiol.*, **131**, 1009–16
23. Thorogood, M. (1993). Oral contraceptives and cardiovascular disease: an epidemiologic overview. *Pharmacoepidemiol. Drug Safety*, **2**, 3–16
24. Croft, P. and Hannaford, P. C. (1989). Risk factors for acute myocardial infarction in women: evidence from the Royal College of General Practitioners' oral contraception study. *Br. Med. J.*, **298**, 165–8
25. Croft, P. and Hannaford, P. C. (1989). Risk factors for acute myocardial infarction in women (Letter). *Br. Med. J.*, **298**, 674
26. Thorogood, M., Mann, J., Murphy, M. and Vessey, M. (1991). Is oral contraceptive use still associated with an increased risk of myocardial infarction? Report of a case–control study. *Br. J. Obstet. Gynaecol.*, **98**, 1245–53
27. Thorogood, M., Mann, J., Murphy, M. and Vessey, M. (1992). Fatal stroke and use of oral contraceptives: findings from a case–control study. *Am. J. Epidemiol.*, **136**, 35–45
28. WHO Collaborative Study of Cardiovascular Disease and Steroid Hormone Contraception (1996). Ischaemic stroke and combined oral contraceptives: results of an international, multicentre, case-control study. *Lancet*, **348**, 498–50
29. WHO Collaborative Study of Cardiovascular Disease and Steroid Hormone Contraception (1996). Haemorrhagic stroke, overall stroke risk, and combined oral contraceptives: results of an international, multicentre, case–control study. *Lancet*, **348**, 505–10

30. Cairns, V., Keil, V., Doering, A. *et al.* (1985). Oral contraceptives and blood pressure in a German metropolitan population. *Int. J. Epidemiol.*, **14**, 389–95
31. Shen, Q., Lin, D., Jiang, X., Li, H. and Zhang, Z. (1994). Blood pressure changes and hormonal contraceptives. *Contraception*, **50**, 131–41
32. La Vecchia, C. (1992). Sex hormones and cardiovascular risk. *Hum. Reprod.*, **7**, 162–7
33. Goldzeiher, J. W. (1994). Are low-dose oral contraceptives safer and better? *Am. J. Obstet. Gynecol.*, **171**, 587–90
34. Hollingworth, B. A. and Guillebaud, J. (1991). Contraception in the perimenopause. *Br. J. Hosp. Med.*, **45**, 213–15
35. Cancer and Steroid Hormone Study of the Centers for Disease Control and the National Institute of Child Health and Human Development (1987). The reduction in risk of ovarian cancer associated with oral-contraceptive use. *N. Engl. J. Med.*, **316**, 650–5
36. Drife, J. O. (1989). The benefits of combined oral contraceptives. *Br. J. Obstet. Gynaecol.*, **96**, 1225–8
37. Rosenberg, L., Palmer, J. R., Zauber, A. G., Warshauer, M. E., Lewis, J. L., Strom, B. L., Harlap, S. and Shapiro, S. (1994). A case–control study of oral contraceptive use and invasive epithelial ovarian cancer. *Am. J. Epidemiol.*, **139**, 654–61
38. Vessey, M. P. and Painter, R. (1995). Endometrial and ovarian cancer and oral contraceptives – findings in a large cohort study. *Br. J. Cancer*, **71**, 1340–2
39. Cancer and Steroid Hormone Study of the Centers for Disease Control and the National Institute of Child Health and Human Development (1987). Combination oral contraceptive use and risk of endometrial cancer. *J. Am. Med. Assoc.*, **257**, 796–800
40. Schlesselman, J. J. (1990). Oral contraceptives and breast cancer. *Am. J. Obstet. Gynecol.*, **163**, 1379–87
41. Romieu, I., Berlin, J. A. and Colditz, G. (1990). Oral contraceptives and breast cancer. *Cancer*, **66**, 2253–63
42. Drife, J. (1989). The contraceptive pill and breast cancer in young women. *Br. Med. J.*, **298**, 1269–70
43. Rushton, L. and Jones, D. R. (1992). Oral contraceptive use and breast cancer risk: a meta-analysis of variations with age at diagnosis, parity and total duration of oral contraceptive use. *Br. J. Obstet. Gynaecol.*, **99**, 239–46
44. Malone, K. E., Daling, J. R. and Weiss, N. S. (1993). Oral contraceptives in relation to breast cancer. *Epidemiol. Rev.*, **15**, 80–97
45. Rookus, M. A. S., van Leeuwen, F. E., for the Netherlands Oral Contraceptives and Breast Cancer Study Group (1994). Oral contraceptives and the risk of breast cancer in women aged 20–54 years. *Lancet*, **344**, 844–51
46. Chilvers, C. E. D., Smith, S. I. and members of the UK National Case–Control Study Group (1994). The effects of patterns of oral contraceptive use on breast cancer risk in young women. *Br. J. Cancer*, **67**, 922–3
47. McPherson, K. and Drife, J. O. (1986). The pill and breast cancer: why the uncertainty? *Br. Med. J.*, **293**, 709–10
48. Chilvers, C. (1994). Oral contraceptives and cancer. *Lancet*, **344**, 1378–9
49. Collaborative Group on Hormonal Factors in Breast Cancer (1996). Breast cancer and hormonal contraceptives: collaborative reanalysis of individual data on 53 297 women with breast cancer and 100 239 women without breast cancer from 54 epidemiological studies. *Lancet*, **347**, 1713–27
50. Masters, J. R. W., Scarisbrick, J. J. and Drife, J. O. (1977). Cyclic variation of DNA synthesis in human breast epithelium. *J. Natl. Cancer Inst.*, **58**, 1263–5
51. Drife, J. (1981). *The Effects of Parity and the Menstrual Cycle on the Normal Mammary Gland and their Possible Relationship to Malignant Change*. MD Thesis, University of Edinburgh
52. Anderson, T. J., Battersby, S., King, R. J. B., McPherson, K. and Going, J. J. (1989). Oral contraceptive use influences resting breast proliferation. *Hum. Pathol.*, **20**, 1139–44
53. Kaunitz, A. M. (1992). Oral contraceptives and gynecologic cancer: an update for the 1990s. *Am. J. Obstet. Gynecol.*, **167**, 1171–6
54. The New Zealand Contraception and Health Study Group (1994). Risk of cervical dysplasia in users of oral contraceptives, intrauterine devices or depot-medroxyprogesterone acetate. *Contraception*, **50**, 431–41
55. Baird, D. T. and Glasier, A. F. (1993). Hormonal contraception. *N. Engl. J. Med.*, **328**, 1543–9
56. Mishell, D. R. (1982). Noncontraceptive health benefits of oral steroidal contraceptives. *Am. J.*

*Obstet. Gynecol.*, **142**, 809–16
57. Vessey, M. P. (1989). Oral contraception and cancer. In Filshie, M. and Guillebaud, J. (eds.) *Contraception: Science and Practice*, pp. 52–68. (London: Butterworths)
58. Davidson, F. and Oates, J. K. (1985). The pill does not cause 'thrush'. *Br. J. Obstet. Gynaecol.*, 92, 1265–6
59. Washington, A. E., Gove, S., Schachter, J. and Sweet, R. (1985). Oral contraceptives, *Chlamydia trachomatis* infection, and pelvic inflammatory disease. *J. Am. Med. Assoc.*, **253**, 2246–50
60. Gall, S. A. (1986). Oral contraceptives and *Chlamydia* infections. *J. Am. Med. Assoc.*, **255**, 38
61. Ross, R. K., Pike, M. C., Vessey, M. P., Bull, D., Yeates, D. and Casagrande, J. T. (1986). Risk factors for uterine fibroids: reduced risk associated with oral contraceptives. *Br. Med. J.*, **293**, 359–62
62. Vessey, M., Metcalfe, A., Wells, C., McPherson, K., Westhoff, C. and Yeates, D. (1987). Ovarian neoplasms, functional ovarian cysts, and oral contraceptives. *Br. Med. J.*, **294**, 1518–20
63. Gebbie, A. E., Glasier, A. and Sweeting, V. (1995). Incidence of ovulation in perimenopausal women before and during hormone replacement therapy. *Contraception*, **52**, 221–2
64. Glasier, A. (1995). Emergency postcoital contraception. In Loudon, N., Glasier, A and Gebbie, A. (eds.) *Handbook of Family Planning and Reproductive Health Care*, 3rd edn, pp. 19–36. (Edinburgh: Churchill Livingstone)
65. Ziebland, S., Maxwell, K. and Greenhall, E. (1996). 'It's a mega dose of hormones, isn't it?' Why women may be reluctant to use emergency contraception. *Br. J. Fam. Plann.*, **22**, 84–6
66. Crosier, A. (1996). Women's knowledge and awareness of emergency contraception. *Br. J. Fam. Plann.*, **22**, 87–91
67. Stevenson, J. (1996). Emergency contraception in the curriculum? *Br. J. Fam. Plann.*, **22**, 75–6
68. Gooder, P. (1996). Knowledge of emergency contraception amongst men and women in the general population and women seeking an abortion. *Br. J. Fam. Plann.*, **22**, 81–3
69. Maxwell, M., Mooney, A. and Wilson, P. (1996). A consumer survey of the availability of hormonal postcoital contraception in the north west region. *Br. J. Fam. Plann.*, **22**, 79–80
70. Hughes, H. and Myres, P. (1996). Women's knowledge and preference about emergency contraception: a survey from a rural general practice. *Br. J. Fam. Plann.*, **22**, 77–8
71. Drife, J. O. (1993). Deregulating emergency contraception. *Br. Med. J.*, **307**, 695–6
72. Kishen, M. and Presho, M. (1996). Emergency contraception – a prescription for change. *Br. J. Fam. Plann.*, **22**, 25–7
73. Fraser, I. (1995). Progestogen-only contraception. In Loudon, N., Glasier, A. and Gebbie, A. (eds.) *Handbook of Family Planning and Reproductive Health Care*, 3rd edn, pp. 19–36. (Edinburgh: Churchill Livingstone)
74. Van Look, P. (1995). Contraceptives of the future. In Loudon, N., Glasier, A. and Gebbie, A. (eds.) *Handbook of Family Planning and Reproductive Health Care*, 3rd edn, pp. 409–34. (Edinburgh: Churchill Livingstone)
75. Newton, J. (1993). Long acting methods of contraception. *Br. Med. Bull.*, **49**, 40–61
76. Fowler, P. (1996). Subdermal implants – still a viable long term contraceptive option? *Br. J. Fam. Plann.*, **22**, 3110–13
77. Newton, J. R. (1996). New hormonal methods of contraception. *Baillière's Clin. Obstet. Gynaecol.*, **10**, 87–102
78. Drife, J. O. (1995). Intrauterine contraceptive devices. In Loudon, N., Glasier, A. and Gebbie, A. (eds.) *Handbook of Family Planning and Reproductive Health Care*, 3rd edn, pp. 19–36. (Edinburgh: Churchill Livingstone)
79. Odlind, V. (1996). Modern intra-uterine devices. *Baillière's Clin. Obstet. Gynaecol.*, **10**, 55–68
80. Fraser, H. M. (1993). GnRH analogues for contraception. *Br. Med. Bull.*, **49**, 62–72
81. Wu, F. C. W. (1996). Male contraception. *Baillière's Clin. Obstet. Gynaecol.*, **10**, 1–24
82. Walsh, J. (1996). Hormonal contraception for men? *Br. J. Fam. Plann.*, **22**, 65–6
83. Baird, D. T. (1993). Antigestogens. *Br. Med. Bull.*, **49**, 73–87
84. Swahn, M. L., Danielsson, K. G. and Bygdeman, M. (1996). Contraception with anti-progesterone. *Baillière's Clin. Obstet. Gynaecol.*, **10**, 43–54
85. Lincoln, D. W. (1993). Contraception for the year 2020. *Br. Med. Bull.*, **49**, 222–36

# Endometriosis

# 23

*Andrew Prentice*

## INTRODUCTION

Endometriosis is one of the commonest benign gynaecological conditions to affect women of reproductive age and is estimated to be present in 10–25% of women presenting to gynaecologists in the UK and USA. It is often described as an enigmatic condition, but it is a major clinical problem with deleterious social, sexual and reproductive consequences. The cynics will say that describing it as an enigma is just an excuse to explain away our apparent poor understanding of the condition. However, the last decade has seen major advances, and advances can often lead to apparent confusion. These advances have come about not only in our understanding of the pathogenesis of this unique condition but also in our realization of what constitutes endometriosis. Progress has also been made in medical and surgical therapies, but the application of these particular advances must be tailored to match our new understanding of the pathology. In this chapter, I will endeavour to describe the advances in our understanding of the pathogenesis of endometriosis and relate these advances to the management of the two main clinical areas, namely endometriosis-associated infertility and the management of symptomatic disease.

## PATHOGENESIS OF ENDOMETRIOSIS

Although endometriosis is a common condition, we have a relatively poor understanding of its pathogenesis and even its aetiology is poorly defined. For many years, the tissue of origin or histogenesis of this condition has engendered much debate but more imporant are the mechanisms by which ectopic tissue can survive. Aetiological factors are also important because they point towards strategies for management.

### Histogenesis of endometriosis

Sampson in 1940[1], reviewing the development of his implantation theory of histogenesis, wrote of endometriosis, 'Its pathogenesis is so tantalisingly alluring and elusive'. This remains true to the present day. One hundred and twenty years have passed since Waldeyer[2] first proposed a theory of histogenesis and suggested that endometriosis arose from the germinal epithelium of the ovary, but it was over 50 years before Sampson first suggested an endometrial origin when he advanced his implantation theory in a series of articles published in the 1920s[3–11]. It would appear from review articles written on histogenesis that Sampson only described his implantation theory, but it is clear from the source documents that he also described vascular dissemination and direct invasion as alternative methods of endometrial dissemination[10,11]. It was left to Javert[12] in the 1940s to unify all the endometrial theories of histogenesis and make the analogy that endometrium can behave in a manner similar to its malignant counterpart.

It is now clear that endometrium can be disseminated by a number of means but tubal regurgitation, as hypothesized by Sampson, is the most common mode. The distribution of endometriotic deposits within the pelvis provides excellent circumstantial evidence to support Sampson's theory. His initial observations have been confirmed by numerous authors[13–18]. The laparoscopic study by Jenkins and her colleagues[18] has the advantage over all other studies of anatomical distribution in that observations were made without disturbing the pelvic organs and relates most closely to current concepts of what is endometriosis (Figure 1). Endometriosis is found most frequently at those sites where endometrial cells will settle undisturbed following retrograde menstruation, most notably on the irregular surface of the ovary and in gravity-dependent pouches in the peritoneal cavity, especially the pouch of Douglas.

*Retrograde menstruation*

It is now well established that retrograde menstruation is a common event but it was not always the case. Novak[19] in 1926, in an attempt to discredit Sampson's theory, examined a large number of Fallopian tubes and was the first to demonstrate fragments of endometrium within their lumen. In a subsequent paper[20], he accepted that retrograde menstruation might occur but questioned why a 'physiological process should frequently give rise to pathology', a question that remains unanswered to the present day.

Menstrual fragments can be an incidental finding in Fallopian tubes removed at the time of menstruation[21] and they may also be carried along the Fallopian tubes by dye insufflation and hysteroscopy[22]. It has also been observed that the dialysate is regularly blood-stained just prior to menstruation in women undergoing peritoneal dialysis[23], an observation which corresponds to the premenstrual symptoms described by many patients. Blood staining of the dialysate is not seen at other times during the menstrual cycle and is rarely seen in either non-menstruating women or men. In fact, retrograde menstruation is an almost ubiquitous phenomenon. In laparoscopic studies, more than 90% of women with patent tubes have evidence of retrograde menstruation[24,25]. Thus we are left with the conundrum, posed by Novak[20], why a ubiquitous event, menstruation, may give rise to a pathological process, endometriosis, the association of ectopic endometrium with symptoms or anatomical distortion.

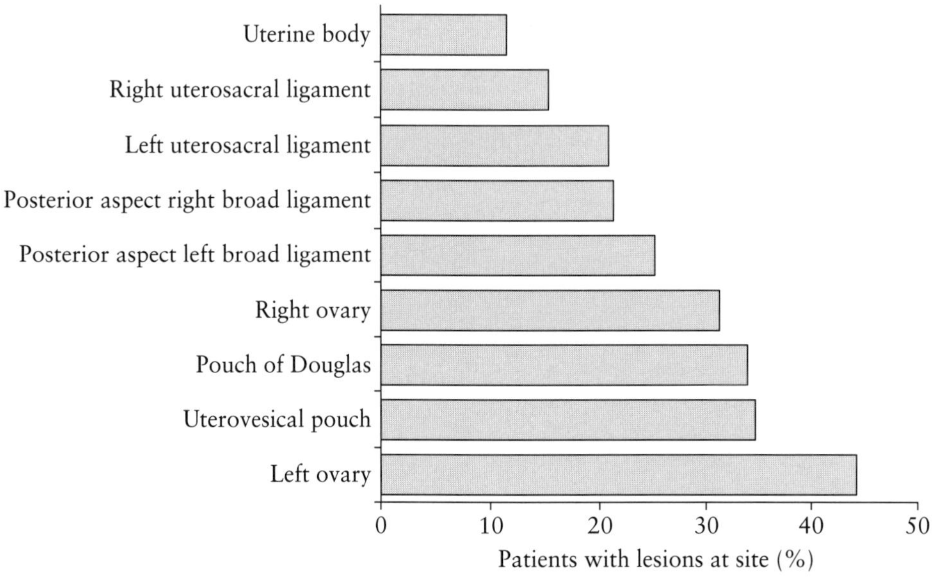


**Figure 1** Graphical representation of the anatomical distribution of endometriotic implants within the pelves of 182 patients undergoing laparoscopy for the investigation of infertility. All other sites, which include the relatively mobile structures of the Fallopian tubes, the sigmoid colon, the ovarian suspensory ligaments and the round ligaments, have rates of involvement of less than 5%. (Modified from Jenkins *et al.*[18])

*Viability of endometrium and ability to implant*
Endometrium is most commonly disseminated at the time of menstruation. If the theory of an endometrial origin is sustainable, the endometrium disseminated at menstruation must be both viable and able to implant.

Many researchers over the years have demonstrated the viability of either the endometrium at the time of menstruation or endometrial cells shed at menstruation. In 1927, Cron and Gey[25] demonstrated that endometrium obtained from the uterine cavity at the time of menstruation could be cultured *in vitro*. This endometrium, however, is not disseminated. Supravital staining of cells from the menstrual fluid indicates that they remain viable[26], and Keettel and Stein in 1951[27] were the first to culture shed endometrium. Thus endometrium shed at the time of menstruation remains viable. It has also been demonstrated that endometrial fragments collected from the pelvis following tubal insufflation may be cultured *in vitro*[28]. Endometrial epithelial colonies have been grown from pellets of cells from peritoneal fluid obtained in the early follicular phase[29].

The endometrium remains viable but can it implant? There is no direct evidence that endometrium can implant when shed at menstruation, but a large body of experimental evidence in both human and other species exists to support an implantation theory. In the 1950s and early 1960s Ridley and Edwards demonstrated both the viability of shed endometrial cells and their potential to survive at ectopic sites[30,31]. They collected menstrual blood and injected it subcutaneously into the adipose tissue of the lower abdominal wall. They identified endometrial tissue when the patients subsequently underwent hysterectomy. In Rhesus monkeys, surgical manipulations to divert the menstrual flow into the peritoneal cavity result in the development of endometriosis[32]. Such experiments are analogous to the development of endometriosis in patients with genital tract anomalies. In these natural experiments, uterine anomalies appear to predispose to the development of endometriosis by obstructing menstrual flow and increasing retrograde menstruation[33]. Human endometrium, and endometriosis, have been successfully transplanted into the lateral abdominal wall of nude mice[34].

Viable endometrium is disseminated by a variety of routes and appears to be able to implant, despite the fact that this has never been observed directly *in vivo*. Nevertheless, there is a large body of opinion to support an endometrial origin for endometriosis.

*Other theories of histogenesis*
If endometriosis is not disseminated endometrium, it must develop *in situ*. There are three theories that propose the concept that endometriosis develops *in situ*. These are:

(1) The Müllerian cell rest theory;

(2) The Wolffian cell rest theory; and

(3) The coelomic metaplasia theory.

If the evidence to support an endometrial origin is circumstantial, then the evidence to support either of the cell rest theories would not justify a court case. The theory of coelomic metaplasia is the best supported of the theories of endometriosis developing from local tissues. It states that endometriosis develops from metaplasia of cells within the coelomic mesothelium which in the pelvis forms the peritoneum. This theory is usually credited to Iwanoff[35] and Meyer[36] but neither article actually proposes such a theory. Thus the origins of this theory remain unclear. The coelomic metaplasia theory assumes that there exist cells within the mesothelium that either retain the potential to differentiate or are undifferentiated.

The rare occurrence of endometriosis in males has been explained as being a consequence of coelomic metaplasia. All cases reported in the literature have occurred in patients with prostatic carcinoma being treated with oestrogen therapy[37–39]. A more probable explanation is that the tissue observed derived from the prostatic utricle, a Müllerian duct-derived structure and the male homologue of the uterus. Indeed, endometrial carcinoma of the prostate arising from the utricle is a well recognized pathology: such carcinomas, responding to the combined endocrine therapies of castration and the administration of exogenous oestrogens, will resemble endometriosis.

Coelomic metaplasia is an intellectually attractive theory and could explain the occurrence of endometriosis at all sites. If endometriosis was a consequence of metaplasia, then we would see a more equal distribution of endometriosis within the peritoneal cavity, and, in addition, should see a universal gender occurrence, increased frequency with age and development of the disease in the absence of the uterus. These characteristics are not associated with endometriosis. There is no substantive evidence that mesothelial cells, or their derivatives, can undergo metaplasia to form endometrial tissue.

### The peritoneal environment in endometriosis

Critical to the validity of an endometrial origin is the phenomenon of retrograde menstruation and implantation of exfoliated endometrium. Much research effort in endometriosis has shown that it contains an ever-increasing array of growth and angiogenic factors[40,41], mainly through detection of the messenger RNA (mRNA) by *in situ* hybridization and protein by immunohistochemical staining. These factors are thought to play a central role in cycling, mitosis, differentiation and vascularization of the endometrium. Therefore, tissue expressing high values of these factors may have a propensity to implant in the pelvis under the correct conditions. Differences between the amount and types of factors found in exfoliated endometrium between women with and without endometriosis may therefore be critical in the pathogenesis of this disease. Expression of such factors may have important implications for the proliferation and vascularization of the ectopic tissue, which is a critical prerequisite for its survival. Although these factors are mainly found in stromal and epithelial cells, in the case of the angiogenic growth factor, vascular endothelial growth factor (VEGF), the greatest level of expression was found in tissue macrophages[42]. The presence of these active cells may provide a source of growth/angiogenic factors deep within the tissue, thereby facilitating the angiogenesis required for survival. Limited data exist on direct comparisons of growth/angiogenic factors between eutopic tissue from patients with and without endometriosis, and ectopic tissue. These studies have failed to show any significant quantitative differences in a number of factors between these groups.

Eutopic and ectopic tissue are both immunopositive for the oestrogen and progesterone receptors[43,44]. It has been demonstrated that staining for both oestrogen and progesterone receptors in both glandular and stromal cells is less in ectopic endometrium. The presence of these receptors explains the hormonal dependency of these tissues and, in turn, provides circumstantial evidence for an endometrial origin for endometriosis; the tissue of origin would be expected to express the ovarian steroid receptors. Nevertheless, the lack of qualitative differences between ectopic and eutopic endometrium suggests that endometriosis is not primarily a disease of the endometrium. Such a conclusion has major implications for our future understanding of this condition.

As first suggested by Javert[12], the implantation of exfoliated endometrium in the peritoneal cavity is analogous to the processes involved in the invasion of tumour cells. Initial adhesion of the viable cells onto peritoneal surfaces is followed by proteolytic digestion of the extracellular matrix and finally the invasion and stabilization of the tissue.

The cell adhesion molecules, integrins and cadherins, are the two determinants of cell–cell and cell–matrix adhesion. The results from a number of studies show that integrins and cadherins are found on the endometrium, menstrual effluent and endometriotic samples[45,46]. However, there appears to be no difference in cell adhesion expression when comparing eutopic and ectopic tissue. The presence of these molecules should enable the tissue to attach. The lack of any difference between these synchronously sampled tissues strengthens the theory that the endometrium is the progenitor of endometriosis. However, the exact subcellular mechanisms by which endometrial cells might attach to the peritoneal serosa are still to be determined.

Metalloproteinases are enzymes responsible for degrading components of the extracellular matrix. It has recently been shown that the three main classes of metalloproteinases are found in normal cycling endometrium and are likely to play a role in endometrial breakdown and remodelling[47]. More important, the presence of these enzymes and their possible maintenance in shed endometrium may be important in the establishment of endometriotic tissue in the pelvis and in the determination of its invasive potential. However, there are no data to indicate whether menstrual effluent or the endometriotic tissue itself maintains these enzymes.

It is clear how endometrium might adhere and begin to invade but how might these deposits maintain themselves? Clinical observations have made clear that endometriosis has myriad appearances and is often associated with hypervascularization[48]. It is assumed that this new blood vessel formation is important in maintenance of the deposits. The cellular and biochemical constituents of the peritoneal fluid are increasingly being seen as important in endometriosis. The peritoneal fluid is in close proximity to peritoneal endometriosis and it is likely to have a direct effect not only on the ability of the ectopic tissue to implant but may also influence the survival, vascularization and progression of the disease. In recent years, our understanding of the constituents of the peritoneal fluid has increased[49]. Peritoneal fluid contains a wide range of growth and angiogenic factors which are important in the proliferation and vascularization of endometrial tissue as well as in the recruitment and activation of the peritoneal macrophages (Figure 2). Recently, in our laboratory, we have shown elevated levels of the potent angiogenic factor VEGF in the peritoneal fluid of women with endometriosis[50]. The highest levels were seen during the proliferative phase of the cycle, a time at which the peritoneum is exposed to the recently regurgitated endometrium.

*Peritoneal macrophages*

There are a number of possible sources for the factors found in the peritoneal fluid. They can originate from the exfoliated endometrium, follicular fluid or peritoneal macrophages. Macrophages are known to be an important

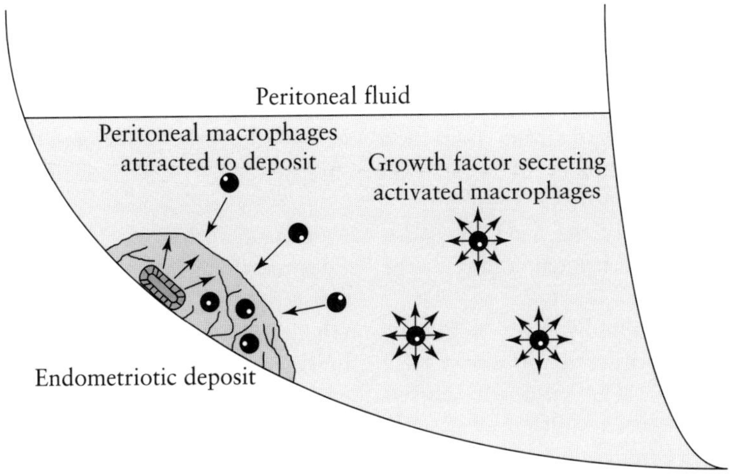


**Figure 2** Schematic representation of the interaction between ectopic endometrium and peritoneal macrophages. The endometriotic deposit is bathed in peritoneal fluid. The fluid is a rich soup of cytokines produced in part by activated macrophages. Macrophages may be activated by the ectopic endometrium or other, undefined, factors. The ectopic endometrium may attract macrophages which become tissue-resident. These macrophages may contribute to the development of a rich vasculature within and around the endometriotic deposit

source of a range of growth and angiogenic factors[51], and it has only been recently that attention has focused on the role of peritoneal macrophages. It has long been known that the largest proportion of cells in the peritoneal fluid are macrophages, and that these cells are increased in number, size and activation status in endometriosis with, as a consequence, increased secretion of a wide range of growth factors. This suggests a direct link between endometriosis, macrophage activation and secretory activity. A major activating stimulus for macrophages is the presence of the endometriotic tissue. However, macrophages can be activated by a range of stimuli and it could be that, in women who develop endometriosis, the macrophages may cause the disease rather than be a consequence of it. Either way, the continued presence of the endometriotic tissue will provide an ongoing powerful activation stimulus for the macrophages and, although their exact role is unclear, their importance in endometriosis is steadily increasing. A consequence of this is the possibility of these cells being future therapeutic targets, possibly through suppression of particular secretory activity by gene therapy and/or selective antagonism.

## Aetiology

A number of factors have been implicated in the aetiology of endometriosis, including genetic and racial predisposition, increased incidence at particular ages and an association with infertility. More important than any of these factors, however, is the role of endogenous oestrogens and peritoneal soiling at the time of menstruation.

Some women undoubtedly have a genetic predispostion to the disorder, as shown by twin and family studies[52,53]. The mode of inheritance has been described as multifactorial with an interplay between environmental and genetic factors. Although there is a genetic component, there appears not to be any significant racial predispostion to endometriosis. Previously, it was believed that Caucasian women were more likely to develop endometriosis than negroid women, although such conclusions were based on comparisons of groups with differing access to health care. At present, the only group of women shown to have an increased incidence appears to be the Japanese[54].

*Endogenous oestrogens*

Strong circumstantial evidence exists to support the dependency of endometriosis on steroid hormones[55]. Endometriosis has not been reported in premenarchal girls and is rare in postmenopausal women. In postmenopausal women, it is usually reported in conjunction with treatment with exogenous oestrogens or when endogenous oestrogen levels remain high. Most instances of endometriosis occur during the reproductive years when the women are exposed to fluctuating but high levels of steroid hormones. Finally, the disease is effectively cured following bilateral oophorectomy. Current treatment regimes rely on this steroid dependency by establishing either a hypoestrogenic environment and/or creating a progestogenic or androgenic environment. Therefore, conditions which alter the oestrogen status may influence the incidence of endometriosis. It has been suggested that smoking and exercise, since they are prone to cause an hypoestrogenic state, are associated with a lower incidence of endometriosis[56]. The association between oestrogens and endometriosis has concentrated research on the endometrium and has resulted in the current endocrine treatments for this disease.

*Peritoneal soiling*

Endometriosis is associated with retrograde menstruation. It is more common in women whose normal menstrual egress is occluded by uterine anomalies and in women who have an earlier menarche, a shorter cycle length and increased duration of menstrual bleeding. In such patients, the degree of peritoneal soiling due to retrograde menstruation is likely to be greater. The number of menstrual periods and the length of time menstruation has been interrupted by childbirth are also important factors. It is interesting to note that the number of menses experienced by women today is greater by a factor of ten than those experienced by their Victorian counterparts and this in part might explain the apparent increased incidence of the disease. All these factors point towards a direct relationship between the degree of menstrual soiling of the pelvis and the appearance of endometriosis. Reducing menstrual soiling, such as is seen in patients using the oral contraceptive pill, is likely to be of benefit in the prevention of both initial and recurrent disease.

## ENDOMETRIOSIS AND INFERTILITY

The association between the occurrence of endometriosis and infertility has long been recognized. Indeed the increased prevalence of endometriosis in women investigated for infertility has led to some suggesting a causal relationship between endometriosis and infertility, although this has been disputed by others. The precise relationship between the two conditions remains unclear and this has led to confusion regarding the optimum management of infertile women with coexistent endometriosis.

### Endometriosis and potential mechanisms of infertility

In women with severe endometriosis, the presence of structural damage, and also ovarian and tubal adhesions, prevents oocyte release, retrieval and transport and leads to a mechanical disruption in fertility. In women with mild endometriosis and no apparent structural damage the aetiological basis for the infertility is unclear. Numerous factors have been investigated to explain how mild endometriosis could affect fertility. These factors include endocrine and immunological abnormalities as well as the development of an autoimmune response and an increase in the incidence of spontaneous abortion.

The endocrine factors implicated in endometriosis-associated infertility include defective folliculogenesis[57–59], anovulation[60], luteinized unruptured follicle syndrome[61], luteal phase defects[62] and hyperprolactinaemia[63]. However, these factors are also found in women with infertility in the absence of endometriosis[64]. In addition, these abnormalities have not been shown to occur in consecutive menstrual cycles or in patients with endometriosis more commonly than in other infertile patients.

In women with endometriosis, inflammatory changes have been observed in the peritoneal fluid. An increase in peritoneal fluid volumes, macrophage numbers, macrophage activity and higher levels of cytokines and prostanoids are observed, as discussed previously. It is thought that the presence of ectopic endometrium in the pelvis provides an antigenic stimulus, resulting in the observed inflammatory changes in the peritoneal fluid. These inflammatory changes are thought to interfere with fertility by a direct cytotoxic effect on the oocyte, spermatozoa and embryo. Studies using peritoneal fluid from women with endometriosis have found impaired ovum penetration[65], decreased sperm motility and velocity[66] and alterations in sperm movement[67]. No improvement in fecundability, however, is seen in women following treatment for endometriosis[60]. Thus, while alterations in the immunological activity of peritoneal fluid appear to affect fertility, their significance and implications remain unclear.

A number of studies have linked an increased miscarriage rate to the presence of mild endometriosis, with one study observing a reduction in this rate following treatment of the endometriosis. However, controlled prospective studies have not confirmed these initial findings and no causal relationship could be demonstrated between endometriosis and spontaneous abortion[68,69]. Should an increased pregnancy loss rate be caused by endometriosis, one might expect to observe it in patients undergoing assisted conception where an early diagnosis of pregnancy is made. Recently, Check and colleagues[70] have demonstrated no difference in the rates of ongoing pregnancies between 'normal' subjects and those with endometriosis, and pregnancy loss rates are not affected by disease stage[71]. Despite extensive research on infertile women with mild endometriosis, there is no evidence for a causal relationsip between these two factors, in contrast with severe endometriosis where mechanical factors can obviously explain the causality of endometriosis in reduced fertility.

### Management of the infertile woman

The dual aims of therapy in the management of endometriosis are to provide symptomatic relief and improve fertility. All current medical therapies are contraceptive. During treatment, therefore, they cannot improve fertility and their use can only be justified if it can be demonstrated that they either prevent disease progression to a stage where anatomical distortion compromises fertility, or increased fecundity can be demonstrated in the period following treatment. The natural history of endometriosis is that it deteriorates in an unpredictable manner, although in a significant proportion of patients it will actually improve[60,72–74]. As the relationship between less severe forms of endometriosis and infertility is unclear, there is little justification in the treatment of endometriosis to prevent disease progression, as for many patients this would be over-treatment. In any case, any improvement as a consequence of medical therapy is likely only to be short-lived, as a delay in a second-look laparoscopy until ovarian and menstrual activity resumes results in a higher rate of diagnosis than if laparoscopy is repeated during ovarian suppression[75]. A more rational approach would be to attempt to achieve a pregnancy before disease progression occurs.

Alternatively, medical treatment could be justified if pregnancy rates following treatment were increased. A number of well-conducted studies, using a variety of treatments, have been published since the early 1980s. Recently, Hughes and his colleagues[76] have published a quantitative overview of all these randomized trials of commonly used treatments for endometriosis-associated infertility. The odds ratio comparing treatment with no treatment was 0.85 (0.95–1.22), thus confirming the conclusions reached from reviewing the trials individually that medical treatment does not bestow any benefit.

All medical therapies, when given continuously, are contraceptive and thus obviously will delay fertility. Overton and colleagues[74] reported the use of luteal-phase, high-dose dydrogesterone in an attempt to provide treatment without compromising fertility. As with previous studies, no improvement in the pregnancy rate was noted, but patients were able to conceive during treatment. They suggest that this mode of treatment may be appropriate for the symptomatic patient who wishes to conceive.

Proven causality between endometriosis and infertility is restricted to those cases with anatomical distortion. Rationally, therefore, restoration of the normal anatomical relationsips should restore fertility. Surgical treatment results in the best pregnancy rates in infertile women with severe pelvic endometriosis and structural damage[77]. When the normal pelvic anatomy can be restored by adhesiolysis and mobilization of the Fallopian tubes and ovaries, pregnancy rates of 50% are observed[78,79]. Recent advances in minimal access surgery suggest that this approach is beneficial. Pregnancy rates between 40 and 81% have been reported (for a review see Sutton, reference 80). The laparoscopic approach, especially when combined with laser adhesiolysis, offers a number of advantages over more conventional approaches. These are:

(1) Precise destruction of lesions and adhesions;

(2) Minimal bleeding, thus minimizing neo-adhesion formation;

(3) Minimal damage to adjacent structures, in particular the Fallopian tube; and

(4) Non-drying of structures that occurs at laparotomy.

With this approach, no increased incidence of adhesion formation has been reported.

How far can we extrapolate these observations relating to minimally invasive surgery and restoration of normal anatomy? It has been suggested that endometriotic implants should be ablated at the time of diagnostic laparoscopy, but would this be any more beneficial than treating medically thereafter? This subject was also considered by Hughes and his colleagues in 1993[76]. They concluded, despite a suggestion of possible benefit, that the studies 'demonstrated such a degree of clinical and statistical heterogeneity that no conclusion could be drawn'. Consequently, properly controlled, randomized trials are required to resolve this important question.

Just as our concepts of the importance of the endometrium have changed with respect to the pathogenesis of endometriosis, so too has the apparent importance of the visual diagnosis of endometriosis in the infertile patient. No longer is it suggested that the mere presence of ectopic endometrium is causal in infertility. It is more likely that the relationship between endometriosis and infertility in most cases is casual. This allows us to adopt a far more dogmatic approach to the infertile patient (Figure 3).

## SYMPTOMATIC ENDOMETRIOSIS

If the significance of the visual diagnosis of ectopic endometrium has been questioned in the asymptomatic infertile patient, then the same questioning should logically occur in the patient with symptoms. There is no doubt that the diagnosis of endometriosis is now made more frequently than previously, but the question is whether this increased frequency of diagnosis is real or apparent. Historically, the diagnosis of endometriosis was made at laparotomy. Sampson's seminal works on the histogenesis of endometriosis gave detailed descriptions of his observations made at laparotomy[3–11]. Nowadays, the diagnosis will most commonly be made at laparoscopy and it is likely that less severe disease will be observed. Even with laparoscopy, the frequency of diagnosis is increasing. In studies published in the late 1970s and early 1980s, prevalences of between 2 and 5% were reported[81,82]. One decade later, prospective studies were suggesting that the diagnosis could be made in almost one in five women[83–86].

Whilst some of the increase in diagnosis can be explained methodologically, in that the latter studies were prospective and designed carefully to inspect the pelvis, over the same period of time reports were published identifying many different visual appearances of endometriotic deposits[87,88]. Further studies utilizing such descriptions of endometriosis have since

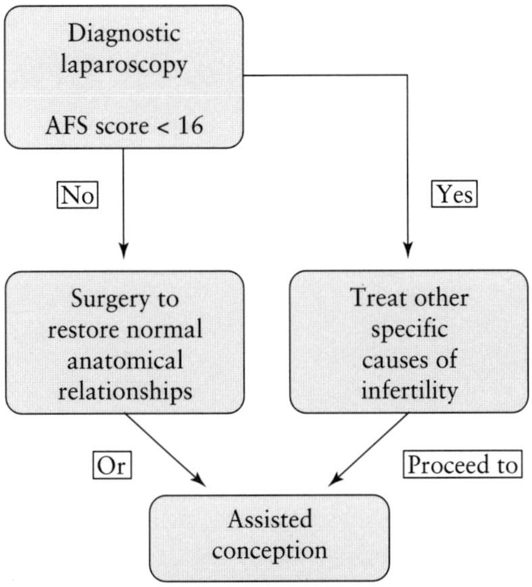


**Figure 3** Flow chart for the management of the patient with endometriosis-associated infertility. AFS, American Fertility Society

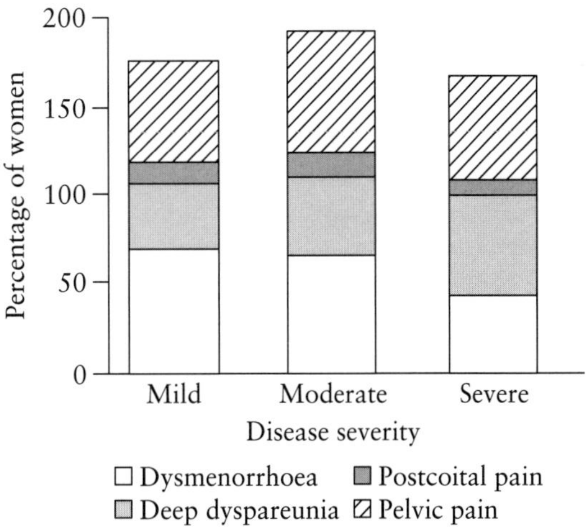


**Figure 4** Proportion of women with symptoms in mild, moderate and severe endometriosis. There are no statistical differences between the groups. (Modified from Mahmood *et al.*[95])

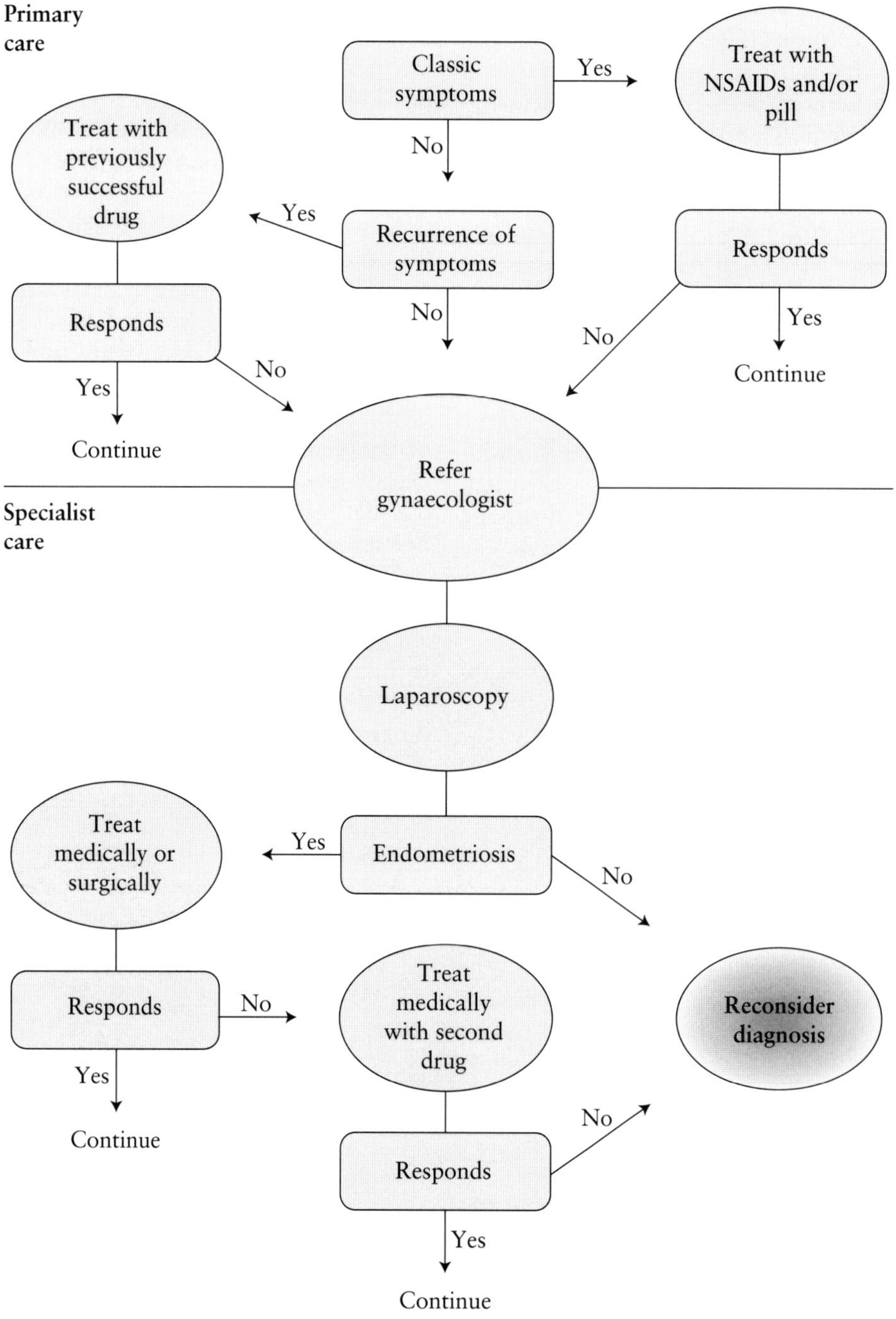


**Figure 5** Flow chart for the proposed management of the patient with suspected endometriosis-associated symptoms. NSAID, non-steroidal anti-inflammatory drug

reported the presence of ectopic endometrium in four out of five women[89,90]. These observations, together with the reported occurrence of endometriosis in visually normal peritoneal peritoneum[87,91], leads to the conclusion that endometriosis is a ubiquitous phenomenon and may, in fact, be the natural consequence of the physiological event, menstruation, rather than pathology *per se*.

If endometriosis is pathological one might expect that it would progress and give rise to symptoms and anatomical distortion. Not all endometriosis is progressive. A limited number of studies have looked at the natural history of this condition[72–74]. In all these studies, progression was noted in between 23 and 47% of cases but, conversely, improvement or resolution was noted in between 27 and 53%. The mechanisms of disease progression, including adhesion formation, are little understood and it is not possible to predict who will develop progressive disease. This further suggests that endometriosis should be redefined as the presence of ectopic endometrium associated with signs of progression or anatomical destruction and not merely the presence of ectopic endometrium[92].

It is often remarked that the severity of symptoms does not correlate with the severity of the endometriosis observed. This phenomenon has been quantified by many authors[93–95] (Figure 4). In addition, many patients, particularly those presenting with infertility, are asymptomatic. Thus, the relationship between the 'disease' and the symptoms is debatable. This is most clearly demonstrated by the observations of Sutton[96]. In a series of 33 patients undergoing second-look laparoscopy for poor response to laser laparoscopy for pelvic pain, over half had no evidence of ectopic endometrium.

Where do these observations lead us therapeutically? There is an obvious danger that, by making the visual diagnosis of endometriosis, we falsely identify the cause for the patient's pain. She may then receive treatment, either medical or surgical at the time of the diagnostic procedure, to which she does not respond. Therapeutically, she may then embark upon a roller coaster of treatments for a gynaecological condition, with perhaps more downs than ups, whilst the underlying problems are not addressed. We should not be too proud to re-examine our original diagnosis when treatment fails. A flow chart for management is suggested in Figure 5. Medical therapies that are employed include the GnRH analogues, danazol, gestrinone and progestogens.

## CONCLUSIONS

Our understanding of the pathogenesis of endometriosis has moved dramatically forward in the last decade. It is now clear that the presence of ectopic endometrium within the pelvis is an ubiquitous and perhaps physiological phenomenon. If this is the case, we should be cautious to ascribe causality to the presence of ectopic endometrium in patients who present with either infertility or symptomatic disease. Failure on our part to exhibit such caution will undoubtedly expose our patients to ineffective over-treatment and divert our attention from their underlying problems.

## REFERENCES

1. Sampson, J. A. (1940). The development of the implantation theory for the origin of peritoneal endometriosis. *Am. J. Obstet. Gynecol.*, **40**, 549–57
2. Waldeyer (1870). Eierstock und Ei, Leipzig. Quoted by Goodall, J. R. (1944). *A Study of Endometriosis*, 2nd edn., p. 2. (Philadelphia: J. B. Lippincott & Co.)
3. Sampson, J. A. (1921). Perforating hemorrhagic (chocolate) cysts of the ovary. Their importance and especially their relation to pelvic adenomas of the endometrial type ('adenomyoma' of the uterus, rectovaginal septum, sigmoid etc). *Arch. Surg.*, **3**, 245–323
4. Sampson, J. A. (1922). Ovarian hematomas of endometrial type (perforating hemorrhagic cysts of the ovary) and implantation adenomas of endometrial type. *Boston Med. Surg. J.*, **186**, 445–56
5. Sampson, J. A. (1922). Intestinal adenomas of endometrial type. Their importance and their relation to ovarian hematomas of endometrial type (perforating hemorrhagic cysts of the ovary). *Arch. Surg.*, **5**, 217–80
6. Sampson, J. A. (1922). The life history of ovarian hematomas (hemorrhagic cysts) of endometrial (Müllerian) type. *Am. J. Obstet. Gynecol.*, **4**, 451–512

7. Sampson, J. A. (1925). Heterotopic or misplaced endometrial tissue. *Am. J. Obstet. Gynecol.*, **10**, 649–64
8. Sampson, J. A. (1925). Inguinal endometriosis (often reported as endometrial tissue in the groin, adenomyoma in the groin, and adenomyoma of the round ligament). *Am. J. Obstet. Gynecol.*, **10**, 462–503
9. Sampson, J. A. (1927). Peritoneal endometriosis due to the menstrual dissemination of endometrial tissue into the peritoneal cavity. *Am. J. Obstet. Gynecol.*, **14**, 422–69
10. Sampson, J. A. (1927). Metastatic or embolic endometriosis, due to the menstrual dissemination of endometrial tissue into the venous circulation. *Am. J. Pathol.*, **3**, 93–109
11. Sampson, J. A. (1928). Endometriosis following salpingectomy. *Am. J. Obstet. Gynecol.*, **16**, 461–99
12. Javert, C. T. (1949). Pathogenesis of endometriosis based on endometrial homeoplasia, direct extension, exfoliation and implantation, lymphatic and hematogenous metastasis (including five case reports of endometrial tissue in pelvic lymph nodes). *Cancer*, **2**, 399–410
13. Fallas, R. and Rosenblum, G. (1940). Endometriosis. A study of 260 private hospital cases. *Am. J. Obstet. Gynecol.*, **39**, 964–75
14. Haydon, G. B. (1942). A study of 569 cases of endometriosis. *Am. J. Obstet. Gynecol.*, **43**, 704–9
15. Holmes, W. R. (1942). Endometriosis. *Am. J. Obstet. Gynecol.*, **43**, 255–64
16. Scott, R. B. and Te Linde, R. W. (1950). External endometriosis – the scourge of the private patient. *Ann. Surg.*, **131**, 697–719
17. Ranney, B. (1971). Endometriosis. III. Complete operations. Reasons, sequelae, treatment. *Am. J. Obstet. Gynecol.*, **109**, 1137–42
18. Jenkins, S., Olive, D. L. and Haney, A. F. (1986). Endometriosis: pathogenetic implications of the anatomic distribution. *Obstet. Gynecol.*, **67**, 335–8
19. Novak, E. (1926). The significance of uterine mucosa in the Fallopian tube, with a discussion of the origin of aberrant endometrium. *Am. J. Obstet. Gynecol.*, **12**, 484–526
20. Novak, E. (1931). Pelvic endometriosis. Spontaneous rupture of endometrial cysts, with a report of three cases. *Am. J. Obstet. Gynecol.*, **22**, 826–37
21. Ridley, J. H. (1968). The histogenesis of endometriosis. A review of facts and fancies. *Obstet. Gynecol. Surv.*, **23**, 1–35
22. Ranta, H., Aine, R., Oksanen, H. and Heinonen, P. K. (1990). Dissemination of endometrial cells during carbon dioxide hysteroscopy and chromotubation among infertile patients. *Fertil. Steril.*, **53**, 751–3
23. Blumenkrantz, M. J., Gallagher, N., Bashore, R. A. and Tenckhoff, H. (1981). Retrograde menstruation in women undergoing chronic peritoneal dialysis. *Obstet. Gynecol.*, **57**, 667–70
24. Halme, J., Hammond, M. G., Hulka, J. F., Raj, S. G. and Talbert, L. M. (1984). Retrograde menstruation in healthy women and in patients with endometriosis. *Obstet. Gynecol.*, **64**, 151–4
25. Cron, R. S. and Gey, G. (1927). The viability of the cast-off menstrual endometrium. *Am. J. Obstet. Gynecol.*, **13**, 645–7
26. Geist, S. H. (1933). The viability of fragments of menstrual endometrium. *Am. J. Obstet. Gynecol.*, **25**, 751
27. Keettel, W. C. and Stein, R. J. (1951). The viability of the cast-off menstrual endometrium. *Am. J. Obstet. Gynecol.*, **61**, 440–2
28. Mungyer, G., Willemsen, W. N. P., Rolland, R., Vemer, H. M., Ramaekers, F. C. S., Jap, P. H. K. and Poels, L. G. (1987). Cells of the mucous membrane of the female genital tract in culture: a comparative study with regard to the histogenesis of endometriosis. *In Vitro*, **23**, 111–17
29. Kruitwagen, R. F. P. M., de Ronde, I. J. Y., Poels, L. G., Jap, P. H. K., Willemsen, W. N. P. and Rolland, R. (1991). Endometrial epithelial cells in peritoneal fluid during the early follicular phase. *Fertil. Steril.*, **55**, 297–303
30. Ridley, J. H. and Edwards, I. K. (1958). Experimental endometriosis in the human. *Am. J. Obstet. Gynecol.*, **76**, 783–9
31. Ridley, J. H. (1961). The validity of Sampson's theory of endometriosis. *Am. J. Obstet. Gynecol.*, **82**, 777–81
32. Scott, R. B., Te Linde, R. W. and Wharton, L. R. (1953). Further studies on experimental endometriosis. *Am. J. Obstet. Gynecol.*, **66**, 1082–103
33. Olive, D. L. and Henderson, D. Y. (1987). Endometriosis and Müllerian anomalies. *Obstet. Gynecol.*, **69**, 412–15

34. Bergqvist, A., Jeppsson, S., Kullander, S. and Ljungberg, O. (1985). Human uterine endometrium and endometriotic tissue transplanted into nude mice. Morphologic effects of various steroid hormones. *Am. J. Pathol.*, **121**, 337–41
35. Iwanoff, N. S. (1898). Drüsiges cysthaltiges uterusfiibromyom compliciert durch sarcom und carcinom (adenofibromyoma cysticum sarcomatodes carcinomatosum). *Monatsschr. Geburtsh. Gynakol.*, **7**, 295
36. Meyer, R. (1919). Über den stand der frage der adenomyositis und adenomyome im allgemeinen und insbesondere über adenomyositis seroepithelialis und adenomyometritis sarcomatosa. *Zentralbl. Gynakol.*, **36**, 745–50
37. Oliker, A. J. and Harris, A. E. (1971). Endometriosis of the bladder in a male patient. *J. Urol.*, **106**, 858–9
38. Pinkert, T. C., Catlow, C. E. and Straus, R. (1979). Endometriosis of the urinary bladder in a man with prostatic carcinoma. *Cancer*, **43**, 1562–7
39. Schrodt,, G. R., Alcorn, M. O. and Ibanez, J. (1980). Endometriosis of the male urinary system: a case report. *J. Urol.*, **124**, 722–3
40. Smith, S. K. (1995). Angiogenic growth factor expression in the uterus. *Hum. Reprod. Update*, **1**, 162–72
41. Tabibzadeh, S. (1991). Human endometrium: an active site of cytokine production and action. *Endocr. Rev.*, **12**, 272–89
42. McLaren, J., Prentice, A., Charnock-Jones, D. S., Millican, S. A., Miller, K. H., Sharkey, A. M. and Smith, S. K. (1996). Vascular endothelial growth factor is produced by peritoneal fluid macrophages in endometriosis and is regulated by ovarian steroids. *J. Clin. Invest.*, in press
43. Prentice, A., Randall, B. J., Weddell, A., McGill, A., Horne, C. H. W. and Thomas, E. J. (1992). Ovarian steroid receptor expression in endometriosis and in two potential parent epithelia: endometrium and peritoneal mesothelium. *Hum. Reprod.*, **7**, 1318–25
44. Nisolle, M., Casanas-Roux, F., Wyns, C., Yvan de Menten, B. S., Mathieu, P.-E. and Donnez, J. (1994). Immunohistochemical analysis of estrogen and progesterone receptors in endometrium and peritoneal endometriosis: a new quantitative method. *Fertil. Steril.*, **62**, 751–9
45. Bridges, J. E., Prentice, A., Roches, W., Englefield, P. and Thomas, E. J. (1994). Expression of integrin adhesion molecules in endometrium and endometriosis. *Br. J. Obstet. Gynaecol.*, **101**, 696–700
46. Van der Linden, P. J. Q., Goeij, A. F. P. M., Dunselman, G. A. J., Van der Linden, E. P. M., Ramaekers, F. C. S. and Evers, J. L. M. (1994). Expression of integrins and E-cadherin in cells from menstrual effluent, endometrium, peritoneal fluid, peritoneum and endometriosis. *Fertil. Steril.*, **61**, 85–90
47. Rodgers, W. H., Matrisian, L. M., Giudice, L. C., Dsupin, B., Cannon, P., Svitek, C., Gorstein, F. and Osteen, K. G. (1994). Patterns of matrix metalloproteinase expression in cycling endometrium imply differential functions and regulation by steroid hormones. *J. Clin. Invest.*, **94**, 946–53
48. Brosens, I. A. (1994). New principles in the management of endometriosis. *Acta Obstet. Gynecol. Scand.*, **159**, 18–21
49. Ramey, J. W. and Archer, D. F. (1993). Peritoneal fluid: its relevance to the development of endometriosis. *Fertil. Steril.*, **60**, 1–14
50. McLaren, J., Prentice, A., Charnock-Jones, D. S. and Smith, S. K. (1996). Vascular endothelial growth factor (VEGF) concentrations are elevated in peritoneal fluid of women with endometriosis. *Hum. Reprod.*, **11**, 220–3
51. Sunderkotter, C., Steinbrink, K., Goebeler, M., Bhardwaj, R. and Sorg, C. (1994). Macrophages and angiogenesis. *J. Leucocyte. Biol.*, **55**, 410–22
52. Malinak, L. R., Buttram, V. C., Elias, S. and Simpson, J. L. (1980). Heritable aspects of endometriosis. II. Clinical aspects of familial endometriosis. *Am. J. Obstet. Gynecol.*, **137**, 332–6
53. Coxhead, D. and Thomas, E. J. (1993). The familial inheritance of endometriosis in a British population: a case control study. *J. Obstet. Gynaecol.*, **13**, 42–4
54. Miyazawa, K. (1976). Incidence of endometriosis among Japanese women. *Obstet. Gynecol.*, **48**, 407–9
55. Haney, A. F. (1991). The pathogenesis and aetiology of endometriosis. In Thomas, E. J. and Rock, J. A. (eds.) *Modern Approaches to Endometriosis*, pp. 3–19. (Lancaster, UK: Kluwer Academic Publishers)
56. Cramer, D. W., Wilson, E., Stillman, R. J. *et al.* (1986). The relation of endometriosis to menstrual characteristics, smoking and exercise. *J. Am. Med. Assoc.*, **255**, 1904–8

57. Ayers, J. W. T., Birenbaum, D. L. and Menon, K. M. L. (1987). Luteal phase dysfunction in endometriosis; elevated progesterone levels in peripheral and ovarian veins during follicular phase. *Fertil. Steril.*, **47**, 925–9
58. Doody, M. C., Gibbons, W. E. and Buttram, V. C. (1988). Linear regression analysis of ultrasound follicular growth series: evidence for an abnormality of follicular growth in endometriosis patients. *Fertil. Steril.*, **49**, 47–51
59. Tummon, I. S., Maclin, V. M., Radwanska, E., Binor, Z. and Dmowski, W. P. (1988). Occult ovulatory dysfunction in women with minimal endometriosis or unexplained infertility. *Fertil. Steril.*, **50**, 716–20
60. Mahmood, T. A. and Templeton, A. (1990). Pathophysiology of mild endometriosis: review of literature. *Hum. Reprod.*, **5**, 765–84
61. Brosens, I. A., Koninckx, P. R. and Corveleyn, P. A. (1978). A study of plasma progesterone, oestradiol 17β, prolactin and LH levels and of the luteal phase appearance of the ovaries in patients with endometriosis and infertility. *Br. J. Obstet. Gynaecol.*, **85**, 246–50
62. Kusuhara, K. (1992). Luteal function in infertile patients with endometriosis. *Am. J. Obstet. Gynecol.*, **167**, 274–7
63. Muse, K., Wilson, E. A. and Jawad, M. J. (1982). Prolactin hyperstimulation in response to thyrotropin-releasing hormone in patients with endometriosis. *Fertil. Steril.*, **38**, 419–22
64. Pepperell, R. J. and McBain, J. C. (1985). Unexplained infertility: a review. *Br. J. Obstet. Gynaecol.*, **92**, 569–80
65. Chacho, K. J., Chacho, M. S., Anderson, B. S. and Scommegna, A. (1986). Peritoneal fluid in patients with and without endometriosis: prostanoids and macrophages and their effect on the spermatozoa penetration assay. *Am. J. Obstet. Gynecol.*, **154**, 1290–9
66. Oak, M. K., Chantler, E. N., Williams, C. A. and Elstein, M. (1985). Sperm survival studies in peritoneal fluid from infertile women with endometriosis and unexplained infertility. *Clin. Reprod. Fertil.*, **3**, 297–303
67. Curtis, P., Lindsay, P., Jackson, A. E. and Shaw, R. W. (1993). Adverse effects on sperm movement characteristics in women with minimal and mild endometriosis. *Br. J. Obstet. Gynaecol.*, **100**, 165–9
68. Metzger, D. A., Olive, D. L., Stohs, G. F. and Franklin, R. R. (1986). Association of endometriosis and spontaneous abortion: effect of control group selection. *Fertil. Steril.*, **45**, 18–23
69. Pittaway, D. E., Vernon, C. and Fayez, J. A. (1988). Spontaneous abortions in women with endometriosis. *Fertil. Steril.*, **50**, 711–15
70. Check, J. H., Lurie, D., O'Shaughnessy, A. and Dietterich, C. (1995). The relationship of endometriosis to endometrial sonographic studies prior to administration of human chorionic gonadotrophin in patients undergoing *in vitro* fertilization and embryo transfer. *Hum. Reprod.*, **10**, 938–41
71. Chedid, S., Camus, M., Smitz, J., Van Steirteghem, A. C. and Devroey, P. (1995). Comparison among different ovarian stimulation regimens for assisted procreation procedures in patients with endometriosis. *Hum. Reprod.*, **10**, 2406–11
72. Telimaa, S., Puolakka, J., Ronnberg, L. and Kaupilla, A. (1987). Placebo-controlled comparison of danazol and high dose medroxyprogesterone acetate in the treatment of endometriosis. *Gynecol. Endocrinol.*, **1**, 13–23
73. Thomas, E. J. and Cooke, I. D. (1987). Impact of gestrinone on the course of asymptomatic endometriosis. *Br. Med. J.*, **294**, 272–4
74. Overton, C. E., Lindsay, P. C., Johal, B., Collins, S. A., Siddle, N. C., Shaw, R. W. and Barlow, D. H. (1994). A randomized, double blind, placebo-controlled study of luteal phase dydrogesterone (Duphaston) in women with minimal to mild endometriosis. *Fertil. Steril.*, **62**, 701–7
75. Evers, J. L. H. (1987). The second look laparoscopy for the evaluation of the results of medical treatment of endometriosis should not be performed during ovarian suppression. *Fertil. Steril.*, **47**, 502–4
76. Hughes, E. G., Fedorkow, D. M. and Collins, J. A. (1993). A quantitative overview of controlled trials in endometriosis-associated infertility. *Fertil. Steril.*, **59**, 963–70
77. Candiani, G. B., Fedele, L. and Vercellini, P. (1989). Laparotomy versus laparoscopy in the surgical treatment of endometriosis: the end of an era? *Acta Eur. Fertil.*, **20**, 163–6
78. Rock, J. A., Guziak, D. S., Sengos, C., Schweditsch, M., Sapp, K. C. and Jones, H. W. (1981). The conservative surgical treatment of endometriosis: evaluation of pregnancy success with respect to the extent of disease as categorized using contemporary classification systems. *Fertil. Steril.*, **35**, 131–7
79. Chong, A. P., Luciano, A. and O'Shaughnessy, A. M. (1990). Laser laparoscopy versus laparotomy in the treatment of infertility patients

with severe endometriosis. *J. Gynecol. Surg.*, **6**, 179–83
80. Sutton, C. J. G. (1993). Minimally invasive surgical approach to endometriosis and adhesiolysis. In Studd, J. and Jardine Brown, C. (eds.) *The Yearbook of The Royal College of Obstetricians and Gynaecologists*, pp. 117–25. (London: RCOG Press)
81. Stock, R. J. (1978). Evaluation of the sequelae of tubal ligation. *Fertil. Steril.*, **29**, 169–74
82. Strathy, R. H., Molgaard, C. A., Coulam, C. B. and Melton, L. J. (1982). Endometriosis and infertility: a laparoscopic study of endometriosis among fertile and infertile women. *Fertil. Steril.*, **38**, 667–72
83. Moen, M. H. (1987). Endometriosis in women at interval sterilisation. *Acta Obstet. Gynaecol. Scand.*, **66**, 451–4
84. Verkauf, B. S. (1987). Incidence, symptoms, and signs of endometriosis in fertile and infertile women. *J. Florida Med. Assoc.*, **74**, 671–5
85. Kirshon, B., Poindexter, A. N. and Fast, J. (1989). Endometriosis in multiparous women. *J. Reprod. Med.*, **34**, 215–17
86. Mahmood, T. A. and Templeton, A. A. (1991). Prevalence and genesis of endometriosis. *Hum. Reprod.*, **6**, 544–9
87. Jansen, R. P. S. and Russell, P. (1986). Non-pigmented endometriosis: clinical, laparoscopic and pathologic definition. *Am. J. Obstet. Gynecol.*, **155**, 1154–9
88. Nisolle, M., Berliëre, M., Paindaveine, B., Casanas-Roux, F., Bourdon, A. and Donnez, J. (1990). Histologic study of peritoneal endometriosis in infertile women. *Fertil. Steril.*, **53**, 984–8
89. Martin, D. C., Hubert, G. D., Van Der Zwaag, R. and El-Zeky, F. A. (1989). Laparoscopic appearance of peritoneal endometriosis. *Fertil. Steril.*, **51**, 63–7
90. Cornillie, F. J., Oosterlynck, D., Lauweryns, J. M. and Koninckx, P. R. (1990). Deeply infiltrating pelvic endometriosis: histology and clinical significance. *Fertil. Steril.*, **53**, 978–83
91. Murphy, A. A., Gren, W. R., Bobbie, D., de la Cruz, A. C. and Rock, J. A. (1986). Unsuspected endometriosis documented by scanning electron microscopy in visually normal peritoneum. *Fertil. Steril.*, **46**, 522–4
92. Thomas, E. J. and Prentice, A. (1992). The aetiology and pathogenesis of endometriosis. *Reprod. Med. Rev.*, **1**, 21–36
93. Buttram, V. C. (1979). Conservative surgery for endometriosis in the infertile female: a study of 206 patients with implications for both medical and surgical therapy. *Fertil. Steril.*, **42**, 117–23
94. Fedele, L., Vercelline, P., Bianchi, S. *et al.* (1990). Stage and localisation of pelvic endometriosis and pain. *Fertil. Steril.*, **53**, 155–8
95. Mahmood, T. A., Templeton, A. A., Thomson, L. and Fraser, C. (1991). Menstrual symptoms in women with pelvic endometriosis. *Br. J. Obstet. Gynaecol.*, **98**, 558–63
96. Sutton, C. J. G. (1991). Laser laparoscopy in the treatment of endometriosis. In Thomas, E. J. and Rock, J. A. (eds.) *Modern Approaches to Endometriosis*, pp. 199–220. (Lancaster, UK: Kluwer Academic Publishers)

# Fibroids

# 24

*Stephen K. Smith*

## INTRODUCTION

Fibroids are the commonest benign tumours arising in women and are blamed for many of the menstrual problems found in women of reproductive age. Every clinician dealing with women in reproductive medicine needs to have a clear understanding about the aetiology of fibroids but more importantly, needs to be familiar with the range of choices that are now available for treating them. The original approaches of abdominal hysterectomy or myomectomy are not the only alternatives available and clinical decisions made in collaboration with the patient need to be undertaken from an informed position. Similarly, the expansion of surgical options complicates these decisions as most surgeons will not have the necessary skills to perform some of the more complicated minimal access procedures. In order that women may receive the best treatment in the future, it is likely that many patients will be cross-referred to practitioners with the required skills. This requires a degree of maturity on behalf of the profession and understanding on behalf of the patients that the increasing complexity of clinical practice, both in the medical and surgical fields, will force changes in the doctor–patient relationship. No longer can women have 'their own gynaecologist' as he/she will no longer have all the skills needed to provide this comprehensive service. This is particularly true in the case of fibroids.

## PATHOPHYSIOLOGY

### Macroscopic

Fibroids appear macroscopically as firm whorled-like benign tumours in the uterus. Their position in the uterus is classified into four areas. *Subserosal* fibroids project from the serosal surface of the uterus and are usually covered by the peritoneum. They may be pedunculated and occasionally can establish an alternative blood supply with omentum. They are of little clinical significance unless they undergo torsion. *Intramural* fibroids lie within the wall of the uterus. They do not project into the uterine cavity. They cause compression of the surrounding myometrial cells which form the false capsule. They are usually served by a large single set of blood vessels[1]. They cause venous congestion and large dilated venules form around the tumour[2]. *Submucosal* fibroids lie just beneath the surface of the endometrium. They distort the uterine cavity and may become pedunculated. Occasionally these growths may pass through the cervix and appear as fibroid polyps. Finally, fibroids may be situated in the cervix.

### Microscopic

Microscopic examination reveals whorls of smooth muscle-like cells and fibroblasts. They are poorly vascularized. Probably in view of this finding, hyaline degeneration may be found within larger fibroids and calcification occurs in older fibroids.

### Aetiology

The cause of uterine fibroids is unknown. However, over the past 10 years increasing evidence has highlighted a range of possible disorders at the endocrine, cellular and molecular levels which have begun to define some differences between the leiomyoma and the surrounding myometrium.

### Clonal development

Individual fibroids are of a monoclonal origin. The initial studies used analysis of X-linked glucose-6-phosphate dehydrogenase (G-6-PD)[3]. This enzyme is present in at least two forms, A and B. As women inherit two X chromosomes, one becomes methylated and inactive. Thus, if fibroids in heterozygous women contain both enzymes, it suggests an individual monoclonal origin of the tumours. This indeed appears to be the case. More recently, analysis of the methylation status of the X-linked androgen receptor has confirmed these findings[4], as have the findings of Hashimoto and co-workers[5] who studied inactivation of the X-chromosome-linked phosphoglycerokinase gene. This suggests that a single myometrial cell undergoes a change in the regulation of its cell cycle which results in a greater rate of mitosis than surrounding myometrial cells. Little is known of the mechanisms that cause this change. Unlike malignant transformation which probably arises after multiple changes, benign transformation is not associated with the development of a malignant phenotype. Recently, however, chromosomal aberrations more often associated with malignant cells have been described.

### Chromosomal aberrations

Most fibroids (50–80%) bear no tumour-specific chromosomal aberrations[6] but a group of cases demonstrating specific gene disorders has now been found. The commonest abnormality is a balanced translocation on chromosome 12, t(12:14) (q13–15;q24)[7–10]. This translocation is also found in other benign solid tumours including lipomas, pleomorphic salivary gland adenomas and pulmonary chondroid hamartomas[6]. Other less frequently identified breakpoints in chromosome 12 include t(12;15) (q15;q24) and ins (12;11) (q14;q21qter). Deletions in chromosome 7 have also been found and occasionally translocations in 7q[11]. Dal Cin and colleagues[12] found chromosomal abnormalities in 52 of 175 leiomyomas and described a new aberration with an interstitial deletion of the long arm of chromosome 3.

### Steroids

The tendency for fibroids to grow during the reproductive years and to regress in the menopause suggests that steroids may be implicated in the pathophysiology of these benign tumours. The absence of gross differences in peripheral levels of steroids between women with fibroids and those without suggests a more local effect in the tissue itself[1].

There has been a suggestion that the induction of a hypo-oestrogenic state reduces fibroid growth. Several studies find higher levels of oestrogen receptor in fibroids compared to adjacent myometrium[13–15], though this has not been found by all researchers[16]. Similarly, there is some confusion about progesterone receptor expression, several studies finding no difference[17] whilst others found higher levels[18]. On balance, the majority of the evidence would suggest higher levels of functional receptor in fibroids. Further confirmation of this is derived from more detailed analysis of receptor expression. Progesterone receptors are now known to be more complex than when most of these studies were undertaken. At least two receptors are identified (PR-A and PR-B) which are derived from a single gene using different initiation codons. Recent studies in our laboratory have shown that PR-A predominates in human fibroids and myometrium and that the levels are higher in fibroids (Viville, personal communication). Similarly, it is clear that there are different forms of the oestrogen receptor and that they may use alternate intracellular signalling mechanisms.

The simplistic view that oestrogen is the most important steroid needs to be challenged[19]. The growth of fibroids during pregnancy suggests that progesterone is the key 'growth hormone' for fibroids. This is supported by the findings that co-existent medroxyprogesterone treatment to women receiving gonadotrophin releasing hormone (GnRH) agonists inhibits fibroid shrinkage[20] and that the antiprogesterone, RU 486, also shrinks fibroids[21].

### Growth factors

Many of the actions of steroids are regulated by their induction of growth factor expression and more recently it seems that growth factors can even enhance steroid regulated gene transcription. Various growth factors have been found in fibroids.

Messenger RNA encoding epidermal growth factor (EGF) is present in both fibroids and myometrium, however, levels are higher in the fibroids but only in the luteal phase of the cycle[22]. Receptors for EGF have been found in mouse and human myometrium and fibroids[23–25]. Oestradiol-17β stimulated EGF expression in mouse uteri[26]. Lower levels of EGF receptor are found after treatment with GnRH analogues[24]. Taken together, these findings implicate EGF in steroid-driven fibroid growth and provide an answer to the stimulation by both oestrogen and progesterone.

Insulin-like growth factor (IGF-1 and -2) are also expressed by fibroids. Messenger RNA for IGF-2 but not IGF-1 is increased in uterine fibroids compared to myometrium[27]. The binding proteins IGF-BP 1, 2 and 3 are also expressed in fibroids but levels of IGF-BP 3 are reduced. This binding protein binds both IGF-1 and IGF-2 so this might explain IGF-induced fibroid growth. As with EGF, oestradiol-17β induces IGF-1 expression in the rat[28,29].

Vascular endothelial growth factor (VEGF), a potent angiogenic growth factor, is also expressed by fibroids but, unlike EGF, expression in the fibroid is not regulated by steroids, though the release from the surrounding myometrium is[30].

## PRESENTATION

### Menorrhagia

Fibroids have been long associated with menorrhagia but there is surprisingly little evidence to substantiate this claim and association is not proven. This apparently simple dilemma has important implications for fully informing patients of their treatment options and in guiding physicians to the correct treatment. The best means of determining the role of fibroids in menorrhagia would be to measure menstrual blood loss before and after myomectomy. No such studies have been reported. Whilst taking the history, a clear distinction should be made between menorrhagia and intermenstrual bleeding (IMB). In certain cases, IMB can be due to a fibroid and removal of the fibroid will remove the symptom. Intracavity fibroids which ulcerate and submucous fibroids which have a poor blood supply may present with IMB. Recently a cervical fibroid was also shown to present with IMB which ceased when the fibroid was lysed with the Nd : YAG laser[31]. Individual cases of disappearance of symptoms following excision of the fibroid would suggest that in a small number of women the fibroid is the cause of menorrhagia. A recent case, in which mean blood loss (MBL) was measured at 1 l per period, was resolved when the patient had hysteroscopic removal of 15 small submucous fibroids (Smith, 1996, personal communication). Nagele and associates[32] found that 30% of women referred with menorrhagia had fibroids on hysteroscopic examination. However, this is the same as the number of women who have fibroids but do not complain of menorrhagia and most women referred for menorrhagia do not have heavy periods[1,33,34].

### Pressure symptoms

Clearly, in women with large fibroids, pressure symptoms may be the cause for presentation. Large fibroids pressing on the bladder may promote frequency and nocturia. Rarely, pressure on the ureter may predispose to recurrent urinary tract infections but cases are so rare that it is difficult to provide evidence to support this case.

Pain may rarely be associated with fibroids, though expulsion of an intrauterine fibroid can present with considerable pain and occasionally torsion of a subserosal fibroid may present as an acute abdomen.

## INVESTIGATION

Most cases will be diagnosed on abdominal and vaginal examination as usually there is more than one fibroid and the masses feel firm and the uterus mobile. Occasionally a single large fibroid can induce uniform enlargement of the uterus. In all cases the mass is mobile unless at around 12 weeks size it is constrained within the pelvis.

### Ultrasound

Ultrasound is indicated in all cases of pelvic masses. The principle aim is to differentiate between the solid fibroid mass and solid/cystic lesions of the ovary. In the majority of cases this is straightforward but there can be difficulty in distinguishing solid ovarian masses and pedunculated fibroids. The presence of ascitic fluid in the pouch of Douglas should be determined, and if there is still confusion, malignancy markers such as CA 125 may be needed. In most centres, nuclear magnetic resonance imaging can provide sufficient discrimination in diagnosis.

In view of the critical importance of having ovarian masses operated on by properly skilled surgeons in centres of oncological excellence, the need to make the correct diagnosis before surgery is very important. Furthermore, in considering the large range of treatment options, the diagnosis may often be made without recourse to surgery. A mistake can be lethal.

### Hysteroscopy

Patients presenting with IMB must have a cervical smear and hysteroscopic examination of the uterine cavity. This permits the exclusion of cervical changes and may identify intrauterine fibroids. Preferably these procedures can be performed as an out-patient[32,35]. The investigation of patients presenting with menorrhagia depends on the initial examination. Women with large fibroids greater than 12 weeks size will probably not benefit from hysteroscopy and women below the age of 40 should be discouraged from having hysteroscopy[36]. Patients over 40 would currently be expected to have a hysteroscopic examination if they complain of menorrhagia and the uterine size is below 12 weeks size.

## TREATMENT

There can be few areas of clinical practice in which there has been such an increase in the treatment options available to patients and their physicians than for uterine fibroids. More precise consideration of the role of fibroids in the symptoms of menstrual dysfunction has altered the 'knee-jerk' response of the past, whilst developments in both medical and surgical treatments have transformed the options available to patients. It is critically important that gynaecologists counselling patients are fully aware of these options and whilst they may not have experience of the newer medical treatments and may not be able to perform the more adventurous surgical treatments they should be prepared to refer patients accordingly.

### Conservative treatment

Undoubtedly, for the majority of women with fibroids, no treatment will be given. Many women will be unaware of the presence of fibroids. Fibroids should not be removed just because 'they are there'. It is the symptoms that dictate treatment, with a reasonable consideration of the possible changes that may arise in the future. This judgemental approach appears to be what happens in practice. Three-fold differences occur in general practitioner (GP) referral rates of patients complaining of menorrhagia[37,38], which is also reflected in referrals of patients known to have fibroids! The chance finding of fibroids should include investigation to make the diagnosis and differentiate it from more dangerous ovarian disease but may not require further intervention. Certainly, women near the menopause who are asymptomatic will probably not require surgery. There is limited information on the effect of hormone replacement therapy on uterine fibroid growth in the postmenopausal years.

The danger of sarcomatous change has, in the past, been used to justify hysterectomy. It seems that the incidence rates of sarcomatous change have been grossly exaggerated. Certain indicators may still be prudent. Rapid growth of fibroids and failure of large fibroids to respond to hypo-oestrogenic treatments should cause some concern.

## Medical treatments

### *GnRH agonists*

In view of the steroidal regulation of uterine growth, the use of GnRH analogues, which down-regulate the pituitary and induce a hypo-oestrogenic state[39,40], provides an obvious approach. Various alterations of the initial decapeptide have been developed which can be administered by a variety of routes, including intranasal, subcutaneous implants, injections and even intramuscular microparticles[41]. In all cases, the agonist promotes an initial stimulation of follicle stimulating hormone (FSH) and luteinizing hormone (LH) release from the pituitary. This is followed by prolonged suppression of pituitary and gonadal function. When the agonist is given in the luteal phase of the menstrual cycle, the ensuing period may be delayed and prolonged. When given in the follicular phase, an additional bleed may occur. However, if given on the first day of bleeding this may not be perceived by the patient to be different from the current period.

The mechanism of action whereby the GnRH agonist reduces fibroid growth is not so clear. Surprisingly, oestradiol receptor levels are increased in fibroids following pituitary down-regulation[13–15]. Possibly steroids act through as yet unidentified oestrogen receptors on the fibroids.

### *GnRH agonist action on uterine fibroids*

There is now substantial agreement that GnRH agonist therapy reduces the growth of fibroids by approximately 35% after 3 months therapy and by 50% after 6 months (reviewed in West[41]). Medication has been given by daily subcutaneous injection[42–47], the intranasal route[44,48,49], subcutaneous infusion[50] or depot preparations[51–53]. Assessment by ultrasound scanning measures either reduction of total uterine volume[44,47,50,53–55] or of the individual fibroid[43,45,48,50]. Reduction of size is variable, there being a tendency for the larger uteri to be reduced the most. Interestingly, the most marked effect on the reduction of uterine size is achieved by shrinkage of the uterus around the fibroid[49,52]. A loose correlation exists between the degree of oestrogen suppression and failed shrinkage[45,53,54]. About 5% of cases fail to respond to the treatment. However, within 6 months of cessation of therapy, fibroids will have 'regrown'[52,56].

*Side-effects and complications* Vasomotor symptoms arising from the loss of oestrogen are the most obvious side-effects occurring in over 80% of cases. Bone loss is of the order of 5–10% after 6–12 months of therapy[53,57–59]. This amount of loss is not important in the short term, but if long-term therapy is needed, various add-back options need to be considered.

Rare complications arise as a consequence of GnRH therapy. Approximately 2% of women may have heavy and persistent bleeding[56,60–62]. This is usually associated with submucosal fibroids. Severe pain may arise with fibroid degeneration[63] and pedunculated fibroids which shrink may pass through the cervix.

### *The use of GnRH agonists in the surgical treatment of fibroids*

As with all medical developments, new options introduce new problems. Gonadotrophin releasing hormone agonist therapy alone cannot be given for more than 12 months because of the deleterious effect on bone. Whilst not documented, it is also likely that prolonged therapy would be detrimental to the cardiovascular system and predispose women to strokes and myocardial infarction. Much attention has focused on the short-term use of these agents in order to facilitate surgery. This is particularly the case when minimal access surgical techniques are to be used. Finally, developments in add-back therapy have raised the prospect of long-term medical treatment of fibroids.

*GnRH agonists and hysterectomy* Preoperative shrinkage of uterine fibroids greater than 12 weeks in size has several clear benefits. First, preoperative haemoglobin levels are maintained[64], thus reducing the number of operative cancellations. Second, operative blood loss is reduced by about 130 ml per case compared to surgery performed on women without pretreatment[65,66]. The use of perioperative blood transfusions is reduced[67] and surgery previously needing to be performed by the abdominal route may be undertaken vaginally[68]. In a study of 50 women with uterine sizes ranging from 14 to 18 weeks, those randomly allocated to preoperative leuprolide acetate therapy achieved a vaginal hysterectomy in 76% of cases, whilst only 16% of the immediate surgery patients could have the operation performed by this route.

However, health economic advantages have not been shown with respect to a reduced incidence of postoperative infection, nor has the length of stay in hospital been altered. Nevertheless, all of the other parameters described above indicate that surgery is easier after preoperative medication. This would suggest that a health economic advantage must exist and that larger studies are needed to count the real cost. This is particularly so where the fibroids are especially large or are situated in difficult situations such as the broad ligament or the cervix. The cost of reparative surgery to the ureters is high but will only occur in a small number of cases. In addition, medical litigation must be added to the cost of not using preoperative medication. On balance, patients should receive GnRH agonist therapy for at least 3 months before surgery.

*GnRH agonists and myomectomy* An alternative to hysterectomy, especially in women who wish to preserve their fertility, is myomectomy performed by the abdominal route. Three studies have examined the benefit of pretreatment on surgical blood loss, two being in favour and one showing no advantage[69–71]. Anecdotal reports suggest a greater difficulty in identification of the 'capsule' in treated patients, resulting in increased difficulty in fibroid enucleation. A further complication is the formation of postoperative adhesions following surgery, particularly occluding the pouch of Douglas or thin filmy adhesions occluding the ovaries. Plication of the round ligaments has been used with no published evidence and fluids instilled into the peritoneal cavity, such as dextran, dexamethasone or normal saline, have similarly been employed to reduce adhesion formation.

*GnRH agonists and minimal access surgery* Developments in both intrauterine and laparoscopic techniques for the surgical removal of intracavity, submucous and intramural fibroids are now well established. A key feature in deciding to use minimal access surgery (MAS) is the size of the fibroid. Not only does the GnRH agonist reduce fibroid size, it reduces the surrounding vasculature and thins the endometrium, making the procedure easier. Randomized studies are rare and placebo-controlled studies non-existent. Anecdotal reports indicate long-term benefit from these procedures but surprisingly, in view of the poor subjective assessment of menstrual blood loss, before and after blood loss studies have not been reported.

*Long-term GnRH therapy*
The bone loss induced by GnRH agonist therapy given alone prevents the use of this treatment for greater than 1 year. However, several groups have now studied the possibility of giving add-back therapy, in which sufficient steroid is replaced to prevent bone loss and even maintain lipid stasis without causing regrowth of the fibroid.

*GnRH agonist and hormone replacement therapy* Two studies treated women for 12 and 24 months, respectively[60,72]. In one, conjugated equine oestrogen (0.3 mg) was given with medroxyprogesterone acetate 5 mg either from day 16 to 25 or continuously. Goserelin implants were the agonist used[72]. Add-back therapy was started after 3 months of agonist alone therapy. Significant regrowth of the fibroid did not occur. Four of ten women on the cyclical therapy were amenorrhoeic and three of ten on the continuous regime continued to bleed.

*GnRH agonist and anti-oestrogens* Combined therapy with a GnRH agonist and anti-oestrogen does not reduce fibroid size, suggesting that tamoxifen has an oestrogenic action on fibroids, as it does with endometrium[73]. This does not appear to be an effective therapy.

*GnRH agonist and progestogens* Medroxyprogesterone acetate (MPA) may cause degenerative changes in fibroids[74] but combined use of GnRH agonist with MPA does not cause shrinkage of fibroids[75]. However, if the progestogen is added after the initial 3 months of treatment with agonist alone, hypo-oestrogenic effects are prevented, and when treatment is stopped there is delayed return to pretreatment size.

These treatments are expensive and it is difficult to justify long-term therapy for all patients. However, sensible selection would identify suitable patients. Clearly, patients with underlying disease for which surgery is contraindicated, e.g. coagulopathies, blood dyscrasias, predisposition to thrombosis, gross obesity and transplants, would benefit from this approach. Perhaps the best group of patients are those near to the menopause for whom only 1 or 2 years therapy is required. Patients with a morbid fear of surgery may also be offered this therapy. Finally, in the modern context, these therapies provide an alternative for women to try. If they find them unacceptable it often makes the decision to undergo surgery easier. This is an important part of decision-making for patients.

*Antiprogestins*

An alternative to GnRH agonist is the use of antiprogestins, based on the newer concept that fibroid growth is at least in part due to progesterone. Murphy and co-workers[21] found on average a 50% reduction of fibroid size with RU 486. The principal complication is the development of hyperplasia of the endometrium. Whilst this prevents treatment currently, the exciting identification of different types of oestrogen receptor may permit combined therapy with newer oestrogens.

*Antifibrinolytics*

Tranexamic acid, which acts to inhibit fibrinolysis by preventing the degradation of plasminogen to plasmin, reduced MBL by about 50% in women with menorrhagia[36]. Surprisingly, Nilsson and Rybo[76] studied 16 women with clinically enlarged uteri. They found that medication with tranexamic acid reduced measured blood loss by the same amount as in women with normal sized uteri. This is clear evidence, albeit in a small sample size, that the association between fibroids and menstrual bleeding is complex. However, for women whose fibroids are smaller than 8 weeks in size, medical treatment may prove to be as effective as that for women with normal sized uteri.

## Surgery

The mainstay of treatment for uterine fibroids remains surgery. In all cases of suspected fibroids, imaging should have been undertaken to confirm the diagnosis and exclude ovarian pathology. Whether hysteroscopy should be performed is less clear. In some women, fibroids will be found in otherwise normal sized uteri during the investigation of menorrhagia or IMB. In these cases intracavity or submucosal fibroids will be present. In women whose uterine size is between 6 and 12 weeks, hysteroscopy may assist the decision to perform surgery, especially if an intracavity fibroid exists, as hysteroscopic removal may be possible. Women whose fibroids exceed 12 weeks in size are unlikely to benefit from hysteroscopy.

*Abdominal hysterectomy*

Access is the first surgical consideration and the rationale for using GnRH agonists preoperatively is that it permits the more frequent use of Pfannensteil incisions as opposed to subumbilical midline procedures. Placing the incision three finger breadths above the symphysis pubis may provide extra access and division of the rectus sheath and ligation of the inferior epigastric vessels may permit still greater access. It may be helpful to perform a myomectomy in cases of large fibroids to gain unhindered access to the cervix. Broad ligament fibroids and those in the cervix are more difficult to deal with than those where the main fibroid is in the body of the uterus. Careful dissection of the broad ligament and positive identification of the ureters is required.

*Abdominal myomectomy*

Blood loss at myomectomy is usually greater than with hysterectomy. It is prudent to advise all patients undergoing myomectomy that in rare cases haemostasis cannot be achieved and that hysterectomy may be required. Consent is a key feature in medical litigation and written consent to perform the ultimate procedure is advised. Clamps have been used to occlude the uterine arteries but are little used in clinical practice today, probably as a consequence of the use of GnRH agonists. The fibroid 'sheath' is incised and the fibroid shelled out. It is usually possible to identify the single major vascular pedicle and this should be clamped, divided and tied before removing the fibroid. This significantly reduces the bleeding from the space. Close attention to the achievement of haemostasis is important to prevent postoperative haemorrhage and to reduce postoperative adhesion formation. Extending the incision into the uterine cavity is associated with higher rates of uterine dehiscence in subsequent pregnancies, an important consideration in women wishing to retain their fertility.

*Hysteroscopic removal of fibroids*

Electrosurgical removal or laser ablation are now well recognized procedures for removing intrauterine fibroids[77,78]. Three aspects are important in deciding whether to use this route. First, the degree of protrusion of the fibroid into the uterine cavity should be considered. The European Society for Hysteroscopy has advocated three categories of fibroid ranging from the pedunculated fibroid to one which has more than 50% of its area within the wall of the uterus. Second, the size of the fibroid, especially if intramural, has an important effect on complications. Finally, the training and experience of the operator is a key factor.

Pedunculated fibroids may be removed by scissor excision of the stalk and resection of the freed fibroid[79,80]. Alternatively, the fibroid can be shaved using the resectoscope and the base diathermied to achieve haemostasis. Difficulties arise with the intramural section of the fibroid. Great care and skill is required in these cases because of the potential for haemorrhage, fluid intravasation, perforation and resection of intra-abdominal structures. Laparoscopy may be employed to reduce the risk of these latter complications.

An alternative to the resectoscope is the use of the laser[77,78,81–83]. In a study of 60 women, Donnez and colleagues[81] were able to remove the fibroid with a single procedure in 48 cases. In the other 12 women, a repeat procedure was undertaken. In this two-step approach, the laser is fired into the fibroid. Following the destruction of part of the fibroid, for reasons which are unclear, the remaining section of the fibroid becomes extruded into the uterine cavity, permitting a definitive procedure some 2 months later. Fibroids up to 12 weeks in size can be dealt with in this fashion. The advantage of the technique is that it minimizes the risk of perforation and damage to abdominal structures. Subjectively good improvements in menorrhagia were achieved with 81% of 92 women[82], and 84% of 94 women followed up 9 years after initial surgery did not require subsequent intervention[83].

*Laparoscopic removal of fibroids*

The laparoscopic removal of fibroids is more controversial than hysteroscopic resection for a number of reasons. First, subserosal fibroids are of no known clinical importance except for the rare cases of torsion. Intramural fibroids cannot be reached by this approach and it is these fibroids which are most likely to cause clinical problems, whether it be menstrual disorders or infertility. The procedure is difficult and requires a high level of skill. The cost of the consumables is greater than for conventional therapy, operative time is longer and postoperative haemostasis harder to achieve[84]. Numerous fibroids (four or more > 3 cm) or a single large fibroid (> 10 cm) are contra-indications for this procedure[85]. However, the removal of large intramural fibroids has been described[86–89].

Incision into the fibroid is made with monopolar or hook diathermy. The fibroid is dissected out of its pseudocapsule using bipolar diathermy to dessicate the blood vessels supplying the fibroid. Great care is needed to identify the vascular pedicle. The gap is closed with sutures.

*Surgical conclusions*

The choice as to which procedure to use depends on the size and site of the fibroid and the skill of the surgeon. Intracavity fibroids below 4 cm, with a well-defined pedicle, should probably be removed hysteroscopically. Fibroids with a greater invasion into the uterine wall may still be removed hysteroscopically but greater care is needed and preoperative scanning may help to define the size of the fibroid. Laparoscopic assistance may reduce the dangers of this procedure. Inspection of the excision site after reduction of pressure of the continuous flow should be performed. Meticulous assessment of infusion fluid will reduce the risks of fluid overload. A blown-up Foley catheter may be retained *in utero* for difficult cases.

Laparoscopic myomectomy or hysterectomy should only be performed by suitably trained individuals. The case for this procedure is less obvious than for hysteroscopic procedures. In the smaller cases with subserosal fibroids, the indication for surgery needs to be questioned. With the larger cases, a very high degree of surgical skill is needed.

The choice to perform abdominal surgery will largely be based on the size of the fibroid and the skill of the surgeon. Cases requiring retention of fertility will require myomectomy. Most surgeons should be competent to perform this procedure.

## CONCLUSION

Fibroids are a very common cause of significant changes in the quality of life in women. The genes which either predispose patients to grow fibroids or which are involved in the process of benign proliferation need to be identified. New techniques would then be available, first to predict patients who would be expected to develop fibroids, and second, to identify novel gene therapies for causing regression of fibroids without recourse to surgery. The management of patients with fibroids has changed dramatically over the past 20 years, particularly when surgical developments are included with the medical changes. The next 20 years are likely to see a significant change in understanding the genomic control of fibroid growth, which will lead to the development of new therapeutic options.

## REFERENCES


1. Buttram, V. C. (1986). Uterine leiomyomata – aetiology, symptomatology, and management. *Prog. Clin. Biol. Res.*, **225**, 275–96
2. Farrer-Brown, G., Beilby, J. O. W. and Tarbit, M. H. (1971). Venous changes in the endometrium of myomatous uteri. *Obstet. Gynecol.*, **38**, 743–51
3. Townsend, D. E., Sparkes, R. S. and McClelland, M. D. (1970). Uncellular histogenesis of uterine leiomyomas as detected by electrophoresis of glucose-6-phosphate dehydrogenase. *Am. J. Obstet. Gynecol.*, **107**, 1168–73
4. Mashal, R. D., Fejzo, M. L. S., Friedman, A. J., Mitchener, N., Nowak, R. A., Rein, M. S., Morton, C. C. and Sklar, J. (1994). Analysis of androgen receptor DNA reveals the independent clonal origins of uterine leiomyomata and the secondary nature of cytogenetic aberrations in the development of leiomyomata. *Gene. Chrom. Can.*, **11**, 1–6
5. Hashimoto, K., Azuma, C., Kamiura, S., Kimura, T., Nobunga, T., Kanai, T., Sawada, M., Noguchi, S. and Saji, F. (1995). Clonal determination of uterine leiomyomas by

analyzing differential inactivation of the X-chromosome-linked phosphoglycerokinase gene. *Gyn. Obstet. Inv.*, **40**, 204–8
6. Nibert, M. and Heim, S. (1990). Uterine leiomyoma cytogenetics. *Gene. Chrom. Can.*, **2**, 3–13
7. Hug, K., Doney, M. K., Tyler, M. J., Grundy, D. A., Soukup, S., Houseal, T. W. and Menon, A. G. (1994). Physical mapping of the uterine leiomyoma t(12;14)(q13-15;q24.1) breakpoint on chromosome 14 between SPTB and D14S77. *Gene. Chrom. Can.*, **11**, 263–6
8. Schoenmakers, E. F. P. M., Mols, R., Wanshura, S., Kools, P. F. J., Geurts, J. M. W., Bartnitzke, S., Bullerdiek, J., Van den Berghe, H. and Van de Ven, W. J. M. (1994). Identification, molecular cloning, and characterization of the chromosome 12 breakpoint cluster region of the uterine leiomyomas. *Gene. Chrom. Can.*, **11**, 106–18
9. Doney, M. K., Gerken, S. C., Lynch, R., Bhugra, B., Hug, K., White, R., Weissenbach, J. and Menon, A. G. (1995). Precise mapping of t(12;14) leiomyoma breakpoint on chromosome 14 between D14S298 and D14S540. *Can. Lett.*, **96**, 245–52
10. Schoenmakers, E. F. P. M., Geurts, J. M. W., Kools, P. F. J., Mols, R., Huysmans, C., Bullerdiek, J., Van den Berghe, H. and Van de Ven, W. J. M. (1995). A 6-Mb yeast artificial chromosome contig and long-range physical map encompassing the region on chromosome 12q15 frequently rearranged in a variety of benign solid tumors. *Genomics*, **29**, 665–78
11. Sargent, M. S., Weremowicz, S., Rein, M. S. and Morton, C. C. (1994). Translocations in 7q22 define a critical region in uterine leiomyomata. *Can. Gene. Cytogen.*, **77**, 65–8
12. Dal Cin, P., Moerman, P., Deprest, J., Brosens, I. and Van den Berghe, H. (1995). A new cytogenetic subgroup in uterine leiomyoma is characterized by a deletion of the long arm of chromosome 3. *Gene. Chrom. Can.*, **13**, 219–20
13. Wilson, E. A., Yang, F. and Rees, E. D. (1980). Estradiol and progesterone binding in uterine leiomyomata and in normal uterine tissue. *Obstet. Gynecol.*, **55**, 20–4
14. Lumsden, M. A., West, C. P., Hawkins, T. A., Bramley, T. A., Rumgay, L. and Baird, D. T. (1989). The binding of steroids to myometrium and leiomyomata (fibroids) in women treated with the gonadotrophin-releasing hormone agonist, Zoladex (ICI 118640). *J. Endocrinol.*, **121**, 389–96
15. Rein, M. S., Friedman, A. J., Stuart, J. M. and MacLaughlin, D. T. (1990). Fibroid and myometrial steroid receptors in women treated with gonadotrophin-releasing hormone agonist leuprolide acetate. *Fertil. Steril.*, **53**, 1018–23
16. Soules, M. R. and McCarty, K. S. (1982). Leiomyomas: steroid receptor content. Variation within normal menstrual cycles. *Am. J. Obstet. Gynecol.*, **143**, 6–11
17. Buchi, K. A. and Keller, P. J. (1983). Cytoplasmic progestin receptors in myomal and myometrial tissues: concentrations and hormonal dependency. *Acta Obstet. Gynecol. Scand.*, **62**, 487–92
18. Tamaya, T., Fujimoto, J. and Okada, H. (1985). Comparison of cellular levels of receptors in uterine leiomyoma and myometrium. *Acta Obstet. Gynecol. Scand.*, **64**, 307–9
19. Smith, S. K. (1993). The regulation of fibroid growth: time for a rethink. *Br. J. Obstet. Gynaecol.*, **100**, 977–8
20. Friedman, A. J., Barbieri, R. L., Doublilet, P. M., Fine, C. and Schiff, I. (1988). A randomised double blind trial of a gonadotrophin releasing hormone agonist (leuprolide) with or without medroxyprogesterone acetate in the treatment of leiomyomata uteri. *Fertil. Steril.*, **49**, 404–9
21. Murphy, A. A., Kettel, L. M., Morales, A. J., Roberts, V. J. and Yen, S. S. C. (1993). Regression of uterine leiomyomata in response to the antiprogesterone RU 486. *J. Clin. Endocrinol. Metab.*, **76**, 513–17
22. Harrison-Woolrych, M. L., Charnock-Jones, D. S. and Smith, S. K. (1994). Quantification of mRNA for epidermal growth factor in human myometrium and leiomyomata using reverse-transcriptase polymerase chain reaction. *J. Clin. Endocrinol. Metab.*, **78**, 1179–84
23. Brown, M. J., Zogg, J. L., Schultz, G. S. and Hilton, F. K. (1989). Increased binding of epidermal growth factor at preimplantation sites. *Endocrinology*, **124**, 2882–8
24. Lumsden, M. A., West, C. P., Bramley, T. A., Rumgay, L. and Baird, D. T. (1988). The binding of epidermal growth factor in human uterine tissue and leiomyomas. *J. Clin. Endocrinol. Metab.*, **58**, 880–4
25. Fayed, Y. M., Tsibris, G. C. M., Langenderg, P. W. and Robertson, A. L. (1989). Human

uterine leiomyoma cells; binding and growth responses to epidermal growth factor, platelet-derived growth factor and insulin. *Lab. Invest.*, **60**, 30–7
26. Murphy, L. J., Gong, Y., Murphy, L. C. and Bhavnani, B. (1991). Growth factors in normal and malignant uterine tissue. *Ann. NY Acad. Sci.*, **662**, 383–91
27. Vollenhoven, B. J., Herington, A. C. and Healy, D. L. (1993). Messenger ribonucleic acid expression of the insulin-like growth factors and their binding proteins in uterine fibroids and myometrium. *J. Clin. Endocrinol. Metab.*, **76**, 1106–10
28. Murphy, L. J., Murphy, L. C. and Friesen, H. G. (1988). Estrogen induces insulin-like growth factor-I expression in rat uterus. *Mol. Endocrinol.*, **1**, 445–52
29. Murphy, L. J. and Friesen, H. G. (1988). Differential effects of estrogen and growth hormone on uterine and hepatic insulin-like growth factor-I (IGF-I) gene expression in the ovariectomized rat. *Endocrinology*, **122**, 325–34
30. Harrison-Woolrych, M. L., Sharkey, A. M., Charnock-Jones, D. S. and Smith, S. K. (1995). Localisation and quantification of vascular endothelial growth factors mRNA in human myometrium and leiomyomata. *J. Clin. Endocrinol. Metab.*, **80**, 1853–8
31. Patient, C., Prentice, A., Sutton, C. J. G. and Smith, S. K. (1996). Myolysis of a cervical fibroid with an Nd:YAG laser. *Br. J. Obstet. Gynaecol.*, **103**, 584–5
32. Nagele, F., O'Connor, H., Davies, A., Badawy, A., Mohamed, H. and Magos, A. (1996). 2500 outpatient diagnostic hysteroscopies. *Obstet. Gynecol.*, **88**, 87–92
33. Cameron, I. T., Haining, R., Lumsden, M.-A., Thomas, V. R. and Smith, S. K. (1990). The effects of mefenamic acid and norethisterone on measured menstrual blood loss. *Obstet. Gynecol.*, **76**, 85–8
34. Deeny, M. and Davies, J. A. (1994). Assessment of menstrual blood loss in women referred for endometrial ablation. *Eur. J. Obstet. Gynaecol.*, **57**, 179–80
35. Lewis, B. V. (1993). Diagnostic dilatation and curettage in young women. *Br. Med. J.*, **306**, 225–6
36. Effective Health Care (1995). *The Management of Menorrhagia*. Department of Health, Bulletin No. 9
37. Coulter, A., Seagroatt, V. and McPherson, K. (1990). Relation between general practices' outpatient referral rates and rates of elective admissions to hospital. *Br. Med. J.*, **301**, 273–6
38. Coulter, A., Bradlow, J., Agass, M., Martin-Bates, C. and Tulloch, A. (1991). Outcomes of referrals to gynaecology outpatient clinics for menstrual problems: an audit of general practice records. *Br. J. Obstet. Gynaecol.*, **98**, 789–96
39. Sandow, J. (1983). Clinical application of LHRH and its analogues. *Clin. Endocrinol.*, **18**, 571–92
40. Fraser, M. H. and Baird, D. T. (1987). Clinical applications of LHRH analogues. *Clin. Endocrinol. Metab.*, **1**, 43–70
41. West, C. P. (1993). GnRH analogues in the treatment of fibroids. *Rep. Med. Rev.*, **2**, 181–97
42. Filicori, M., Hall, D. A., Loughlin, J. S., Rivier, J., Vale, W. and Crowley, W. F. (1983). A conservative approach to the management of uterine leiomyomata: pituitary desensitisation by a luteinizing hormone-releasing hormone analogue. *Am. J. Obstet. Gynecol.*, **147**, 726–7
43. Maheux, R., Guilloteau, C., Lemay, A., Bastide, A. and Fazekas, A. T. (1985). Luteinizing hormone-releasing hormone agonist and uterine leiomyoma: a pilot study. *Am. J. Obstet. Gynecol.*, **152**, 1034–8
44. Friedman, A. J., Barbieri, R. L., Benacerraf, B. R. and Schiff, I. (1987). Treatment of leiomyomata with intranasal or subcutaneous leuprolide, a gonadotropin-releasing hormone agonist. *Fertil. Steril.*, **48**, 560–4
45. Perl, V., Marquez, J., Schally, A. V. *et al.* (1987). Treatment of leiomyomata uteri with D-Trp-6-luteinizing hormone-releasing hormone. *Fertil. Steril.*, **48**, 383–9
46. Kessel, B., Liu, J., Berga, S. and Ywen, S. S. C. (1988). Treatment of uterine fibroids with agonist analogues of gonadotropin-releasing hormone. *Fertil. Steril.*, **49**, 538–41
47. Lettrie, G. S., Coddington, C. C., Winkel, C. A., Shawker, T. H., Loriaux, D. L. and Colline, R. L. (1989). Efficacy of a gonadotropin-releasing hormone agonist in the treatment of uterine leiomyomata: long-term follow-up. *Fertil. Steril.*, **51**, 951–6
48. Maheux, R., Lemay, A. and Merat, P. (1987). Use of intranasal luteinizing hormone-releasing hormone agonist in uterine leiomyomas. *Fertil. Steril.*, **7**, 229–33

49. Andreyko, J. L., Blumenfeld, Z., Marshall, A., Monroe, S. E., Hricak, H. and Jaffe, R. B. (1988). Use of an agonist analog of gonadotropin-releasing hormone (nafarelin) to treat leiomyomas: assessment of magnetic resonance imaging. *Am. J. Obstet. Gynecol.*, **158**, 903–10
50. Healy, D. L., Lawson, S. R., Abbott, M., Baird, D. T. and Fraser, H. M. (1986). Towards removing uterine fibroids without surgery: subcutaneous infusion of a luteinizing hormone-releasing hormone agonist commencing in the luteal phase. *J. Clin. Endocrinol. Metab.*, **63**, 619–25
51. Golan, A., Bukovsky, I., Schneider, D., Ron-El, R., Harman, A. and Caspi, E. (1989). D-Trp-6 luteinizing hormone-releasing hormone microcapsules in the treatment of uterine leiomyomas. *Fertil. Steril.*, **52**, 406–11
52. Schlaff, W. D., Zernouni, E. A., Huth, J., Chan, J., Damewood, M. D. and Rock, J. A. (1989). A placebo-controlled trial of a depot gonadotropin-releasing hormone analog (leuprolide) in the treatment of uterine leiomyomata. *Obstet. Gynecol.*, **74**, 856–62
53. Friedman, A. J., Hoffman, C. I., Comite, F., Browneller, R. W. and Miller, J. D. (1991). Treatment of leiomyomata uteri with leuprolide acetate depot: a double-blind, placebo-controlled, multicenter study. The leuprolide study group. *Obstet. Gynecol.*, **77**, 720–5
54. West, C. P., Lumsden, M. A., Lawson, S., Williamson, J. and Baird, D. T. (1987). Shrinkage of uterine fibroids during therapy with goserelin (Zoladex): a luteinizing hormone-releasing hormone agonist administered as a monthly subcutaneous depot. *Fertil. Steril.*, **48**, 45–51
55. Matta, W. H. M., Shaw, R. W. and Nye, M. (1989). Long term follow-up of patients with uterine fibroids after treatment with the LHRH agonist buserelin. *Br. J. Obstet. Gynaecol.*, **96**, 200–6
56. Vollenhoven, B. J., Shekleton, P., McDonald, J. and Healy, D. L. (1990). Clinical predictors of buserelin acetate treatment of uterine fibroids: a prospective study of 40 women. *Fertil. Steril.*, **54**, 1032–8
57. Matta, W. H., Shaw, R. W., Hesp, R. and Katz, D. (1987). Hypogonadism induced by luteinizing hormone releasing hormone agonist analogues: effects on bone density in premenopausal women. *Br. Med. J.*, **294**, 1523–4
58. Dawood, M. J., Lewis, V. and Ramos, J. (1989). Cortical and trabecular bone mineral content in women with endometriosis: effects of gonadotropin-releasing hormone agonist and danazol. *Fertil. Steril.*, **52**, 21–6
59. Johansen, J. S., Riis, B. J., Hassanger, C., Moen, M., Jacobson, J. and Christiansen, C. (1988). The effect of a gonadotropin-releasing hormone agonist analogue (nafarelin) on bone metabolism. *J. Clin. Endocrinol. Metab.*, **67**, 701–6
60. Friedman, A. J. (1989). Vaginal haemorrhage associated with degenerating submucous leiomyomata during leuprolide acetate treatment. *Fertil. Steril.*, **52**, 152–4
61. Thorp, J. M. and Katz, V. L. (1991). Submucous myomas treated with gonadotropin-releasing hormone agonist and resulting in vaginal haemorrhage – a case report. *J. Reprod. Med.*, **36**, 625–6
62. Healy, D. L. and Vollenhoven, B. J. (1992). The role of GnRH agonists in the treatment of uterine fibroids. *Br. J. Obstet. Gynaecol.*, **99** (Suppl. 7), 23–6
63. Chipato, T., Vollenhoven, B. J., Buckler, H. M. and Healy, D. L. (1991). Pelvic pain complicating LHRH agonist treatment of fibroids. *Aust. NZ J. Obstet. Gynaecol.*, **31**, 383–4
64. Candiani, G. B., Vercellini, P., Arcaini, L., Bianchi, S. and Candiani, M. (1990). Use of goserelin depot, a gonadotropin-releasing hormone agonist for the treatment of menorrhagia and severe anaemia in women with leiomyomata uteri. *Acta Obstet. Gynaecol. Scand.*, **69**, 413–15
65. Lumsden, M. A., Thomas, E., Coutts, J. R. T., West, C. P. and Baird, D. T. (1990). Goserelin pretreatment facilitates abdominal hysterectomy for the removal of uterine leiomyomata (fibroids). *Gynecol. Endocrinol.*, **4** (Suppl. 2), 41
66. West, C. P., Lumsden, M. A. and Baird, D. T. (1992). Goserelin (Zoladex) in the treatment of fibroids. *Br. J. Obstet. Gynaecol.*, **99** (Suppl. 7), 27–30
67. Fedele, L., Bianchi, S., Baglioni, A., Arcaini, L., Marchini, M. and Bocciolone, L. (1991). Intranasal buserelin versus surgery in the treatment of uterine leiomyomata: long-term follow-up. *Eur. J. Obstet. Gynecol. Reprod. Biol.*, **38**, 53–7
68. Stovall, T. G., Ling, F. W., Henry, L. C. and Woodruff, R. A. (1991). A randomised trial

evaluating leuprolide acetate before hysterectomy as treatment for leiomyomas. *Am. J. Obstet. Gynecol.*, **164**, 1420–3

69. Gardner, R. L. and Shaw, R. W. (1992). GnRH agonists and blood loss at surgery. In Shaw, R. W. (ed.) *Uterine Fibroids: Time for Review*, pp. 123–4. (Carnforth, UK: The Parthenon Publishing Group)
70. Fedele, L., Vercellini, P., Bianchi, S., Briuoschi, D. and Dorta, M. (1990). Treatment with GnRH agonists before myomectomy and the risk of short-term myoma recurrence. *Br. J. Obstet. Gynaecol.*, **97**, 393–6
71. Friedman, A. J., Daly, M., Juneau-Norcross, M., Fine, C. and Rein, M. S. (1992). Recurrence of myomas after myomectomy in women pretreated with leuprolide acetate depot or placebo. *Fertil. Steril.*, **59**, 205–8
72. Maheux, R. and Lemay, A. (1992). Treatment of perimenopausal women: potential long-term therapy with a depot GnRH agonist combined with hormone replacement therapy. *Br. J. Obstet. Gynaecol.*, **99** (Suppl. 7), 13–17
73. Lumsden, M. A., West, C. P., Hillier, H. and Baird, D. T. (1989). Estrogenic action of tamoxifen in women treated with luteinizing hormone-releasing hormone agonists (goserelin) – a lack of shrinkage of uterine fibroids. *Fertil. Steril.*, **52**, 924–9
74. Goldzieher, J. W., Maqueo, M., Ricard, L., Aquilar, J. A. and Canales, E. (1966). Induction of degenerative changes in uterine myomas by high dose progestin therapy. *Am. J. Obstet. Gynecol.*, **96**, 1078–87
75. West, C. P., Lumsden, M. A., Hillier, H., Sweeting, V. and Baird, D. T. (1992). Potential role for medroxyprogesterone acetate as an adjunct to goserelin (Zoladex) in the medical management of uterine fibroids. *Hum. Reprod.*, **7**, 328–32
76. Nilsson, L. and Rybo, G. (1971). Treatment of menorrhagia. *Am. J. Obstet. Gynecol.*, **110**, 713–20
77. Neuwirth, R. S. (1983). Hysteroscopic management of symptomatic submucous uterine fibroids. *Obstet. Gynecol.*, **62**, 509–11
78. Donnez, J., Schrurs, B., Gillerot, S., Sandow, J. and Clerckx, F. (1989). Treatment of uterine fibroids with implants of gonadotropin-releasing hormone agonist: assessment by hysterography. *Fertil. Steril.*, **51**, 947–50
79. Neuwirth, R. S. and Amin, H. K. (1976). Excision of submucous fibroids with hysteroscopic control. *Am. J. Obstet. Gynecol.*, **176**, 95–9
80. Neuwirth, R. S. (1978). A new technique for an additional experience with hysteroscopic resection of submucous fibroids. *Am. J. Obstet. Gynecol.*, **131**, 91–4
81. Donnez, J., Gillerot, S., Bourgonjon, D., Clerckx, F. and Nisolle, M. (1990). Neodymium: YAG laser hysteroscopy in large submucous fibroids. *Fertil. Steril.*, **54**, 999–1003
82. Donnez, J., Nisolle, M., Grandjean, P., Gillerot, S. and Clerckx, F. (1991). The place of GnRH agonists in the treatment of endometriosis and fibroids by advanced hysteroscopic techniques. *Br. J. Obstet. Gynaecol.*, **99** (Suppl. 7), 31–33
83. Derman, S. G., Rehnstrom, J. and Neuwirth, R. S. (1991). The long-term effectiveness of hysteroscopic treatment of menorrhagia and leiomyomas. *Obstet. Gynecol.*, **77**, 591–4
84. Dicker, D., Dekel, A., Orvieto, R., Bar-Hava, I., Peleg, D. and Ben-Rafael, Z. (1996). The controversy of laparoscopic myomectomy. *Hum. Reprod.*, **11**, 935–7
85. Dubuisson, J. B., Lecuru, F., Foulot, H. *et al.* (1992). Gonadotrophin-releasing hormone agonist and laparoscopic myomectomy. *Clin. Ther.*, **14**, 51–5
86. Nehzat, C., Nezhat, F., Silfen, S. L. *et al.* (1991). Laparoscopic myomectomy. *Int. J. Fertil.*, **36**, 275–80
87. Hasson, H. M., Rotman, C., Rana, N. *et al.* (1992). Laparoscopic myomectomy. *Obstet. Gynecol.*, **80**, 884–8
88. Dubuisson, J. B., Chapron, C., Mouly, M. *et al.* (1993). Laparoscopic myomectomy. *Gynaecol. Endosc.*, **2**, 171–3
89. Reich, H. (1995). Laparoscopic myomectomy. *Obstet. Gynecol. Clin. North Am.*, **22**, 757–80

# Minimal access surgery 25

*Roger Hart and Adam Magos*

## INTRODUCTION

As in many other specialties, the advent of minimal access surgery has revolutionized gynaecological practice. Advantages such as small abdominal scars, decreased patient discomfort, reduced hospital stay and faster time to return to functional activity have meant that it has become a rapidly advancing field. The lack of major external trauma does not, however, mean that these operations should be considered as minor. It is essential that surgery is performed by operators trained and skilled at their task, and that patients are aware of the possible complications and the occasional requirement to proceed to traditional surgical techniques.

## LAPAROSCOPIC SURGERY

For many years gynaecologists were the primary users of laparoscopy for the investigation of pelvic pain and infertility, and for female sterilization. In the last decade, however, a major change has occurred, and operative laparoscopy for conditions as diverse as ectopic pregnancy and fibroids has been widely introduced. There is now little in the female pelvis which is not amenable to the laparoscopic surgeon, and the limits of surgery are forever being rewritten. It would be true to say that, provided the pathology is not massive or an extensive malignancy, laparoscopic surgery may well represent an alternative to laparotomy. This is not to say that laparoscopic surgery should replace laparotomy in all these situations, but more that the advantages and disadvantages of the two approaches should be considered and the better offered to our patients.

### Equipment

Basic equipment for modern laparoscopic procedures includes a high-flow carbon dioxide ($CO_2$) insufflator, a cold light fountain rated at least 250 W, light lead, a chip camera linked to a high-resolution colour monitor, 10 mm 0° or 30° laparoscope, and a variety of 5 and 10 mm ports and instruments such as grasping forceps, scissors, bipolar electrosurgical forceps and suction/irrigation cannulae. Ideally, back-up equipment should be available in case of equipment failure during surgery. It is vital that all the theatre staff understand the mechanics and care of the various instruments and that regular service checks are made. The surgeon should also check the equipment prior to surgery and should have a standard arrangement of trolleys, etc. to which all staff are accustomed.

The patient should be placed in a Trendelenburg tilt of 15–30° with the legs abducted, hips straight and the knees flexed at 90°; flexion at the hip would obstruct the movement of suprapubic instruments and is not recommended for all but the most minor of laparoscopic procedures. Following bladder catheterization, a $CO_2$ pneumoperitoneum is produced using a Veress needle placed subumbilically. When the intra-abdominal pressure reaches 12–15 mmHg, the trochar for the laparoscope is inserted, usually subumbilically, in a Z-shaped manner to reduce the risk of a subsequent incisional hernia. The laparoscope and attachments are introduced through the trochar. It is useful for educational purposes to record each procedure on video tape.

All ancillary ports should be inserted under direct vision to prevent accidental vascular or bowel trauma. A single suprapubic cannula should be sufficient for diagnostic laparoscopy, but further 5 or 10 mm ports are required if surgery is to be performed, and these are best placed lateral to the inferior epigastric vessels above the uterine fundus for optimum access to the pelvis. The ability to control the position of the uterus is essential in all cases, and this is easily achieved by an intrauterine sound inserted via the vagina and cervix; it is often useful forcibly to antevert the uterus if it is naturally retroverted, as this greatly improves the view of the pouch of Douglas.

### Electrosurgery

Surgical diathermy employs alternating current and is characterized by its power output and frequency modulation (the number of times per second that the current changes direction). Cutting is facilitated by a low-voltage continuous waveform and coagulation by a high-voltage, non-continuous waveform[1]. Any waveform will desiccate when the electrode is in contact with the tissue. Current is converted into heat in the tissue for the purposes of cutting and coagulation. Tissue necrosis starts at 44°C and, above 70°C, coagulation begins by activation of the clotting mechanism and the denaturation of collagen. Tissue desiccation starts above 90°C and vaporization above 100°C.

Monopolar diathermy uses one electrical pole at the site of application and a dispersive plate is attached to the patient for the other pole, usually on the thigh. Bipolar diathermy requires much less power than the monopolar mode, as there is only a small distance between the electrodes and it is only this tissue which is affected by the current flowing. The current will flow until the tissue is electrodesiccated, at which point it ceases, a phenomenon which can be detected using an ammeter. Generally, monopolar electrodes are used for cutting and bipolar for coagulation and desiccation.

Monopolar coagulation current is modulated so that it is on for only 6% of the time and uses voltages in excess of ten times that of cutting current, with the result that it can arc a distance of up to 2 mm[2]. Electrosurgical injury can also occur out of the surgeon's field of view due to capacitative coupling and insulation failure. The former is minimized by avoiding hybrid plastic/metal trochar sleeves, and the latter by regular equipment checks and the use of sensitive monitors to detect insulation failure. Other areas for concern are unintended contact with other metal instruments in the abdomen (direct coupling), energy transfer through the tissue from the point of desiccation, and non-electrical burns when a recently activated electrode accidentally touches tissue whilst still hot. The patient may also receive a burn due to a fault at the site of the dispersive patient return electrode (e.g. partial detachment or a manufacturing error leading to a high power density at the point of skin contact). The relatively large size of these plates and built-in safety features such as the return electrode monitor greatly minimize this risk.

Great care has to be taken when using electrosurgical instruments. They should only be activated by the surgeon under direct vision, and the lowest power output should be utilized which produces the desired tissue effect. The electrodes should be stored in an insulated holster when not in use. Provided these points are remembered, electrosurgery has proved itself to be a most useful aid to the laparoscopic surgeon.

### Lasers

The mechanism of action and propagation of laser energy will not be discussed here. Carbon dioxide laser energy is transmitted down straight tubes or mirrors and, as it is invisible, an aiming beam of helium and neon is required. The energy is absorbed rapidly by fluids so $CO_2$ lasers are generally not used for hysteroscopic surgery. Carbon dioxide is essentially a cutting laser and has poor coagulating properties; tissue penetration is as little as 0.1 mm, and the amount of carbonization produced is less than with electrosurgery. The neodymium–yttrium–aluminium–garnet laser (Nd:YAG) is a visible fibre laser which has greater tissue penetration and is able to seal blood vessels up to

0.5 cm in diameter; it can also be utilized for cutting when fitted with a conical tip. The potassium–titanyl–phosphate (KTP) and the argon lasers have similar properties and wavelengths, the former being a better cutting instrument and the latter an effective photocoagulator.

### Complications of laparoscopic surgery

Laparoscopic surgery has the advantage of small operative scars and early patient discharge, but all operations can have complications and patients should be well aware of the risks. Most injuries occur on creating a pneumoperitoneum and inserting the first trochar.

Injuries on inserting the Veress needle are caused in the obese patient due to a reduced awareness of the sensation of entering the peritoneal cavity, and in the thin patient due to close proximity of the major vessels, and in patients with previous surgery due to visceral adherence to abdominal scars. Insertion of the trochar should be performed in a Z manner through the abdominal wall to minimize the chances of formation of a postoperative hernia. The risk of vascular injury is 1 per 1000 cases[3] and an immediate laparotomy should be performed with the trochar still in place to locate the injured vessel and apply pressure until a vascular surgeon arrives. Bowel injury occurs slightly more frequently but only 60% are recognized during surgery[3]. The classical injury incurred with the second trochar is laceration of the inferior epigastric artery, but this should be avoided by insertion under direct vision. Injury may be repaired by sutures or inflating a Foley catheter to cause tamponade when secured externally. Bladder injuries can be repaired by laparoscopic sutures and prolonged catheterization. Overall, only 62% of all visceral injuries are recognized at the time of initial procedure[4] and hence patients must be instructed to seek medical advice postoperatively if they develop any unexplained symptoms such as abdominal pain or vomiting.

Complications are partly operator-dependent and rely on the surgeon's expertise, knowledge of the equipment used and instruments being used. Training in laparoscopic surgery is essential and concern that inadequately trained surgeons were performing these procedures led the Royal College of Obstetricians and Gynaecologists in London to set up a Working Party in 1993 to look at the implications and development of gynaecological endoscopic surgery. Attendance at recognized workshops and practice on simulator models or animals are essential. Ideally, training should include a period of proctorship whereby an experienced surgeon supervises one less experienced during the initial cases. Despite these plans, no formal system of certification exists at present.

Anaesthetic complications peculiar to laparoscopic surgery are those of gas embolus producing the characteristic 'millwheel murmur'. The abdomen should be deflated immediately, the patient placed in the left lateral position, administered oxygen and central aspiration of the embolus is then performed. Other complications include bradycardia/asystole induced by peritoneal stimulation, and over-distension of the abdomen leading to hypotension and decreased lung compliance.

### Diagnostic laparoscopy

After inserting the laparoscope, the abdomen is inspected to ensure that no injury occurred during initial instrumentation. The upper abdomen is inspected for evidence of the perihepatic adhesions characteristic of the Fitz–Hugh–Curtis syndrome and for bowel adhesions. Then systematic inspection of the pelvic organs can begin. This is facilitated by an intrauterine manipulator and by a suprapubically placed probe. Inspection of the pelvis should elicit the size, shape and mobility of the uterus, swelling, distortion and occlusion of the Fallopian tubes, the state of the fimbriae, the size, mobility and presence of any cysts or adhesions on the ovaries. The peritoneum is inspected in a systematic manner for any evidence of adhesions or endometriosis, starting with the pouch of Douglas.

Chromopertubation is performed in infertility cases by injecting a dilute methylene blue solution through the cervix via a cervical cannula. The Fallopian tubes are inspected for the free flow of dye, and, in cases where there is no fimbrial spill of dye, the level of obstruction is determined and evidence of hydrosalpinges and salpingitis isthmica nodosa sought. Salpingoscopy using a narrow rigid endoscope inserted through the operating channel of an operating laparoscope enables visualization of the ampullary mucosa of the Fallopian tubes.

### Female sterilization

Laparoscopic techniques of tubal ligation consist of thermal destruction, mechanical obstruction with clips or rings at the isthmus of the Fallopian tube, and salpingectomy.

The original technique of thermal destruction to affect tubal ligation used monopolar electrocoagulation. This technique should not now be employed routinely due to the frequent occurrence of accidental thermal injury to adjacent viscera. Bipolar electrocoagulation relies on the blades of the forceps being placed completely to occlude the Fallopian tube, then current being applied until an area 2 cm wide is desiccated. Transection of the Fallopian tube is not necessary. Due to direct transmission of heat, injury to adjacent structures is still a possibility.

Clips used for tubal occlusion include the Filshie clip, consisting of a silastic lining in a titanium clip, and the Hulka-Clemens clip made of plastic with a steel hinge and spring. These techniques rely on proximal closure with a special applicator. It is essential to check that the tube is completely occluded, the clip is locked, and no other trauma has been incurred. The Fallope ring relies on a technique of drawing up a loop of tube into an applicator and then pushing the silastic ring over the Fallopian tube to occlude it. Partial salpingectomy is not widely used but can easily be performed using laparoscopic endoloops (see under *Ectopic pregnancy*).

### Ectopic pregnancy

The first reported laparoscopic salpingectomy was performed in 1973 by Shapiro and Alder[5], and Bruhat and colleagues described laparoscopic salpingotomy in 1980[6]. Many studies have been published since then, mostly descriptive series but several prospective randomized trials have also been carried out. In a large study, for instance, Tuomivaara and Kauppila reported a pregnancy rate of 80% after conservative surgery and 82% after salpingectomy, with repeat ectopic pregnancy rates of 14% and 13%, respectively[7]. No studies show any real difference in subsequent fertility rates after salpingotomy as compared to salpingectomy, despite the fact that tubal patency rates after laparoscopic salpingotomy approach 100%[8].

The only absolute contraindication to laparoscopic surgery in this situation is evidence of shock, as bleeding can be stopped more quickly at laparotomy. Relative contraindications depend on the experience of the surgeon and include the presence of a cornual pregnancy, a grossly distended ampullary ectopic gestation and severe pelvic adhesions.

Salpingectomy for an ectopic gestation is performed when there is an irreparably damaged ruptured Fallopian tube, when there is considerable bleeding after attempted conservative surgery, when it is felt there is a very significant chance of a repeat tubal pregnancy, and if a future pregnancy is not desired. A therapeutic scoring system has been devised to aid decision-making, ranging from conservative management to radical laparoscopic treatment and contralateral tubal sterilization and subsequent *in vitro* fertilization (IVF) treatment[9]. Caution is advised in interpreting the latter, as access to IVF provision is not the same in the UK as it is in some other countries.

Salpingectomy is performed after initial irrigation and removal of blood clots. Several techniques can be used, the simplest being the use of special pre-tied endoloop sutures to snare the affected Fallopian tube prior to excision. Alternatively, bipolar electrosurgery and scissors, Nd:YAG laser or staplers can be used to transect the tube and mesosalpinx up to the infundibulopelvic ligament. In cases of a very dilated Fallopian tube, it may be necessary to perform a salpingotomy initially to extrude the ectopic gestation and facilitate the salpingectomy. Pelvic lavage is performed at the end of the procedure to remove any remaining blood clots.

For salpingotomy, some endoscopists infiltrate the Fallopian tube on either side of the ectopic pregnancy or along the mesosalpinx with dilute vasopressin to diminish intraoperative bleeding. After stabilization of the Fallopian tube, monopolar electrocautery or laser is used to make an incision approximately 1 cm long on the anti-mesenteric border of the Fallopian tube over the ectopic gestation. This enables extrusion of the ectopic gestation either spontaneously or by suction and irrigation. The ectopic bed should then be thoroughly checked to remove any residual trophoblastic tissue. Closure of the salpingotomy is not necessary unless the incision is over-long. The procedure of milking the ectopic pregnancy is not recommended in view of the high incidence of persistent trophoblastic tissue, up to 16% in one series[10].

Postoperative management is routine. Some centres advocate monitoring serum β-human chorionic gonadotrophin (β-hCG) levels in view of the 5% rate of persistence of trophoblastic activity, detection of treatment failure being possible after the third or fourth postoperative day[11]. However, other authors do not monitor the decline in β-hCG levels as there is no difference in persistence whether the procedure is performed laparoscopically or at laparotomy, and monitoring is not routine after open surgery. To reduce the chance of persistence of trophoblastic activity, Pouly and associates recommend salpingectomy if initial β-hCG levels exceed 20 000 IU/l[12].

The laparoscopic approach to dealing with ectopic pregnancies is highly effective in that it gives better future fertility results than those after open surgery[13] but with the advantages of a significantly shorter hospital stay, operating time, postoperative analgesic requirements, convalescence and health service costs[14,15].

Newer techniques for managing ectopic pregnancies include the systemic and/or local injection of methotrexate[16,17] and the local injection of hyperosmolar glucose and other solutions[18]. Although they give good tubal patency rates, patient selection is very important; β-hCG levels should be less than 2000 IU/l and the pregnancy should not be larger than 2 cm, as outside these limits there is a significant failure rate and the long-term future reproductive outcome has not been assessed. The local administration of prostaglandin $F_{2\alpha}$ has also been studied in carefully selected patients and has been shown to have a reasonable success rate. In one series, however, 7.5% of patients required a subsequent laparotomy[19]. The use of the antiprogesterone RU 486 has not as yet proved successful in the management of ectopic pregnancies as it has for therapeutic abortion.

**Pelvic sepsis and adhesiolysis**

Pelvic adhesions have been implicated in the causation of infertility, pelvic pain and bowel obstruction. The cause of adhesion formation is usually a healing process from some irritant stimulus such as sepsis, devascularization, haemorrhage, reaction to endometriosis or to a foreign stimulus such as suture material. Peritoneal injury, in particular drying of the serosa in the presence of blood, produces peritoneal adhesions[20].

The role of laparoscopy in acute salpingitis is as an aid to diagnosis, to grade the adhesions and to establish a prognosis[21]. Not all patients with acute salpingitis undergo laparoscopy, as they may be treated solely by their general practitioner or laparoscopy is felt not to be warranted, but most commonly the diagnosis is missed altogether. Laparoscopy is an invasive procedure and this needs to be taken into account. However, establishing a firm diagnosis of salpingitis is important for the woman as it has a bearing on her future fertility and it also prevents women without pelvic inflammatory disease being labelled as such.

At laparoscopy, it is possible to take samples for bacteriological and histological assessment.

Special transport media will be required for the culture of chlamydia and mycoplasma. Freshly forming adhesions can be broken down, purulent fluid aspirated and the pelvis thoroughly irrigated. The procedure must be performed with antibiotic prophylaxis once bacteriological samples have been taken. There is a case for a 'second-look' laparoscopy 3 months later if fertility is desired. The risk of infertility after treatment for acute pelvic inflammatory disease is 19.2% after one episode, 31% after two and 60% after three or more episodes of infection in a woman aged 24–34 years[22]; the rates for women aged 15–24 years are lower. The risk of subfertility also relates to the timing of treatment; those treated in the acute phase are much more likely to conceive than those with long-standing abscesses. In one study, 11 of 13 patients treated for bilateral acute abscesses became pregnant compared to one of seven managed for long-term abscesses[21].

The more usual situation in the treatment of pelvic adhesions is the discovery of adhesions during a diagnostic laparoscopy for pelvic pain or infertility. Adhesiolysis can be performed at the initial procedure if the patient had received prior counselling. Scissors, monopolar electrosurgery or laser energy can be used depending on the availability of equipment and the vascularity of the adhesions. The aim of salpingolysis is to mobilize the Fallopian tubes, particularly the fimbriae, and in ovariolysis to provide for adequate oocyte release. The principles of microsurgery should be adhered to, such as limiting tissue handling to a minimum and irrigating the pelvis to prevent tissue drying as well as to act as a backstop for laser surgery.

It is usual to leave fluid in the pelvis to prevent adhesion reformation after surgery, but only a hypertonic solution such as 32% dextran 70 will be present in the pelvic cavity for a significant length of time[23–26]. The use of dextran, however, is occasionally associated with side-effects such as anaphylaxis, pleural effusion and pulmonary oedema. Prospects for the future include the potential use of synthetic absorbable sheets placed laparoscopically to cover the deperitonealized surfaces created by adhesiolysis.

Several series have reported on pregnancy rates after laparoscopic adhesiolysis. As an example, 64% of infertile patients with filmy and avascular adhesions and 50% of those with dense and vascular adhesions conceived within 18 months of laparoscopic $CO_2$ laser adhesiolysis[27]. The success rate is considerably worse in cases with extensive tubal damage and these women should be advised that *in vitro* fertilization may be a more appropriate course of action. The value of adhesiolysis in the management of pelvic pain is not clearly demonstrated, particularly as adhesions are a common incidental finding in asymptomatic women. It is thought that, in some, pain is related to the limitation of mobility of viscera and the stimulation of nociceptors[28]. In one study, adhesiolysis resulted in alleviation of pain in up to 84% of women during a 1–5 year follow-up[29]. Another trial, in which women with 'chronic pain syndrome' were excluded, noted improvement in 75%[28]. A randomized, prospective, double-blind trial is required to prove the efficacy of adhesiolysis in the management of pelvic pain.

### Endometriosis

Endometriosis is a disease of the pelvic mesenchyme in which tissue with epithelial and stromal characteristics of endometrium develops in situations other than in the uterine mucosa[30] (see Chapter 21). Although many women with endometriosis are asymptomatic, most present with dysmenorrhoea, pelvic pain, deep dyspareunia or infertility. The only way to be certain of the diagnosis is at laparoscopy. It is essential to perform a thorough and systematic examination of the pelvis and the peritoneum, with particular attention being paid to the pouch of Douglas, including aspiration of any peritoneal fluid to enable full visualization. Small chocolate-coloured or blood-filled cysts are characteristic of endometriosis, but Jansen and Russell identified other non-pigmented peritoneal lesions such as white opacification, gland-like growths, flame-like lesions and other unexplained adhesions and peritoneal defects[31]. An attempt to document the appearance should be made by staging the disease according to the modified American Fertility Society classification[32], and photographing or preferably videotaping the procedure to enable the response to treatment to be assessed. After a diagnosis of endometriosis is made on visual inspection, some advise biopsy of the peritoneum to confirm the presence of endometriosis histologically.

A treatment strategy should then be drawn up. Treatment is generally recommended in symptomatic patients, although those patients having a laparoscopy and in whom endometriosis is identified coincidentally should be counselled regarding the findings in view of the progressive nature of endometriosis. Medical management of endometriosis is often the first line of treatment, but, in severe disease or in women not responding to medical management or unable to tolerate the many side-effects, surgery is the course of action. There is a growing tendency to treat at the initial laparoscopy.

A wide variety of surgical procedures may be required, all of which can be performed laparoscopically: excision of endometrioma, adhesiolysis, tubal repair, dissection of the pouch of Douglas or the rectovaginal septum, oophorectomy, and hysterectomy with bilateral oophorectomy. Two specific techniques used in endometriosis include the ablation of endometriotic deposits and laparoscopic uterosacral nerve ablation.

Modalities to treat endometriosis consist chiefly of electrocautery or laser vaporization. The most frequently used therapy is with $CO_2$ laser, which, with a depth of penetration of 0.1 mm or less, can destroy endometriotic deposits whilst minimizing the risk to underlying structures. A focused beam can also be used to divide adhesions and incise endometriomas. After aspiration of the cystic fluid, a defocused beam can vaporize the cyst wall. Problems with the use of the $CO_2$ laser are those of the generation of large volumes of smoke (plume) and a lack of a coagulating effect in cases of bleeding.

Nowroozi and colleagues found that the pregnancy rate after cauterization of mild endometriosis was significantly higher than after expectant management alone[33]. Aspiration of peritoneal fluid in the pouch of Douglas may in itself be beneficial, as this fluid contains many macrophages which have been implicated as a potential source of infertility[34]. Interestingly, a large meta-analysis reported that, in cases of minimal and mild endometriosis associated with infertility, surgery or expectant management produced better 3-year pregnancy rates than medical management alone[35]. Women with moderate or severe disease are usually treated by surgery, and evidence suggests that laparoscopic surgery is as effective as laparotomy, even in cases with endometriomas and cul-de-sac obliteration. Results in 100 patients with complete or partial cul-de-sac obliteration demonstrated a viable intrauterine pregnancy rate of 70% in those desiring fertility[36]. The results of laparoscopic laser treatment and electrocautery for infertility are similar[36], so the type of treatment used is usually determined by the modality with which the operator is more experienced.

The results of laparoscopic treatment of pelvic pain and dysmenorrhoea attributable to endometriosis demonstrate it to be effective with few side-effects. In a prospective randomized, double-blind, controlled trial of laser laparoscopy in the treatment of pelvic pain associated with minimal, mild and moderate endometriosis, Sutton and co-workers demonstrated that, at 6 months after surgery, 62.5% of patients allocated to laser treatment and laparoscopic uterine nerve ablation reported an improvement or resolution of their symptomatology compared to 22.6% in the control group[37]. Of women with mild and moderate disease, 73.7% noted an improvement after laser surgery. Patients with severe disease were excluded from the study, as it was felt unethical to withhold treatment.

Laparoscopic uterine nerve ablation, involving transection of the uterine nerves running in the uterosacral ligaments just proximal to the cervix, has been successful in the treatment of pelvic pain and dysmenorrhoea. Feste reported significant relief from menstrual pain in 70% of over 300 women[38]. In another trial, 81% of women with dysmenorrhoea unresponsive to analgesics reported significant relief of their symptoms[39].

A further procedure aimed at interrupting afferent nerve fibres to the uterus, known as laparoscopic presacral neurectomy, can also be performed in women with intractable pelvic pain and severe dysmenorrhoea. Nezhat and Nezhat described their procedure in which the presacral nerves and the superior hypogastric plexus are cauterized and excised using $CO_2$ laser[40]. They reported a 94% success rate in pain relief and 92% of women noted a reduction in dysmenorrhoea. Problems reported include the risk of 'painless labour' in a subsequent pregnancy, although some would surely describe this as an advantage.

In conclusion, while minimally invasive surgery can assist in the management of endometriosis, there is a paucity of large prospective randomized trials to compare new treatments with more traditional methods of management.

### Polycystic ovarian syndrome

Polycystic ovarian syndrome was first reported by Stein and Leventhal in 1935[41]. In 1964[42], Stein reported a series of 108 women who had undergone bilateral ovarian wedge resection over a period of 34 years, of whom 95% returned to cyclical menstruation, and 85% of the 83 women desiring fertility had conceived[42]. However, a later study looking at women who failed to conceive after wedge resection found significant pelvic adhesions which did not predate their surgery[43]. The use of surgery for the treatment of polycystic ovaries tended to drop out of favour after this report.

Treatment since then has relied on the use of clomiphene citrate and gonadotrophins in resistant cases. Both of these methods run the risks of multiple pregnancy and ovarian hyperstimulation. This has led to the re-emergence of a surgical approach to the problem, this time laparoscopically. In 1984, Gjonnaess used electrosurgery to destroy atretic follicles[44]. This technique has gained wide acceptance, as has the use of endoscopic lasers, in the treatment of clomiphene-resistant polycystic ovarian syndrome. The principle with all these methods is to drill 10–15 holes into atretic androgen-secreting follicles on each ovary[44] (Figure 1).

Laparoscopic surgery is highly effective as demonstrated by the rapid resumption of regular menstrual cycles. In Gjonnaess' original series, three women became pregnant within 7 weeks and 86% of 59 patients developed regular menstrual cycles after electrocautery[44]. In women with anovulation refractory to medical treatment, the use of ovarian electrocautery or laser vaporization can lead to spontaneous ovulation rates of up to 92%[45] and pregnancy rates averaging 55%[46], with up to 84% in a large series by Gjonnaess[45]. Of those that did not conceive, treatment with clomiphene citrate increased this figure to 89%[45]. The response to electrocautery was shown to be influenced by body weight.

The method by which ovarian surgery interferes with polycystic ovarian syndrome is thought to be by a correction of disturbed ovarian–pituitary feedback, as treatment of only one ovary is effective at restoring ovulation from both ovaries[47]. It is thought that it is the reduction of the intraovarian androgens in wedge resection which leads to a resumption of ovulation[48]. In fact, levels of androstenedione, testosterone and dihydrotestosterone fall in the early postoperative period[49,50], and the postoperative effect depends on the number of sites cauterized[44]. The effect on gonadotrophins is to reduce the characteristically raised luteinizing hormone (LH)[49,50] and increase follicle stimulating hormone (FSH)[45], thus reversing the classical abnormally elevated LH : FSH ratio.

The long-term follow-up of these patients confirms laparoscopy as a beneficial treatment modality. Naether and colleagues followed 206 women for up to 72 months and found that 145 previously anovulatory women achieved a total of 211 conceptions, a rate of 70%; 18% of the women miscarried; and there were two late pregnancy losses and three ectopic pregnancies[51].

As with laparotomy, a problem that has been encountered is that of postoperative adhesion formation. However, at short-interval

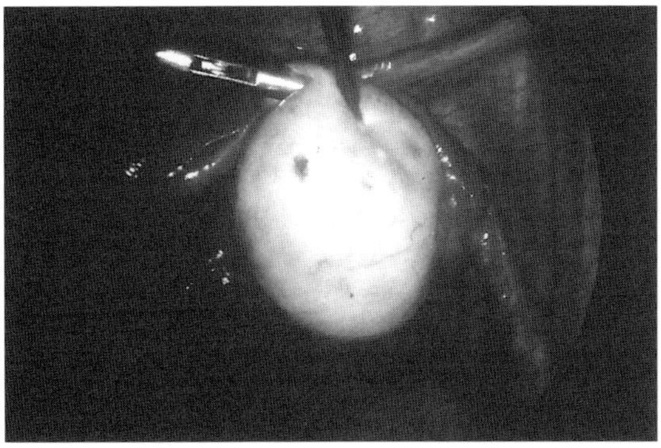

**Figure 1** Laparoscopic ovarian drilling

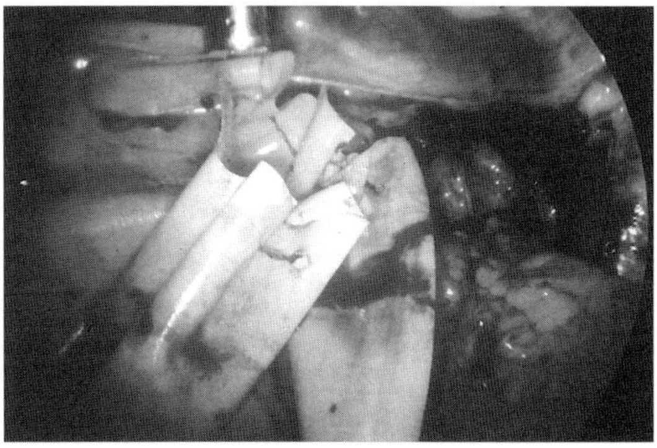

**Figure 2** The drawstring of a laparoscopic bag being pulled to complete an oophorectomy

second-look laparoscopy, these adhesions are usually amenable to laparoscopic lysis and the possibility exists to use agents such as Interceed® or a laparoscopically instilled fluid as an adjunct to diminish adhesion formation.

In summary, laparoscopic surgical treatment of polycystic ovary syndrome is effective in restoring regular ovulation and menstruation and its effects are similar to gonadotrophin stimulation[52] with advantages in terms of treatment cost savings, reduced patient monitoring, avoidance of ovarian hyperstimulation or multiple gestation, and the prospect of a higher live birth rate due to an apparent lower risk of miscarriage[46].

### Ovarian cysts

Ovarian masses are one of the commonest indications for laparoscopy in recent years (13 739 in USA in 1990)[53]. Laparoscopy provides the opportunity to visualize the pelvis clearly and perform aspiration, fenestration (biopsy) or cyst enucleation if required without sacrificing the ability to convert to laparotomy if the situation necessitates this. The use of vaginal ultrasound, colour flow Doppler and serum tumour markers can assist with the pre-operative work-up of the patient and counselling, but these tests are not able as yet to replace the need for a histological diagnosis. The inability to be 100% certain of the diagnosis prior to surgery has led to the concern that the prognosis of women found to have ovarian cancer may be worsened by intraoperative cyst rupture, but this has been refuted in patients managed adequately by laparotomy[54].

Surgeons differ in their criteria for laparoscopic management in terms of cyst size and patient age. Laparoscopic surgery has been reported even in cases of large cysts measuring 25 cm in diameter following drainage under ultrasound control[55], and in carefully selected postmenopausal women[56]. All agree, however, that ultrasonically suspicious masses with overt signs of malignancy are indications for laparotomy. The procedure for laparoscopy is as previously described, although initial $CO_2$ insufflation via the Veress needle may be necessary in the left hypochondrium to avoid accidental cyst rupture. As at laparotomy, peritoneal washings should be taken prior to surgery and signs of ovarian capsule invasion or evidence of metastases sought. If present, the procedure should be converted to a laparotomy.

Aspiration of ovarian cysts is simply performed using an aspiration needle or trochar followed by irrigation to wash the cavity[57]. The inside of the cyst should be inspected by 'cystoscopy', either through a small endoscope inserted through the trochar or by extending the cyst wall incision with scissors; vegetations and other signs of malignancy are an indication for laparotomy. Most surgeons continue to complete excision of the cyst as, even when it is thought that clinically the cyst is functional in origin, the laparoscopic diagnosis is wrong in approximately 10% of cases[57]. There is, therefore, the risk of missing an organic cyst, with an up to 30% chance of cyst re-accumulation.

Ovarian cystectomy should be performed on the anti-mesenteric surface of the ovary away from the hilum and as far as possible from the tubal fimbriae. A dissection plane is established and the cyst is separated from the ovarian cortex using atraumatic grasping forceps; adherent surfaces may require sharp or hydro-dissection to assist in cleavage. Bipolar coagulation is used for haemostasis, and the ovarian cortex is generally left open, rather than being sutured, to reduce postoperative adhesion formation. The recent introduction of laparoscopic bags enables cyst puncture and dissection to occur without contaminating the pelvis and enables withdrawal of the capsule without the risk of seeding to the abdominal wall[58] (see Figure 2).

If the procedure to be performed is oophorectomy (or salpingo-oophorectomy), either in view of the patient's age or if the cyst completely fills the ovary, this can be performed using either laparoscopic sutures, bipolar coagulation or a linear stapler. The specimen is removed via a larger (10–12 mm) cannula, by extending one of the port incisions, or via a posterior colpotomy using a bag as for cystectomy.

Laparoscopic surgery has potentially a very important role in the management of benign adnexal masses and patients treated this way appear to retain normal fertility; in one series of 38 cases, for instance, the intrauterine pregnancy rate was 92%, with one ectopic pregnancy[59]. The use of laparoscopic surgery for the management of early ovarian cancer is still being evaluated[60].

## Uterine fibroids

Uterine fibroids are very common, occurring in up to 25% of women of reproductive age[61]. Many do not produce symptoms, and these should be left alone, but those associated with menorrhagia, infertility, urinary frequency, pelvic discomfort or abdominal distension may well need surgery. Open myomectomy has been performed for many years as an alternative to hysterectomy in women desirous of future fertility, resulting in a conception rate of around 40% and a reduction in the spontaneous abortion rate[61]. The recent advances in laparoscopic surgery have meant that some women with uterine myomata have become suitable for minimally invasive surgery.

Myomata may be subserous, intramural or submucous. Submucous fibroids can be excised hysteroscopically and laparoscopic techniques are used to remove intramural and subserous fibroids. As with ovarian cysts, the limit of what it is reasonable to attempt laparoscopically has yet to be defined, but most would agree that the fibroids should be neither too numerous (< 3–4) nor too large (< 10 cm diameter)[62]. Larger fibroids may be reduced in size by up to 40% by prior treatment with gonadotrophin-releasing hormone agonists for 3 months[63]. Studies at the time of laparotomy have shown that such pretreatment also reduces intraoperative blood loss, although it can make enucleation of the fibroid more difficult[64]. Another technique to reduce intraoperative blood loss is the local injection of vasoconstrictors.

Prior to surgery, a pelvic ultrasound is essential to assess the size and exact location of the fibroids, and a diagnostic hysteroscopy is useful to assess the extent of any intracavity lesions. Subserous fibroids are removed by stabilization of the fibroid with grasping forceps, followed by bipolar or monopolar electrocautery to the pedicle which is then cut. For subserous fibroids with a large implantation surface and for intramural fibroids, the uterus is incised with a monopolar electrode over the myoma without opening the uterine cavity. The incision should penetrate the capsule of the fibroid, recognizable by its characteristic pearly-white appearance. The fibroid is then fixed by a grasping forceps and dissected away from the myometrium using counter-traction on the uterus. The vascular pedicle of the fibroid should be identified and desiccated with bipolar diathermy prior to transecting. Constant pelvic irrigation with normal saline is performed throughout the procedure. Prior to suturing the uterine defect with interrupted sutures, meticulous haemostasis is achieved with electrocoagulation. The operative site is thoroughly irrigated to reduce postoperative adhesion formation.

The fibroid should be removed from the peritoneal cavity to avoid peritoneal implantation. A morcellator can be used to divide up the specimen and facilitate its removal, either via one of the suprapubic puncture sites, extension of one of the incisions or via a posterior colpotomy.

Apart from a relatively long operating time, up to 7 h in one series[65], reported complications of the procedure are rare provided the patient is well selected. Particular care has to be taken to avoid damage to adjacent organs. Attempts to remove numerous or over-large and deep fibroids will be associated with excessive bleeding which is more difficult to control laparoscopically than at laparotomy. Repair of deep uterine incisions is also more problematic laparoscopically. Perhaps as an indication of this, two instances of uterine rupture in a subsequent pregnancy have been reported to date, both occurring prior to full term[66,67].

The obvious technical limits and potential difficulties of laparoscopic myomectomy led to the development of another approach to treatment, namely myolysis. Large fibroids can be reduced in size after preoperative treatment with gonadotrophin-releasing hormone agonists for 3 months and then holes are drilled in the tissue using the Nd : YAG laser or electrosurgery. This provokes devascularization and hence ischaemic necrosis. The procedure produces a significant reduction in fibroid size with no recurrence at up to 14 months of follow-up[68]. Due to the necrotic process, however, adhesion formation is common[69]. A recent technique which may reduce the requirement for laparoscopic myomectomy is that of vaginal myomectomy[70].

The recurrence rate of fibroids after conventional myomectomy is about 15%[61], but there are as yet no data regarding the laparoscopic approach; neither do we know whether there are any advantages to minimal access surgery with respect to postoperative adhesion formation and fertility.

### Tubal surgery

The principles involved in minimal access tubal surgery are the same as those employed at laparotomy. These consist of minimal tissue trauma, keeping the surfaces moist with irrigating solutions, meticulous haemostasis, and the use of fine instruments with the assistance of magnification, conditions which are ideally met by laparoscopic surgery. One area which is understandably difficult laparoscopically is the use of fine microsurgical sutures, but alternative techniques exist which generally make suturing unnecessary.

The patient is prepared for the operating theatre as previously described, with the addition of antibiotic cover for the surgery. The cervix is cannulated and hydrotubation performed to establish the site of tubal disease. This has usually been previously documented at a diagnostic laparoscopy and the point of occlusion located by a hysterosalpingogram. Initially, it may be necessary to divide pelvic adhesions to gain access and adequate visualization of the pelvis.

The first tubal surgery performed after surveying the pelvis is salpingo-ovariolysis. This consists of freeing the Fallopian tubes and the ovaries from adhesions which may prevent conception occurring. Scissors, monopolar electrosurgery or laser can be used. It is essential to be sure what structures lie behind the adhesions to prevent accidental damage, and here the technique of hydrodissection is very useful to separate the surfaces, particularly if they are cohesive. This is achieved by cutting a small window in the adhesion and applying short bursts of irrigation fluid under high pressure. Dissection of adhesions continues until the normal anatomy is restored.

Fimbrioplasty is the restitution of patency by reconstruction of a distally occluded or partially occluded Fallopian tube. If the distal Fallopian tube is phimotic with agglutinated fimbriae, it may initially be necessary to incise any fibrous bands of tissue and perform salpingo-ovariolysis. The agglutinated fimbriae can be separated by introducing a pointed, closed atraumatic forceps through the phimotic opening and withdrawing whilst concurrently opening its jaws to separate the fimbriae. An additional incision may be required on the antimesosalpingeal border of the Fallopian tube to a point proximal to the stenosis. Haemostasis is achieved by electrocoagulation and constant irrigation of the operative site.

In the presence of a hydrosalpinx or a completely occluded Fallopian tube, the procedure of salpingostomy (neosalpingostomy) is performed. After distension of the Fallopian tube and freeing of adhesions, a cruciate incision is made over the stenosed area with scissors, needle electrosurgery or laser. The stoma is further opened by additional longitudinal cuts into non-vascular areas representing agglutinated fimbriae. Finally, eversion is effected by either employing a defocused laser or desiccation with low-power electrosurgery to the proximal serosa. Fine sutures can be applied to produce a similar result.

Salpingoscopy should ideally be performed prior to salpingostomy, as the presence of a thick-walled ampulla and adhesions characteristic of chronic salpingitis are associated with a high chance of continuing infertility or an ectopic pregnancy occurring. In a study to assess the prognostic role of laparoscopic salpingoscopy of the only remaining tube after contralateral ectopic pregnancy, Marana and associates demonstrated that eight of the 13 women with a normal mucosa conceived an intrauterine pregnancy, while three of the five with intra-ampullary adhesions had further ectopic pregnancies[71].

Thorough pelvic irrigation is essential throughout laparoscopic tubal surgery and at the end of the procedure, most surgeons leave fluid in the peritoneal cavity to prevent serosal drying and adhesion formation. Substances range from isotonic saline and Ringer's solution to hypertonic Dextran 70, and various adjuvants including heparin, intraperitoneal steroids and systemic steroids or antihistamines. Hypertonic solutions are known to stay in the pelvis for a significant length of time[23–25], while Hart and Magos demonstrated that an isotonic solution is only present in the peritoneal cavity for up to 16 h[26], perhaps not long enough to prevent adhesion formation. A large trial, however, could show no significant difference in adhesion formation and pregnancy rate between several of the above-mentioned modalities[72].

In a recent large series to assess the treatment of complete distal tubal occlusion or moderate-to-severe tubal phimosis, 113 patients underwent neosalpingostomy[73]. The overall pregnancy rate was 20.4%, with a monthly fecundity rate of 2.6%, and there were six ectopic pregnancies. Patients in this series of women, with total or near total tubal blockage with endometriosis and no other infertility factors, had significantly better cumulative pregnancy rates compared to those with other infertility factors but no endometriosis, and patients with complete bilateral distal tubal occlusion fared significantly worse than those with near total occlusion. However, no randomized controlled trials comparing microsurgery with laparoscopic surgery have been performed. Similarly, there are no comparative data about laparoscopic and open reversal of clip tubal sterilization.

### Laparoscopic hysterectomy

The first reported hysterectomy performed laparoscopically was by Reich in 1988[74]. The aim of laparoscopic hysterectomy is to convert an abdominal hysterectomy into a laparoscopic/vaginal procedure, therefore deriving the advantages of reduced morbidity, discomfort, hospital stay and earlier return to work. The extent to which the operation is performed laparoscopically depends on the surgeon and the procedure is staged accordingly[75]. Most gynaecologists carry out a combination of laparoscopic and vaginal dissection, so called laparoscopically assisted vaginal hysterectomy (LAVH). Women who are candidates for LAVH have usually had previous pelvic surgery, endometriosis, pelvic sepsis, fibroids or need concurrent oophorectomy.

Usual instrumentation is performed, the pelvis is assessed and the extent of the laparoscopic component of the procedure planned. After adhesiolysis, the upper pedicles can be secured with biopolar diathermy, with linear staples or by sutures and transected using scissors. The peritoneum over the bladder is then opened and the bladder reflected caudally. The uterine arteries are identified, secured with sutures, staples or by desiccation and then transected. Identification of the ureters is essential and some surgeons use transilluminating ureteric stents to assist them at this stage. The operation is usually completed vaginally, but in total laparoscopic hysterectomy the vaginal vault is opened laparoscopically, the uterus removed and the vagina closed and reperitonealized with laparoscopic sutures. From the point of view of operating time, there is no advantage in doing the whole operation laparoscopically, and indeed Richardson and colleagues clearly showed that the operation should be converted to a vaginal procedure as early as possible to reduce the duration of the procedure[76].

A variation on total hysterectomy is laparoscopic supracervical (subtotal) hysterectomy. Here, the cervix is not excised, and, to minimize the risk of subsequent cervical neoplasia, the transformation zone is often reamed out. The uterus is either morcellated to allow delivery through an extended abdominal wall incision or removed via a posterior colpotomy. The advantages of this procedure are postulated to be less risk of injury to the ureter intraoperatively (as the main trunk of uterine vessels does not have to be ligated), and reduced incidence of vault haematoma postoperatively[77]. The effect of supracervical hysterectomy on the chances of subsequent vault prolapse and orgasmic function remains purely theoretical and should not be a reason to select this procedure in preference to total hysterectomy[78].

Randomized trials of laparoscopic hysterectomy and abdominal hysterectomy have all come to the same conclusion, namely that the laparoscopic procedure is considerably slower and has comparable complication rates, but has advantages in terms of analgesia requirements, hospital stay and recovery times[79,80]. Similar comparisons with vaginal hysterectomy demonstrated that laparoscopic hysterectomy is the slower and more costly procedure with no advantages in terms of complications, post-operative discomfort or recovery time[76,81]. The main consequence of laparoscopic hysterectomy may well prove to be a resurgence in the use of vaginal hysterectomy without laparoscopy; Kovac, for instance, demonstrated that over 90% of hysterectomies for benign indications could be performed vaginally[82]. Other studies have shown that absence of uterine prolapse, the presence of fibroids, or the need for oophorectomy should not be considered as contraindications to vaginal hysterectomy[83,84].

## HYSTEROSCOPIC SURGERY

The developments in laparoscopic surgery have been paralleled in hysteroscopy. Modern hysteroscopes provide an excellent view of the uterine cavity, and surgical procedures also become a possibility. Blind curettage of the uterus has been rendered obsolete. The treatment of uterine septae, adhesions and submucous fibroids has been revolutionized. In many cases, hysterectomy for menorrhagia can now be avoided by endometrial ablation.

### Equipment

The equipment for diagnostic hysteroscopy includes a 0–30° hysteroscope, most commonly 4 mm in diameter, an insufflation sheath, a fibre-optic cable and cold light source, and a distension medium such as $CO_2$ or isotonic saline. Carbon dioxide is administered via a hysteroflator at a maximum pressure of 150 mmHg and flow rate of up to 100 ml/min. Normal saline can be run in under gravity or more usually with a pressure cuff, and has the advantage that it does not cause bubbles or shoulder pain and provides a good view even in the presence of bleeding[85]. The hysteroscope can be fitted with an operating sheath to enable small biopsies to be taken or scissors introduced to cut off the stalk of polyps or divide minor adhesions.

For more extensive intrauterine surgery, it is necessary to use an operating hysteroscope. Saline as distension medium is dangerous with electrosurgery in view of its electrical conductive properties, and $CO_2$ is not suitable as the view will be obscured by smoke. Solutions such as 1.5% glycine are usually used with electrosurgery, although excessive intravasation can produce cardiac failure and encephalopathy. Fluid can be instilled into the uterine cavity under gravity but more usually it is administered via a pump. Surgery is usually performed with a fibre Nd : YAG laser rated at 60–100 W of power and a depth of penetration of approximately 4 mm, or a continuous flow resectoscope fitted with a cutting loop, rollerball or knife electrode. The resectoscope uses monopolar cutting and coagulating currents, typically between 75 and 100 W. As for laparoscopy, the procedures should be video-recorded for future reference and teaching purposes.

Operative hysteroscopy is usually performed under general anaesthesia, although one of the authors has published a series of endometrial resections performed under local anaesthesia and intravenous sedation[86].

### Complications of hysteroscopic surgery

Complications in hysteroscopic surgery can be divided in a similar manner to those in laparoscopy: equipment-related, operator-related and procedure-related. The first two can be minimized by regular checks of the equipment and by adequate training. Hysteroscopy should initially be carried out under general anaesthesia before progressing to local anaesthesia, and diagnostic hysteroscopy must be mastered before undertaking the more minor operative procedures. As for laparoscopy, attendance at workshops, practice on models and proctoring are the best ways to master diagnostic and operative hysteroscopy.

Technical problems can still arise. A very tight cervix which is difficult to dilatate sufficiently may be overcome by the prior administration of vaginal prostaglandins. Problems related to the distension media are those of cardiorespiratory collapse after $CO_2$ embolism if the insufflation pressure exceeds 200 mmHg, anaphylaxis with Dextran 70, and fluid overload if there is excessive intravasation of fluid. Uterine perforation can occur during cervical dilatation or as the hysteroscope is being guided into the uterine cavity, although the latter should not happen when the endoscope is inserted under direct vision rather than with an obturator.

Potentially much more serious is uterine perforation while a laser hysteroscope or resectoscope is being used, when major vascular, bowel and urinary tract trauma can occur. While observation may be sufficient in other cases, in this situation immediate laparoscopy and even laparotomy is mandatory to assess and treat any extrauterine trauma. Haemorrhage is not often seen during hysteroscopic surgery and can usually be stopped by laser or electrosurgical coagulation of the bleeding vessels. More generalized bleeding at the end of surgery, typically after endometrial ablation or hysteroscopic myomectomy, may require tamponade using a 20–30 ml balloon catheter left *in situ* for 6–8 h. Rarely is laparotomy or hysterectomy required.

### Diagnostic hysteroscopy

Diagnostic hysteroscopy is ideally suited to the out-patient setting. The patient is placed in a lithotomy position and should be attended by a nurse for reassurance; the patient can observe the procedure on the video monitor if she desires. Local anaesthesia is only needed by a minority, and generally the cervix requires no dilatation as the pressure of the distension medium is enough to open the cervical canal ahead of the hysteroscope[87]. The anterior lip of the cervix may be grasped with a tenaculum but this is often not necessary. When using a 30° fore-oblique optic, allowance has to be made for angulation of the view as the optic is advanced towards the uterine cavity to prevent trauma to the cervix. If at any time the view is obscured, then gentle withdrawal of the hysteroscope enables the cervix to be distended again and the cervical canal to be identified. Once in the uterus, the cavity can be systematically inspected for any endometrial abnormalities or focal lesions. The endocervical canal is best assessed as the hysteroscope is being withdrawn. An endometrial biopsy is generally taken even in the absence of any obvious abnormalities to ensure that pathology is not missed.

Lesions which may be identified at diagnostic hysteroscopy include endometrial hyperplasia, atypia and frank malignancy, polyps, submucous fibroids, intrauterine adhesions and anatomical abnormalities such as uterine septae. Hysteroscopy is also useful in locating and removing lost intrauterine contraceptive devices. In our experience, almost all diagnostic hysteroscopies can be performed without the need for a general anaesthetic, with the result that a 'one-stop' approach to diagnosis and treatment, involving consultation, vaginal ultrasound and diagnostic hysteroscopy with biopsy, becomes a reality[88].

### Polypectomy

Polyps are a common finding in women with menorrhagia, irregular periods, and intermenstrual or postmenopausal bleeding. They are often missed at dilatation and curettage but are reliably diagnosed at hysteroscopy. Hysteroscopy is also the most reliable technique for excising endometrial and endocervical polyps. Scissors are adequate for small polyps, but resectoscopic polypectomy is both fast and most suitable for larger lesions[89].

### Myomectomy

The hysteroscopic excision of submucous fibroids was first reported in 1976 by Neuwirth and Amin[90], and 2 years later Neuwirth described the use of the resectoscope for excising deeper fibroids[91]. The Nd : YAG laser can also be used[92]. Essentially, only fibroids which are more than 50% in the uterine cavity and less than 5 cm in diameter are suitable for hysteroscopic surgery, as attempts at excising deeper or larger fibroids risk uterine perforation and fluid overload. Surgery is facilitated by pretreatment with danazol or a gonadotrophin releasing analogue for 6–12 weeks to thin the endometrium and shrink the fibroid. Care should be taken to avoid damaging the surrounding endometrium, particularly if fertility is desired[93]. Deeper fibroids may be amenable to a two-stage procedure involving excision of the superficial portion of the fibroid, coagulation of the deep blood supply (myolysis), continued gonadotrophin releasing hormone treatment followed by repeat hysteroscopic surgery for the residual portion after a few months[92].

Several observation series with long-term follow-up have shown that hysteroscopic myomectomy is effective in relieving menorrhagia and offering many women the chance to avoid hysterectomy[94,95]. Objective measures of menstrual blood loss have confirmed these results[96]. Hysteroscopic myomectomy can also be valuable in cases of infertility, with pregnancy rates of up to 66% following surgery[92,97]. When myomectomy is performed prior to *in vitro* fertilization, it does not adversely affect the reproductive outcome[98]. There are no randomized studies comparing the effects of abdominal versus hysteroscopic myomectomy and, in the light of our current knowledge, it would be difficult to justify such a trial.

### Sterilization

Attempts at hysteroscopic sterilization have been made for many years using various designs of tubal plugs, sclerosant injections, or coagulation of the cornual portion of the Fallopian tube with monopolar electrosurgery and, more recently, laser energy. None has proved successful. Currently, most attention is being focused on an injectable silicone plug, and, in those cases where bilateral application is possible, early results have been promising, with a Pearl index of 0.12–0.84[99]. A postoperative hysterosalpingogram is required to ensure that the plugs have not migrated. Removal of the plug does not necessarily produce a patent tube, as it provokes tubal closure and hence cannot be used as a form of pregnancy spacing. More work needs to be carried out before hysteroscopic sterilization can replace laparoscopic methods.

### Metroplasty

Uterine septa can cause recurrent miscarriage. It is essential to fully evaluate the uterus by either ultrasound or laparoscopy prior to metroplasty as it is impossible to exclude a bicornuate uterus at hysteroscopy. The septum needs to be divided rather than excised, and scissors, the knife electrode or laser can be used for this. It is important not to extend the incision too far, and it is better to leave the fundus slightly convex rather than concave at the end of the procedure. If there is any uncertainty, the metroplasty can be controlled by simultaneous laparoscopy or, even better, by ultrasound, ensuring that the fundal myometrium measures at least 1.5 cm in depth. Some surgeons leave an intrauterine contraceptive device in place and administer oral oestrogens to stimulate endometrial proliferation and healing, and to prevent adhesion formation, but there is little scientific support for either. A second-look hysteroscopy 2–3 months after surgery is useful to assess the end result, and any filmy adhesions which might have formed can be broken down at the same time.

Hysteroscopic metroplasty has become the treatment of choice for the septate uterus associated with reproductive failure[100–102]. It is associated with shorter operating time, hospital stay and time taken to conceive, and pregnancy rates are slightly better than those achieved following laparotomy. Cervical cerclage early in the second trimester should be considered if the septum is close to the internal cervical os. There is, however, no necessity for elective Caesarean delivery, although there are reports in the literature of uterine dehiscence in a subsequent pregnancy[103]. A prospective trial looking at the use of an intrauterine contraceptive device and concomitant treatment with oestrogen after metroplasty demonstrated no difference in intrauterine adhesions at repeat hysteroscopy as compared to those patients who received neither[104].

### Adhesiolysis

Intrauterine adhesions typical of Asherman's syndrome are increasingly being recognized as hysteroscopy becomes a routine procedure. They may be classified into mild, moderate or severe, depending on their extent and nature, myofibrous adhesions with obliteration of the uterine cavity being the most extreme case (Figure 3). Filmy endometrial adhesions can be divided by the blunt end of the hysteroscope, but their clinical significance is doubtful. Denser and more extensive adhesions require hysteroscopic scissors, although some surgeons use the knife electrode or Nd : YAG laser. Extreme care has to be taken to avoid uterine perforation, and simultaneous laparoscopy is mandatory if the uterine fundus cannot be seen at the start of surgery. The treatment of severe Asherman's syndrome is one of the most difficult of hysteroscopic procedures. There is a little more logic to the use of exogenous oestrogens following surgery, and, as after metroplasty, hysteroscopy a few months after adhesiolysis is useful to check for fresh adhesions which are generally easily divided at this time.

The menstrual and fertility outcomes after hysteroscopic adhesiolysis very much depend on the extent of the uterine damage. In women with intrauterine adhesions undergoing hysteroscopic resection, 90% of women resumed menstruation[105]. Of 187 women treated, there was an overall term pregnancy rate of 80%, but, in cases of severe connective tissue adhesions, this fell to 32%. Poor placentation,

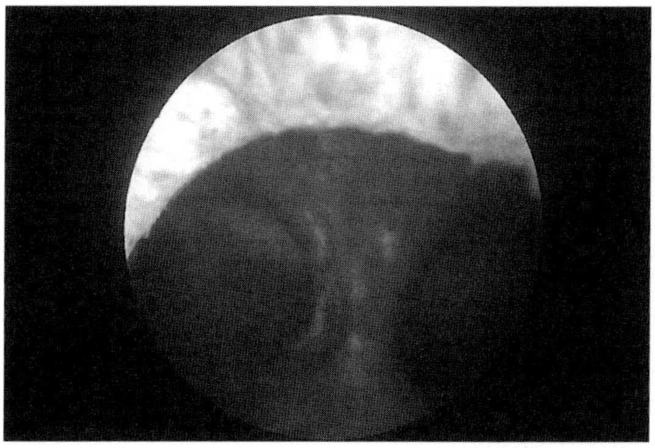

**Figure 3** A fibrous endometrial adhesion in Asherman's syndrome

premature delivery and retained placenta are some of the obstetric problems which can affect women who have undergone adhesiolysis.

### Endometrial ablation

Attempts have long been made to destroy the endometrium and thus offer women with menorrhagia an alternative to prolonged drug treatment or hysterectomy. The early, blind methods of endometrial ablation were largely abandoned by the time Goldrath and associates described hysteroscopic laser ablation of the endometrium in 1981[106]. Two years later, a resectoscopic technique was introduced for cases of uncontrollable uterine haemorrhage in women unfit for hysterectomy[107], but it was several years before it was adapted for the wider treatment of menorrhagia[108] (Figure 4). Endometrial resection has remained the more popular technique of endometrial ablation in Europe, whereas rollerball coagulation is the most common procedure in the USA[109].

Irrespective of the instrumentation, the principles of hysteroscopic endometrial ablation are similar. The endometrium is systematically excised with a cutting loop or destroyed with the rollerball or laser from the fundus to the endocervical canal. Surgery can be combined with hysteroscopic myomectomy in cases with submucous myoma, and, as with myomectomy, prior endometrial thinning facilitates surgery. Particular care has to be taken when treating the cornual areas where the thickness of the myometrium is as little as 4 mm and 7 mm at the isthmic region of the uterus adjacent to the uterine artery and ureter[110], bearing in mind that the area of thermal necrosis under a blended 7 mm electroresection loop is 0.69–0.76 mm[111]. The penetration of the Nd : YAG laser is approximately 6 mm.

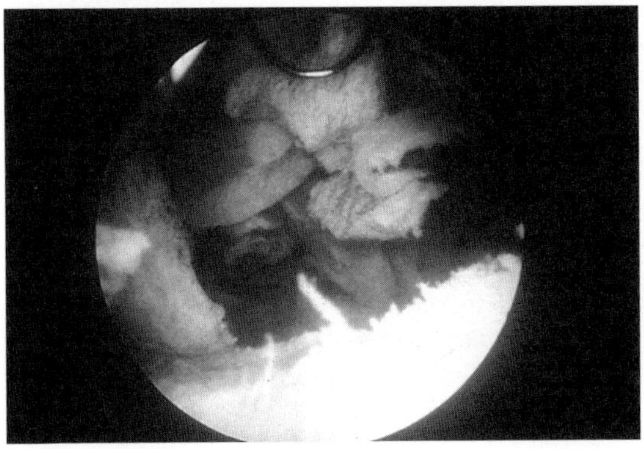

**Figure 4** The process of endometrial resection

Endometrial ablation can be highly effective, provided women are carefully selected and those with gross pelvic pathology are not offered this treatment. For instance, a recent analysis of women undergoing endometrial resection in our unit demonstrated that over 90% avoid hysterectomy in the first 5 years after surgery, and 80% avoid any further surgical intervention[112]. Amenorrhoea is the end result in approximately one-third of patients. Randomized studies have confirmed that hysteroscopic surgery is associated with a shorter operating time, fewer complications, less analgesic requirement and faster resumption of normal activities and return to work than hysterectomy[113–116]. However, after a mean follow-up of 2.8 years, women randomized to hysterectomy reported higher rates of satisfaction than those treated hysteroscopically[117]. Nonetheless, the treatment costs of endometrial ablation were still considerably less than those of hysterectomy[117].

Endometrial ablation is clearly not the answer for every woman with menorrhagia, but the results of surgery are sufficiently good for it to represent an important treatment modality for those women who wish to avoid hysterectomy.

## SUMMARY

Minimal access surgery offers many advantages over traditional treatments. There is little argument about the short-term advantages over conventional surgery, but many questions remain unanswered regarding longer-term outcome. Unlike new drug therapies, most endoscopic procedures have not been subjected to the rigours of randomized controlled trials. The new surgery is a constantly changing field but our natural enthusiasm must be tempered by the need for safety, adequate research and training.

## REFERENCES


1. McAnena, O. J. and Willson, P. D. (1993). Diathermy in laparoscopic surgery. *Br. J. Surg.*, **80**, 1094–6
2. Reich, H. and Maher, P. J. (1994). Instruments and equipment used in operative laparoscopy. In Wood, C., Hill, D. J. and Maher, R. J. (eds.) *Ballière's Clinical Obstetrics and Gynaecology*, pp. 687–705. (London: Ballière Tindall)
3. Hill, D. J. (1994). Complications of the laparoscopic approach. In Wood, C., Hill, D. J. and Maher, P. J. (eds./) *Ballière's Clinical Obstetrics and Gynaecology*, pp. 865–79. (London: Ballière Tindall)
4. Querleu, D., Chevallier, L., Chapron, C. and Bruhat, M. A. (1993). Complications of gynaecological laparoscopic surgery. A French multicentre collaborative study. *Gynaecol. Endosc.*, **2**, 3–6
5. Shapiro, H. I. and Adler, D. L. N. (1973). Excision of an ectopic pregnancy through the laparoscope. *Am. J. Obstet. Gynecol.*, **117**, 290–1
6. Bruhat, M. A., Manhes, H., Mage, G. and Pouly, J. L. (1980). Treatment of ectopic pregnancy by means of laparoscopy. *Fertil. Steril.*, **33**, 411–14
7. Tuomivaara, L. and Kauppila, A. (1988). Radical or conservative surgery for ectopic pregnancy? A follow-up study of fertility of 323 patients. *Fertil. Steril.*, **50**, 580–3
8. Valle, J. A. and Lifchez, A. S. (1983). Reproductive outcome following conservative surgery for tubal pregnancy in women with a single Fallopian tube. *Fertil. Steril.*, **39**, 316–20
9. Pouly, J. L., Chapron, C., Manhes, H., Canis, M., Wattiez, A. and Bruhat, M. A. (1991). Multifactorial analysis of fertility after conservative laparoscopic treatment of ectopic pregnancy in a series of 223 patients. *Fertil. Steril.*, **56**, 453–60
10. Pouly, J. L., Manhes, H., Mage, G., Canis, M. and Bruhat, M. A. (1986). Conservative laparoscopic treatment of 321 ectopic pregnancies. *Fertil. Steril.*, **46**, 1093–7
11. Pouly, J. L., Mage, G., Gachon, F., Gaillard, G. and Bruhat, M. A. (1987). Decrease in HCG levels after conservative laparoscopic treatment of extra-uterine pregnancy. *J. Gynecol. Obstet. Biol. Reprod. Paris*, **16**, 195–9
12. Pouly, J. L., Chapron, C. and Wattiez, A. (1993). Ectopic pregnancy. In Sutton, C. and Diamond, M. P. (eds.) In *Endoscopic Surgery for Gynaecologists*, pp. 105–12. (London: W.B. Saunders)
13. Koninckx, P. R., Witters, K., Brosens, J., Stemers, N., Oosterinck, D. and Meuleman, C. (1991). Conservative laparoscopic treatment of ectopic pregnancies using the $CO_2$ laser. *Br. J. Obstet. Gynaecol.*, **98**, 1254–9
14. Brumsted, J., Kessel, C., Gibson, C., Nakajima, S., Riddick, D. H. and Gibson, M. (1988). A comparison of laparoscopy and laparotomy for the treatment of ectopic pregnancy. *Obstet. Gynecol.*, **71**, 889–92
15. Baumann, R., Magos, A. L. and Turnbull, A. C. (1991). Prospective comparison of videopelviscopy with laparotomy for ectopic pregnancy. *Br. J. Obstet. Gynaecol.*, **98**, 765–71
16. Shalev, E., Peleg, D., Bustan, M., Romano, S. and Tsabari, A. (1995). Limited role of intratubal methotrexate treatment of ectopic pregnancy. *Fertil. Steril.*, **63**, 20–4
17. Fernandez, H., Pauthier, S., Doumerc, S., Lelaidier, C., Olivennes, F., Ville, Y. and Frydman, R. (1995). Ultrasound-guided injection of methotrexate versus laparoscopic salpingotomy in ectopic pregnancy. *Fertil. Steril.*, **63**, 25–9
18. Yeko, T. R., Mayer, J. C., Parsons, A. K. and Maroulis, G. B. (1995). A prospective series of unruptured ectopic pregnancies treated by intratubal injection with hyperosmolar glucose. *Obstet. Gynecol.*, **85**, 265–8
19. Paulsson, G., Kvint, S., Labecker, B. M., Lofstrand, T. and Linblom, B. (1995). Laparoscopic prostaglandin injection in ectopic pregnancy: success rates according to endocrine activity. *Fertil. Steril.*, **63**, 473–7
20. Ryan, G. B., Grobetsky, J. and Majno, G. (1971). Postoperative peritoneal adhesions. *Am. J. Pathol.*, **65**, 117
21. Henry-Suchet, J. and Tesquier, L. (1994). Role of laparoscopy in the management of pelvic adhesions and pelvic sepsis. In Wood, C., Hill, D. J. and Maher, P. J. (eds.) *Ballière's Clinical Obstetrics and Gynaecology*, **8**, 759–72. (London: Ballière Tindall)
22. Westrom, L. (1980). Incidence, prevalence and trends of acute pelvic inflammatory disease and its consequences in industrialized countries. *Am. J. Obstet. Gynecol.*, **138**, 880–91

23. DiZerega, G. S. and Hodgen, G. D. (1980). Prevention of postsurgical adhesions: comparative study of commonly used agents. *Am. J. Obstet. Gynecol.*, **136**, 173
24. Krinsky, A. H., Haseltine, F. P. and DeCherney, A. (1984). Peritoneal fluid accumulation with dextran 70 instilled at the time of laparoscopy. *Fertil. Steril.*, **41**, 647–9
25. Rose, B. I., MacNeill, C., Larrain, R. and Kopreski, M. M. (1991). Abdominal instillation of high-molecular-weight dextran or lactated Ringer's solution after laparoscopic surgery. A randomized comparison of the effect on weight change. *J. Reprod. Med.*, **36**, 537–9
26. Hart, R. J. and Magos, A. L. (1996). Laparoscopically instilled fluid: the rate of absorption and the effects on patient discomfort and fluid balance. *Gynaecol. Endosc.*, in press
27. Donnez, J., Nissolle-Pochet, M. and Casnas, F. (1989). $CO_2$ laser laparoscopy in infertile women with adnexal adhesions and women with tubal occlusion. *J. Gynecol. Surg.*, **5**, 47–53
28. Steege, J. F. and Stout, A. L. (1991). Resolution of chronic pelvic pain after laparoscopic lysis of adhesions. *Am. J. Obstet. Gynecol.*, **165**, 278–83
29. Sutton, C. and MacDonald, R. (1990). Laser laparoscopic adhesiolysis. *J. Gynecol. Surg.*, **6**, 155–9
30. Sampson, J. A. (1940). The development of the implantation theory for the origin of peritoneal endometriosis. *Am. J. Obstet. Gynecol.*, **40**, 549–57
31. Jansen, R. and Russell, P. (1986). Nonpigmented endometriosis: clinical, laparoscopic and pathological definition. *Am. J. Obstet. Gynecol.*, **155**, 1154–9
32. American Fertility Society (1985). Classification of endometriosis. *Fertil. Steril.*, **43**, 351–2
33. Nowroozi, K., Chase, J. S., Check, J. H. and Wu, C. H. (1987). The importance of laparoscopic coagulation of mild endometriosis in infertile women. *Int. J. Fertil.*, **32**, 442–4
34. Haney, A. F., Muscato, J. J. and Weinberg, J. B. (1981). Peritoneal fluid cell populations in infertility patients. *Fertil. Steril.*, **35**, 696–8
35. Adamson, G. D. and Pasta, D. J. (1994). Surgical treatment of endometriosis-associated infertility: meta-analysis compared with survival analysis. *Am. J. Obstet. Gynecol.*, **171**, 1488–504
36. Reich, H., McGlynn, F. and Salvat, J. (1991). Laparoscopic treatment of cul-de-sac obliteration secondary to retrocervical deep fibrotic endometriosis. *J. Reprod. Med.*, **36**, 516–22
37. Sutton, C. J., Ewen, S. P., Whitelaw, N. and Haines, P. (1994). Prospective randomized double-blind, controlled trial of laser laparoscopy in the treatment of pelvic pain associated with minimal, mild and moderate endometriosis. *Fertil. Steril.*, **62**, 696–700
38. Feste, J. R. (1985). Laser laparoscopy. A new modality. *J. Reprod. Med.*, **30**, 413–17
39. Lichten, E. M. and Bombard, J. (1987). Surgical treatment of primary dysmenorrhea with laparoscopic uterine nerve ablation. *J. Reprod. Med.*, **32**, 37–41
40. Nezhat, C. and Nezhat, F. (1992). A simplified method of presacral neurectomy for the treatment of central pelvic pain due to endometriosis. *Br. J. Obstet. Gynaecol.*, **99**, 659–63
41. Stein, F. I. and Leventhal, M. L. (1935). Amenorrhea associated with bilateral polycystic ovaries. *Am. J. Obstet. Gynecol.*, **46**, 23–8
42. Stein, F. I. (1964). Duration of fertility following ovarian wedge resection–Stein–Leventhal syndrome. *West. J. Surg. Obstet. Gynaecol.*, **78**, 237
43. Toaff, R., Toaff, M. E. and Peyser, M. R. (1976). Infertility following wedge resection of the ovaries. *Am. J. Obstet. Gynecol.*, **124**, 92–6
44. Gjonnaess, H. (1984). Polycystic ovarian syndrome treated by ovarian electrocautery through the laparoscope. *Fertil. Steril.*, **41**, 20–5
45. Gjonnaess, H. (1994). Ovarian electrocautery in the treatment of women with polycystic ovary syndrome (PCOS). Factors affecting the results. *Acta Obstet. Gynecol. Scand.*, **73**, 407–12
46. Donesky, B. W. and Adashi, E. Y. (1995). Surgically induced ovulation in the polycystic ovary syndrome: wedge resection revisited in the age of laparoscopy. *Fertil. Steril.*, **63**, 439–63
47. Balen, A. H. and Jacobs, H. S. (1994). A prospective study comparing unilateral and bilateral laparoscopic ovarian diathermy in women with the polycystic ovary syndrome. *Fertil. Steril.*, **62**, 921–5

48. Katz, M., Carr, P., Cohan, B. and Millar, R. (1978). Hormonal effects of wedge resection of polycystic ovaries. *Obstet. Gynecol.*, **41**, 437–44
49. Aakvaag, A. and Gjonnaess, H. (1985). Hormonal response to electrocautery of the ovary in patients with polycystic ovarian disease. *Br. J. Obstet. Gynaecol.*, **92**, 1258–64
50. Greenblatt, E. and Casper, R. F. (1987). Endocrine changes after laparoscopic ovarian cautery in the polycystic ovarian syndrome. *Am. J. Obstet. Gynecol.*, **156**, 279–85
51. Naether, O. G., Baukloh, V., Fischer, R. and Kowalczyk, T. (1994). Long-term follow-up in 206 infertility patients with polycystic ovarian syndrome after laparoscopic electrocautery of the ovarian surface. *Hum. Reprod.*, **9**, 2342–9
52. Abel-Gadir, A., Mowafi, R. S., Alnaser, H. M., Alrashid, A. H., Alonezi, O. M. and Shaw, R. W. (1990). Ovarian electrocautery versus human menopausal gonadotrophins and pure follicle stimulating hormone therapy in the treatment of patients with polycystic ovarian disease. *Clin. Endocrinol.*, **33**, 585–92
53. Hulka, J. F., Parker, W. H., Surrey, M. W. and Phillips, J. M. (1992). Management of ovarian masses. American Association of Gynecologic Laparoscopists 1990 Survey. *J. Reprod. Med.*, **37**, 599–602
54. Dembo, A. J., Davy, M., Stenwig, A. E., Berle, E. J., Bush, R. S. and Kjorstad, K. (1990). Prognostic factors in patients with stage I epithelial ovarian cancer. *Obstet. Gynecol.*, **75**, 263–73
55. Nagele, F. and Magos, A. L. (1996). Combined ultrasound drainage and laparoscopic excision of a large ovarian cyst. *Am. J. Obstet. Gynecol.*, in press
56. Parker, W. and Berek, J. (1990). Management of selected cystic adnexal masses in postmenopausal women by operative laparoscopy: pilot study. *Am. J. Obstet. Gynecol.*, **163**, 1574–7
57. Canis, M., Mage, G., Pouly, J. L., Wattiez, A., Manhes, H. and Bruhat, M. A. (1994). Laparoscopic diagnosis of adnexal cystic masses: a 12 year experience with long term follow-up. *Obstet. Gynecol.*, **83**, 707–12
58. Amso, N. N., Broadbent, J. A. M., Hill, N. C. W. and Magos, A. L. (1992). Laparoscopic 'oophorectomy-in-a-bag' for removal of ovarian tumours of uncertain origin. *Gynaecol. Endosc.*, **1**, 85–9
59. Canis, M., Bassil, S., Wattiez, A., Pouly, J. L., Manhes, H., Mage, G. and Bruhat, M. A. (1992). Fertility following laparoscopic management of benign adnexal cysts. *Hum. Reprod.*, **7**, 529–31
60. Pomel, C., Provencher, D., Dauplat, J., Gauthier, P., LeBouedec, G., Drouin, P., Audet-Lapointe, P. and Dubuc-Lissoir, J. (1995). Laparoscopic staging of early ovarian cancer. *Gynaecol. Oncol.*, **58**, 301–6
61. Buttram, V. C. and Reiter, R. C. (1981). Uterine leiomyomata: etiology, symptomatiology and management. *Fertil. Steril.*, **36**, 433–45
62. Dubuisson, J. B., Lecuru, F., Foulot, H., Mandelbrot, L., Aubriot, F. X. and Mouly, M. (1991). Myomectomy by laparoscopy: a preliminary report of 43 cases. *Fertil. Steril.*, **56**, 827–30
63. Friedman, A. J., Harrison-Atlas, D., Barbieri, R. L., Benacerraf, B., Gleason, R. and Schiff, I. (1989). A randomized, placebo-controlled, double-blind study evaluating the efficacy of leuprolide acetate depot in the treatment of uterine leiomyomata. *Fertil. Steril.*, **51**, 251–6
64. Shaw, R. W. (1989). Mechanism of LHRH analogue action in uterine fibroids. *Horm. Res.*, **32** (Suppl.), 150–3
65. Hassan, H. M., Rotman, C., Ronan, N., Sistos, F. and Dmowski, W. P. (1992). Laparoscopic myomectomy. *Obstet. Gynecol.*, **80**, 884–8
66. Harris, W. J. (1992). Uterine dehiscence following laparoscopic myomectomy. *Obstet. Gynecol.*, **80**, 545–6
67. Dubuisson, J. B., Chavet, X., Chapron, C., Gregorakis, S. S. and Morice, P. (1995). Uterine rupture during pregnancy after laparoscopic myomectomy. *Hum. Reprod.*, **10**, 1475–7
68. Goldfarb, H. A. (1992). Nd:YAG laser laparoscopic coagulation of symptomatic myomas. *J. Reprod. Med.*, **37**, 636–8
69. Nisolle, M., Smets, M., Malvaux, V., Anaf, V. and Donnez, J. (1993). Laparoscopic myolysis with the Nd:YAG laser. *J. Gynecol. Surg.*, **9**, 95–9
70. Magos, A. L., Bournas, N., Sinha, R., Richardson, R. E. and O'Connor, H. (1994). Vaginal myomectomy. *Br. J. Obstet. Gynaecol.*, **101**, 1092–4
71. Marana, R., Muzii, L., Rizzi, M., dell'Acqua, S. and Mancuso, S. (1995). Prognostic role of laparoscopic salpingoscopy of the only remaining tube after contralateral ectopic pregnancy. *Fertil. Steril.*, **63**, 303–6

72. Fayez, J. A. and Schneider, P. J. (1987). Prevention of pelvic adhesion formation by different modalities of treatment. *Am. J. Obstet. Gynecol.*, **157**(5), 1184–8
73. Dlugi, A. M., Reddy, S., Saleh, W. A., Mersol-Barg, M. S. and Jacobsen, G. (1994). Pregnancy rates after operative endoscopic treatment of total (neosalpingostomy) or near total (salpingostomy) distal tubal occlusion. *Fertil. Steril.*, **62**, 913–20
74. Reich, H., De Capria, J. and McGlynn, F. (1989). Laparoscopic hysterectomy. *J. Gynecol. Surg.*, **5**, 213–16
75. Johns, D. A. (1993). Laparoscopic assisted vaginal hysterectomy (LAVH). In Sutton, C. and Diamond, M. (eds.) *Endoscopic Surgery for Gynaecologists*, pp. 179–86. (London: W. B. Saunders)
76. Richardson, R. E., Bournas, N. and Magos, A. L. (1995). Is laparoscopic hysterectomy a waste of time? *Lancet*, **345**, 36–41
77. Drife, J. (1994). Conserving the cervix at hysterectomy. *Br. J. Obstet. Gynecol.*, **101**, 563–4
78. Sutton, C. (1995). Laparoscopic hysterectomy. *Curr. Obstet. Gynecol.*, **5**, 142–6
79. Phipps, J. H., John, M. and Nayak, S. (1993). Comparison of laparoscopically assisted vaginal hysterectomy and bilateral salpingo-oophorectomy with conventional abdominal hysterectomy and bilateral salpingo-oophorectomy. *Br. J. Obstet. Gynaecol.*, **100**, 698–700
80. Raju, K. S. and Auld, B. J. (1994). A randomised prospective study of laparoscopic vaginal hysterectomy versus abdominal hysterectomy each with bilateral salpingo-oophorectomy. *Br. J. Obstet. Gynaecol.*, **101**, 1068–71
81. Summitt, R. L. Jr, Stovall, T. G., Lipscomb, G. H. and Ling, F. W. (1992). Randomized comparison of laparoscopy-assisted vaginal hysterectomy with standard vaginal hysterectomy in an out-patient setting. *Obstet. Gynecol.*, **80**, 895–901
82. Kovac, S. R. (1995). Guidelines to determine the route of hysterectomy. *Obstet. Gynecol.*, **85**, 18–23
83. Magos, A. L., Bournas, N., Sinha, R. and O'Connor, H. (1996). Vaginal hysterectomy for the large uterus. *Br. J. Obstet. Gynaecol.*, **103**, 246–51
84. Davies, A., Bournas, N., Richardson, R. E., O'Connor, H. and Magos, A. L. (1996). A prospective study to evaluate oophorectomy at the time of vaginal hysterectomy. *Br. J. Obstet. Gynaecol.*, in press
85. Nagele, F., Broadbent, M., Bournas, N., Richardson, R., O'Connor, H. and Magos, A. (1996). Comparison of carbon dioxide and normal saline for uterine distension media in out-patient hysteroscopy. *Fertil. Steril.*, **65**, 305–9
86. Magos, A. L., Baumann, R., Lockwood, G. M. and Turnbull, A. C. (1991). Experience with the first 250 endometrial resections for menhorrhagia. *Lancet*, **337**, 1074–8
87. Nagele, F., Richardson, R. E., O'Connor, H. and Magos, A. L. (1996). 2500 out-patient diagnostic hysteroscopies. *Obstet. Gynecol.*, in press
88. Baskett, T. F., O'Connor, H. and Magos, A. L. (1996). A comprehensive one-stop menstrual problem clinic for the diagnosis and management of abnormal uterine bleeding. *Br. J. Obstet. Gynaecol.*, **103**, 76–7
89. Nagele, F., Mane, S., Chandrasekaran, P., Rubinger, T. and Magos, A. L. (1996). How successful is hysteroscopic polypectomy. *Gynaecol. Endosc.*, **5**, 137–40
90. Neuwirth, R. S. and Amin, H. K. (1976). Excision of submucous fibroids with hysteroscopic control. *Am. J. Obstet. Gynecol.*, **126**, 95–9
91. Neuwirth, R. S. (1978). A new technique for and additional experience with hysteroscopic resection of submucous fibroids. *Am. J. Obstet. Gynecol.*, **131**, 91–4
92. Donnez, J., Gillerot, S., Bourgonjon, D., Clerckx, F. and Nisolle, M. (1990). Neodymium:YAG laser hysteroscopy in large submucous fibroids. *Fertil. Steril.*, **54**, 999–1003
93. Hallez, J. P., Netter, A. and Cartier, R. (1987). Methodical intrauterine resection. *Am. J. Obstet. Gynecol.*, **156**, 1080–4
94. Derman, S. G., Rehnstrom, J. and Neuwirth, R. S. (1991). The long term effectiveness of hysteroscopic treatment of menorrhagia and leiomyomas. *Obstet. Gynecol.*, **77**, 591–4
95. Hallez, J. P. (1995). Single-stage total hysteroscopic myomectomies: indications, techniques and results. *Fertil. Steril.*, **63**, 703–8
96. Broadbent, J. A. M. and Magos, A. L. (1995). Menstrual blood loss after hysteroscopic myomectomy. *Gynaecol. Endosc.*, **4**, 41–4
97. Goldenberg, M., Sivan, E., Sharabi, Z., Bider, D., Rabinovici, J. and Seidman, D. S. (1995). Outcome of hysteroscopic resection of

submucous myomas for infertility. *Fertil. Steril.*, **64**, 714–16

98. Seoud, M. A., Patterson, R., Muasher, S. J. and Coddington, C. C. 3rd (1992). Effects of myomas or prior myomectomy on *in vitro* fertilisation (IVF) performance. *J. Assist. Reprod. Genet.*, **9**, 217–21
99. Loffer, F. D. (1993). Hysteroscopic tubal occlusion. In Sutton, C. and Diamond, M. P. (eds.) *Endoscopic Surgery for Gynaecologists*, pp. 105–12. (London: W. B. Saunders)
100. Fayez, J. A. (1986). Comparison between abdominal and hysteroscopic metroplasty. *Obstet. Gynecol.*, **68**, 399–403
101. March, C. M. and Israel, R. (1987). Hysteroscopic management of recurrent abortion caused by septate uterus. *Am. J. Obstet. Gynecol.*, **156**, 834–42
102. Elchalal, U. and Schenker, J. G. (1994). Hysteroscopic resection of uterus septus versus abdominal metroplasty. *J. Am. Coll. Surg.*, **178**, 637–44
103. Halvorson, L. M., Askerkoff, R. D. and Oskowitz, S. P. (1993). Spontaneous uterine rupture after hysteroscopic metroplasty with uterine perforation. A case report. *J. Reprod. Med.*, **38**, 236–8
104. Vercellini, P., Fedele, L., Arcaini, L., Rognoni, M. T. and Candiani, G. B. (1989). Value of intrauterine device insertion and estrogen administration after hysteroscopic metroplasty. *J. Reprod. Med.*, **34**, 447–50
105. Valle, R. F. and Sciarra, J. J. (1988). Intrauterine adhesions: hysteroscopic diagnosis, classification treatment and reproductive outcome. *Am. J. Obstet. Gynecol.*, **158**, 1459–70
106. Goldrath, M. H., Fuller, T. A. and Segal, S. (1981). Laser photovaporization of endometrium for the treatment of menorrhagia. *Am. J. Obstet. Gynecol.*, **140**, 14–19
107. DeCherney, A. H. and Polan, M. L. (1983). Hysteroscopic management of intrauterine lesions and intractable uterine bleeding. *Obstet. Gynecol.*, **61**, 392–7
108. Magos, A. L., Baumann, R. and Turnbull, A. C. (1989). Transcervical resection of the endometrium in women with menorrhagia. *Br. Med. J.*, **298**, 1209–12
109. Vancaillie, T. G. (1989). Electrocoagulation of the endometrium with the ball-end resectoscope. *Obstet. Gynecol.*, **74**, 425–7
110. Duffy, S., Reid, P. C., Smith, J. H. F. and Sharp, F. (1991). *In vitro* studies of uterine electrosurgery. *Obstet. Gynecol.*, **78**, 213–20
111. Duffy, S., Reid, P. C. and Sharp, F. (1992). *In vivo* studies of uterine electrosurgery. *Br. J. Obstet. Gynaecol.*, **99**, 579–82
112. O'Connor, H. and Magos, A. L. (1996). Endometrial resection for the treatment of menorrhagia. *N. Engl. J. Med.*, **335**, 151–6
113. O'Connor, H., Broadbent, M., Richardson, R., Bournas, N. and Magos, A. (1994). Interim reort on the Medical Research Council trial of transcervical resection of the endometrium vs. hysterectomy in the treatment of menorrhagia. Presented at the *European Congress of Gynecologic Endoscopic Surgery*, June, Rome, Italy
114. Dwyer, N., Hutton, J. and Stirrat, G. M. (1993). Randomised controlled trial comparing endometrial resection with abdominal hysterectomy for the surgical treatment of menorrhagia. *Br. J. Obstet. Gynaecol.*, **100**, 237–43
115. Pinion, S. B., Parkin, D. E., Abramovich, D. R., Naji, A., Alexander, D. A., Russell, I. T. and Kitchener, H. C. (1994). Randomised trial of hysterectomy, endometrial laser ablation, and transcervical endometrial resection for dysfunctional uterine bleeding. *Br. Med. J.*, **309**, 979–83
116. Sculpher, M. J., Dwyer, N., Byford, S. and Stirrat, G. M. (1996). Randomised trial comparing hysterectomy and transcervical endometrial resection: effect on health related quality of life and costs two years after surgery. *Br. J. Obstet. Gynaecol.*, **103**, 142–9
117. Sculpher, M. J., Bryan, S., Dwyer, N., Hutton, J. and Stirrat, G. M. (1993). An economic evaluation of transcervical endometrial resection versus abdominal hysterectomy for the treatment of menorrhagia. *Br. J. Obstet. Gynaecol.*, **100**, 244–52

# Menorrhagia and dysfunctional uterine bleeding

# 26

*David A. Viniker*

## INTRODUCTION

Excessive menstrual blood loss can be a debilitating problem causing more than the usual inconvenience of menstruation and at times it can lead to social embarrassment. Modern couples in western society generally limit their family size by the use of effective contraception, such as the combined oral contraceptive pill, which has only been available for a few decades. With a reduction in the number of pregnancies and a tendency to less breast feeding, a woman can now expect to see a nine-fold increase in the number of menstrual cycles in her lifetime when compared to earlier generations[1]. Menorrhagia (from the Greek: men, month + rhegnunai, to burst forth), or heavy periods, is a common problem; one woman in 20, aged 25–44, attends her general practitioner each year for this problem[2]. Heavy periods may be associated with:

(1) Pelvic pathology, e.g. congenital uterine anomaly, endometrial polyps, fibroids, endometriosis;

(2) Traditional intrauterine contraceptive devices;

(3) Medical problems, e.g. coagulation abnormality, hypothyroidism;

(4) Unexplained – dysfunctional uterine bleeding.

There is no difference in the bleeding pattern of women undergoing laparoscopic sterilization, when compared to women whose husbands have had a vasectomy[3]. Women may have heavy menstruation suppressed by the combined oral contraceptive pill; when they stop taking the pill, following sterilization of either partner, they may then report increased menstrual flow.

## ASSESSMENT OF MENSTRUAL LOSS

The diagnosis of dysfunctional uterine bleeding is reached after taking a full history and examination and carrying out appropriate investigations. From a routine clinical point of view the diagnosis of heavy periods is assumed from the patient's history. Generally, the patient is aware of an increase in flow using her own experience as the reference. Normally, the menstrual blood clots in the uterus and is then broken down by fibrinolysins to produce the characteristic fluid loss. Fibrinolytic activity in the uterus is increased in patients with dysfunctional uterine bleeding[4]. When the flow is excessive, blood passes into the vagina where it coagulates and results in the patient observing a change from a fluid loss to blood clots. An increase in the requirements of sanitary wear and the need for extra protection are further indicators of increased flow, although the number of pads used and measured blood loss show no direct correlation[5].

Laboratory methods of measuring menstrual loss require collection of sanitary wear and an extraction procedure such as the alkaline haematin method. This is unpleasant for patients and staff so that it has only found a place in units undertaking research. Modifications to improve the accuracy of the haematin method have been described[6]. From the classic studies of Hallberg and colleagues[7] and Cole and associates[8], a loss of greater than 80 ml each period tends to be associated with iron deficiency anaemia and this is regarded as excessive loss. Many women are not aware that they have heavy periods. In a group of 20 women with iron deficiency anaemia, only three reported heavy menstrual loss. Measurement of menstrual loss with the alkaline haematin method demonstrated heavy loss in 12 of these women (296 ± 45 ml per cycle)[9]. Serum ferritin concentrations are reduced in patients with menorrhagia, although haemoglobin concentration and mean corpuscular volume may be maintained[10]. Some women presenting with a complaint of heavy periods may have relatively little menstrual disturbance but a tendency to depression[11].

In a study to establish the relationship between blood and total fluid loss during menstruation, 28 volunteers collected all their sanitary wear on a daily basis throughout one menstrual period. The percentage contribution of blood to the total fluid volume loss varied greatly from individual to individual. The mean blood loss to total volume loss was 36.1% with a range from 1.6–81.7%[12]. The ratio for an individual remained stable for each day. It would seem probable that some of the debilitating symptoms reported by some patients may relate to the total fluid loss rather than to just blood loss alone.

Scientific assessment of menstrual loss has demonstrated a remarkable variation between an individual woman's assessment of her loss compared to objective measurement[5,13]. A variety of methods have been used to enhance the evaluation of a patient's menstrual loss. A vaginally placed latex seal has been described to determine suitability in women with normal and heavy flow. It proved to be simple to insert but unacceptably 'messy' to remove and it did not adequately control menstrual blood loss[14]. Accurate determination of blood loss is essential when conducting trials to evaluate the efficacy of menorrhagia therapy. A pictorial blood loss assessment chart provides an objective, cheap and acceptably accurate method for assessing menstrual blood loss in clinical practice[15,16].

Patients with menorrhagia should have a full blood count including a blood film. This will show evidence of anaemia with a microcytic picture if there is iron deficiency. Iron deficiency may sometimes be confirmed by serum ferritin levels but this should not be a routine investigation. A coagulation screen is indicated if the history suggests a tendency to bruise or bleed excessively.

## DYSFUNCTIONAL UTERINE BLEEDING

Although dysfunctional uterine bleeding is generally regarded as unexplained menorrhagia, there have been a variety of hypotheses put forward. The majority of patients are anovulatory or have abnormal local production of prostaglandins. The concept of increased endometrial surface area has been refuted[13]. Daily measurements of follicle stimulating hormone (FSH), luteinizing hormone (LH), oestradiol and progesterone in women with proven menstrual flow greater than 80 ml, and in a control group of women with normal loss have shown no relationship between ovarian and pituitary hormones and menstrual loss[17].

The vascular ultrastructure of the endometrium appears abnormal in patients with dysfunctional uterine bleeding[18]. There is evidence of increased prostaglandin E receptors in the endometrium of patients with dysfunctional uterine bleeding[19] and abnormal uptake of prostaglandin precursor by endometrial cells in patients with menorrhagia[20]. Endometrial concentrations of prostaglandins are increased in patients with dysfunctional uterine bleeding[21,22]. Endothelins, which have powerful vasoconstrictive activity, have been identified in the human endometrium and probably play an important role in the regulation of menstrual flow[23].

Dysfunctional uterine bleeding is more common in the first cycles after the menarche and the last cycles before the menopause[24]; these cycles are typically anovulatory.

Traditionally, the endometrium has been evaluated by dilatation of the cervix and curettage of the endometrium (D & C). This procedure is essentially diagnostic rather than therapeutic, unless there are endometrial polyps that can be avulsed. The most important function of the D & C has been the exclusion of premalignant or malignant pathology. Typically, endometrial malignancy presents with irregular bleeding rather than regular heavy bleeding. Endometrial curettage is associated with a reduction in measured blood flow in the following period but this improvement is not sustained[25]. It has been recognized that there are few indications for D & C in women under the age of 40, although the exceptions include failure of uterine bleeding to respond to medical therapy or persistent intermenstrual bleeding[26].

Direct visualization of the endometrial cavity with the hysteroscope enhances diagnostic accuracy and facilitates directed endometrial biopsy. Approximately half the women who are thought to have dysfunctional uterine bleeding clinically prove to have organic disease[27].

Endometrial sampling in the office environment has become more popular with the development of disposable instruments such as the Pipelle (Figure 1). The accuracy of endometrial samples with the Pipelle has been reported to be equivalent to the traditional Novak curette[28,29] but others have recorded occasional failure of the Pipelle to pick up hyperplasia[30]. In one study of 37 women known to have endometrial carcinoma, there was a 33% failure to detect the tumour with the Pipelle[31] so that caution should be exercised. Patients find the Pipelle less painful than the Novak curette[28,29] but 50% report delayed dysmenorrhoea-type pain starting 2–3 h after the procedure and persisting for 2 or 3 h which may require mild analgesia[32].

Ultrasound scanning of the pelvic organs, increasingly undertaken with the vaginal probe, often provides valuable information (Chapter 13). Structural abnormalities of the uterus were identified in 31% of a series of patients with heavy periods compared to 9% identified by clinical examination; evidence of anovulation could also be detected[33]. Vaginal ultrasonography may provide useful guidance in planning treatment[34].

## MEDICAL TREATMENT

### Combined oral contraceptive pill

It is a frequent observation that progestogens in combination with oestrogens, generally prescribed as oral contraceptive pills, significantly reduce menstrual flow, although there are surprisingly few studies in the literature[35–37]. In a group of 164 women with a mean blood loss of 157 ml before treatment, menstrual loss was reduced to a mean loss of 74.7 ml with treatment but rapidly returned to pretreatment levels once the pill was withdrawn[36].

### Progestogens

Progestogens are frequently prescribed for menorrhagia. When there is evidence of anovulation or endometrial hyperplasia, progestogens can be beneficial[38–40] but when there is evidence of ovulation, the efficacy of progestogens to reduce blood loss is generally considered to be limited. There have been reports of reduction in measured menstrual blood loss in ovulatory and anovulatory women with dysfunctional uterine bleeding[39]. Others have reported an increased flow in association with progestogen therapy[40]. Norethisterone is associated with a reduction in oestradiol, FSH, LH, sex hormone binding globulin (SHBG) and high density lipoprotein (HDL) cholesterol; micronized progesterone has less effect on biochemistry and has been advocated for premenopausal bleeding disorders[38]. Cyclical progestogens undoubtedly have a role to play in the management of intermenstrual bleeding and irregular menstruation.

The endometrium shows an atrophic pattern in oral contraceptive users and this must be associated with the low-dose progestogen which is taken for 21 days with a 7-day gap. The oestrogen in the pill suppresses endogenous oestrogen production. It would be interesting to know whether low-dose progestogens, taken days 5–26 of the cycle without oestrogen administration, would be effective. In one small study[39], ten ovulatory women received norethisterone 5 mg t.d.s. from days 5–26 of the

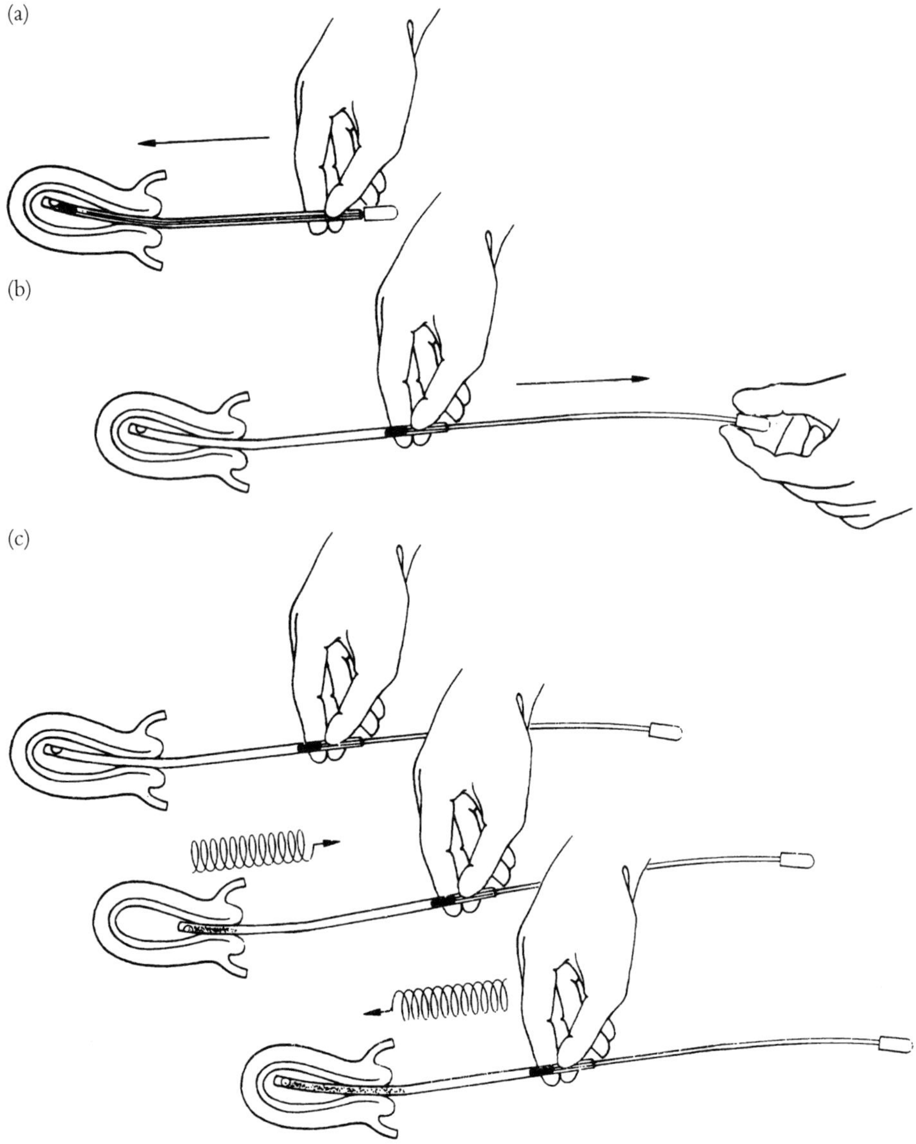


**Figure 1** Endometrial sampling with the Pipelle. (a) With piston fully advanced within sheath, insert Pipelle through cervical canal into uterine cavity until resistance is felt. (Prior determination of uterine depth and direction with a uterine sound is recommended); (b) while holding sheath, pull piston back completely and without interruption to proximal piston stop, thus creating maximum negative pressure within sheath. Leave piston fully retracted; (c) simultaneously roll (twirl) sheath between fingers while moving sheath laterally and back and forth (in and out) between the fundus and internal os three or four times to obtain sample

menstrual cycle. Menstrual blood loss was reduced from 113 ml to 71 ml. Although such regimens are mentioned in the literature, there have been no major studies. It may be that irregular bleeding might be a problem as endogenous oestrogen would not be suppressed.

### Tranexamic acid

Fibrinolytic activity in the uterus of women with dysfunctional uterine bleeding is reduced by tranexamic acid (Cyklokapron®, Pharmacia) administration[41]. Reduction in blood loss of 58% has been reported[42] and heavy periods can be reduced to normal[40]. In a comparison of tranexamic acid with the prostaglandin synthesis inhibitor diclofenac sodium, tranexamic acid provided better blood loss reduction but was associated more frequently with side-effects[43].

The pharmacodynamics of tranexamic acid are such that frequent administration varying from 1 to 1.5 g 6–8 hourly is recommended. An ester prodrug of tranexamic acid (Kabi 2161) is under investigation. Initial results show good patient tolerance and effect with just twice daily administration[44].

### Prostaglandin synthetase inhibitors

Mefenamic acid, a prostaglandin synthetase inhibitor, significantly reduces excessive menstrual blood loss[21,22,45]. The mechanisms of action by which mefenamic acid is effective in reducing heavy periods may be by increased platelet aggregation and vasoconstriction as well as in the reduction of local endometrial prostaglandin concentrations[46]. Blood loss is reduced by about 40% with mefenamic acid 500 mg three times daily during menstruation[46], although with severe menorrhagia the reduction in blood loss may be greater[47].

Danazol 100 mg twice daily for 60 days was found to be more efficacious than mefenamic acid 500 mg three times daily during menstruation in terms of blood loss reduction but adverse side-effects were less common with the mefenamic acid[41]. Tranexamic acid has proven to be more effective in reducing heavy menstrual flow than flurbiprofen[48], another prostaglandin synthetase inhibitor. The clinical value of prostaglandin inhibitors in the management of menstrual disturbance lies not only in reducing blood loss but also in controlling dysmenorrhoea which often accompanies menorrhagia.

Mefenamic acid 500 mg three times daily during menstruation or norethisterone 5 mg twice daily from the 19th to the 26th day of the cycle was randomly allocated to 32 women with ovulatory menorrhagia[49]. The duration of the period was reduced by the mefenamic acid only but otherwise the two regimens proved equally beneficial.

### Gonadotrophin releasing hormone agonists

Long-acting gonadotrophin releasing hormones, after an initial flare of increased endogenous gonadotrophin, depress FSH, LH and subsequently oestrogen. Gonadotrophin releasing hormone (GnRH) agonists have been shown to produce amenorrhoea in patients with severe menorrhagia, allowing their haematological indices to return to normal[50] and avoiding the need for blood transfusion. The temporary hypogonadism induced by GnRH analogues is likely to be associated with unacceptable side-effects for some patients. Cyclical hormone replacement therapy (HRT) in combination with GnRH analogues increases patient acceptability[51], although economic considerations may at this time limit the use of GnRH for dysfunctional uterine bleeding. From a theoretical point of view, GnRH agonists could be used with continuous combined HRT. Howell and her colleagues[52] have reported that GnRH used in combination with continuous combined HRT over 20 weeks for the treatment of endometriosis had no deleterious effect on treatment but there were less adverse hypo-oestrogenic problems.

### Hormone replacement therapy

The author would agree with Rees[53] that many patients in their menopausal years, presenting with oestrogen deficiency symptoms and also heavy periods, report improvement in their menses with cyclical HRT. It is probably the cyclical administration of progestogen in the HRT that is improving the periods in the anovulatory cycles before the menopause.

These patients require investigation of the endometrium before commencing hormonal therapy. Whilst we are not aware of any objective studies evaluating menstrual blood loss with HRT in premenopausal women, measurement of withdrawal bleeds in postmenopausal women on cyclical HRT has demonstrated median blood loss of less than 30 ml but 13% of patients had heavy loss (> 80 ml blood loss per cycle)[54].

### Danazol

Danazol is a gonadotrophin releasing inhibitor and suppresses ovulation and reduces oestradiol concentrations. Fertility may not be completely suppressed and a barrier method should be recommended. Evaluation of danazol 100 or 200 mg taken daily, in the luteal phase or during menstruation showed that the 200 mg daily regimen proved to be clinically the most appropriate; by the 3rd month, blood loss was reduced from a mean of 183 ml to 26 ml. Although a dose of 100 mg daily proved to reduce flow, many patients had irregular bleeding[55]. Others have confirmed a significant fall in blood loss with danazol 200 mg daily but considered that the side-effects of treatment would limit its use for long-term treatment[56].

### Gestrinone

Gestrinone 2.5 mg twice weekly inhibits gonadotrophin release and is marketed for the treatment of endometriosis. It has been demonstrated to reduce menstrual flow significantly[57] but it is expensive.

### Ethamsylate

Ethamsylate is believed to maintain capillary integrity, possibly by reducing prostaglandin synthesis. Ethamsylate produced a similar reduction in blood loss to mefenamic acid in one double-blind trial[58]. The benefits with ethamsylate gradually increased with time and there were fewer side-effects with this agent.

## LEVONORGESTREL-RELEASING INTRAUTERINE CONTRACEPTIVE DEVICE

The levonorgestrel-releasing intrauterine contraceptive device (Mirena®, Pharmacia-Leiras) has been developed primarily for contraception. This new device has the benefit of being associated with a significantly reduced menstrual blood loss. The reduction in menstrual flow with Mirena proved to be significantly greater than with tranexamic acid or flurbiprofen, a prostaglandin synthetase inhibitor[59]. There may be initial spotting but this settles within a few weeks. Patient acceptance seems high and the device would seem to be a valuable alternative for the treatment of dysfunctional uterine bleeding in women who do not wish to have a hysterectomy[60]. We have found that several women have chosen this device as treatment of dysfunctional uterine bleeding. It can be introduced in the clinic or at completion of hysteroscopy and D & C. Most patients tolerate initial spotting but this can be a problem particularly if spotting precludes sexual activity for personal or cultural reasons.

## SURGICAL TREATMENT

### Hysterectomy

For more than a generation, the definitive surgical treatment of dysfunctional uterine bleeding for a woman who has completed her family has been hysterectomy. Abdominal hysterectomy has been the most popular route, although many have advocated vaginal hysterectomy even in the absence of prolapse. In the United States 625 000 hysterectomies are performed annually[61].

In the UK, 90 000 women have a hysterectomy each year. Following hysterectomy with conservation of the ovaries, Siddle and coworkers[62] found that the mean age of ovarian failure is brought forward by an average of 6 years. There has been increasing evidence that ovarian function fails relatively early if hysterectomy is undertaken with ovarian conservation[63]. The risk of a woman developing ovarian carcinoma if the ovaries are conserved is 1 in 250. One woman in 20 undergoing hysterectomy with adnexal conservation will require subsequent oophorectomy for pain.

Following bilateral oophorectomy, there is a need for HRT. Women electing to have hysterectomy with ovarian conservation should be encouraged to have regular hormone studies at yearly intervals to detect evidence of ovarian failure rather than to await symptoms. Using a comprehensive mathematical model, it has been hypothesized that bilateral oophorectomy may have a substantial protective effect on breast cancer risk, even allowing for the possible risks of HRT. Women with a family history of ovarian or breast cancer undergoing hysterectomy should therefore seriously consider bilateral oophorectomy when undergoing hysterectomy[64].

All women with pelvic pain should be offered bilateral salpingo-oophorectomy at the time of hysterectomy, particularly in the presence of endometriosis or pelvic inflammatory disease. Ultimately, it must be for the informed woman to make her choice but, from the medical point of view, oophorectomy with hormone replacement would seem to be justifiable[63].

It has been estimated that 20% of British women will have had a hysterectomy by the age of 55[65]. Despite thousands of procedures with minimally invasive surgery, there has been no obvious reduction in the numbers of hysterectomies being performed, suggesting that many endometrial ablations and resections are additional procedures rather than replacing hysterectomy[66].

There has been debate about the psychological effects of hysterectomy and this has been intensified with the arrival of minimal access surgery. In a carefully conducted randomized trial of 204 women with dysfunctional uterine bleeding, 99 were allocated to hysterectomy, 52 to transcervical resection and 53 to laser ablation of the endometrium[67]. No evidence was found to suggest that hysterectomy leads to psychiatric illness. Increased sexual interest was reported by 50 women and 46 had reduced sexual interest, with no obvious differences between the groups.

We should also recognize that there is a tendency to reduce hospitalization following traditional major abdominal surgery. Many maternity units are now discharging mothers by the 4th day following Caesarean section and these women have a baby to cope with as well as their own post-operative recovery. In the United states, medical insurance companies are 'encouraging' discharge from hospital within 48 h of Caesarean section; such recommendations after abdominal hysterectomy are likely to follow. At Whipps Cross Hospital, we have recently started to introduce 'hospital-at-home' care. Patients can be discharged home usually 48 h after major gynaecological surgery and they are seen daily as required by one of our nurses.

Supravaginal hysterectomy reduces the operating time and has been reported to be associated with better sexual satisfaction than total abdominal hysterectomy[68]. In the UK, we have traditionally followed the course of total abdominal hysterectomy. The arguments in favour of removing the cervix have been as follows:

(1) There is a substantial risk of cervical cancer;

(2) The cervix may continue to produce symptoms including pain and discharge;

(3) Increased chance of pelvic haematoma;

(4) Increased risk of vault prolapse.

Nwosu and Atlay[69] have found counter-arguments to all these points and believe that subtotal hysterectomy is associated with less damage to the urinary and gastrointestinal tracts and patients enjoy greater sexual satisfaction. From his extensive experience with minimally invasive surgery, Sutton[70] now considers subtotal hysterectomy to be a more logical approach, as retaining the cervix but removing the transformation zone reduces the chance of damage to the urinary tract and results in little or no impairment of sexual satisfaction.

### Hysterectomy or minimally invasive surgery?

If patients are advised before admission, that they can expect to be discharged within 2 or 3 days of abdominal hysterectomy, all domestic arrangements can be planned accordingly. This is consistent with the current trend towards reduced hospitalization[71]. Many patients requiring hysterectomy are suitable for minilaparotomy and the majority of these can safely be discharged within 48 h[72]. The economic argument may yet tilt back in favour of traditional surgery rather than the newer techniques.

A full discussion of minimally invasive surgery is presented in Chapter 25. In an environment that seems to be veering increasingly towards economic consideration, comparison of the costs of the new surgical techniques would suggest that they may have a slight advantage. Even with relatively short follow-up, however, it is becoming apparent that a significant number of patients undergoing transcervical resection require further surgery, thereby reducing the apparent financial benefit[73,74]. In a randomized trial comparing hysterectomy with transcervical endometrial resection, the effect on health-related quality of life at an average of 2.8 years after surgery was evaluated. Women randomized to hysterectomy had better scores in seven out of eight parameters, with the greatest difference being for pain. Of those randomized to endometrial resection, 12% had a repeat procedure and 16% came to hysterectomy, so that 28% had sufficient problems to require a second surgical procedure. In general, there was superior health-related quality of life amongst hysterectomy patients[75]. Laparoscopic hysterectomy may reduce postoperative pain and convalescent time but increases the operative time by 1 h[76].

We are now faced not only with the difficult prospect of comparing the new techniques with the gold standard of hysterectomy but also trying to compare the various new techniques with each other. Furthermore, there are new developments appearing almost annually and some may prove to be simple to use. Neuwirth and colleagues[77], for example, have described a latex balloon which can be introduced transcervically into the uterine cavity. The balloon houses a shielded heating element which raises the temperature of the fluid in the balloon to 92°C.

## MENORRHAGIA: INVESTIGATION AND TREATMENT GUIDELINES

### Investigation

Figure 2 is a flowchart outlining the investigation and treatment of menorrhagia. We take a conventional history in the clinic with the benefit of a proforma. Special attention is given to the effect that the menstrual disturbance is having on the patient's lifestyle and the response to any previous treatment. It should be possible to establish early whether the patient is seeking reduction in her menstrual loss or just reassurance that there is no serious pathology. Details of the obstetric history, future fertility requirements and family planning are recorded together with a general medical history. General and pelvic examination are performed.

A full blood count is requested and a ferrous preparation prescribed if there is a suggestion of iron deficiency. Ultrasound of the pelvis is commonly performed and often provides reassurance for the patient that her pelvic organs are normal. It may be advantageous to schedule the ultrasound examination for the 12th day of the cycle to establish normal follicular development. Ultrasound is of particular value in young or obese patients.

On occasion, LH and FSH estimations in the mid-follicular phase may be requested as indicators for polycystic ovary syndrome or impending menopause, respectively, and a progesterone estimation between 4 and 10 days before an expected period may indicate anovulation. Thyroid function tests are of little value in the routine investigation of menorrhagia but they should be considered if there is other clinical evidence of thyroid dysfunction. Coagulation screening should be considered in young

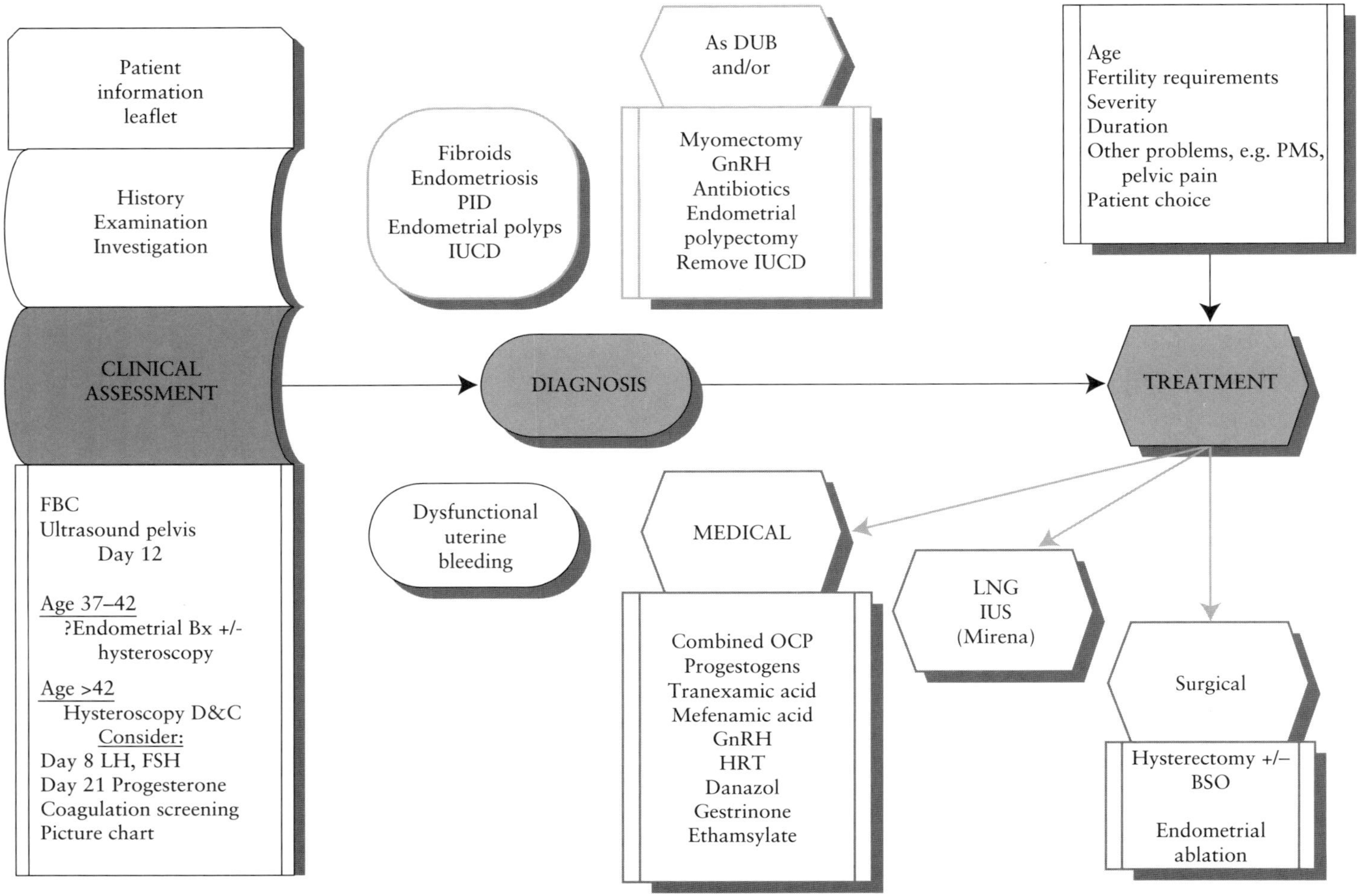


**Figure 2** Flowchart for the investigation and treatment of menorrhagia. FBC = full blood count; D & C = dilatation and curettage; LH = luteinizing hormone; FSH = follicle-stimulating hormone; PID = pelvic inflammatory disease; IUCD = intrauterine contraceptive device; DUB = dysfunctional uterine bleeding; GnRH = gonadotrophin releasing hormone; OCP = oral contraceptive pill; HRT = hormone replacement therapy; PMS = premenstrual syndrome; LNG = levonorgestrel; IUS = intrauterine system; BSO, bilateral salpingo-oophorectomy

patients and any woman with a tendency to bleeding or bruising problems. Picture charts undoubtedly reflect blood loss and may be helpful with some patients. However, the symptoms of excess flow reported by some patients may be due to fluid that is only in part blood and in this respect such charts may not fully reflect patients' difficulties.

There has been a trend to reduce the indications for cervical dilatation and endometrial curettage in gynaecological investigation. Some patients still believe that it has a therapeutic 'cleansing' effect. However, unless there are endometrial polyps which can be avulsed at the time of curettage, D & C should be recognized as being purely a diagnostic procedure. Endometrial biopsy or curettage in the second half of the menstrual cycle allows assessment of ovulation as indicated by secretory changes. Hysteroscopy enhances diagnostic accuracy. There is probably no value in submitting younger women to D & C and the age of 40 years has become a useful criterion. Depending on the severity and duration of the problem and response to medical treatment, we tend to consider outpatient endometrial biopsy from approximately age 37 and invariably hysteroscopy with D & C from age 42. Managerial and contract guidelines are increasingly influencing clinical practice but there must remain an appreciation for clinical judgement.

### Treatment

Treatment is dependent on the underlying diagnosis and will be influenced by the age, fertility requirements, severity and duration of the menorrhagia. Concurrent problems such as premenstrual syndrome and pelvic pain may influence clinical advice but ultimately much will depend on patient choice.

Dysfunctional uterine bleeding will generally respond to medical treatment. For younger women, the combined oral contraceptive pill is frequently a valuable first choice, particularly when there is a need for contraception. Adolescent girls frequently have anovulatory cycles and luteal phase progestogens may be favoured by parents who have reservations about the pill. Tranexamic acid 1–1.5 g three or four times daily, to be taken either as required or on the usual heavy period days, is otherwise a reliable first choice. Accompanying dysmenorrhoea would indicate a non-steroidal anti-inflammatory agent which may have analgesic as well as flow-reducing properties; mefanamic acid 500 mg three times daily is a popular selection. Irregular, heavy periods may respond to progestogens, particularly at the extremes of the reproductive years. When ovulation is thought to be occurring, we find that progestogens administered from day 5 to day 26 of the menstrual cycle may be effective. Older women with heavy periods and menopausal symptoms often report improvement of their periods when introduced to cyclical hormone replacement therapy.

Gonadotrophin releasing hormone agonists are expensive and cannot be used for more than a few months; they should be considered before myomectomy or hysterectomy when there is significant anaemia and blood transfusion is unacceptable to the patient. Danazol can be effective but side-effects are common which reduces patient compliance.

The levonorgestrel intrauterine system provides effective contraception and reduction of menstrual flow. It provides an alternative to conventional intrauterine contraceptive devices when they are associated with menstrual problems. The levonorgestrel intrauterine system offers an additional choice when medical treatments fail and surgical options are not appropriate although at the time of writing, this intrauterine system is only licensed for contraception.

Hysterectomy has been the treatment of choice for women with menorrhagia who have completed their family and for whom medical treatment fails to suffice. In the presence of uterine prolapse, vaginal hysterectomy and pelvic floor repair may solve two problems. Some schools have advocated the vaginal approach, even in the absence of uterine descent, and, for those with an interest in minimally invasive surgery, laparoscopically assisted vaginal hysterectomy may have a place. Destruction of the endometrium by laser ablation, resection or other methods accommodates those who wish to have surgical treatment whilst conserving the uterus.

Fibroids and endometriosis are discussed elsewhere (Chapters 21 and 22). Fibroids, endometriosis or an intrauterine contraceptive device may be found in association with menorrhagia but we should not necessarily assume that they are unequivocally the cause of increased menstrual flow in every patient. Submucous fibroids are more likely to be the cause of menorrhagia than subserous fibroids, so that myomectomy, for these latter fibroids, is less likely to resolve the problem. When an apparent causative factor is found, skilled judgement may be required in deciding whether to recommend specific treatment such as myomectomy, or GnRH agonist therapy for endometriosis. The other option would be to employ treatment regimens described for dysfunctional uterine bleeding.

Patient information leaflets should be provided to enhance patient understanding of investigation and treatment options. Gynaecologists are learning to accept change in their clinical practice at an unprecedented rate. We each have our personal preferences which result from a combination of education, subspecialty interests and inherent skills. The current trend towards a consultant-based service is likely to lead to an increase in subspecialization. We must ensure that our patients are provided with relevant contemporary information so that they can make an informed choice from the full set of options available to them (Chapter 2). There is a need for systematic reviews on the treatment of menstrual disorders and the formation of a Cochrane collaborative review group addressing this issue is to be welcomed[78].

## REFERENCES


1. Short, R. V. (1976). The evolution of human reproduction. *Proc. R. Soc. London B*, **195**, 3–24
2. Anonymous (1994). Surgical management of menorrhagia. *Drug Ther. Bull.*, **32**, 70–2
3. Sapire, K. E. and Davey, D. A. (1980). The effect of sterilization by bipolar cautery and falope ring on menstrual bleeding patterns. *S. Afr. Med. J.*, **58**, 889–90
4. Dockeray, C. J., Sheppard, B. L., Daly, L. and Bonnar, J. (1987). The fibrinolytic enzyme system in normal menstruation and excessive uterine bleeding and the effect of tranexamic acid. *Eur. J. Obstet. Gynaecol. Reprod. Biol.*, **24**, 309–18
5. Fraser, I. S., McCarron, G. and Markham, R. (1984). A preliminary study of factors influencing perception of menstrual blood loss volume. *Am. J. Obstet. Gynecol.*, **149**, 788–93
6. van Eijkeren, M. A., Scholten, P. C., Christiaens, G. C., Alsbach, G. P. and Haspels, A. A. (1986). The alkaline hematin method for measuring menstrual blood loss – a modification and its clinical use in menorrhagia. *Eur. J. Obstet. Gynaecol. Reprod. Biol.*, **22**, 345–51
7. Hallberg, L., Hogdahl, A. M., Nilsson, L. and Rybo, G. (1966). Menstrual blood loss – a population study. Variation at different ages and attempts to define normality. *Acta Obstet. Gynecol. Scand.*, **45**, 320–51
8. Cole, S. K., Billewicz, W. Z. and Thompson, A. M. (1971). Sources of variation in menstrual blood loss. *J. Obstet. Gynaecol. Br. Commwlth.*, **78**, 933–9
9. McKenna, D. M., Dockeray, C. J. and McCann, S. R. (1989). Iron deficiency in premenopausal females. *Ir. Med. J.*, **82**, 69–70
10. Lewis, G. J. (1982). Do women with menorrhagia need iron? *Br. Med. J.*, **284**, 1158
11. Greenberg, M. (1983). The meaning of menorrhagia: an investigation into the association between the complaint of menorrhagia and depression. *J. Psychosom. Res.*, **27**, 209–14
12. Fraser, I. S., McCarron, G., Markham, R. and Resta, T. (1985). Blood and total fluid content of menstrual discharge. *Obstet. Gynecol.*, **65**, 194–8
13. Chimbira, T. H., Anderson, A. B. and Turnbull, A. C. (1980). Relation between measured blood loss and patient's subjective assessment of loss, duration of bleeding, number of sanitary towels used, uterine weight and endometrial surface area. *Br. J. Obstet. Gynaecol.*, **87**, 603–9
14. Gleeson, N., Devitt, M., Buggy, F. and Bonnar, J. (1993). Menstrual blood loss measurement with gynaeseal. *Aust. N. Z. J. Obstet. Gynaecol.*, **33**, 79–80

15. Higham, J. M., O'Brien, P. M. and Shaw, R. W. (1990). Assessment of menstrual loss using a pictorial chart. *Br. J. Obstet. Gynaecol.*, **97**, 734–9
16. Janssen, C. A., Scholten, P. C. and Heintz, A. P. (1995). A simple visual assessment technique to discriminate between menorrhagia and normal menstrual blood loss. *Obstet. Gynecol.*, **85**, 977–82
17. Eldred, J. M. and Thomas, E. J. (1994). Pituitary and ovarian hormone levels in unexplained menorrhagia. *Obstet. Gynecol.*, **84**, 775–8
18. Hourihan, H. M., Sheppard, B. L. and Bonnar, J. (1989). The morphologic characteristics of menstrual hemostasis in patients with unexplained menorrhagia. *Int. J. Gynecol. Pathol.*, 8, 221–9
19. Adelantado, J. M., Rees, M. C., Lopez Bernal, A. and Turnbull, A. C. (1988). Increased uterine prostaglandin E receptors in menorrhagic women. *Br. J. Obstet. Gynaecol.*, **95**, 162–5
20. Downing, I., Hutchon, D. J. and Poyser, N. L. (1983). Uptake of [$^3$H]-arachidonic acid by human endometrium. Differences between normal and menorrhagic tissue. *Prostaglandins*, **26**, 55–69
21. Haynes, P. J., Flint, A. P., Hodgson, H., Anderson, A. B., Dray, F. and Turnbull, A. C. (1980). Studies in menorrhagia: (a) mefanamic acid, (b) endometrial prostaglandin concentrations. *Int. J. Gynaecol. Obstet.*, **17**, 567–72
22. Tsang, B. K., Domingo, M. T., Spence, J. E., Garner, P. R., Dudley, D. K. and Oxorn, H. (1987). Endometrial prostaglandins and menorrhagia: influence of a prostaglandin synthetase inhibitor *in vivo*. *Can. J. Physiol. Pharmacol.*, **65**, 2081–4
23. Cameron, I. T., Plumpton, C., Champeney, R., van Papendorp, C., Ashy, M. J. and Davenport, A. P. (1993). Identification of endothelin-1, endothelin-2 and endothelin-3 in human endometrium. *J. Reprod. Fertil.*, **98**, 251–5
24. Wilbush, J. (1988). Menorrhagia and menopause: a historical review. *Maturitas*, **10**, 5–26
25. Haynes, P. J., Hodgson, H., Anderson, A. B. and Turnbull, A. C. (1977). Measurement of menstrual blood loss in patients complaining of menorrhagia. *Br. J. Obstet. Gynaecol.*, **84**, 763–8
26. RCOG Guidelines (1994). *In-patient Treatment – D & C in Women Age 40 or Less.* (London: Royal College of Obstetricians and Gynaecologists)
27. Fraser, I.S. (1990). Hysteroscopy and laparoscopy in women with menorrhagia. *Am. J. Obstet. Gynecol.*, **165**, 1264–9
28. Silver, M. M., Miles, P. and Rosa, C. (1991). Comparison of Novak and Pipelle endometrial biopsy instruments. *Obstet. Gynecol.*, **78**, 828–30
29. Stovall, T. G., Ling, F. W. and Morgan, P. L. (1991). A prospective, randomized comparison of the Pipelle endometrial sampling device with the Novak curette. *Am. J. Obstet. Gynecol.*, **165**, 1287–90
30. Goldschmit, R., Katz, Z., Blickstein, I., Caspi, B. and Dgani, R. (1993). The accuracy of endometrial Pipelle sampling with and without sonographic measurement of endometrial thickness. *Obstet. Gynecol.*, **82**, 727–30
31. Ferry, J., Farnsworth, A., Webster, M. and Wren, B. (1993). The efficacy of the pipelle endometrial biopsy in detecting endometrial carcinoma. *Aust. N. Z. J. Obstet. Gynaecol.*, **33**, 76–8
32. Li, T. C. and Cooke, I. D. (1990). Delayed abdominal pain after outpatient endometrial biopsy in the luteal phase. *Int. J. Gynaecol. Obstet.*, **32**, 267–8
33. Dodson, M. G. (1994). Use of transvaginal ultrasound in diagnosing the etiology of menometrorrhagia. *J. Reprod. Med.*, **39**, 362–72
34. Wood, C., Hurley, V. A., Hurley, V. A. and Leoni, M. (1993). The value of vaginal ultrasound in the management of menorrhagia. *Aust. N. Z. J. Obstet. Gynaecol.*, **33**, 198–200
35. Vasiliu, V. and Filipescu, D. (1960). Oral contraceptives in the treatment of the meno-metrorrhagia of the solitary ovary syndrome after unilateral castration. *Bull. Fed. Soc. Gynecol. Obstet. Lang. Fr.*, **20** Suppl., 485–6
36. Nilsson, L. and Rybo, G. (1971). Treatment of menorrhagia. *Am. J. Obstet. Gynecol.*, **110**, 713–20
37. Nygren, K. G. and Rybo, G. (1983). Prostaglandins and menorrhagia. *Acta Obstet. Gynecol. Scand. Suppl.*, **113**, 101–3
38. Saarikoski, S., Yliskoski, M. and Penttila, I. (1990). Sequential use of norethisterone and natural progesterone in pre-menopausal bleeding disorders. *Maturitas*, **12**, 89–97
39. Fraser, I. S. (1990). Treatment of ovulatory and anovulatory dysfunctional uterine bleeding

with oral progestogens. *Aust. N. Z. J. Obstet. Gynaecol.*, **30**, 353–6
40. Preston, J. T., Cameron, I. T., Adams, E. J. and Smith, S. K. (1995). Comparative study of tranexamic acid and norethisterone in the treatment of ovulatory menorrhagia. *Br. J. Obstet. Gynaecol.*, **102**, 401–6
41. Dockeray, C. J., Sheppard, B. L. and Bonnar, J. (1989). Comparison between mefenamic acid and danazol in the treatment of established menorrhagia. *Br. J. Obstet. Gynaecol.*, **96**, 840–4
42. Gleeson, N. C., Buggy, F., Sheppard, B. L. and Bonnar, J. (1994). The effect of tranexamic acid on measured menstrual loss and endometrial fibrinolytic enzymes in dysfunctional uterine bleeding. *Acta Obstet. Gynecol. Scand.*, **73**, 274–7
43. Ylikorkala, O. and Vinnikka, L. (1983). Comparison between antifibrinolytic and antiprostaglandin treatment in the reduction of increased menstrual blood loss in women with intrauterine contraceptive devices. *Br. J. Obstet. Gynaecol.*, **90**, 78–83
44. Edlund, M., Andersson, K., Rybo, G., Lindoff, C., Astedt, B. and von Schoultz, B. (1995). Reduction of menstrual blood loss in women suffering from idiopathic menorrhagia with a novel antifibrinolytic drug (Kabi 2161). *Br. J. Obstet. Gynaecol.*, **102**, 913–17
45. Fraser, I. S., McCarron, G., Markham, R., Robinson, M. and Smythe, E. (1983). Long-term treatment of menorrhagia with mefanamic acid. *Obstet. Gynecol.*, **61**, 109–12
46. van Eijkeren, M. A., Christiaens, G. C., Geuze, H. J., Haspels, A. A. and Sixma, J. J. (1992). Effects of mefenamic acid on menstrual hemostasis in essential menorrhagia. *Am. J. Obstet. Gynecol.*, **166**, 1419–28
47. Fraser, I. S., Pearse, C., Shearman, R. P., Elliott, P. M., McIlveen, J. and Markham, R. (1981). Efficacy of mefenamic acid in patients with a complaint of menorrhagia. *Obstet. Gynecol.*, **58**, 543–51
48. Andersch, B., Milsom, I. and Rybo, G. (1988). An objective evaluation of flurbiprofen and tranexamic acid in the treatment of idiopathic menorrhagia. *Acta Obstet. Gynecol. Scand.*, **67**, 645–8
49. Cameron, I. T., Haining, R., Lumsden, M. A., Thomas, V. R. and Smith, S. K. (1990). The effects of mefenamic acid and norethisterone on measured menstrual blood loss. *Obstet. Gynecol.*, **76**, 85–8
50. Vercellini, P., Fedele, L., Maggi, R., Vendola, N., Bocciolone, L. and Colombo, A. (1993). Gonadotrophin releasing hormone agonist for chronic anovulatory uterine bleeding and severe anaemia. *J. Reprod. Med.*, **38**, 127–9
51. Thomas, E. J., Okuda, K. J. and Thomas, N. M. (1991). The combination of a depot gonadotrophin releasing hormone agonist and cyclical hormone replacement therapy for dysfunctional uterine bleeding. *Br. J. Obstet. Gynaecol.*, **98**, 1155–9
52. Howell, R., Edmonds, D. K., Dowsett, M., Crook, D., Lees, B. and Stevenson, J. C. (1995). Gonadotropin-releasing hormone analogue (goserelin) plus hormone replacement therapy for the treatment of endometriosis: a randomized controlled trial. *Fertil. Steril.*, **64**, 474–81
53. Rees, M. C. P. (1992). Modern management of menorrhagia. *Hospital Update*, **18**, 353–61
54. Rees, M. C. P. and Barlow, D. H. (1991). Quantitation of hormone replacement induced withdrawal bleeds. *Br. J. Obstet. Gynaecol.*, **98**, 106–7
55. Chimbira, T. H., Anderson, A. B., Naish, C., Cope, E. and Turnbull, A. C. (1980). Reduction of menstrual blood loss by danazol in unexplained menorrhagia: lack of effect of placebo. *Br. J. Obstet. Gynaecol.*, **87**, 1152–8
56. Fraser, I. S. (1995). Treatment of dysfunctional uterine bleeding with danazol. *Aust. N. Z. J. Obstet. Gynaecol.*, **25**, 224–6
57. Turnbull, A. C. and Rees, M. C. (1990). Gestrinone in the treatment of menorrhagia. *Br. J. Obstet. Gynaecol.*, **97**, 713–15
58. Chamberlain, G., Freemand, R., Price, F., Kennedy, A., Green, D. and Eve, L. (1991). A comparative study of ethamsylate and mefenamic acid in dysfunctional uterine bleeding. *Br. J. Obstet. Gynaecol.*, **98**, 707–11
59. Milsom, I., Anderson, K., Andersch, B. and Rybo, G. (1991). A comparison of flurbiprofen, tranexamic acid, and a levonorgestrel-releasing intrauterine contraceptive device in the treatment of idiopathic menorrhagia. *Am. J. Obstet. Gynecol.*, **164**, 879–83
60. Tang, G. W. and Lo, S. S. (1995). Levonorgestrel intrauterine device in the treatment of menorrhagia in Chinese women: effi-

cacy versus acceptability. *Contraception*, **51**, 231–5
61. Lalonde, A. (1994). Evaluation of surgical options in menorrhagia. *Br. J. Obstet. Gynaecol.*, **101** (Suppl. 11), 8–14
62. Siddle, N., Sarrel, P. and Whitehead, M. (1987). The effect of hysterectomy on the age at ovarian failure: identification of a subgroup of women with premature loss of ovarian function and literature review. *Fertil. Steril.*, **47**, 94–100
63. Quinn, A. J., Barrett, T., Kingdom, J. C. P. and Murray, G. D. (1994). Relation between hysterectomy and subsequent ovarian function in a district hospital population. *J. Obstet. Gynaecol.*, **14**, 103–7
64. Meijer, W. J. and van Lindert, A. C. (1992). Prophylactic oophorectomy. *Eur. J. Obstet. Gynaecol. Reprod. Biol.*, **47**, 59–65
65. Vessey, M. P., Villard-Mackintosh, L., McPherson, K., Coulter, A. and Yeates, D. (1992). The epidemiology of hysterectomy: findings in a large cohort study. *Br. J. Obstet. Gynaecol.*, **99**, 402–7
66. Smith, R. N. J., Mould, T. A. J., Cockell, A. and Coltart, T. M. (1994). Endometrial resection increases demand for surgical treatment of menorrhagia. *J. Obstet. Gynaecol.*, **14**, 115–16
67. Alexander, D. A., Naji, A. A., Pinion, S. B., Mollison, J., Kitchener, H. C., Parkin, D. E., Abromovich, D. R. and Russell, I. T. (1996). Randomised trial comparing hysterectomy with endometrial ablation for dysfunctional uterine bleeding: psychiatric and psychosocial aspects. *Br. Med. J.*, **312**, 280–4
68. Ruoss, C. F. (1995). Supravaginal hysterectomy – a less invasive procedure. *J. Obstet. Gynaecol.*, **15**, 406–9
69. Nwosu, E. and Atlay, R. (1995). Subtotal hysterectomy. *Diplomate*, **2**, 203–7
70. Sutton, C. (1995). Subtotal hysterectomy revisited. *Endosc. Surg. Allied Technol.*, **3**, 105–8
71. MacKenzie, I. Z. (1996). Reducing hospital stay after abdominal hysterectomy. *Br. J. Obstet. Gynaecol.*, **103**, 175–8
72. Youssif, S. N. M. (1995). Early discharge after hysterectomy for benign diseases by minilaparotomy. *J. Obstet. Gynaecol.*, **15**, 401–5
73. Sculpher, M. J., Bryan, S., Dwyer, N., Hutton, J. and Stirrat, G. M. (1993). An economic evaluation of transcervical endometrial resection versus abdominal hysterectomy for the treatment of menorrhagia. *Br. J. Obstet. Gynaecol.*, **100**, 244–52
74. Brooks, P. G., Clouse, J. and Morris, L. S. (1994). Hysterectomy vs. resectoscopic endometrial ablation for the control of abnormal uterine bleeding. A cost-comparative study. *J. Reprod. Med.*, **39**, 755–60
75. Sculpher, M. J., Dwyer, N., Byford, S. and Stirrat, G. M. (1996). Randomised trial comparing hysterectomy and transcervical endometrial resection: effect on health related quality of life and costs two years after surgery. *Br. J. Obstet. Gynaecol.*, **103**, 142–9
76. Olsson, J., Ellstrom, M. and Hahlin, M. (1996). A randomised prospective trial comparing laparoscopic and abdominal hysterectomy. *Br. J. Obstet. Gynaecol.*, **103**, 345–50
77. Neuwirth, R. S., Duran, A. A., Singer, A., MacDonald, R. and Bolduc, L. (1994). The endometrial ablator: a new instrument. *Obstet. Gynecol.*, **83**, 792–6
78. Farquahar, C. M. (1996). The need for systematic reviews in the treatment of menstrual disorders – another Cochrane collaborative review group is born. *Br. J. Obstet. Gynaecol.*, **103**, 497–500

# The premenstrual syndrome 27

*P. M. Shaughn O'Brien*

## INTRODUCTION

The structure and function of the ovary vary dramatically throughout life. The ovum, as the central component of the Graafian follicle and resulting corpus luteum, is responsible for the production of female sex steroids and significant changes occur in the number and function of these ova between fetal life and death. In fetal life, there are some 2 million ova in the ovaries. By birth, this has reduced significantly and, by puberty, there are probably only in the region of 250 000 ova remaining. Throughout reproductive life, the development of several ova are initiated during each cycle and, though there are only some 200–300 ovulations during reproductive life, the number diminishes far more than this by the time of the menopause. At the menopause, few functioning ova remain and these become unresponsive to gonadotrophin stimulation.

During the ovulatory cycles of reproductive life, several disorders can arise. They may be due to a breakdown in the hypothalamo–pituitary–ovarian axis and ovulatory function, resulting in conditions such as infertility, anovulation and amenorrhoea. However, there are many disorders which exist in the presence of a normally functioning ovarian cycle. Such disorders include dysmenorrhoea, menorrhagia, endometriosis, cyclical mastalgia and the premenstrual syndrome. Psychological and somatic disturbances occur as a normal physiological component of menstrual cycles in most women. When these changes are exaggerated, they can result in severe psychological disturbance and behavioural abnormalities. When these are of such severity as to disrupt the patient's normal functioning, then they are termed premenstrual syndrome.

In the past, the role of sex steroids in human behaviour has probably been underestimated. Testosterone, for instance, certainly appears to have a major influence on aggressive behaviour and normal or abnormal sexual behaviour in women and men. Oestrogen and progesterone levels clearly have a significant effect around the time of puberty, during reproductive cycles and around the time of and following the menopause. Premenstrual syndrome results in some way from the combined effect of oestrogen and progesterone on the central nervous system and other sites within the body. Even so, the aetiology remains obscure and, therefore, the treatment of premenstrual syndrome poses many therapeutic difficulties.

The importance of premenstrual syndrome has been dismissed by many members of the medical profession. It is likely that this is because their experiences of the disorder relate to their observations of female partners and colleagues. Mild physiological symptoms probably occur in as many as 95% of women of reproductive age. A small percentage, possibly 5%, are totally free from symptoms. Five per cent of women fall into the group complaining of symptoms of such severity as to have a major impact on their lives. The most distressing symptoms are psychological and behavioural. In rare instances, they may be so severe as to lead to suicide or acts of aggression. Premenstrual syndrome has even been cited in legal defence in cases of murder.

## DEFINITION AND DIAGNOSIS

Women who present to the gynaecologist, psychiatrist or general practitioner with premenstrual syndrome are very often self-diagnosed and it is important that the diagnosis is not too readily accepted. The range of differential diagnoses in such patients is wide. They may be organic and must be distinguished from such disorders as endometriosis, thyrotoxicosis, dysmenorrhoea and migraine. The actual diagnosis may be a psychological disorder which is unrelated to the menstrual cycle. This group of patients is particularly important. They may present with symptoms which are extremely similar to those of premenstrual syndrome but bear no relationship to the menstrual cycle. It is important that these patients are excluded at an early stage, as the treatment methods appropriate to premenstrual syndrome will not usually be appropriate for these patients.

### Physiological symptoms

A large percentage of patients presenting may actually have only the mild 'physiological' premenstrual symptoms and it is important that these patients are distinguished from those with severe premenstrual syndrome as few of them justify medical intervention.

### True premenstrual syndrome

The premenstrual syndrome is defined as the cyclical recurrence of psychological, behavioural or physical symptoms during the luteal phase of the menstrual cycle. The symptoms should resolve completely by the end of menstruation and women should be free of symptoms for at least a week between menstruation and ovulation. The symptoms must be sufficiently severe to interfere with normal functioning or inter-personal relationships.

Although there are several characteristic symptoms of premenstrual syndrome, these represent only a few of the large number that have been reported. In any case, the nature of the symptoms is less important than the timing of the symptoms. The definition states that any combination of psychological, somatic or behavioural symptoms occurs specifically during the luteal phase of the cycle. What is perhaps more important is the resolution of the symptoms by the end of menstruation. In cases of doubt, it may be necessary to eliminate the ovarian cycle component of the disorder so as to determine the components of the patient's symptoms that are related to her underlying psychopathology and the ovarian cycle (see goserelin test below).

### Secondary premenstrual syndrome

There is a group of patients who have a combination of true premenstrual syndrome coexisting with underlying psychopathology. In these cases, the resolution of symptoms after menstruation will only be partial.

## AETIOLOGY OF PREMENSTRUAL SYNDROME

The underlying cause of premenstrual syndrome is unknown. There have been an enormous number of theories. Many of these relate to abnormalities and imbalances of ovarian steroids, whilst others relate to abnormalities in central nervous neurotransmitter function. The truth is that premenstrual syndrome is probably the product of both of these.

### Neurotransmitter function in premenstrual syndrome

All gonadal steroids are fat soluble and, thus, easily enter nerve cells and bind to specific receptor proteins, either within the cell nucleolus or in the cellular cytoplasm. The receptor hormone complexes attach themselves to specific regulatory sequences of DNA, which in turn either enhance or diminish the expression of specific protein encoding genes. Oestrogen and progesterone may also act directly on neurotransmitter systems. There is now increasing evidence that central nervous system disorders, such as schizophrenia, depression and epilepsy, have close relationships with ovarian endocrine cyclicity.

There are several possible mediators of ovarian steroid action within the brain. These include the endogenous opioid peptides (endorphins), encephalins, γ-aminobutyric acid, prostaglandins, monoamines and serotonin. During the menstrual cycle, lowered levels of β-endorphin have been demonstrated during the luteal phase of women with premenstrual syndrome[1] and modulation of β-endorphin concentration by means of naltrexone appears to reduce symptoms. More recently, interest has been focused on serotoninergic activity in endogenous depression and in premenstrual syndrome. Lowered levels of whole blood serotonin concentration and platelet serotonin have been demonstrated in women with premenstrual syndrome[2]. Additionally, several serotonin re-uptake inhibitors have now been shown to improve the symptoms of premenstrual syndrome. These include clomipramine, paroxetine and fluoxetine[3–5].

## Ovarian function in premenstrual syndrome

Many of the early theories of premenstrual syndrome relate to oestrogen excess or progesterone deficiency[6]. There is no convincing evidence to support theories of excess or deficiency of either oestrogen or progesterone[7]. The combination of endogenous oestrogen with cyclical ovulatory progesterone is considered to be the underlying trigger mechanism for premenstrual syndrome for several reasons. Elimination of cyclical ovarian function by hysterectomy and bilateral oophorectomy[8] or by medical suppression of the cycle, using danazol[9] or, more convincingly, using gonadotrophin releasing hormone agonist analogues[10,11], results in complete suppression of premenstrual syndrome symptoms. Conversely, in women who receive oestrogen replacement therapy with cyclical progestogen, premenstrual syndrome-like symptoms are regenerated during the progestogen phase of therapy. Not all women receiving cyclical hormone replacement therapy develop these premenstrual syndrome symptoms, even though they receive identical dose schedules. This suggests a differential response to the same levels of steroids in specific women.

In a recent research study[12], women who had undergone hysterectomy and bilateral salpingo-oophorectomy for gynaecological pathology were recruited to an endocrine challenge test. Women who had previously been defined as having severe premenstrual syndrome were recruited. Following surgery these women were prescribed unopposed oestrogen therapy and then given cyclical progesterone experimentally. During the oestrogen-only phase of therapy, no premenstrual syndrome symptoms were demonstrated. However, during the progesterone phase of therapy, premenstrual syndrome-like symptoms re-developed (Figure 1). The combination of these facts suggests that cyclical ovarian steroid function is the trigger for premenstrual syndrome in women who have an exaggerated response to either endogenous or exogenously administered oestrogen and cyclical progesterone. Future research into the aetiology of premenstrual syndrome should centre around determination of the cause of this increased responsiveness to hormone, rather than seeking an oestrogen or progesterone imbalance. Abnormal neurotransmitter function would appear to be the most likely explanation for the enhanced sensitivity for the psychological manifestation of premenstrual syndrome.

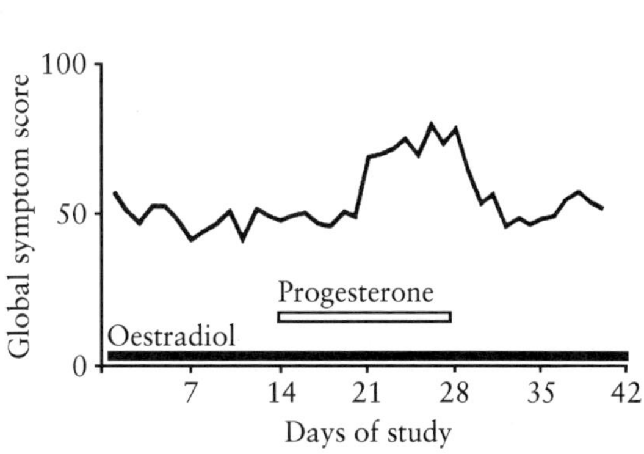


**Figure 1** Simulation of premenstrual syndrome by progesterone therapy. Reproduced with permission from O'Brien, P. M. S. (1993). Helping women with premenstrual syndrome. *Br. Med. J.*, 307, 1471–5

There have been many other proposed mechanisms for premenstrual syndrome but many of these have been largely discounted by the lack of supportive evidence. For instance, recent research has demonstrated the improbability of the theory of sodium and water retention[13]. In a group of women who experienced significant premenstrual bloatedness and abdominal distention, no premenstrual increases have been demonstrated in total body water or total exchangeable body sodium.

The popular theory of release of a 'menotoxin' is excluded because symptoms can be regenerated in patients receiving cyclical oestrogen and progesterone following removal of the uterus.

Thus, the current hypothesis, that cyclical oestrogen and progesterone provide the trigger in women who have a central nervous susceptibility due to abnormal endorphin or serotonin function, appears to be the most credible explanation at present.

## SYMPTOMS AND THEIR MEASUREMENT

Characteristic physical symptoms include abdominal bloatedness and the sensation of weight increase which, as we have seen, appears to be unrelated to sodium and water retention. Severe cyclical mastalgia is also a common complaint and may be seen in association with, or separately from, premenstrual syndrome. Premenstrual pelvic pain may need to be distinguished from that of endometriosis by laparoscopy. Premenstrual headache or migraine is also common but, again, it is important to distinguish those patients with true menstrual migraine from those whose migraine occasionally coincides with events in the menstrual cycle.

Psychological symptoms include aggression, depression, tension and, perhaps most distressingly of all, the feeling of loss of control. These symptoms comprise only a few of the many symptoms which have been documented in the literature.

### Measurement of premenstrual syndrome symptoms

Many rating scales have been devised for premenstrual syndrome. Most of these are complex, having been developed for research, and are too cumbersome for use in a clinical setting. Simple premenstrual syndrome charts are limited. They define the character of symptoms and their timing but they do not identify the severity of symptoms nor do they determine the impact of these symptoms on the patient's quality of life.

The author has recently developed and is currently validating a new simple computerised method of measuring the important components of premenstrual syndrome. The device utilizes a commercially available hand-held computer with a touch-sensitive screen. This enables the recording of questionnaire data for underlying psychopathology, and visual analogue scales (measured on the touch-sensitive screen) to record the typical symptoms on a daily basis. The device also incorporates a questionnaire to measure the quality of life. The instrument is capable of recording data for an individual patient for up to 1 year and this can be readily transferred to the database of a personal computer. The method utilizes the most sensitive method of measuring premenstrual syndrome, the visual analogue scale, but avoids the extremely tedious process of measuring visual analogue scales by hand.

Whatever the technique employed to quantify premenstrual syndrome, it is important that the rating scales are administered prospectively since retrospective assessment of premenstrual syndrome results in over-reporting of symptoms.

### Goserelin test

Gonadotrophin releasing hormone agonist analogues, such as goserelin and buserelin, can be used to produce 'a medical oophorectomy' where ovarian cyclicity is suppressed completely. When a clinician is confronted with a patient whose symptoms do not obviously fall into one of the diagnostic categories above, the goserelin test may be used to assist this distinction. Goserelin is administered monthly for a total of 3 months. By the 3rd month, the ovarian cycle will be suppressed along with those symptoms directly related to ovarian function. Symptoms which persist will be related to the patient's underlying psychopathology. This test will enable the distinction between those patients with a continuous non-cyclical disorder and those with pure premenstrual syndrome; it will also identify the proportion of ovarian and underlying psychological components of those patients who have co-existing disorders.

The goserelin test will also assist in identifying those patients in whom the ovaries should be removed at the time of hysterectomy. For patients undergoing hysterectomy for gynaecological pathology, their counselling would normally include the need to conserve or remove ovaries. If a patient has significant premenstrual syndrome in addition to her gynaecological problem, then it may be justifiable to remove the ovaries; the likely success of bilateral oophorectomy in such cases can be predetermined by this goserelin test.

### Objective tests for premenstrual syndrome

Unfortunately, no objective method for distinguishing premenstrual syndrome from other disorders exists. Although many blood tests have been proposed, including oestrogen estimation, sex hormone binding globulin, progesterone and thyroid function tests, none of these has any value in diagnosing premenstrual syndrome.

## MANAGEMENT OF PREMENSTRUAL SYNDROME

Two groups of patients are relatively easy to manage. Patients with mild premenstrual symptoms often need no more than reassurance as to the normality of their symptoms. Patients with very severe premenstrual syndrome are usually easy to manage because invasive approaches such as hormonal manipulation or even surgical intervention can be justified. The patients with moderately severe symptoms are much more difficult to manage as the less invasive therapies are less predictable and have been less well proven in scientific studies. In general, a hierarchical approach is best utilized for the majority of patients (Figure 2).

The range of proposed treatment methods described since the first description of premenstrual syndrome in the 1930s has included approaches as diverse as psychotherapy, radiotherapy, acupuncture, dietary supplementation, minimally invasive surgery, pelvic clearance and administration of virtually every sex steroid.

### Non-medical management

The cause of premenstrual syndrome is complex and the underlying neuroendocrine status in a patient can have many influences. These include environmental, dietary, general health, stress, psychosocial factors, personal factors, personality, self-esteem and general well-being. Which is the cause, or which is the result of the neuroendocrine differences cannot be determined. However, it is probably a patient's threshold to deal with the challenge of the premenstrual phase of the cycle that is most potentially treatable by non-medical interventions. Such interventions should be considered long before endocrine therapy, psychiatric consultation or surgery. Indeed, it is likely that gynaecologists and psychiatrists should only be consulted when such measures have failed.

Counselling, relaxation therapy, formalized stress management and improvement in coping skills can be appropriate for many patients. Reassurance is also important. The nature of the relaxation therapy will vary from patient to patient. Hypnotherapy, yoga, acupuncture, exercise therapy and, more recently, aromatherapy will be appropriate for different types of patients. The only formal psychotherapeutic intervention that has been demonstrated to be effective is cognitive therapy[14].

General improvement in a patient's health, effected through exercise, vitamin therapy and dietary interventions, may improve her ability to tolerate premenstrual syndrome symptoms.

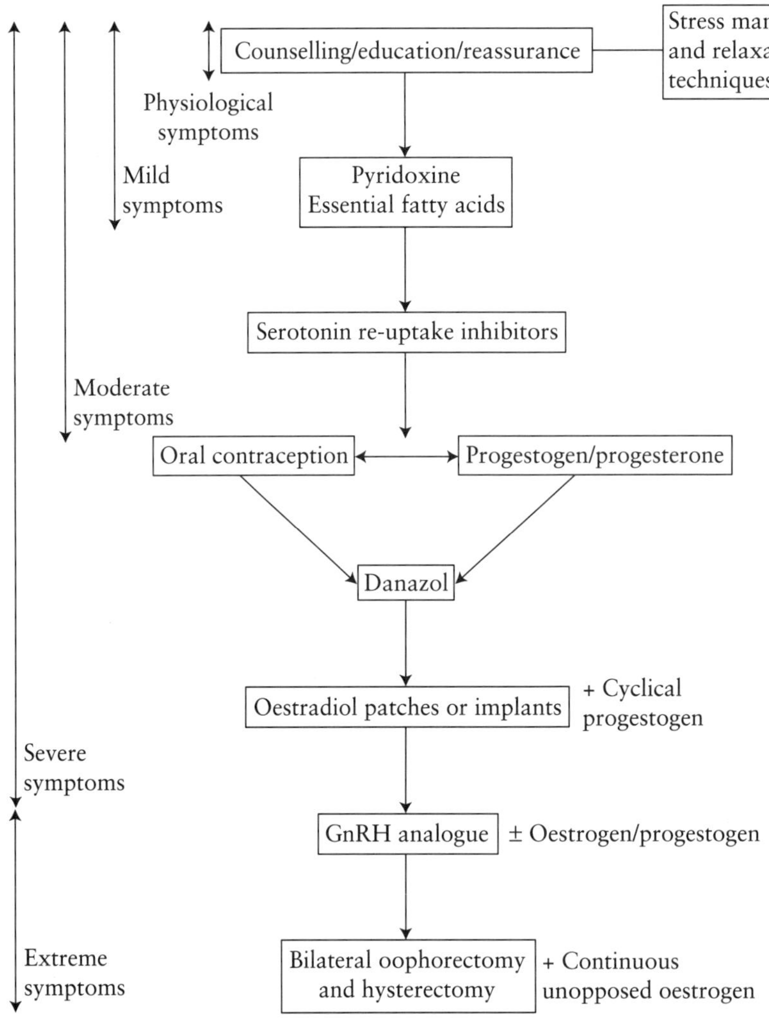


**Figure 2** Hierarchical approach to the management of premenstrual syndrome. Reproduced with permission from O'Brien, P. M. S. (1993). Helping women with premenstrual syndrome. *Br. Med. J.*, **307**, 1471–5

There is no current evidence to support the use of specific dietary interventions, particularly the taking of frequent carbohydrate meals to prevent premenstrual hypoglycaemia. (Low plasma glucose has never been demonstrated in patients with so-called premenstrual hypoglycaemia.)

Many vitamins have been proposed to manage premenstrual syndrome, though there is little evidence for the effectiveness of any of these from randomized controlled trials. Pyridoxine (vitamin B6) and magnesium have been shown to be only a little better than placebo in one or two trials, despite the logical basis to these approaches to treatment in that they are cofactors in the synthesis of various neurotransmitters from tryptophan.

The use of evening primrose oil, which contains gamolenic acid, has been advocated to the extent that evening primrose oil is marketed extensively for premenstrual syndrome. However, the evidence for the use of evening primrose oil in premenstrual syndrome is very limited and benefit has only been clearly demonstrated to be superior to placebo in the management of cyclical mastalgia[15]. For the remaining symptoms of premenstrual syndrome, further research work is necessary before such treatment can be advocated[16,17].

### Medical management: non-hormonal

*Psychotrophic drugs*
Despite the fact that the dominant symptomatology of premenstrual syndrome is of a psychological nature, there are relatively few studies of psychotropic interventions.

Benzodiazepines, antidepressants, monoamine-oxidase inhibitors and lithium have all been used or assessed from time to time, but none of these has been demonstrated to have benefit over and above placebo. The newer selective serotonin re-uptake inhibitors (SSRIs) have been assessed or are being assessed in current clinical trials[3–5]. Fluoxetine has been shown in several trials to be superior to placebo, as has clomipramine. Paroxetine has been shown to be effective in uncontrolled trials and is the subject of several current double-blind studies. As with many psychotherapeutic drugs, there is a delay in the onset of action of SSRIs and it is probably not appropriate to give these drugs cyclically. Side-effects and dependency do not appear to be particular problems, although reduction in libido has been reported.

*Diuretics*
Sodium and water retention have not been demonstrated in the majority of women with premenstrual syndrome[13]. Even patients with marked bloatedness do not appear to retain fluid, though there is a small proportion of women who have idiopathic oedema which may occasionally coincide with the menstrual cycle[7]. These patients need to be identified as being separate from those with premenstrual syndrome and managed separately by an appropriate physician. The small proportion of women who gain weight premenstrually may be retaining fluid and may respond to diuretic therapy. These drugs can be administered in the luteal phase. The loop diuretics should be avoided as they can produce secondary aldosteronism and it is more appropriate to give an aldosterone antagonist such as triamterene or spironolactone. Spironolactone has been shown to be effective in controlled studies and reduces weight increase and the sensation of bloatedness. Patients should be selected only if measurable premenstrual weight increase has been demonstrated[7].

### Medical management: hormonal

Given that no differences have been demonstrated in the endogenous hormone levels of women with premenstrual syndrome, regimens which are claimed to correct hormone deficiency are not supported. However, it may be argued that disruption of the endogenous cycle or even complete elimination of the ovarian cycle may be effective. Methods of suppressing the ovarian cycle may be hormonal or surgical (Table 1).

**Table 1** Methods to suppress ovarian function

| |
|---|
| Continuous combined pill |
| Progestogen, continuous |
| Oestrogen |
| Danazol |
| GnRH agonist analogues |
| Bilateral oophorectomy (usually with hysterectomy) |

*Oral contraception*
Conventional oral contraceptive therapy suppresses ovulation but introduces a new cyclicity which may produce associated cyclical symptoms. In practice, many patients do have relief of their premenstrual syndrome with oral contraceptive therapy, though, conversely, many patients will actually develop premenstrual syndrome symptoms for the first time[18]. The logical approach to the management of premenstrual syndrome with oral contraceptive therapy would be to give continuous combined oral contraception. This does not appear to be effective in general clinical use and there are no published studies evaluating its efficacy. In the management of young patients requiring contraception, this may be an appropriate and empirical approach to treatment.

*Progestogens*
Cyclical progestogens such as norethisterone and dydrogesterone are licensed for the management of premenstrual syndrome but this is based on very scanty scientific evidence. There is no rationale for their use but again an empirical approach to therapy may be reasonable. Both of these would be given cyclically in the luteal phase of the cycle. High doses of continuous progestogen would suppress ovulation, but this approach is rarely followed and there is no evidence to support its use. Depot preparations of medroxyprogesterone acetate, as given for contraception, are often tried in general practice. Again, there is no scientific evidence currently available to support its use.

*Progesterone*
It is the theory of progesterone deficiency and progesterone therapy that brought the subject of premenstrual syndrome to light in the 1950s and 1960s[6]. It has already been stated that there is no evidence for progesterone deficiency. Similarly, there is extremely limited evidence to support the use of progesterone[19]. However, there are far more studies demonstrating that there is no effect of progesterone over and above that of placebo[20].

We will see later that the use of oestrogen is of value in premenstrual syndrome and also, of course, in hormone replacement therapy. The use of oestrogen requires that a progestogen is given cyclically in women who still have a uterus. We have also seen that the administration of progesterone re-stimulates premenstrual syndrome. In a proportion of patients, there is evidence to suggest that dydrogesterone, medroxyprogesterone acetate and progesterone are less likely to stimulate premenstrual syndrome-like symptoms than many of the other progestogens available.

*Danazol*
Danazol is clearly effective in the management of symptoms of premenstrual syndrome and cyclical mastalgia. This effect is certainly seen when the menstrual cycle is suppressed using 400 mg, but also seems to be apparent when lower doses are used[21]. It is surprising that danazol is not utilized more frequently for premenstrual syndrome, but this is probably due to reluctance on the part of doctors to prescribe it in view of the perceived incidence of side-effects. Danazol can produce masculinization of the patient, including voice change, weight gain and deterioration in the lipid profile. It can also cause masculinization of her fetus should pregnancy arise. Recent attempts to reduce the overall dose of danazol have been assessed by the author. A dose of 200 mg of danazol has been given in the luteal phase only of the menstrual cycle. This study demonstrated that the general symptoms of premenstrual syndrome were not improved in comparison with placebo, whilst cyclical mastalgia was significantly improved in comparison with placebo.

*Bromocriptine*
Although theories of prolactin excess have been addressed in the past, no differences in prolactin or cyclicity of prolactin have been demonstrated. Bromocriptine has been clearly shown to be effective for the management of cyclical mastalgia[15]. Again, there are significant side-effects with bromocriptine.

Breast symptoms can evidently be managed in several different ways and, again, a hierarchical approach can be used, beginning with evening primrose oil therapy, progressing through cyclical danazol to continuous danazol to cyclical bromocriptine. The majority of patients will be effectively treated by such an approach.

*Oestrogen*
Oestrogen can be administered in several ways including oral tablets, transdermal patches, transdermal gel and subcutaneous implants. Oral therapy appears to be generally ineffective. Oestrogen gel has not been assessed adequately. Transdermal patches have been assessed fairly rigorously and both 200 μg and 100 μg patches appear to be effective in controlling symptoms[22]. Oestradiol implants of 100 mg appear effective and probably are the most effective[23]. However, there are several problems associated with these and perhaps such therapy should be reserved for patients in

whom other oestrogen methods have failed. Tachyphylaxis is an important problem and should always be considered when treatment appears effective initially and then ceases. Although unopposed oestrogen will suppress ovulation and reduce the symptoms of premenstrual syndrome, in women who still have a uterus this approach to therapy is not appropriate: it is necessary to give a progestogen to prevent the risk of endometrial hyperplasia and endometrial adenocarcinoma. Various progestogens are effective for this purpose but, of course, we have already stated that this results in the regeneration of premenstrual syndrome symptoms in a significant proportion of patients. Trials of different progestogen regimens may be helpful, remembering that reduction in the dose and reduction in the duration of progestogen increases the likelihood of endometrial hyperplasia. One potential avenue of research will be the use of the levonorgestrel-containing intrauterine contraceptive device (Mirena-IUS) as an alternative to oral progestogen. This device delivers progestogen directly to the endometrium without resulting in significant absorption of progestogen into the blood. Protection of the endometrium is thus achieved without stimulation of the central nervous system. No properly controlled trials are currently available to support this regimen and it would, for the time being, need to be tried empirically on a named patient basis.

*GnRH agonist analogues*

All disorders relating to the ovarian cycle can be effectively eliminated by giving gonadotrophin releasing hormone (GnRH) agonist analogues such as goserelin and buserelin. There are controlled trials to demonstrate the efficacy of these analogues in premenstrual syndrome[10,11]. It is important to appreciate that these are agonists and, therefore, will begin their action by stimulating the ovary before achieving suppression. It must also be appreciated that long-term therapy with this type of treatment is inappropriate because of the creation of the pseudomenopause. This, of course, has short- and medium-term effects but, more worryingly, the long-term risks of osteoporosis and the increase in cardiovascular disease exist. The use of GnRH agonist analogues, whilst probably being the most effective medical form of treatment, is not suitable for long-term therapy. On discontinuation of therapy, unlike GnRH treatment of endometriosis, the symptoms return immediately[11].

The use of these analogues is restricted to:

(1) The diagnostic test;

(2) Short-term therapy which can be extremely valuable in patients whose quality of life has significantly deteriorated;

(3) Demonstration to the patient and her family and employers that her problem has a biological basis;

(4) As a test prior to hysterectomy to determine the potential benefit of bilateral oophorectomy.

Occasionally, it may be appropriate to suppress the cycle with these analogues and provide protection with conventional hormone replacement therapy[24].

## Surgery

*Hysterectomy and bilateral salpingo-oophorectomy*

It is difficult to justify surgery for a psychological disorder in which the normal ovaries and uterus are removed. However, there is a small group of women whose lives can be transformed by such an approach. The removal of the uterus and ovaries will clearly eliminate all premenstrual symptoms proved to be related to the ovarian cycle[8]. The effects of the menopause can then be counteracted by giving unopposed oestrogen replacement therapy. Progesterone therapy is no longer necessary after the endometrium has been removed.

*Minimal access surgery*

Laparoscopic oophorectomy may be effective for premenstrual syndrome. However, oestrogen replacement would be required and, again, it would be necessary to protect the endometrium with progestogen. Laparoscopically assisted vaginal hysterectomy and bilateral oophorectomy will be appropriate in the same instances as the equivalent abdominal procedure. Endometrial ablation should not logically have any effect on premenstrual syndrome and, where claims have been made for such a procedure, this has been part of a research report where the premenstrual syndrome has only been casually addressed. There are no specific controlled studies of endometrial resection and premenstrual syndrome. Logically, one would not expect this to be an effective therapy since ovarian cyclicity persists.

## CONCLUSIONS

Adherence to a hierarchical approach, where the invasiveness of the procedure relates directly to the severity of the premenstrual syndrome and the failure of non-invasive treatment, is probably the best compromise approach available to management at the present time. It is important to take into account aspects of the patient's history such as desire for pregnancy, age and the co-existence of other symptoms. For instance, a patient who also requires contraception may benefit from the use of combined continuous oral contraception or the Mirena-IUS to protect the endometrium during oestrogen replacement. Patients who are older and who have flushing as one of their symptoms may benefit from an early resort to oestrogen replacement therapy. It must be remembered that some of the preparations used are contraindicated, in some circumstances, for instance, in pregnant women. Patients receiving danazol and gonadotrophin releasing hormone agonist analogue should be advised to take additional mechanical forms of contraception. Patients should also be aware that treatment regimes for premenstrual syndrome (apart from the oral contraceptive pill, depo-Provera and the Mirena-IUS) are not guaranteed to be contraceptive. Several legal claims have been made by patients suffering from premenstrual syndrome who claim that their gynaecologist has guaranteed the contraceptive efficacy of various techniques.

It is often suggested that gynaecologists will not consider premenstrual syndrome to be a gynaecological disorder until an easily performed surgical option exists. It is important that we do not embark on unnecessary and unproven operative procedures such as endometrial ablation and laparoscopic oophorectomy until research has clarified the role of these treatments in premenstrual syndrome.

## REFERENCES

1. Choung, C. J., Coulam, C. B., Kao, P. C., Bergstalh, E. J. and Go, V. L. W. (1985). Neuropeptide levels in premenstrual syndrome. *Fertil. Steril.*, **44**, 760–5
2. Rapkin, A. J. (1992). The role of serotonin in premenstrual syndrome. *Clin. Obstet. Gynecol.*, **35**, 629–36
3. Menkes, D. B., Ebrahim, T., Mason, P. A., Spears, G. F. S. and Howard, R. C. (1992). Fluoxetine treatment of severe premenstrual syndrome. *Br. Med. J.*, **305**, 346–7
4. Wood, S. H., Mortola, J. F., Chan, Y. F., Moossazadeh, F. and Yen, S. S. (1992). Treatment of premenstrual syndrome with fluoxetine: a double-blind, placebo-controlled crossover study. *Obstet. Gynecol.*, **80**, 339–44
5. Steiner, M., Steinberg, S., Stewart, D., Canter, D., Berger, C., Reid, R. *et al.* (1995). Fluoxetine treatment of premenstrual dysphoria. *N. Engl. J. Med.*, **333**, 1529–34
6. Dalton, K. (1984). *The Premenstrual Syndrome and Progesterone Therapy.* (London: William Heinemann)
7. O'Brien, P. M. S. (1987). *Premenstrual Syndrome.* (Oxford: Blackwell Scientific)
8. Casson, P., Hahn, P. M., van Vugt, D. A. and Reid, R. L. (1990). Lasting response to ovariectomy in severe intractable premenstrual syndrome. *Am. J. Obstet. Gynecol.*, **162**, 99–105
9. Halbreich, U., Rojansky, N. and Palter, S. (1990). Elimination of ovulation and menstrual cyclicity (with danazol) improves dysphoric premenstrual syndrome. *Fertil. Steril.*, **56**, 1066
10. Muse, K. (1992). Hormonal manipulation in the treatment of premenstrual syndrome. *Clin. Obstet. Gynecol.*, **35**, 658–66
11. Hussain, S. Y., Massil, J. H., Matta, W. H., Shaw, R. W. and O'Brien, P. M. S. (1992). Buserelin in premenstrual syndrome. *Gynecol. Endocrinol.*, **6**, 57–64

12. Henshaw, C., Foreman, D., Belcher, J., Cox, J. and O'Brien, P. M. S. (1996). Can one induce premenstrual symptomatology in women with prior hysterectomy and bilateral oophorectomy? *J. Psychosom. Obstet. Gynecol.*, **17**, 21–8
13. Hussain, S. Y. (1993). Compartmental distribution of fluid and electrolytes in the menstrual cycle and premenstrual syndrome. University of London, PhD Thesis
14. Johnson, S. (1992). Clinician's approach to the diagnosis and management of premenstrual syndrome. *Clin. Obstet. Gynecol.*, **35**, 637–57
15. Pye, J. K., Mansel, R. E. and Hughes, L. E. (1985). Clinical experience of drug treatments for mastalgia. *Lancet*, **2**, 373–7
16. O'Brien, P. M. S. and Massil, H. (1990). Premenstrual syndrome: clinical studies on essential fatty acids. In Horrobin, D. (ed.) *Omega-6 Essential Fatty Acids. Pathophysiology and Role in Clinical Medicine*, pp. 523–45. (New York: Wiley-Liss)
17. Khoo, S. K., Munro, C. and Battistutta, D. (1990). Evening primrose oil and treatment of premenstrual syndrome. *Med. J. Aust.*, **153**, 189–92
18. Backstrom, T., Hansson-Malmstorm, Y., Lindhe, B. A., Cavilli-Bjorkman, B. and Nordenstorm, S. (1992). Oral contraceptives in premenstrual syndrome: a randomised comparison of triphasic and monophasic preparations. *Contraception*, **46**, 253–68
19. Magill, P. J. (1995). Investigation of the efficacy of progesterone pessaries in the relief of symptoms of premenstrual syndrome. *Br. J. Gen. Pract.*, **45**, 589–93
20. Freeman, E., Rickel, K., Soundheimer, S. J. and Polansky, M. (1990). Ineffectiveness of progesterone suppository treatment for premenstrual syndrome. *J. Am. Med. Assoc.*, **264**, 349–53
21. Deeny, M., Hawthorn, R. and McKay Hart, D. (1991). Low dose danazol treatment of the premenstrual syndrome. *Postgrad. Med. J.*, **67**, 450–4
22. Watson, N. R., Studd, J. W. W., Savvas, M., Garnett, T. and Baber, R. J. (1989). Treatment of severe premenstrual syndrome with oestradiol patches and cyclical oral norethisterone. *Lancet*, **2**, 730–2
23. Watson, N. R., Studd, J. W. W., Savvas, M. and Baber, R. J. (1990). The long-term effects of oestradiol implant therapy for the treatment of premenstrual syndrome. *Gynecol. Endocrinol.*, **4**, 99–107
24. Mortola, J. F., Girton, L. and Fischer, U. (1991). Successful treatment of premenstrual syndrome by combined use of gonadotrophin releasing hormone agonist and estrogen/progestin. *J. Endocrinol. Metab.*, **72**, 252A–F

# The climacteric and hormone replacement therapy

# 28

*David A. Viniker*

## INTRODUCTION

The objective of hormone replacement therapy is to alleviate or minimize the morbidity and mortality associated with the menopause whilst ensuring that our patients are fully informed of the possible consequences of treatment and that they are involved in decision making. During reproductive years, the ovary secretes oestrogens, progestogen and testosterone; after the menopause, there is significantly reduced production of each of these. Hormone replacement therapy is the term most frequently associated with oestrogen replacement and certainly oestrogen replacement receives the greatest attention in the literature relating to the menopause. Progesterone and testosterone deficiency and replacement should also be considered.

The menopause is defined as the final natural menstruation and compares to the menarche which is the first menstruation. Just as the menarche is one event in the plethora of physical and emotional changes associated with puberty, so the menopause is just one event in the climacteric when a woman ceases to have natural reproductive capability. In association with the climacteric or perimenopause, the majority of women encounter a variety of physical and emotional symptoms which generally respond to hormone replacement therapy (HRT). There is good evidence that, as a result of ovarian failure which produces a deficiency of reproductive steroids, degenerative pathology of the arterial and skeletal systems is exacerbated. Hormone replacement therapy may reduce the rate of these degenerative processes, and possibly reverse them, leading to reduced morbidity and mortality.

Whereas the age at menarche has shown a downward trend in industrialized countries[1], Caucasian women reach the menopause on average at 50.5 years and this has probably not changed through the last 100 years. The majority of studies, however, have accepted self-reported age at last menstruation, which is subject to recall bias[2].

The age at menarche and the number of pregnancies do not seem to influence the age at menopause. Women who smoke tend to have an earlier menopause[2,3]. Poor education and low income are associated with earlier menopause but marital status, parity, weight, height and use of oestrogens in the pill or hormone replacement therapy are not related[2]. There is a tendency for early menopause to be familial[4]. Premature menopause occurs spontaneously in 1% of women and just less than 10% will be menopausal before the age of 46 years.

The life expectancy of women in England and Wales in 1900 was 50.1 years. By 1950, it had risen to 71.1 years and it reached 79.2 years in 1990. This 60% increase in life expectancy is typical of data throughout industrialized countries[5]. A woman currently aged 60 has a life expectancy of a further 22.6 years. Improved nutrition is probably the most significant factor. Most women will spend one-third of their life beyond the menopause. There are now an estimated 10 million postmenopausal women in the United Kingdom.

The menopause is characterized by a significant reduction of endogenous oestrogens, with correspondingly elevated gonadotrophin levels as the pituitary attempts to achieve a response from ovaries that have run out of an adequate number of oocytes. The monthly shedding of the endometrium, menstruation, stops as it is no longer under the influence of cyclical oestrogens and progesterone. The menopause is endocrinologically termed 'hypergonadotrophic hypogonadism'.

After the menopause, there is still a small amount of oestrogen production; this is mostly derived from peripheral conversion of androgen precursors, although the ovaries and adrenals provide a tiny contribution[6].

Biennial examinations of 1686 women in the Framingham study[7] have demonstrated a rise in serum cholesterol in association with spontaneous or surgical menopause but blood pressure, blood glucose and weight are not significantly altered.

Although several authorities suggest that 1 year of amenorrhoea in the late forties or beyond provides confirmatory evidence of ovarian failure, there is no absolute clinical or endocrinological test that can unequivocally confirm that the ovaries have completely run out of functional oocytes. It is a regular clinical observation that women present with a period-like bleed having previously fulfilled the criteria for the menopause. Often, they will experience typical premenstrual symptoms before the bleed. Adequate clinical examination and investigation must be pursued. Transvaginal or transrectal ultrasound of the endometrium can often exclude pathology[8]. There is a variation in the recommended upper limit of normal for the endometrial thickness; we have accepted 5 mm and are not aware of any resulting problems. It should be stressed that the endometrium should appear homogeneous and the radiographer should see all areas of the endometrium. If these criteria are not fulfilled, then hysteroscopy with endometrial curettage, or possibly an endometrial biopsy, should be carried out. It would seem logical to accept that women are often correct in their belief that they have experienced menstruation again; this must, presumably, follow recruitment of an oocyte scheduled to commence maturation a year or more after the previous period (Chapter 2).

A 49-year-old lady, who presented with menorrhagia, provides a case example of the difficulty in determining when the menopause has occurred. A dilatation and curettage (D & C) was performed and she was treated medically for dysfunctional uterine bleeding. Within a year she became amenorrhoeic and developed menopausal symptoms; her follicle stimulating hormone (FSH) was elevated on two occasions. Cyclical HRT was commenced but the withdrawal bleeds were heavy. When the HRT was withdrawn, she continued to have heavy periods and her FSH continued at premenopausal levels. The menorrhagia was inadequately controlled by medication and she came to total abdominal hysterectomy, bilateral salpingo-oophorectomy and an oestradiol implant.

A total abdominal hysterectomy was performed for a 40-year-old lady who presented with abdominal distension and an ultrasound picture consistent with ovarian malignancy. The histopathologist reported the tumour to be a granulosa cell tumour with a high mitotic rate. Her preoperative FSH was 4.2 mmol/l and on the 6th postoperative day her oestradiol had fallen to less than 100 pmol/l with an FSH of 40.5 nmol/l. It has been shown that, in patients on the combined oral contraceptive pill, FSH levels tend to become clearly elevated by the 7th pill-free day in those women who have probably reached the menopause[9].

Ovarian biopsy to estimate the number of follicles may accurately predict the timing of the menopause for an individual woman[10].

### Local symptoms

The majority of women experience vaginal dryness, local discomfort and superficial dyspareunia around the menopause. Atrophic changes related to oestrogen deficiency are common and respond quickly to local oestrogen or systemic HRT. For those patients who require local therapy only, there is a choice of vaginal tablets, creams or a ring, which slowly releases oestrogen.

### Vasomotor symptoms

Hot flushes, sweats during the night, headaches, giddiness and palpitations are the most common of the multitude of symptoms that can occur at the menopause. These are probably directly related to oestrogen deficiency and they respond to hormone replacement therapy within 10 days. Similarly, fatigue and exhaustion, which may accompany sleep disturbance, should respond quickly to treatment.

### Urological problems

The lower urinary tract, in common with the genital tract, develops from the primitive urogenital sinus. Oestrogen receptor sites have been demonstrated in the urethra. Urinary symptoms are more common after the menopause and there is an extensive literature describing the effects of oestrogen therapy. The Hormones and Urogenital Therapy Committee have undertaken a meta-analysis of the subject[11]. They found 166 papers of which 23 were clinical trials. Subjectively, oestrogen has a beneficial effect on postmenopausal urinary incontinence, which is greater for detrusor instability than for stress incontinence. There is evidence that the maximum urethral closure pressure is significantly increased. Urgency of micturition, urge incontinence, frequency and nocturia may improve with oestrogen administration.

### Psychological problems

Psychological problems during the perimenopause are common and may respond to HRT. The wise clinician must recognize that the arrival of the menopause serves as a reminder to the patient that the vitality of youth, and perhaps half her adult years, have been completed. For many menopausal women, early ambitions, aspirations and dreams are not progressing towards fulfilment. Children have attained adulthood and may be the source of ever-increasing anxiety and stress. Parents are ageing and making increasing demands. Medication cannot cure the stresses and strains of life but often the administration of HRT decreases sleep disturbance and increases energy and well-being to a major degree. Clinicians thrive by watching their patients' health improve with the treatments that they prescribe. For a clinician treating menopause problems, the administration of HRT is a rewarding exercise. The clinician should seek to achieve the best results from HRT for symptoms attributable to hormone insufficiency. Sympathy, understanding and support are an essential part of the clinician's armamentarium.

A relationship between psychological symptoms and alteration in hormone concentrations is commonly encountered premenstrually, postnatally, and around the time of the menopause. In a controlled study, Montgomery and colleagues[12] demonstrated significant improvement in anxiety and depression with oestradiol or combined oestradiol and testosterone implants. The improvement only occurred in those women approaching the menopause. Frequently premenstrual syndrome, which typically has a cyclical nature, insidiously alters to include symptoms that do not have a cyclical component as the menopause approaches.

Psychiatrists have emphasized the need to distinguish between depressed mood and depressive disorder. Low spirits, despondency and demoralization are common symptoms, typical of depressed mood, that most people have experienced at times. Depressive disorder is more severe. Depressed mood is accompanied by 'loss' symptoms such as loss of energy, interest, sex drive, appetite and the capacity for enjoyment. There is evidence that depressed mood may respond to HRT[13,14] but psychiatrists regard depressive disorders to be generally outside hormonal influence.

A beneficial effect on cognitive function has been demonstrated in a crossover-designed trial of oestrogen and/or androgen therapy compared with placebo in surgically menopausal women[15]. The patients had tests of short-term memory, a test of long-term memory and a logical reasoning test. There was a significant improvement in patients receiving treatment in all groups compared to placebo. Oestrogen proved to be better than placebo for headache, memory, anxiety and insomnia[16]. Ditkoff and co-workers[17], in a double-blind study, found that oestrogen had a beneficial effect in postmenopausal women on adaptation to life and it also reduced depression. Psychological well-being tends to improve with HRT[18].

There are significant differences in responses to psychological stress between premenopausal and postmenopausal women; oestrogen replacement therapy reduces the biophysical and neuroendocrine responses to stress[19].

## PROPHYLACTIC HORMONE REPLACEMENT THERAPY

### Ischaemic heart disease

Oestrogens protect women from ischaemic heart disease. The relatively high risk ratio between males and females at age 50 rapidly falls in the fifties and sixties and one study showed equal risk by age 70[20]. Surgical menopause accelerates development of atherosclerosis and its clinical sequelae[21]. In a review of the literature, Ross and associates[22] found nearly 20 studies all consistently demonstrating cardioprotection associated with HRT. Low-density lipoprotein (LDL) is associated with increased risk of coronary heart disease whereas high-density lipoprotein (HDL) levels are inversely related; low levels of HDL are associated with increased mortality[23]. Higher HDL-cholesterol and decreased LDL-cholesterol are seen in women during reproductive years, when compared with men of the same age. This biochemical protection is lost after the menopause. Hormone replacement therapy does not elevate systolic or diastolic blood pressure[16].

In 1952, Barr and co-workers[24] demonstrated reversal of menopausal trends in lipoproteins by the replacement of oestrogen. Postmenopausal women who are taking HRT have higher HDL-cholesterol than matched controls[25]. HRT significantly reduces total cholesterol[13].

Bush and Miller[26] found alterations in lipoprotein levels according to the available literature, as shown in Table 1.

Hormone replacement therapy may have additional effects including vascular dilatation as a result of altered prostaglandin/thromboxane levels[27], a reduction of platelet aggregation and increased fibrinolytic activity[28]. Evidence from the American Nurses Health Study[29] has shown that HRT is associated with a reduced incidence of coronary heart disease and reduced mortality from cardiovascular disease. A total of 48 470 postmenopausal women aged 30–63, who did not have a history of cancer or cardiovascular disease on entry to the study, were followed up for 10 years. There was no associated change in the risk for stroke.

One problem in evaluating studies is the possible bias in favour of HRT by excluding therapy from high-risk patients; in the past, patients with risk factors such as previous coronary insufficiency, significant family history and obesity may have been advised that HRT was contraindicated. In a study designed to minimize this bias, Rosenberg and colleagues[30] undertook a case–control analysis of 858 cases of first myocardial infarction among women aged 45–69 during 1986–90. The results indicated that unopposed oestrogen use may reduce the risk of first myocardial infarction. The degree of protection was related to the duration of HRT. For past users, protection gradually diminished with amount of time since last taking HRT.

There are insufficient epidemiological data to establish a clear relationship between cardioprotection and either strength of HRT or duration of use[22]. In a recent review of the literature, Samsioe[31] found that the risk of myocardial infarction may be halved by HRT.

**Table 1** Alterations in lipoprotein levels following administration of oestrogen

| *Conjugated equine oestrogen* | *HDL-cholesterol (% increase)* | *LDL-cholesterol (% decrease)* |
|---|---|---|
| 0.625 mg daily | 10 | 4 |
| 1.25 mg daily | 14 | 8 |

Women with high risk factors for coronary artery disease, including family history, hypertension and abnormal lipid profiles, may receive even greater benefit. For those women who had previously sustained a myocardial infarction, the relative risk may be reduced to 0.2 by HRT administration.

Progestogens used in combination with oestrogens may partly offset the cardiovascular benefits. This has been more noticeable with androgenic progestogens, such as norethisterone or levonorgestrel[32]. Medroxyprogesterone acetate and the newer progestins do not seem to have any detrimental action on lipid profiles[33].

### Cerebrovascular disease

Paganini-Hill and co-workers[34] reported a 50% reduction in stroke mortality in women on HRT. It is possible that oestrogen deficiency is a factor in the aetiology of Alzheimer's disease in women and there has been some research showing improvement in affected women following HRT. In a prospective study, 8879 women in Leisure World Laguna Hills, a retirement community in California, were enrolled in 1981. At the time of enrolment, their past and current use of HRT was recorded. Between 1981 and 1992, 138 women of this group had Alzheimer's disease or senile dementia mentioned on their death certificate. The relative risk of developing Alzheimer's was 0.69 for those who had taken HRT and the risk decreased with increasing dose and duration of use[35]. There is some early evidence that long-term, low-dose HRT improves cognitive functions and daily activity in women with mild to moderate Alzheimer's disease[36].

### Osteoporosis

Osteoporosis has been defined as a skeletal condition in which bone mass is sufficiently reduced to the extent that there is an increased risk of fracture with minimal or even no trauma. There is an exponential increase in hip fractures with age and this is more common in women. Following the menopause, the rate of bone loss is accelerated; this can be reduced by the administration of oestrogen. Hip fracture is thought to account for 30 000 deaths each year in the USA. By 1984, hip fractures were costing $7 billion.

Crush fractures of the vertebrae are common in the elderly and are thought to be three times more common than hip fractures. Half of these fractures are not associated with pain. The increasing curvature of the spine results in loss of height and difficulty looking up which is demoralizing and reduces self-esteem.

A woman at the menopause has a lifetime risk of 15% for having a hip fracture, which is equivalent to the combined risk for breast, uterine and ovarian cancer. Bone density measurement at the menopause provides a reasonable prediction of skeletal prognosis with age. There are now several advanced techniques for measuring bone density accurately and allowing serial scans to assess effectiveness of therapy[37]. A 50-year-old patient was referred by her general practitioner who found a cervical polyp when taking a routine smear. Her menopause had occurred at the age of 40 and she had never considered HRT. Her bone density scan showed that she was at risk. Figure 1 shows her serial scan results since commencing HRT (oestradiol 2 mg and medroxyprogesterone acetate 2.5 mg daily).

Oestrogen replacement therapy, with cyclical progestogens when required, provides effective prophylaxis against postmenopausal bone loss. In the Framingham study[38], the relative risk of hip fracture was 0.65 for those who had taken HRT at some time and 0.34 for those who had been taking HRT within the last 2 years. The minimum effective doses of oestrogens are 25 μg ethinyloestradiol, 0.625 mg conjugated oestrogens or 2 mg 17β-oestradiol daily. Treatment should be commenced early and continued for at least 10 years.

Generally, 25 mg implants of oestradiol are effective for the prevention of postmenopausal bone loss[39]. In a study to determine whether there is a dose–response effect of oestradiol implants, 45 postmenopausal women were randomized to receive 25 mg, 50 mg or 75 mg implants. There were significant correlations

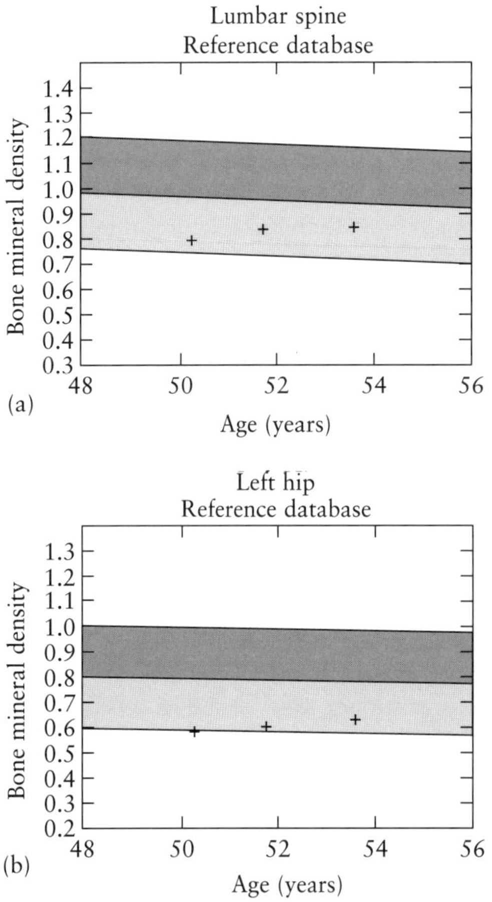


**Figure 1** Serial bone scan results since commencing hormone replacement therapy in a 50-year-old menopausal lady. (a) Lumbar spine; (b) left hip

between the plasma oestradiol levels and the rate of increase in bone density. Three women in the group receiving 25 mg had reduced bone density over the study period. Bone density in the spine and femoral neck was maintained, provided serum oestradiol levels were above 300 pmol/l[40]. Implants would seem to be more effective for increasing bone density than oral oestrogen. Twenty postmenopausal women were receiving long-term oral oestrogen therapy. Ten were changed to oestradiol and testosterone implants whilst the other ten continued with oral oestrogen. Bone density increased by 5.7% at the spine and 5.2% at the neck of the femur in the group receiving the implants but the bone density did not change in those continuing with oral therapy[41].

Felson and colleagues[42] assessed elderly women to determine whether bone mass was affected by earlier oestrogen therapy and how long women needed to take it to obtain a beneficial effect in later life. For long-term preservation of bone mineral density, at least 7 years of oestrogen was required. Women under the age of 75 who had taken oestrogen for more than 7 years had bone densities averaging 11.2% greater than controls. The bone density was just 3.2% higher for women aged 75 or more, who had taken oestrogen for more than 7 years following the menopause, but who had stopped taking it for some years. This study suggests that the benefits on bone density may not be completely sustained for many years after the HRT has been discontinued.

A variety of new medications for the treatment and prevention of osteoporosis, such as the bisphosphonates, are becoming available but HRT remains the first-line treatment[43].

## BENEFITS COMPARED TO RISKS OF HORMONE REPLACEMENT THERAPY

Hormone replacement therapy is indicated to treat symptoms attributable to oestrogen deficiency and to reduce long-term morbidity and mortality that are likely to arise as a result of postmenopausal oestrogen deficiency. Clearly, we need to consider the possible disadvantages, if any, of HRT to establish a balance between benefits and risks. The organs that are sensitive to sex steroids have been the subject of numerous epidemiological studies to evaluate any possible increased risk associated with HRT. Cancers of the breast, uterus and ovaries are common and were common before the advent of HRT. Breast carcinoma is the most common malignancy in women. One woman in 12 will develop the condition during her life. A 50-year-old woman has a 10% chance of breast carcinoma developing. A small increase in relative risk of breast carcinoma would potentially affect a large number of women. The question to be addressed is whether HRT alters the incidence and outcome of these tumours.

### Carcinoma of the breast

There is conflicting epidemiological evidence on the relationship between HRT and breast carcinoma. Many of the studies have not been adequately controlled for factors already known to influence the risk of breast cancer. There are many factors that need to be evaluated. These include the duration of therapy, natural or surgical menopause, and presence of benign breast disease before treatment is commenced.

Epidemiological studies demonstrate that natural events can influence the risk of breast malignancy. Several possible risk factors relate to endogenous sex steroid hormones. Nulliparity and late first pregnancy are associated with increased risk; early first pregnancy, multiparity and lactation serve to reduce the risk. These associations suggest a plausible link between oestrogen and breast cancer. Surgical menopause before age 35 reduces the risk of subsequent breast cancer developing 30 or more years later by more than 60%[44]. There is a doubling of the risk of breast carcinoma for women who have their menopause at age 55 years or later compared to those who have a natural menopause before aged 45 years. The relative risk is greatest after age 70[44]. In contrast, a girl reaching her menarche before the age of 13 has twice the risk of developing breast cancer in later life when compared to other girls[45]. This would suggest that, although increased exposure to oestrogen may increase the risk of breast cancer, the risk is more substantial from exposure in early life rather than in later years. In developed countries, the menarche has tended to occur earlier[1].

There is a tendency for breast malignancy to be familial. The risk ratio for developing breast cancer is 1.9 if the mother has been affected and 2.3 if a sister is affected[46]. The impact on risk for more distant relatives is minimal. It has been estimated that only in a quarter of patients developing breast cancer can a known risk factor be identified[47].

Assessing the possible effects of HRT on the risk of breast cancer is complicated by the variety of confounding factors. Even when considering natural risk factors, there is a lack of consistency between epidemiological studies. For example, Unger and associates[48] found no correlation between early menarche or late menopause and the risk of breast malignancy. Colditz and co-workers[49] observed no increase in the risk of breast cancer when related to the family history of the condition. In addition to the natural factors described above, consideration should be given to the age of commencing HRT, duration of therapy, type of therapy and dosage.

Many patients wish to take HRT for short-term symptomatic relief only. Most investigators conclude that, when used for less than 5 years, the probability is that HRT does not increase the risk[50]. A meta-analysis of the literature found an overall risk of breast cancer associated with HRT to be 1.07[51].

There is a tendency for studies, including the American Nurses Health Study, to suggest that, when HRT is used for more than 10 years, there may be an increased risk of about 30–50%[50,52,53]. It is noteworthy that the apparent increased risk relates to current users. The American Nurses Health Study recruited 121 700 female registered nurses aged 30–55 years in 1976. Nurses who discontinued HRT after 10 years were not at increased risk[53].

Women who are diagnosed as having breast cancer whilst taking HRT, tend to have relatively early-stage disease[54]. This may be a reflection of increased surveillance among those taking therapy and also by those prescribing it. Mortality from breast cancer in patients who have taken HRT seems to be decreased, with risk ratios varying from 0.5 to 0.8[50]. Current users of HRT who have been taking it for more than 15 years have a 40% reduction in overall mortality from atherosclerosis and cancer[55]. It will be a number of years yet before such large ongoing studies, such as the American Nurses Health Study, will provide us with the absolute risks and benefits of HRT.

Patients taking HRT, who have not had a hysterectomy, should receive a progestogen to prevent endometrial hyperplasia and malignancy. Progestogens are not generally considered to protect against breast carcinoma. In an early prospective study[56], there was a lower incidence of breast cancer in HRT users compared to an untreated group. The protective effect was enhanced in the combined oestrogen–progestogen user group. Badwe and colleagues[57] found a significantly better outcome for premenopausal women having surgery for breast cancer in the luteal phase of the cycle compared to those undergoing surgery in the proliferative phase. This group of researchers conjectured that, in perimenopausal women, intervention might be of value to counteract prolonged low but unopposed oestrogen secretion. From a theoretical point of view, however, it has been suggested that progestogens are unlikely to reduce the risks of breast malignancy. A second evaluation of the effects of progestogens with oestrogen replacement therapy concluded that progestogens might marginally increase the risk[58]. Recent analysis from the Nurses Health Study would suggest that the addition of progestogens to oestrogen replacement therapy does not reduce the risk of breast cancer among postmenopausal women[53].

For women who have had breast cancer, HRT has generally been considered to be contraindicated. Progestogens, such as medroxyprogesterone acetate 10–50 mg daily, may alleviate flushes, and vaginal moisturisers (e.g. Replens®, Winthrop) may overcome symptoms of vaginal atrophy. Topical vaginal oestrogen preparations that are poorly absorbed may also be used if vaginal problems persist. For patients with continuing distressing symptoms, HRT may be considered if quality of life is a major problem. There are some early reassuring data to suggest that, for these women, continuous combined HRT may have a lower risk of tumour recurrence than previously anticipated[59]. There is a trend for oncologists to recognize that the case against HRT for patients with a history of breast carcinoma has probably been overstated. There is probably, however, a small but unmeasured increased risk. When we counsel a patient who has a history of breast cancer, it is a matter of policy to liaise with her other clinicians, before prescribing treatment. This serves to ensure that the patient receives consistent and concerted advice. This policy would also apply to any other condition where there might possibly be a conflict of medical opinion where HRT is concerned.

A gene mutation has been identified which predisposes to both cancer of the ovary and breast. It may be that gene probing for increased risk of these cancers will become available for screening the population in general[60].

### Hormone replacement therapy and mastalgia

Mastalgia may occur in 8% of women commencing HRT. Paradoxically, it would seem that postmenopausal women troubled by mastalgia before HRT, tend to report an improvement after commencing treatment[61]. We have observed that mastalgia appears to be a particular problem when starting HRT after several years of oestrogen deficiency. In these circumstances, we often introduce the oestrogen slowly with an escalating regimen. A 40-year-old lady, who had a total abdominal hysterectomy and right salpingo-oophorectomy at the age of 30, presented with reduced energy and other menopausal symptoms. Before her hysterectomy, cyclical mastalgia had been a major problem. Oestradiol valerate 1 mg on alternate days for 2 weeks and then daily was prescribed. She reported no side-effects. For women starting HRT several years after ovarian failure, particularly when they are aged 60 or more, we often start oestrogen replacement with just one tablet weekly and gradually increase the frequency in step-wise fashion.

### Hormone replacement therapy and endometrial malignancy

In the early days of HRT, many women who had not undergone hysterectomy were given unopposed oestrogen. These women proved to have an eight-fold increased chance of developing endometrial carcinoma. Interestingly, the association between oestrogen replacement therapy and endometrial carcinoma was for local disease rather than advanced malignancy[62]. The administration of progestogens for 10 days each month in combination with oestrogen replacement therapy has been clearly shown to prevent any increased risk of endometrial carcinoma[63].

### Hormone replacement therapy and ovarian malignancy

Combined oral contraceptives reduce the incidence of ovarian carcinoma, probably by inhibiting ovulation and suppressing gonadotrophins. There is conflicting evidence as to whether HRT is associated with a decreased incidence of ovarian cancer[64] or a small increased risk[65]. Hormone replacement therapy does not appear to have a detrimental effect on the prognosis of patients with ovarian malignancy[66].

### Hormone replacement therapy and thromboembolism

A history of thromboembolism is no longer regarded as a contraindication to HRT. Three papers recently published in *The Lancet*[67–69] have indicated a small increased risk of thromboembolism in current HRT users. The risk of thromboembolism in non-users is 1 in 10 000 per year (mortality 1 in a million) and for HRT users it is 3 in 10 000 per year (mortality 3 in a million). The Committee on Safety of Medicines has commented that the new data do not change the overall positive balance between the benefits and risks of treatment for most women.

Should a patient develop a thromboembolism, HRT should be withheld during the acute phase. Patients who are considered to be at high risk from their medical or family history should be screened for thrombophilia. A 50-year-old lady was referred by her general practitioner for consideration of HRT. The patient, who went through the menopause at the age of 43 and who had five episodes of deep venous thrombosis before the age of 40, had menopausal symptoms. She proved to be protein S deficient and also resistant to activated protein C, which predisposed her to thrombosis. Our haematologists recommended formal anticoagulation with warfarin and she has subsequently commenced continuous combined HRT.

### Hormone replacement therapy and weight gain

A common anxiety of patients contemplating HRT is weight gain. Reubinoff and his colleagues[70] studied 63 early postmenopausal women attending their menopause clinic. Continuous combined oral conjugated oestrogens and medroxyprogesterone acetate 2.5 mg daily were given to 34 women who accepted HRT; 29 women who declined HRT provided the controls. Age, menopausal status, weight, body mass index, fat mass, waist-to-hip ratios, and daily calorie intake were similar in the two groups. The body weight and fat mass increased by 2.35 kg in the treatment group and by 2.06 kg in the control group over 12 months; there was no significant difference in the weight gain between the two groups. Serial measurements of the waist-to-hip ratio demonstrated a significant change from a gynaecoid to an android fat distribution in the control group but not in the treatment group.

### Hormone replacement therapy and life expectancy

There is evidence that HRT increases life expectancy. After 7.5 years of follow-up of the original 8881 postmenopausal women in the Leisure World Laguna Hills study[71], there had been 1447 deaths. Those women with a history of oestrogen use had a 20% reduction in mortality compared to non-users. Mortality decreased with increasing duration of use but the advantages were less pronounced for those women who had not recently taken HRT. There was a 40% reduction in overall mortality for current users taking HRT for more than 15 years. Women in the HRT group were less likely to die from cancer.

From an analysis of the available literature, Grady and her colleagues[72] calculated the lifetime probabilities of a 50-year-old woman with varying situations developing coronary heart disease, stroke, hip fracture, breast cancer, endometrial cancer and also her overall life expectancy. In general, there was a net gain of 1 year for women taking HRT. For women at risk of coronary heart disease, HRT provides a gain of 2 years. For women at risk of breast cancer, HRT was still calculated to provide a net gain of nearly 1 year.

The long-term studies described above, which look at the risks and benefits of HRT, have many years to run before they reach completion. It is still a matter of conjecture as to whether HRT will be conclusively proven to provide increased longevity, although commentators believe that this is likely to be the case[73,74].

## PRESCRIBING HORMONE REPLACEMENT THERAPY: GUIDELINES

A brief questionnaire, which the patient completes just before her initial consultation listing her symptoms and her views about HRT, seems helpful. A full history is recorded with the benefit of a proforma. Specific attention is given to the family history of heart, bone and breast disease. A full physical examination of the patient is performed.

If the patient has a medical problem that would need considerable caution before prescribing HRT, such as breast cancer, we liaise with the other clinicians involved in her care before prescribing. Such correspondence and co-operation ensure that the patient receives consistent advice.

The advantages and possible risks of HRT in general and for the individual patient in particular are discussed with her and information leaflets supplied for further clarification (see Chapter 2). Each patient receives a choice of therapy.

Figure 2 is a flow chart to assist decision-making in prescribing hormone therapy. There are four questions to consider.

### Question 1: Has the patient had a hysterectomy?

If the uterus has been removed then, in general, hormone replacement can be provided by oestrogen alone (letter A in Figure 2); occasionally, if there has been significant endometriosis, additional low-dose continuous progestogen may be indicated. Oestrogen can be administered by mouth, transdermally or subcutaneously. A variety of oral oestrogen preparations are available (Table 2).

Physicians tend to have personal preference for their first-choice preparation. As with prescribing combined oral contraceptive pills, patient acceptance of the various formulations is unpredictable. It is probably wise to start with a low dose initially to reduce the likelihood of side-effects. Women who have been deprived of oestrogen for any length of time seem

**Table 2** Oral oestrogen preparations

| *Oestrogen* | *Dose* (mg) | *Preparation* | *Manufacturer* |
|---|---|---|---|
| Oestradiol | 1 and 2 | Climaval | Sandoz |
| | 1 and 2 | Progynova | Schering |
| | 2 | Zumenon | Duphar |
| | 1 and 2 | Elleste Solo | Searle |
| Conjugated oestrogens | 0.625 | Premarin | Wyeth |
| | 1.25 | | |
| Oestrone | 1.5 | Harmogen | Abbott |
| Oestriol/oestrone/oestradiol | 0.27/1.4/0.6 | Hormonin | Shire |

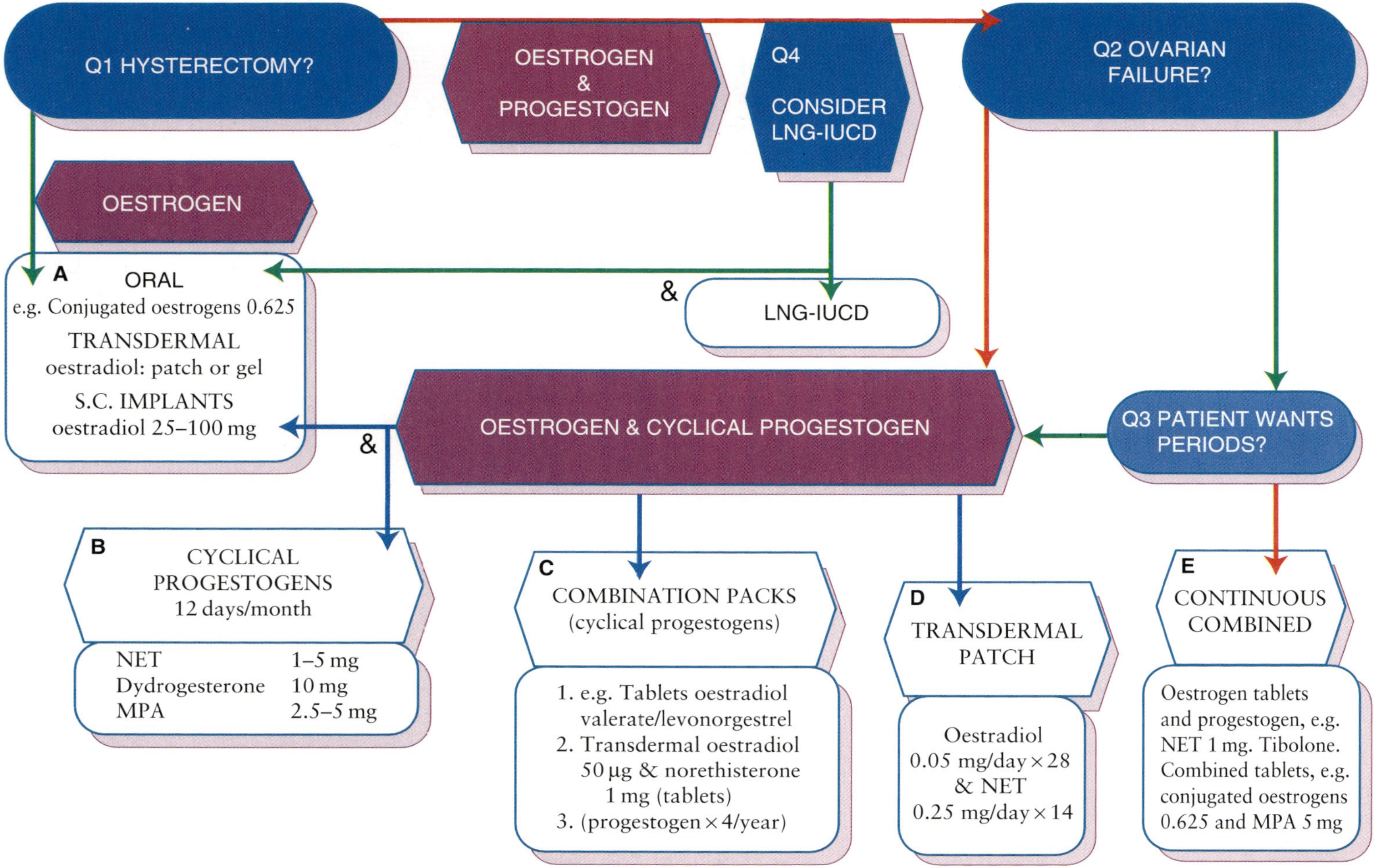


**Figure 2** Flow chart to assist decision-making in prescribing hormone replacement therapy. MPA = medroxyprogesterone acetate; NET = norethisterone acetate; LNG-IUCD = levonorgestrel intrauterine contraceptive device. Green arrows represent 'yes' or a positive result, red arrows 'no' or a negative result, blue arrows options

to be more prone to side-effects and mastalgia may be particularly distressing. In some circumstances, particularly if there is a history of mastalgia, it may be prudent to start with one tablet every few days and slowly increase to a daily regimen.

Orally administered oestrogens are metabolized in the intestine and liver. It has been suggested that some side-effects of oestrogen therapy can be reduced by percutaneous or subcutaneous administration. Oestrogen skin patches are available to release oestradiol 25–100 μg/24 h (Estraderm, Ciba; Evorel, Cilag; Fematrix, Solvay; Menorest, Rhone-Poulenc Rorer). A new patch is applied twice weekly to a fresh area of healthy skin below the waistline. Patches that are active for 1 week are becoming available (Progynova TS, Schering and Femseven, Merck). These patches can be temporarily removed during bathing.

An oestrogen gel (Oestrogel: Hoechst Roussel) containing 0.75 mg oestradiol per measure has become available in the UK. Two to four measures daily are rubbed gently into the upper arms, shoulders or thighs usually after bathing. Beneficial effects on bone density have been demonstrated[75].

Oestradiol implants are introduced subcutaneously at abdominal hysterectomy and bilateral salpingo-oophorectomy, or in the outpatient clinic under local anaesthetic. Oestradiol implants are available at 25, 50 and 100 mg strengths.

Concern has been expressed about the supraphysiological concentrations of oestradiol that can occur with implants, particularly after several have been used[76]. Garnett and associates[77] observed supraphysiological oestradiol levels in just 3% of long-term users; this was particularly evident with short intervals and high-dose implants. Higher-dose implants are associated with a greater difference in peak and trough plasma concentrations of oestradiol. Patients may return early after an implant complaining of symptoms apparently typical of oestrogen deficiency. Some of the symptoms may be attributable to the rapid rate of decline in oestradiol concentration[78]. Owen and coworkers[78] concluded that the initial dose should be 25 mg pellets. Buckler and colleagues[79] advocated 50 mg oestradiol implants and generally found no justification for introducing implants more frequently than once each year. They found that this achieved physiological levels of oestradiol and good symptomatic relief.

In our department, we introduce 800 oestradiol implants annually. About half of our patients have 100 mg implants and half 50 mg. One woman in four is also given testosterone. If symptoms return early, the plasma oestradiol is estimated. If this proves to be supraphysiological, a 25 mg implant is introduced. Occasionally, it might be prudent to check the serum oestradiol level as this is directly related to the beneficial effect on bone[40]. Patients show a wide variation in serum oestradiol concentrations for a given implant[40]. The range of oestradiol levels with 25 mg implants ranged from 114 to 853 pmol/l after 1 year.

**Question 2: If the patient has not had a hysterectomy, has she reached the menopause?**

If the uterus is *in situ*, it is imperative that a progestogen is also prescribed; this virtually abolishes the risks of endometrial hyperplasia and malignancy. Many premenopausal women experience symptom relief with HRT; they require cyclical progestogens to produce adequate endometrial shedding (A and B, C or D, Figure 2). The progestogen may be prescribed separately from the oestrogen of choice (A and B). Medroxyprogesterone 5 mg, dydrogesterone 10 mg or norethisterone 1–5 mg daily for 12 days each cycle should suffice. Commercial preparations (Micronor HRT, norethisterone 1 mg; Duphaston HRT, dydrogesterone 10 mg) are available; patients should be advised that, despite their name, these agents are not the HRT but essential supplements to be taken with HRT. The dosage of progestogen should be titrated against cycle control and side-effects. There may be variation in endometrial response. Dydrogesterone 10 or 20 mg daily for 14 days each cycle protects the endometrium against hyperplasia. With the lower dosage, irregular bleeding problems may occur[80].

For convenience, several pharmaceutical companies provide packages of oral oestrogen with cyclical progestogen tablets for 12 days (C, Table 3). There are three preparations with varying amounts of oestrogen through the month. In one preparation, oestradiol 1 mg and oestriol 0.5 mg for 6 days and then 2 mg and 1 mg, respectively, for 22 days is combined with norethisterone 1 mg for the last 12 days of the 28-day cycle (Trisequens, Novo Nordisk). The oestrogens are available in double strength with norethisterone 1 mg for 12 days (Trisequens forte). The third preparation has varying quantities of both oestrogens and progestogen (Menophase, Syntex). The oestrogen is mestranol starting with 12.5 µg daily and peaking at 50 µg; norethisterone is given for 13 days with a maximum of 1.5 mg.

For those women who prefer not to take tablets of any sort, transdermal patches with oestradiol 50 µg daily and norethisterone 250 µg daily for 14 days each month can be prescribed (D) (Estracombi, Ciba).

One disadvantage of all the combined oestrogen and progestogen packages is cycle adjustment for social convenience. This is particularly difficult when the package has varying amounts of oestrogen and progestogen through the month.

The cyclical administration of progestogens prescribed in combination with HRT may be associated occasionally with distressing symptoms typical of the premenstrual syndrome. In some circumstances, it may be necessary to reduce the number of days of progestogen administration. Ettinger and co-workers[81] studied 214 postmenopausal women who were initially taking conjugated oestrogens 0.625 mg and medroxyprogesterone 5 or 10 mg cyclically each month. The frequency of medroxyprogesterone was reduced to 10 mg/day for 14 days every 3 months for 1 year. Endometrial biopsies were examined before and after treatment; there was no significant increase of hyperplasia. Although there was increased duration and quantity of flow, and also more unscheduled bleeding, 80% of the patients preferred the quarterly regimen. Tridestra (Winthrop) has 91 tablets in three blister packs with a regimen for periods every 3 months for perimenopausal women. The first 70 tablets contain oestradiol valerate 2 mg. The next 14 tablets have oestradiol acetate 2 mg and medroxyprogesterone acetate 20 mg and there are then seven placebo tablets. Unscheduled and heavy withdrawal bleeds were more common in women who were less than 3 years beyond their menopause[82]. Continuous oestrogen replacement by transdermal patch with transdermal norethisterone acetate administered every other month may be

**Table 3** Oral oestrogen and cyclical progestogen preparations

| *Oestrogen/progestogen* | *Dose* (mg) | *Preparation* | *Manufacturer* |
|---|---|---|---|
| Oestradiol/levonorgestrel | 1/75 µg | Nuvelle | Schering |
| Oestradiol/norethisterone | 1/1 | Climagest 1 mg | Sandoz |
| | 2/1 | Climagest 2 mg | Sandoz |
| | 50 µg/24 h/1 | Estrapak | Ciba |
| | 50 µg/24 h/1 | Evorel-Pak | Ortho |
| | 2/1 | Elleste Duet | Searle |
| Conjugated oestrogens/norgestrel | 0.625/0.15 | Prempak-C 0.625 | Wyeth |
| | 1.25/0.15 | Prempak-C 1.25 | Wyeth |
| Conjugated oestrogens/ medroxyprogesterone acetate | 0.625/10 | Premique cycle | Wyeth |
| Oestropipate/medroxyprogesterone acetate | 1.5/10 | Improvera | Upjohn |

an alternative to monthly bleeds in postmenopausal women[83].

Cooper and Whitehead[84] have recommended caution when considering long-cycle hormone replacement therapy as the risk of endometrial hyperplasia increases with the duration of oestrogen treatment. They recommend more long-term studies before incorporating long-cycle hormone replacement therapy into routine clinical use. A study by Kemp and his colleagues[85] provides a degree of reassurance. Eighty-five postmenopausal women received conjugated oestrogens for 6 months and then a 10-day course of norethisterone 0.35 mg. This was repeated for 4 years. The endometria were sampled and no patient developed carcinoma.

### Question 3: If the patient has not had a hysterectomy and has reached the menopause, does she wish to have periods when taking hormone replacement therapy?

Postmenopausal women who have not had a hysterectomy have a choice as to whether they would wish to see a withdrawal bleed or not. Younger women, particularly those who have had a premature menopause, are more likely to feel happier with a cyclical regimen. It is prudent to remember that there have been sporadic reports of spontaneous pregnancy in these younger women even when there may have been endocrinological evidence of ovarian failure. The majority of postmenopausal women, however, prefer to have the benefits of HRT without the inconvenience of withdrawal bleeds (E).

Sporrong and associates[86] treated 60 women with micronized oestradiol 2 mg and one of four continuous progestogen regimens (norethisterone acetate 1 mg; norethisterone acetate 0.5 mg; megestrol acetate 5 mg or megestrol acetate 2.5 mg). The endometrium was atrophic in the majority of biopsies. Irregular bleeding was confined to the first few weeks of therapy in all groups.

In a 1-year prospective, double-blind, randomized, multicentre study of 1724 postmenopausal women, five groups of women all received conjugated oestrogens (0.625 mg) daily. Groups A and B received 2.5 and 5 mg medroxyprogesterone acetate daily and groups C and D received 5 and 10 mg for 14 days every 28 days. Of these women, 1385 had endometrial biopsies. The group receiving oestrogen alone had a 20% incidence of endometrial hyperplasia. The maximum incidence of endometrial hyperplasia in the groups receiving medroxyprogesterone acetate was 1%; none of the patients receiving 5 mg medroxyprogesterone daily or 10 mg cyclically developed endometrial hyperplasia[87].

Tibolone (Livial, Organon) is a synthetic steroid that seems to have oestrogenic and progestogenic properties. This allows the benefits of continuous treatment for menopausal symptoms in women who are 1 year beyond the menopause, without planned bleeds. The role of tibolone in osteoporosis and coronary heart disease has yet to be conclusively defined. A minority of postmenopausal women, particularly those who are relatively young or only recently menopausal, bleed whilst taking tibolone[88].

For the last few years, we have prescribed continuous combined HRT for postmenopausal women who do not wish to be bothered by bleeds. The oestrogen has always been from the oral group (E) together with a low-dose progestogen. This has allowed fine-tuning of therapy to suit the individual patient's requirements. Combined tablets have become available as shown in Table 4. It may be prudent to consider the economic implications of the various options.

### Question 4: Is there an indication for a levonorgestrel intrauterine contraceptive device to provide continuous progestogen to the endometrium?

The levonorgestrel intrauterine system (Mirena, Pharmacia-Leiras) was released in the UK in 1995. It provides sufficient progestogen locally to maintain endometrial suppression for the postmenopausal woman on HRT. For the patient in her later reproductive years, it will provide excellent contraception with reduced

**Table 4** Continuous combined oestrogen/progestogen tablet preparations

| *Oestrogen/progestogen* | *Dose* (mg) | *Preparation* | *Manufacturer* |
|---|---|---|---|
| Oestradiol valerate | 1/0.7 | Climesse | Sandoz |
| Conjugated oestrogens/ medroxyprogesterone acetate | 0.625/5 | Premique | Wyeth |
| Oestradiol/norethisterone acetate | 2/1 | Kliofem | Novo Nordisk |
| Tibolone | 2.5 | Livial | Organon |

menstrual loss, with the additional advantage that no cyclical progestogens are required. Initial reports indicate that, for some perimenopausal women taking HRT, this may prove to be a valuable alternative and an acceptable method of continuous progestogen administration with oral oestrogen[89], transdermal oestrogen patches[90] or subcutaneous oestradiol implants[91].

**Table 5** Local oestrogen preparations

| *Oestrogen* | *Manufacturer* |
|---|---|
| Dienoestrol cream | Ortho |
| Ortho-Gynest pessaries/ cream | Ortho |
| Ovestin cream | Organon |
| Tampovagan pessaries | Norgine |
| Vagifem pessaries | Novo Nordisk |
| Estring ring | Pharmacia-Leiras |
| Premarin | Wyeth |

### Local oestrogens

A variety of oestrogen creams and pessaries are available for local treatment of atrophic vaginitis (Table 5). A synthetic soft rubber ring (Estring) releasing oestradiol may be introduced into the vagina and changed at 3-monthly intervals; if the uterus is still present, intermittent courses of progestogen should be considered to encourage endometrial shedding. This ring has proven to be as effective as vaginal oestrogen creams but more readily accepted by patients[92].

## PROGESTERONE REPLACEMENT THERAPY

Lee[93] correctly points out that ovarian failure is associated with progesterone deficiency as well as oestrogen deficiency. He has described his experience with 'natural progesterone cream' applied to the skin. The progesterone is in fact converted in the laboratory from diosgenin extracted from the Mexican yam. A large variety of clinical benefits from the product are claimed, including increased bone density, relief of benign breast disease, enhanced libido and relief from the premenstrual syndrome. Lee noted that others had used progesterone in capsule form or rectal suppositories but found the transdermal route to be acceptable to his patients. Controlled studies would be required to confirm these observations.

The half-life of progesterone taken orally is short and it is therefore not effective. Micronized progesterone has recently been shown to be well absorbed and can be used in postmenopausal hormone replacement therapy[94].

## TESTOSTERONE REPLACEMENT THERAPY

Testosterone implants may have a role for women with reduced libido or insufficient energy when oestrogen replacement therapy does not adequately resolve these problems. Five aspects of sexual behaviour were monitored in three groups of women 4 years after total abdominal hysterectomy and bilateral salpingo-oophorectomy for benign disease[95]. One group were receiving oestrogen alone, the second group combined oestrogen and androgen and the third group had no hormonal therapy. Rates of coitus and orgasm were higher in the group receiving combined oestrogen and androgen. Rates of coitus and orgasm could be related to testosterone levels. Experience has shown that virilizing side-effects, such as hirsutism, occur rarely and disappear if further implants are withheld[96]. The importance of androgen replacement therapy for women with deficiency symptoms has been emphasized[97].

## NON-HORMONAL THERAPY OF MENOPAUSAL SYMPTOMS

Some patients with menopausal symptoms may not be able to take oestrogen but other treatments may provide a degree of symptomatic relief. Clonidine significantly reduces the frequency of hot flushes.

For patients with vaginal symptoms including discomfort and dyspareunia, a bioadhesive vaginal moisturizer (Replens, Unipath) may be an effective alternative to local oestrogens[98]. Progestogens can increase bone density[99,100] and reduce hot flushes. Veralipride, an anti-dopaminergic, reduces hot flushes associated with GnRH therapy[101] and may be considered for postmenopausal flushes.

Tamoxifen, which is commonly prescribed for breast cancer as an oestrogen antagonist, also has oestrogen agonist actions. It has an HRT-type action on the genital tract and there is an increased risk of endometrial carcinoma. As with oestrogen replacement therapy, cyclical progestogens probably have a part to play in the prevention of endometrial carcinoma for patients with a uterus receiving long-term tamoxifen therapy[102]. Lipids are reduced which may decrease coronary heart disease and there is also a beneficial effect on bone density. It may be an alternative to HRT for women who have had a history of breast cancer or who are at risk of breast cancer[103].

A 46-year-old patient presented with hot flushes and more troublesome night sweats whilst taking tamoxifen 20 mg daily. Three years earlier she had had a breast lumpectomy and radiotherapy. There was a strong family history of osteoporosis. Medroxyprogesterone acetate 5 mg each morning and 10 mg at night for 21 days with a 7-day gap resolved her vasomotor symptoms.

## MONITORING PATIENTS TAKING HORMONE REPLACEMENT THERAPY

Opinion varies as to the frequency that physical examination should be undertaken for patients receiving HRT. Some would suggest that pelvic examinations should be performed only at the time of taking routine cervical smears which is usually at 3–5 year intervals[104]. Others recommend pelvic examinations once or twice each year[105].

A 72-year-old lady presented in November 1995 with heavy vaginal bleeding whilst taking HRT. She had been on HRT from 1968. In 1992, she had had a D & C by a consultant colleague to investigate heavy withdrawal bleeds with cyclical HRT; cervical biopsy was performed at the same time as the cervix was enlarged. The histology was benign. No vaginal examination had been performed for more than 2 years before her recent presentation. We found a 14 cm fibroid arising from the cervix and attempting to come through the os. Oestrogen was withheld for 2 months and a total abdominal hysterectomy, bilateral salpingo-oophorectomy was performed (Figure 3). Hormone replacement therapy may be associated with enlargement of uterine fibroids[106]. Whilst this case is unusual, it is the author's view that those looking after women's health should undertake breast and pelvic examination at least annually to exclude the development of obvious pathology.

Endometrial hyperplasia with cytological atypia has at least a 30% chance of becoming malignant. Irregular bleeding can be investigated by transvaginal ultrasonography, hysteroscopy or endometrial curettage or sampling (e.g. Pipelle). In general, HRT with progestogen is associated with a reduced incidence of endometrial malignancy. Irregular bleeding beyond

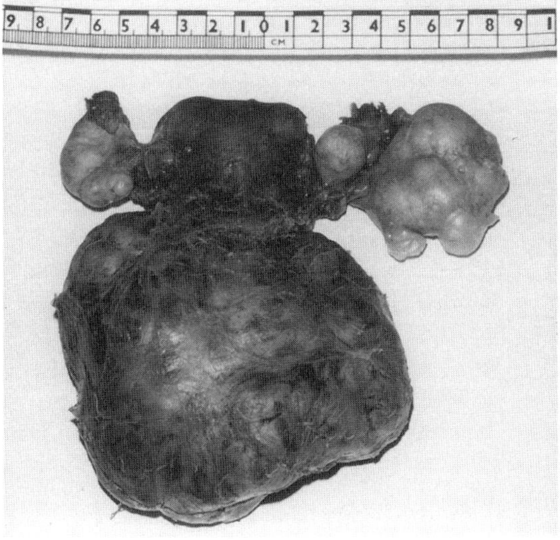

Figure 3 Cervical fibroid measuring 14 cm with body of uterus and adnexae from a 72-year-old lady who had been taking hormone replacement therapy for 27 years

the initial treatment cycles requires investigation.

A 48-year-old lady with depression initially showed some benefit with oestradiol skin patches. When her symptoms increased again, the dose was increased without benefit. Her plasma oestradiol proved to be just 73 pmol/l. A 50 mg oestradiol implant was introduced and proved to be successful. We tend to use oestradiol estimations only when symptoms are proving unexpectedly difficult to control. Testosterone estimations are generally reassuring for patients receiving testosterone tablets or implants and can assist in adjusting individual patient treatment regimens.

Breast screening is gradually becoming routine in some countries[107]. Hormone replacement therapy can be associated with increased glandular tissue and, as always, it is essential that the radiologist is advised about the patient's medication. The radiologist might occasionally recommend supplementary screening including ultrasound. We would advocate regular mammography for postmenopausal women and, for women who have been on HRT for more than 10 years, annual screening is probably appropriate.

## PATIENT COMPLIANCE WITH HORMONE REPLACEMENT THERAPY

Ultimately it is for the individual patient, with an unbiased summary of the available information provided by her doctor, to decide whether she wishes to take HRT. The media, which seem to be increasingly interested in controversy rather than harmony, tend to highlight those individuals who may have developed problems whilst taking medication. With risk ratios for an association between HRT and pathology hovering around 1.0, it is impossible to determine for any individual whether the pathology is related to treatment. Unfortunately, clinicians, who believe that there is persuasive statistical evidence of reduced mortality and morbidity with HRT, can only present the statistics: we cannot identify those specific individuals who have been spared illness and premature death.

Although it is now recognized that HRT is probably the most important recent advance in preventative medicine, patient compliance is variable. Patients may stop their HRT because of fear of breast cancer, mastalgia or weight gain[108]. In practice, many patients insist that they are gaining weight despite records showing that their weight has not changed. It may be that some of this weight gain is a change in self-perception rather than physical change.

Ravnikar[109] found that only 40% of women started on HRT continue taking it reliably after 9 months. Failure to involve patients in their choice of HRT, fears of cancer, headaches, mastalgia and heavy periods are the major contributing factors in poor patient compliance. Reassurance, patient involvement in decision making, information leaflets, encouraging continuous combined preparations after the menopause, and regular review encourage patients to enjoy the long-term benefits of HRT[110]. Clinicians should be willing to adjust treatment when problems arise.

## CONCLUSION

During reproductive years, most oestrogens are produced by the Graffian follicles and corpora lutea. The human newborn, although destined to have a mentality and dexterity greatly superior to any other species, is delivered at a relatively early stage of development and is totally reliant on parental care. Nature has arranged for a woman to lose her reproductive capability 20 or 30 years ahead of her life expectancy, although, provided she remains healthy, she should continue to have the physical and mental ability to care for, and enjoy, her family.

The menopause heralds the arrival of a naturally induced sex steroid deficiency state in otherwise healthy women. It may be associated with distressing symptoms in the short-term. In the long-term, there is a significant risk of severe morbidity and mortality that can be reduced by hormone replacement therapy. On current evidence, the benefits outweigh the risks. To withhold vitamin supplements, in such deficiency states as pernicious anaemia or scurvy, would be unthinkable. To withhold hormone replacement such as thyroxin for patients with hypothyroidism, corticosteroids for patients with Addison's disease or insulin for diabetes mellitus would be unethical.

In northern Italy, women who had received formal education for 12 years or more were three times more likely to take hormone replacement therapy than those with less than 7 years' formal education, and HRT acceptance was also strongly related to social class[111]. The majority of menopausal women doctors in the United Kingdom have taken hormone replacement therapy and most seem to be taking it for more than 5 years[112]. Hormonal replacement therapy should be offered to the majority of postmenopausal women, and also to perimenopausal women with oestrogen deficiency symptoms.

## REFERENCES


1. Short, R. V. (1976). The evolution of human reproduction. *Proc. R. Soc. London B*, **195**, 3–24
2. Brambilla, D. J. and McKinley, S. M. (1989). A prospective study of factors affecting age at menopause. *J. Clin. Epidemiol.*, **42**, 1031–9
3. Kaufman, D. W., Slone, D., Rosenberg, L., Miettinen, O. S. and Shapiro, S. (1980). Cigarette smoking and age at natural menopause. *Am. J. Public Health*, **70**, 420–2
4. Cramer, D. W., Xu, H. and Harlow, B. L. (1995). Family history as a predictor of early menopause. *Fertil. Steril.*, **64**, 740–5
5. Kinsella, K. G. (1992). Changes in life expectancy 1900–1990. *Am. J. Clin. Nutr.*, **55**, 1196–920S
6. Baird, D. T. (1990). Biology of the menopause. In Drife, J. O. and Studd, J. W. W. (eds.) *HRT and Osteoporosis*, pp. 3–10. (London: Springer-Verlag)
7. Hjortland, M. C., McNamara, P. M. and Kannel, W. B. (1976). Some atherogenic concomitants of menopause: the Framingham Study. *Am. J. Epidemiol.*, **103**, 304–11
8. Nasri, M. N. (1992). Transvaginal versus transrectal sonography in postmenopausal women. *Br. J. Obstet. Gynaecol.*, **99**, 932–3
9. Castracane, V. D., Gimpel, T. and Goldzieher, J. W. (1993). Oral contraception in women over 40; diagnostic tests for the menopausal transition. In *Abstracts of the Scientific Oral and Poster Sessions of the American Society for Reproductive Medicine*, Programme Supplement, November 1993, Montreal, S37
10. Gosden, R. G. and Faddy, M. J. (1995). Mathematical models for predicting the timing of the menopause. In Asch, R. and Studd, J. (eds.) *Progress in Reproductive Medicine*, Vol. II, pp. 95–102. (New York and London: The Parthenon Publishing Group)
11. Fantl, J. A., Cardoza, L. D. and McClish, D. K. (1994). Oestrogen therapy in the management of urinary incontinence in postmenopausal women: a meta-analysis. First Report of the Hormones and Urological Therapy Committee. *Obstet. Gynecol.*, **83**, 12–18
12. Montgomery, J. C., Appleby, L., Brincat, M., Versi, E., Tapp, A., Fenwick, P. B. and Studd, J. W. (1987). Effect of oestrogen and testosterone implants on psychological disorders in the climacteric. *Lancet,* **1**, 297–9
13. Furuhjelm, M., Karlgren, E. and Carlstrom, K. (1984). The effect of oestrogen therapy on somatic and psychical symptoms in postmenopausal women. *Acta Obstet. Gynecol. Scand.*, **63**, 655–61
14. Sherwin, B. B. (1988). Affective changes with oestrogen and androgen replacement therapy

in surgically menopausal women. *J. Affect. Disord.*, **14**, 177–87
15. Sherwin, B. B. (1988). Oestrogen and/or androgen replacement therapy and cognitive functioning in surgically menopausal women. *Psychoneuroendocrinology*, **13**, 345–57
16. Campbell, S. and Whitehead, M. (1977). Oestrogen therapy and the menopausal syndrome. *Clin. Obstet. Gynaecol.*, **4**, 31–7
17. Ditkoff, E. C., Crary, W. G., Cristo, M. and Lobo, R. A. (1991). Oestrogen improves psychological function in asymptomatic postmenopausal women. *Obstet. Gynecol.*, **78**, 991–5
18. Purdie, D. W., Empson, J. A. C., Crichton, C. and MacDonald, L. (1995). Hormone replacement therapy, sleep quality and psychological wellbeing. *Br. J. Obstet. Gynaecol.*, **102**, 735–9
19. Lindheim, S. R., Legro, R. S., Bernstein, L., Stanczyk, F. Z., Vijod, M. A., Presser, S. C. and Lobo, R. A. (1992). Behavioural stress responses in premenopausal and postmenopausal women and the effect of oestrogen. *Am. J. Obstet. Gynecol.*, **167**, 1831–6
20. Kannel, W. B., Hjortland, M. C., McNamara, P. M. and Gordon, T. (1976). Menopause and the risk of cardiovascular disease: the Framingham study. *Ann. Intern. Med.*, **85**, 447–52
21. Parrish, H. M., Carr, C. A., Hall, D. G. and King, T. M. (1967). Time interval from castration in premenopausal women to development of excessive coronary atherosclerosis. *Am. J. Obstet. Gynecol.*, **99**, 155–62
22. Ross, R. K., Pike, M. C., Mack, T. M. and Henderson, B. E. (1990). Oestrogen replacement therapy and cardiovascular disease. In Drife, J. O. and Studd, J. W. W. (eds.) *HRT and Osteoporosis*, pp. 209–22. (London: Springer-Verlag)
23. Wilson, P. W., Abbott, R. D. and Castelli, W. P. (1988). High density lipoprotein cholesterol and mortality. The Framingham Heart Study. *Arteriosclerosis*, **8**, 737–41
24. Barr, D. P., Russ, E. M. and Eder, H. A. (1952). Influence of oestrogens on lipoproteins in atherosclerosis. *Trans. Assoc. Am. Physicians*, **65**, 102–13
25. Wilson, P. W., Garrison, R. J. and Castelli, W. P. (1985). Postmenopausal oestrogen use, cigarette smoking and cardiovascular morbidity in women over 50. The Framingham Study. *N. Engl. J. Med.*, **313**, 1038–43
26. Bush, T. L. and Miller, V. T. (1987). Effects of pharmacologic agents used during menopause: impact on lipids and lipoproteins. In Mishell, D. R. (ed.) *Menopause, Physiology and Pharmacology*, pp. 187–208. (Chicago and London: Yearbook Medical Publishers)
27. Ylikorkala, O., Puolakka, J. and Viinikka, L. (1984). Vasoconstrictory thromboxane A2 and vasodilatory prostacyclin in climacteric women: effect of oestrogen-progestogen therapy. *Maturitas*, **5**, 201–5
28. Gebara, O. C., Mittleman, M. A., Sutherland, P., Lipinska, I., Matheney, T., Xu, P., Welty, F. K., Wilson, P. W., Levy, D. and Muller, J. E. (1995). Association between increased oestrogen status and increased fibrinolytic potential in the Framingham Offspring Study. *Circulation*, **91**, 1952–8
29. Stampfer, M. J., Colditz, G. A., Willett, W. C., Manson, J. E., Rosner, B., Speizer, F. E. and Hennekens, C. H. (1991). Postmenopausal oestrogen therapy and cardiovascular disease. Ten-year follow-up from the nurses' health study. *N. Engl. J. Med.*, **325**, 756–62
30. Rosenberg, L., Palmer, J. R. and Shapiro, S. (1993). A case control study of myocardial infarction in relation to use of oestrogen supplements. *Am. J. Epidemiol.*, **137**, 54–63
31. Samsioe, G. (1995). Cardioprotection by hormone replacement therapy. *Contemp. Rev. Obstet. Gynaecol.*, **7**, 118–24
32. Studd, J. W. W., Watson, N. R. and Henderson, A. (1990). Symptoms and metabolic sequelae of the menopause. In Drife, J. O. and Studd, J. W. W. (eds.) *HRT and Osteoporosis*, pp. 23–33. (London: Springer-Verlag)
33. Kuusi, T., Nikkila, E. A., Tikkanen, M. J. and Sipenen, S. (1985). Effects of two progestins with different androgenic properties on hepatic endothelial lipase and high density lipoprotein 2. *Atherosclerosis*, **54**, 251–62
34. Paganini-Hill, A., Ross, R. K. and Henderson, B. E. (1988). Postmenopausal oestrogen treatment and stroke: a prospective study. *Br. Med. J.*, **297**, 519–22
35. Paganini-Hill, A. and Henderson, V. W. (1994). Oestrogen deficiency and risk of Alzheimer's disease in women. *Am. J. Epidemiol.*, **140**, 256–61
36. Ohkura, T., Isse, K., Akazawa, K., Hamamoto, M., Yaoi, Y. and Hagino, N. (1995). Long-term oestrogen replacement therapy in female

patients with dementia of the Alzheimer type: 7 case reports. *Dementia*, **6**, 99–107

37. Kanis, J. A. McCloskey, E. V., Eyres, K. S., O'Doherty, D. V. and Aaron, J. (1990). Screening techniques in the evaluation of osteoporosis. In Drife, J. O. and Studd, J. W. W. (eds.) *HRT and Osteoporosis*, pp. 135–47. (London: Springer-Verlag)
38. Kiel, D. P., Felson, D. T., Anderson, J. J., Wilson, P. W. and Moskowitz, M. A. (1987). Hip fracture and the use of oestrogens in postmenopausal women. The Framingham Study. *N. Engl. J. Med.*, **317**, 1169–74
39. Holland, E. F., Leather, A. T. and Studd, J. W. (1994). The effect of 25 mg percutaneous oestradiol implants on the bone mass of postmenopausal women. *Obstet. Gynecol.*, **83**, 43–46
40. Studd, J. W., Holland, E. F., Leather, A. T. and Smith, R. N. (1994). The dose-response of percutaneous implants on the skeletons of postmenopausal women. *Br. J. Obstet. Gynaecol.*, **101**, 787–91
41. Savvas, M., Studd, J. W., Norman, S., Leather, A. T., Garnett, T. J. and Fogelman, I. (1992). Increase in bone mass after one year of percutaneous ooestradiol and testosterone implants in post-menopausal women who have previously received long-term oral oestrogens. *Br. J. Obstet. Gynaecol.*, **99**, 757–60
42. Felson, D. T., Zhang, Y., Hannan, M. T., Kiel, D. P., Wilson, P. W. and Anderson, J. J. (1993). The effect of postmenopausal oestrogen therapy on bone density in elderly women. *N. Engl. J. Med.*, **329**, 1141–6
43. Stevenson, R. C., Hillard, R. C. and Ellerington, M. (1990). Prevention and treatment of osteoporosis. In Drife, J. O. and Studd, J. W. W. (eds.) *HRT and Osteoporosis*, pp. 315–21. (London: Springer-Verlag)
44. Trichopoulos, D., MacMahon, B. and Cole, P. (1972). Menopause and breast cancer risk. *J. Natl. Cancer Inst.*, **48**, 605–13
45. Henderson, I. C. (1993). Risk factors for breast cancer development. *Cancer*, **71** (Suppl.), 2127–40
46. Byrne, C., Brinton, L. A., Haile, R. W. and Schairer, C. (1991). Heterogenicity of the effect of family history on breast cancer risk. *Epidemiology*, **2**, 276–84
47. Hulka, B. S., Liu, E. T. and Lininger, R. A. (1994). Steroid hormones and risk of breast cancer. *Cancer*, **74** (Suppl.), 1111–24
48. Unger, C., Rageth, J. C., Wyss, P., Spillman, M. and Hochuli, E. (1991). Risk factors in breast carcinoma. *Schweiz. Med. Wochenschr.*, **121**, 30–6
49. Colditz, G. A., Egan, K. M. and Stamfer, M. J. (1993). Hormone replacement therapy and risk of breast cancer: results from epidemiologic studies. *Am. J. Obstet. Gynecol.*, **168**, 1473–80
50. Brinton, L. A. and Schairer, C. (1993). Oestrogen replacement therapy and breast cancer risk. *Epidemiol. Rev.*, **15**, 66–79
51. Dupont, W. D. and Page, D. L. (1991). Menopausal oestrogen replacement therapy and breast cancer. *Arch. Intern. Med.*, **151**, 67–72
52. Steinberg, K. K., Thacker, S. B., Smith, S. J., Stroup, D. F., Zack, M. M., Flanders, W. D. and Berkelman, R. L. (1991). A meta-analysis of the effect of oestrogen replacement therapy on the risk of breast cancer. *J. Am. Med. Assoc.*, **265**, 1985–90
53. Colditz, G. A., Hankinson, S. E., Hunter, D. J., Willett, W. C., Manson, J. E., Stampfer, M. J., Hennekens, C., Rosner, B. and Speizer, F. E. (1995). The use of oestrogens and progestins and the risk of breast cancer in postmenopausal women. *N. Engl. J. Med.*, **332**, 1589–93
54. Schairer, C., Byrne, C., Keyl, P. M., Brinton, L. A., Sturgeion, S. R. and Hoover, R. N. (1994). Menopausal oestrogen and oestrogen-progestin replacement therapy and risk of breast cancer. *Cancer Causes Control*, **56**, 491–500
55. Cummings, S. R. (1991). Evaluating the benefits of postmenopausal hormone therapy. *Am. J. Med.*, **91**, 14–18S
56. Gambrell, R. D., Maier, R. C. and Sanders, B. I. (1983). Decreased incidence of breast cancer in postmenopausal oestrogen-progestogen users. *Obstet. Gynecol.*, **62**, 435–43
57. Badwe, R. A., Gregory, W. M., Chaudary, M. A., Richards, M. A., Bentley, A. E., Rubens, R. D. and Fentiman, I. S. (1991). Timing of surgery during menstrual cycle and survival of premenopausal women with operable breast cancer. *Lancet*, **337**, 1261–4
58. Bergkvist, L., Adami, H. O., Persson, I., Hoover, R. and Schairer, C. (1989). The risk of breast cancer after oestrogen and oestrogen-progestin replacement. *N. Engl. J. Med.*, **321**, 293–7
59. Eden, J. A. (1995). The use of hormone replacement therapy in women previously

treated for breast cancer. *Contemp. Rev. Obstet. Gynaecol.*, 7, 20–4
60. Narod, S. A. (1994). Genetics of breast and ovarian cancer. *Br. Med. Bull.*, **50**, 656–76
61. Marsh, M. S., Whitcroft, S. and Whitehead, M. I. (1994). Paradoxical effects of hormone replacement therapy on breast tenderness in postmenopausal women. *Maturitas*, **19**, 97–102
62. Cramer, D. W. and Knapp, R. C. (1979). Review of epidemiologic studies of endometrial cancer and exogenous oestrogen. *Obstet. Gynecol.*, **54**, 521–6
63. Voigt, L. F., Weiss, N. S., Chu, J., Daling, J. R., McNight, B. and van Belle, G. (1991). Progestagen supplementation of exogenous oestrogens and risk of endometrial cancer. *Lancet*, **338**, 274–7
64. Hartge, P., Hoover, R., McGowan, L., Lesher, L. and Norris, H. J. (1988). Menopause and ovarian cancer. *Am. J. Epidemiol.*, **127**, 990–8
65. Rodriguez, C., Calle, E. E., Coates, R. J., Miracle-McMahill, H. L., Thun, M. J. and Heath, C. W. Jr (1990). Oestrogen replacement therapy and fatal ovarian cancer. *Am. J. Epidemiol.*, **141**, 828–35
66. Eeles, R. A., Tan, S., Wiltshaw, E., Fryatt, I., A'Hern, R. P., Shepherd, J. H., Harmer, C. L., Blake, P. R. and Chilvers, C. E. (1991). Hormone replacement therapy and survival after surgery for ovarian cancer. *Br. Med. J.*, **302**, 259–62
67. Daly, E., Vessey, M. P., Hawkins, M. M., Carson, J. L., Gough, P. and Marsh, S. (1996). Risk of venous thromboembolism in users of hormone replacement therapy. *Lancet,* **348**, 977–80
68. Jick, H., Derby, L. E., Myers, M. W., Vasilakis, C. and Newton, M. (1996). Risk of hospital admission for idiopathic venous thromboembolism among users of postmenopausal oestrogens. *Lancet,* **348**, 981–3
69. Grodstein, F., Stampfer, M. J., Goldhaber, S. Z., Manson, J. E., Colditz, G. A., Speizer, F. E., Willett, W. C. and Hennekens, C. H. (1996). Prospective study of exogenous hormones and risk of pulmonary embolism in women. *Lancet,* **348**, 983–7
70. Reubinoff, B. E., Wurtman, J., Rojansky, N., Adler, D., Stein, P., Schenker, J. G. and Brzezinski, A. (1995). Effects of hormone replacement therapy on weight, body composition, fat distribution, and food intake in early postmenopausal women: a prospective study. *Fertil., Steril.*, **64**, 963–8
71. Henderson, B. E., Paganini-Hill, A. and Ross, R. K. (1991). Decreased mortality in users of oestrogen replacement therapy. *Arch. Int. Med.*, **151**, 75–8
72. Grady, D., Rubin, S. M., Petitti, D. B., Fox, C. S., Black, D., Ettinger, B., Ernster, V. L. and Cummings, S. R. (1992). Hormone therapy to prevent disease and prolong life in postmenopausal women. *Ann. Intern. Med.*, **117**, 1016–37
73. McPherson, K. (1995). Breast cancer and hormonal supplements in postmenopausal women. *Br. Med. J.*, **311**, 699–700
74. Viniker, D. A. (1995). Breast cancer and hormonal supplements in postmenopausal women: benefits probably outweigh risks. (Correspondence). *Br. Med. J.*, **311**, 1504–5
75. Riis, B. J., Thomsen, K., Strom, V. and Christiansen, C. (1987). The effect of percutaneous oestradiol and natural progesterone on postmenopausal bone loss. *Am. J. Obstet. Gynecol.*, **156**, 61–5
76. Gangar, K., Cust, M. and Whitehead, M. I. (1989). Symptoms of oestrogen deficiency associated with supraphysiological plasma ooestradiol concentrations in women with ooestradiol implants. *Br. Med. J.*, **299**, 601–2
77. Garnett, T., Studd, J. W., Henderson, A., Watson, N., Savvas, M. and Leather, A. (1990). Hormone implants and tachyphylaxis. *Br. J. Obstet. Gynaecol.*, **97**, 917–21
78. Owen, E. J., Siddle, N. C., McGarrigle, H. T. and Pugh, M. A. (1992). 25 mg ooestradiol implants – the dosage of first choice for subcutaneous oestrogen replacement therapy? *Br. J. Obstet. Gynaecol.*, **99**, 671–4
79. Buckler, H. M., Kalsi, P. K., Cantrill, J. A. and Anderson, D. C. (1995). An audit of ooestradiol levels and implant frequency in women undergoing subcutaneous implant therapy. *Clin. Endocrinol. (Oxford)*, **42**, 445–50
80. Rees, M., Leather, A., Pryse-Davies, J., Collins, S. A., Barlow, D. H. and Studd, J. W. (1991). A first study to compare two dosages of dydrogesterone in opposing the 50 mg ooestradiol implant. *Maturitas*, **14**, 9–15
81. Ettinger, B., Selby, J., Citron, J. T., Vangessel, A., Ettinger, V. M. and Hendrickson, M. R. (1994). Cyclic hormone replacement therapy using quarterly progestin. *Obstet. Gynecol.*, **83**, 693–700

82. Hirvonen, E., Salmi, T., Puolakka, J., Heikkinen, J., Granfors, E., Hulkko, S., Makarainen, L., Nummi, S., Pekonen, F., Rautio, A., Sundstrom, H., Telimaa, S., Wilen-Rosenqvist, G., Virkkunen, A. and Wahlstrom, T. (1995). Can progestin be limited to every third month only in postmenopausal women taking oestrogen? *Maturitas*, **21**, 39–44
83. Lindgren, R., Risberg, B., Hammar, M. and Berg, G. (1995). Transdermal hormonal replacement therapy with transdermal progestin every second month. *Maturitas*, **22**, 25–30
84. Cooper, A. and Whitehead, M. (1995). Menopause: refining benefits and risks of hormone replacement therapy. *Curr. Opin. Obstet. Gynecol.*, **7**, 214–19
85. Kemp, J. F., Fryer, J. A. and Baber, R. J. (1989). An alternative regimen of hormone replacement therapy to improve patient compliance. *Aust. N. Z. J. Obstet. Gynaecol.*, **29**, 66–9
86. Sporrong, T., Hellgren, M., Samsioe, G. and Matteson, L. A. (1988). Comparison of four continuously administered progestogen plus ooestradiol combinations for climacteric complaints. *Br. J. Obstet. Gynaecol.*, **95**, 1042–8
87. Woodruff, J. D. and Pickar, J. H. (1994). Incidence of endometrial hyperplasia in postmenopausal women taking conjugated oestrogens (Premarin) with medroxyprogesterone acetate or conjugated oestrogens alone. *Am. J. Obstet. Gynecol.*, **170**, 1213–23
88. Rymer, J., Fogelman, I. and Chapman, M. G. (1994). The incidence of vaginal bleeding with tibolone treatment. *Br. J. Obstet. Gynaecol.*, **101**, 53–6
89. Andersson, K., Mattsson, L., Rybo, G. and Stadberg, E. (1992). Intrauterine release of levonorgestrel – a new way of adding progestogen in hormone replacement therapy. *Obstet. Gynecol.*, **79**, 963–7
90. Raudaskoski, T. H., Lahti, E. I., Kauppila, A. J., Apaja-Sarkkinen, M. A. and Laatikainen, T. J. (1995). Transdermal oestrogen with a levonorgestrel-releasing intrauterine device for climacteric complaints: clinical and endometrial responses. *Am. J. Obstet. Gynecol.*, **172**, 114–19
91. Suhonen, S. P., Holmstrom, T., Allonen, H. O. and Lahteenmaki, P. (1995). Intrauterine and subdermal progestin administration in postmenopausal hormone replacement therapy. *Fertil. Steril.*, **63**, 336
92. Ayton, R. A., Darling, G. M., Murkies, A. L., Farrell, E. A., Weisberg, E., Selinus, I. and Fraser, I. S. (1996). A comparative study of safety and efficacy of continuous low dose ooestradiol released from a vaginal ring compared with conjugated equine oestrogen vaginal cream in the treatment of postmenopausal urogenital atrophy. *Br. J. Obstet. Gynaecol.*, **103**, 351–8
93. Lee, J. R. (1993). *Natural Progesterone: The Multiple Roles of a Remarkable Hormone.* (Sebastopol: BLL Publishing)
94. Darj, E., Axelsson, O., Lennernas, H. and Nilsson, S. (1995). Natural micronized progesterone orally administered in postmenopausal hormone replacement therapy. *Eur. Menopause J.*, **2**, 16–20
95. Sherwin, B. B. and Gelfand, M. M. (1987). The role of androgen in the maintenance of sexual functioning in oophorectomized women. *Psychosom. Med.*, **49**, 397–409
96. Whitehead, M. and Godfree, V. (1992). *Hormone Replacement Therapy: Your Questions Answered*, p. 107. (Edinburgh: Churchill Livingstone)
97. Gelfand, M. M. (1995). Oestrogen-androgen hormone replacement therapy. *Eur. Menopause J.*, **2**, 22–6
98. Nachtigall, L. E. (1994). Comparative study: Replens versus local oestrogen in menopausal women. *Fertil. Steril.*, **61**, 178–80
99. Abdalla, H. I., Hart, D. M., Lindsay, R., Leggate, I. and Hooke, A. (1985). Prevention of bone mineral loss in postmenopausal women by norethisterone. *Obstet. Gynecol.*, **66**, 789–92
100. McNeeley, S. G., Schinfeld, J. S., Stovall, T. G., Ling, F. W. and Buxton, B. H. (1991). Prevention of osteoporosis by medroxyprogesterone acetate in postmenopausal women. *Int. J. Gynecol. Obstet.*, **34**, 253–6
101. Vercellini, P., Vendola, N., Colombo, A., Passadore, C., Trespidi, L. and Crosignani, P. G. (1992). Veralipride for hot flushes during gonadotropin-releasing hormone agonist treatment. *Gynecol. Obstet. Invest.*, **34**, 102–4
102. Neven, P., De Muylder, X., Van Belle, Y., Campo, R. and Vanderick, G. (1994). Tamoxifen and the uterus. *Br. Med. J.*, **309**, 1313–14
103. Neven, P., Shepherd, J. H. and Lowe, D. G. (1993). Tamoxifen and the gynaecologist. *Br. J. Obstet. Gynaecol.*, **100**, 893–7

104. Whitehead, M. and Godfree, V. (1992). *Hormone Replacement Therapy: Your Questions Answered*, p. 177. (Edinburgh: Churchill Livingstone)
105. Shoupe, D. and Mishell, D. R. (1987). Therapeutic regimens. In Mishell, D. R. (ed.) *Menopause, Physiology and Pharmacology*, pp. 335–51. (Chicago and London: Yearbook Medical Publishers)
106. Sener, A. B., Seckin, N. C., Ozmen, S., Gokmen, O., Dogu, N. and Ekici, E. (1996). The effects of hormone replacement therapy on uterine fibroids in postmenopausal women. *Fertil. Steril.*, **65**, 354–7
107. Marugg, R. C. and Van Der Mooren, M. J. (1995). Mammography with or without hormonal replacement therapy. *Eur. Menopause J.*, **2**, 27–30
108. Castelo-Branco, C., Duran, M., Puig, L. and Vanrell, J. A. (1995). Compliance with hormone replacement therapy at the menopause. *J. Obstet. Gynaecol.*, **15**, 204–5
109. Ravnikar, V. A. (1987). Compliance with hormone therapy. *Am. J. Obstet. Gynecol.*, **156**, 1332–4
110. Nachtigall, L. E. (1990). Enhancing patient compliance with hormone replacement therapy at menopause. *Obstet. Gynecol.*, **75**, 77–80S
111. Parazzini, F., La Vechia, C., Negri, E., Bianchi, C. and Fedele, L. (1993). Determinants of oestrogen replacement therapy use in northern Italy. *Rev. Epidemiol. Sante Publique*, **41**, 53–8
112. Isaacs, A. J., Britton, A. R. and McPherson, K. (1995). Utilisation of hormone replacement therapy by women doctors. *Br. Med. J.*, **311**, 1399–401

# Gonadotrophins into the next century: the research and development of Puregon®

# 29

*T. B. Paul Geurts, Marjo J. H. Peters, Hans G. C. van Bruggen, Willem de Boer and Henk-Yan Out*

## INTRODUCTION

Follicle stimulating hormone (FSH) is produced and secreted by the anterior lobe of the pituitary. It is a glycoprotein hormone with a relative molecular mass of approximately 35 000. FSH is indispensable in normal female and male gamete growth and maturation, as well as in gonadal steroid production. Consequently, deficient endogenous production of FSH can cause infertility; studies have indicated that in developed countries about 15% of couples will experience infertility at some time during their reproductive lives[1]. The already firmly established role for gonadotrophins in the treatment of infertility continues to be confirmed and extended as a result of new technological developments, such as the use of assisted reproduction.

Gonadotrophin preparations are derived from the urine of postmenopausal women containing FSH only (urofollitrophin), or both FSH and luteinizing hormone (LH) activity (human menopausal gonadotrophin, hMG). They have been on the market for about 10 and 30 years, respectively. They have proven to be effective and safe in the treatment of female as well as male infertility. However, use of traditional urinary preparations is associated with a number of disadvantages, including low purity, no absolute source control, cumbersome urine collection, LH contamination in 'pure' FSH preparations, risk of batch-to-batch inconsistency, and low specific activity. Recently, recombinant DNA technology has made it possible to produce unlimited quantities of formerly scarce biological products. This technology was used to develop recombinant human FSH (hFSH) by transfecting a Chinese hamster ovary (CHO) cell line with a plasmid containing the two subunit genes encoding FSH (Figure 1)[2].

The recombinant hFSH preparation Puregon® (originally coded Org 32489), produced by Organon, is almost identical to natural hFSH. Structural and conformational analyses showed that the amino acid sequence and structure are indistinguishable from those of natural hFSH. In addition, the oligosaccharide side-chains are very similar to those reported for natural hFSH. The small

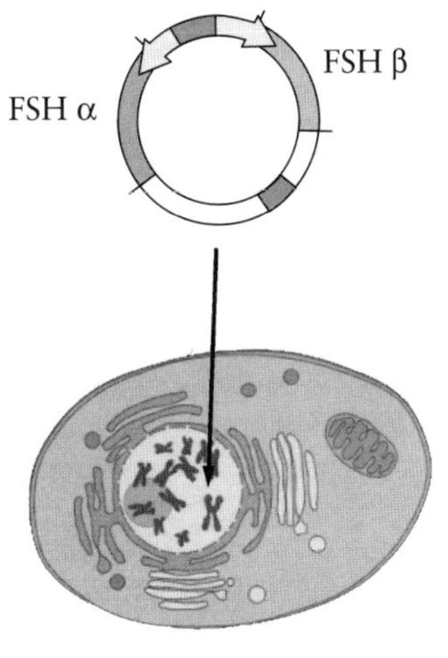


**Figure 1** Transfection of genes: introduction of the human FSH genes into the host cell chromosomes takes place with the aid of a so-called vector, in this case a plasmid

differences do not affect the degree of charge heterogeneity, receptor binding affinity, or the *in vitro* and *in vivo* bioactivities of Puregon as compared to natural hFSH. Consequently, Puregon is expected to be safe and effective in ovarian stimulation in anovulatory infertility, in controlled ovarian hyperstimulation in medically assisted reproduction, and probably in the treatment of infertility associated with male hypogonadotrophic hypogonadism.

## PRECLINICAL INFORMATION

### Animal pharmacology

Follicle stimulating hormone exerts its biological effects via binding to specific high-affinity hormone receptors present in the target cell membrane. As a consequence of hormone–receptor complex formation, the synthesis of intracellular second messenger molecules such as cyclic AMP is stimulated, resulting in the stimulation of steroidogenesis and the expression of differentiation-related genes[3,4].

*FSH receptor binding*

The receptor binding capacity of Puregon was examined in receptor displacement studies using calf testis membranes and $^{125}$I-iodinated pituitary hFSH. Puregon inhibited the receptor binding of iodinated FSH in a dose-dependent manner. The displacement curves of Puregon and three reference preparations, IS 83/575 (an international pituitary-derived reference preparation for gonadotrophins), Metrodin® (Serono, Geneva, Switzerland) and Humegon®, (NV Organon, Oss, The Netherlands) were parallel[5]. This indicates comparable dose dependencies for all preparations tested. The receptor binding affinity of Puregon was 2–3-fold higher than that of the three reference preparations when these preparations were added on the basis of their declared *in vivo* bioactivity, as determined by the rat ovarian weight augmentation assay. When added in terms of immunoreactive FSH, the affinities of Puregon and Metrodin were similar[5], indicating that the *in vivo* bioactivity/immunoreactivity ratio (B/I) varied between preparations. The apparent discrepancy between the receptor binding affinities using the declared *in vivo* bioactivity, as described above, is ascribed to isohormone profile differences between the gonadotrophin preparations.

*Aromatase induction*

Induction of aromatase activity in Sertoli cells or granulosa cells obtained from immature rats is a good indicator of the *in vitro* biological activity of FSH-containing preparations[6,7]. Puregon induced dose responses parallel to those obtained for the reference preparations IS 70/45 (urine-derived), IS 83/575 (pituitary-derived) and Metrodin[5]. The maximal responses obtained with Puregon, Metrodin and the international reference FSH preparations were comparable.

The inhibition of *in vitro* bioactivity by three different monoclonal antibodies directed against either an α- or β-subunit-specific epitope or an α/β-subunit-specific conformational epitope was investigated in a comparative study with Puregon, reference preparation IS 83/575 and Metrodin[5]. The amount of each antibody required to neutralize the *in vitro* bioactivity was similar for all three preparations. Although this is not absolute proof of identity, it may be concluded that the FSH proteins in all preparations shared a close structural and functional similarity.

*Intrinsic LH activity*

Most commercially available FSH-containing preparations also contain small or considerable quantities of LH activity due to the presence of hLH, human chorionic gonadotrophin (hCG)-like material originating from the pituitary, and/or placental hCG[8–10]. As a consequence of the biotechnological manufacturing process, Puregon cannot contain LH activity ascribed to the physical presence of any of these hormones.

The capability of Puregon to induce LH-specific biological responses was assayed in the mouse *in vitro* Leydig cell test for the induction of testosterone synthesis. Puregon induced a relatively small increase in testosterone production, and at 75 IU/ml a maximal response only 30% of that obtained with Metrodin (at 10 IU/ml) was found[5]. This effect is most likely induced by a non-specific interaction of recombinant hFSH with the LH receptor at supraphysiological concentrations. The calculated *in vitro* LH activity of Puregon per IU *in vivo* bioactive FSH was less than 0.025 mIU per IU FSH, which is approximately 100-fold lower than 2.4 mIU of Metrodin per IU FSH. Therefore, the intrinsic LH bioactivity of Puregon must be considered negligible.

*In vivo bioactivity in rats*

In the rat ovarian weight gain assay (Steelman–Pohley test), Puregon induced a dose response parallel to that of a calibrated urinary in-house reference preparation. The specific bioactivity of Puregon (relative to the IS 70/45) was approximately 10 000 IU/mg protein, the mass of protein being measured by the Moore and Stein assay[11].

To investigate the effect of Puregon on ovarian activity, the drug was administered to immature hypophysectomized rats. This animal model can be considered analogous to infertile human subjects with low endogenous FSH and LH levels. Subcutaneous administration of Puregon produced a significant dose-dependent increase in ovarian weight and aromatase activity when given for 4 days as a cumulative dose of FSH between 5 and 40 IU (in terms of IS 70/45 *in vivo* bioactivity units). Maximal increases were found with total doses between 20 and 40 IU. Within the dose range applied, Puregon given alone did not affect the plasma oestradiol concentration, indicating that circulating androgen levels were too low to act as a substrate for the aromatase enzyme complex.

The efficacy of Puregon was also assessed by gross histological examination of the ovaries. After treatment with a cumulative dose of 2.5–10 IU Puregon, a dose-dependent increase in the number of large follicles and a gradual shift of small antral to large preovulatory follicles were observed. The latter ovulated after a bolus injection of 10 IU of hCG. In comparison to hypophysectomized vehicle-treated animals, the incidence of atresia diminished, especially in the smallest size class of antral follicles[5,12]. The number of atretic follicles reduced with increasing doses of Puregon[12,13]. In the same animal model, the supportive effect of LH activity on the FSH bioactivity of Puregon was assessed by the co-administration of increasing quantities of hCG[5,12,13]. When Puregon, at a total dose of 40 IU, was supplemented with 0.1–10 IU of hCG, a further increase in ovarian weight was observed. This augmentation was significant and hCG dose-dependent. In addition, concomitant administration of hCG had a dramatic, hCG-dependent effect in increasing plasma oestradiol. It was shown that minute quantities of LH activity (< 2.5 mIU hCG per IU FSH) are sufficient to stimulate the production of significant quantities of androgens, which can subsequently be converted to oestrogens.

## Animal pharmacokinetics

Follicle stimulating hormone and LH (like other glycoprotein hormones) occur in a spectrum of isohormones, all with similar immunoreactivity but with varying intrinsic bioactivity and plasma residence time. Gonadotrophin concentrations in serum can be assessed either by immunoassay or by *in vitro* bioassay. Whereas an immunoassay only gives information on the mere presence of molecules (quantity), an *in vitro* bioassay gives an indication of the overall intrinsic bioactivity present (quantity and quality). The *in vivo* bioactivity is determined by the intrinsic (*in vitro*) bioactivity and the plasma residence time (reflected by $t_{1/2}$).

Pharmacokinetic studies on Puregon were performed in rats and dogs. Animals were dosed with FSH based on the declared *in vivo* bioactivity (in terms of IU) as determined in the rat Steelman–Pohley assay.

Pharmacokinetic parameters of immunoreactive FSH (Delfia® Pharmacia, The Netherlands) in the rat were very similar for Puregon and Metrodin. Single-dose intravenous administration (50 IU/kg) revealed no differences in terms of elimination half-life ($t_{1/2elim}$) (approximately 6 h) and area under the curve (AUC; approximately 1000 IU h/l). No dose-related effects on pharmacokinetics (immunoreactive dose-normalized $C_{max}$ and half-life) were found when comparing intravenous administration of 50 and 250 IU/kg.

In the dog, $C_{max}$ values and terminal $t_{1/2elim}$ (approximately 30 h) for Puregon and Metrodin were also similar after intravenous injection of 25 IU/kg. The much slower elimination rates in dogs compared to rats are most likely related to differences in renal clearance of the compounds. In dogs, the AUC after single-dose intravenous administration was significantly lower for Puregon than for Metrodin. The observed difference in clearance rates (0.0122 and 0.0076 l/h/kg for Puregon and Metrodin, respectively) is attributed to the difference in isohormone composition of the two preparations.

After a single intramuscular dose in rats (50 IU/kg), Puregon displayed slow absorption into the circulation. The plasma immunoreactive FSH peaked between 6 and 8 h after injection. No dose-related effects on absorption were found in rats after injection of 50 IU/kg and 250 IU/kg, as $C_{max}$ values (2.7 vs. 2.9 IU/l) normalized for the injected immunoreactive FSH (real) dose and $t_{max}$ values (7.5 vs. 8.3 h) were similar. Similar $t_{max}$ and $C_{max}$ values were also obtained after single-dose intramuscular injection of the reference preparations Metrodin and Humegon (50 IU/kg). Likewise the extent of absorption was the same. Values of AUC were 498, 488 and 466 IU h/l for Metrodin, Humegon and Puregon, respectively. Absolute bioavailability after single-dose intramuscular administration ranged from 42% to 49%. Therefore the three preparations can be considered to be bioequivalent. Thus Puregon, Metrodin and Humegon administered to rats as a single intramuscular dose of equal *in vivo* bioactive quantities of FSH display the same pharmacokinetics. This is not surprising since the different preparations have been calibrated in the rat *in vivo* bioassay.

However, when normalizing the $C_{max}$ and AUC values for the immunoreactive dose, significantly lower values for Puregon emerge. This is due to the fact that Puregon is less acidic than Metrodin and thus higher quantities of immunoreactive hormone are needed for Puregon to achieve the same *in vivo* biological activity. A similar significant difference between the dose-normalized AUC of Gonal-F® (Serono, Geneva, Switzerland) (another recombinant hFSH preparation) and Metrodin has recently been reported[14]. Comparison of a single-dose intramuscular and intravenous administration in rats revealed that $t_{1/2elim}$ differed approximately two-fold, the latter being faster (11 h vs. 6 h). This was also found for urinary-derived hFSH (Metrodin and Humegon). It is assumed that the terminal declining phase in the plasma level vs. time curve intramuscular dosing does not reflect true elimination but rather relatively slow absorption of FSH from the injection site (so-called flip-flop effect). When 50 IU/kg intramuscular Puregon was repeatedly administered to rats for 3 weeks, plasma immunoreactive FSH levels were undetectable after the dosing period and no pharmacokinetic parameters could be calculated. The inability to detect recombinant hFSH was probably related to the induction of anti-recombinant hFSH antibodies which most likely interfered with the immunoassay used to quantify FSH. When Metrodin was repeatedly administered intramuscularly (50 IU/kg, once daily for 3 weeks) to rats, plasma FSH levels showed a profile very similar to that obtained after single-dose intramuscular administration, as evidenced by the immunoreacive dose-normalized $C_{max}$ (6.4 vs. 4.1 IU/l), $t_{max}$ (8.4 vs. 6.3 h) and immunoreactive dose-normalized AUC (95 vs. 73 IU h/l) values (Table 1).

Plasma levels of Puregon were also determined in dogs after repeated intramuscular dosing of 20 IU/kg for 8 days and after intramuscular dosing of successively 25, 50 and 75 IU/kg each for 5 days. Steady-state levels of recombinant hFSH were reached within 5 days of treatment.

Clearance of FSH after repeated dosing was higher than after a single dose. The immunoreactive AUC after repeated administration (4255 IU h/l) was lower than the expected value of at least three times the AUC after single-dose administration. Accordingly, the immunoreactive dose-normalized AUC values were slightly different. From these

**Table 1** Follicle stimulating hormone pharmacokinetics after single intramuscular dosing of 300 IU Puregon or Metrodin (mean ± SD)

| | *Male* | | *Female* | | *Probability from ANOVA* | |
|---|---|---|---|---|---|---|
| *Parameter* | *Puregon* ($n$ = 6) | *Metrodin* ($n$ = 4) | *Puregon* ($n$ = 8) | *Metrodin* ($n$ = 5) | *Male vs. female* | *Puregon vs. Metrodin* |
| $C_{max}$ (IU/l) | 7.4 ± 2.8 | 11.6 ± 1.7 | 4.3 ± 1.7 | 7.2 ± 2.3 | 0.0072 | 0.0002 |
| $t_{max}$ (h) | 14.3 ± 7.5 | 9.2 ± 2.1 | 26.9 ± 5.4 | 21.1 ± 10.9 | 0.0004 | 0.3778 |
| $t_{1/2}$ (h) | 32.1 ± 11.6 | 43.9 ± 9.9 | 43.9 ± 14.1 | 37.2 ± 9.3 | 0.2685 | 0.2785 |
| $AUC_{0-\infty}$ (IU h/l) | 452 ± 183 | 764 ± 190 | 339 ± 105 | 547 ± 127 | 0.0582 | 0.0001 |

observations, it was concluded that repeated dosing does lead to accumulation of FSH, but only of the relatively acidic and not of the relatively basic isohormones. Thus, relatively basic isoforms will not give a major contribution to steady-state hormone levels.

The pharmacokinetics of Puregon in dogs were also studied after subcutaneous, intramuscular and intravenous administration. Absorption via the subcutaneous and intramuscular routes were similar in terms of (normalized) $C_{max}$ and $t_{max}$. Absolute bioavailability in dogs was not significantly different for the intramuscular and subcutaneous routes being 85% and 74%, respectively. These values were not significantly different from those for the intravenous route. Likewise, clearance of Puregon in dogs was independent of the route of administration, as demonstrated by the identical clearance values of approximately 0.01 l/h/kg. Terminal $t_{1/2elim}$ values were also not different between the three routes (about 30 h), and were in all cases probably determined by the same proportion of relatively acidic isohormones.

Glycoproteins are thought to be removed from the circulation by binding to one of the following types of receptors, depending on the terminal sugar residue of the carbohydrate chains: the asialo-galactose receptor in hepatocytes, the $SO_4$-GalNAc receptor in liver Kupffer and endothelial cells, the ubiquitous mannose phosphate receptor and the mannose receptor in macrophages and liver endothelial cells[15]. The removal of recombinant hFSH was studied after a single dose of intravenously administered Puregon by measuring the plasma disappearance of immunoreactive FSH in intact, nephrectomized and ovariectomized rats. The removal of FSH after administration of Metrodin served as a comparison. It was shown that FSH (recombinant or urinary), given intravenously to rats, is distributed into a central volume of distribution of 30–50 ml/kg. Since this value is close to the total plasma volume of the rat and was not affected by surgery, it is concluded that the distribution of the hormone is limited to the plasma water compartment of the animal. After administration of a single intravenous dose to nephrectomized rats, a similar, approximately 2–3-fold increase in the AUC was observed with both preparations, indicating that the kidney is indeed very important in the clearance of FSH. Removal of the ovaries did not alter pharmacokinetic parameters, indicating the limited role of this organ in the clearance process.

## CLINICAL INFORMATION

### Human pharmacokinetics

*Single-dose pharmacokinetics*

In a cross-over design, gonadotrophin-deficient, but otherwise healthy subjects were treated intramuscularly with 300 IU Puregon and 300 IU Metrodin[16]. The values of $C_{max}$, $t_{max}$, $t_{1/2elim}$ and AUC were calculated for each treatment on the basis of immunoreactive FSH plasma levels (Table 1).

Serum FSH concentrations in the range of $C_{max}$ were reached within 12 h after administration, remaining on that level for 24–48 h. There was a statistically significant difference in the rate of absorption between male and female subjects: in males, $C_{max}$ is reached in about half the time needed to reach $C_{max}$ in women, and the mean $C_{max}$ is about 70% higher than in women. No significant sex differences could be established with respect to $t_{1/2}$ and AUC. Gender differences in drug absorption after administration of aqueous solutions, specifically into the gluteus maximus, have been described. They are thought to be related to gluteal fat thickness in women, which exceeds that in men[17]. The extent of absorption of immunoreactive FSH was significantly higher for Metrodin than for Puregon ($C_{max}$ and AUC both about 65% of those after Metrodin). The differences with respect to $t_{max}$ and $t_{1/2}$ were not statistically significant.

*Multiple-dose pharmacokinetics*

The pharmacokinetics of Puregon after repeated intramuscular administration were investigated in open group-comparative studies. In the first study, Puregon was administered in weekly rising doses of 75, 150 and 225 IU in gonadotrophin-deficient but otherwise healthy volunteers. From the individual data, it appears that relatively high concentrations of FSH were reached within about 12 h after administration. Serum FSH increased dose-proportionally in the course of treatment and the steady-state for each dose level was reached after three to five daily doses. As expected, serum LH concentrations did not increase during the study, confirming that Puregon lacks intrinsic LH activity. Due to the relatively long $t_{1/2elim}$, serum concentrations of FSH at steady-state were higher than after single administration. Based on $C_{min}$ (FSH concentration just prior to each dosing), a cumulation factor of approximately 1.5–2.5 could be estimated. In gonadotrophin-deficient subjects, significantly different disappearance half-lives were found between female and male volunteers ($t_{1/2elim}$, 39 and 48 h, respectively)[18,19].

The second multiple-dose pharmacokinetic study was performed in four groups of nine healthy female volunteers, whose endogenous gonadotrophin production was suppressed by a high-dose contraceptive pill (Lyndiol®, NV Organon, Oss, The Netherlands), and who received 75, 150 or 225 IU Puregon or 150 IU Metrodin (Table 2).

Statistical analysis based on ANOVA indicated dose proportionality for the 75 and 150 IU Puregon treatments. Based on $C_{max}$ and AUD (AUC of one dosing interval), the relative availability after dosing of 225 IU Puregon seemed to be lower, although the mean (dose-normalized) $C_{min}$ levels were reported to be dose-proportional. In contrast to the data obtained after single administration, the bioavailability of immunoreactive FSH (reflected by AUD and $C_{max}$) after repeated administration of 150 IU Puregon and Metrodin were in the same range, although bioequivalence could

**Table 2** Follicle stimulating hormone pharmacokinetics after repeated intramuscular dosing of Puregon or Metrodin in healthy female volunteers (mean ± SD)

| *Parameter* | *Puregon* 75 IU ($n$ = 9) | *Puregon* 150 IU ($n$ = 7) | *Puregon* 225 IU ($n$ = 8) | *Metrodin* 150 IU ($n$ = 8) |
|---|---|---|---|---|
| $C_{max}$ (IU/l)† | 4.7 ± 1.5 | 9.5 ± 2.6 | 11.3 ± 1.8 | 10.7 ± 2.2 |
| $t_{max}$ (h)† | 8.2 ± 4.3 | 10.9 ± 6.3 | 11.3 ± 8.0 | 4.8 ± 3.0 |
| $AUD_{0–24}$(IU h/l)‡ | 97 ± 22 | 204 ± 49 | 242 ± 44 | 231 ± 44 |
| $t_{1/2}$ (h)† | 26.9 ± 7.8 | 30.1 ± 6.2 | 28.9 ± 6.5 | 30.3 ± 4.1 |
| Clearance (l/h/kg) | 0.011 ± 0.002 | 0.010 ± 0.002 | 0.013 ± 0.002 | 0.010 ± 0.001 |

†Measured after the last injection (for $t_{1/2}$ during the linear phase of the curve); ‡determined after the last injection by using the trapezoidal rule; AUD = AUC of one dosing interval

not be proven due to a high variability. With respect to $t_{1/2elim}$ and clearance, Puregon and Metrodin proved to be bioequivalent.

*Bioavailability*
To assess the absolute bioavailability of Puregon in healthy female volunteers of reproductive age, pituitary suppression is required to prevent interference of endogenous FSH with the determination of exogenous FSH. Pituitary suppression was obtained by using a high-dose oral contraceptive pill (Lyndiol). In an open, randomized, three-way, cross-over study, the absolute bioavailability was assessed after single-dose intramuscular (buttock) and subcutaneous (abdominal wall) administration of 300 IU Puregon to healthy female subjects. Based on serum immunoreactive FSH, $C_{max}$, $t_{max}$, AUC and the absolute bioavailability were calculated (Table 3).

With respect to the extent of absorption, measured by the AUC of immunoreactive FSH, intramuscular and subcutaneous administration proved to be bioequivalent. For both routes, the absolute bioavailability was found to be about 77%. Although the means were almost identical, no bioequivalence could be proven with respect to $C_{max}$ and $t_{max}$. For the latter, this may have been caused by the high intra-subject variability. The inter-subject variability in $C_{max}$ after intramuscular administration was higher than after subcutaneous administration (43% vs. 13%). This may be attributable to the high variation between subjects with respect to the presence of gluteal fat. Although bioequivalence could only be proven with respect to the extent of absorption, these data indicate that single-dose intramuscular and subcutaneous administration lead to highly similar immunoreactive FSH serum concentration curves.

## Clinical trials

In 1992, the first pregnancy and birth of a healthy baby after treatment with Puregon in controlled ovarian hyperstimulation with *in vitro* fertilization/embryo transfer (IVF/ET)[20,21], as well as in ovulation induction[22,23], were achieved. Clinical studies performed since then have confirmed that Puregon is a safe and efficacious drug.

*Controlled ovarian hyperstimulation*
A pilot efficacy study was carried out to evaluate whether Puregon may be combined with various gonadotrophin releasing hormone agonist (GnRHa) treatment regimens, inducing various degrees of pituitary suppression[24]. Eligible subjects were allocated to five different treatment groups. GnRH agonist treatment with buserelin (Suprecur®, Hoechst) in both a 'long' and 'short' GnRHa protocol, or triptorelin (Decapeptyl®, Ferring) in a 'long' protocol intramuscularly or subcutaneously, was started at day 1 of the menstrual cycle. During the first treatment days, the Puregon dose was fixed at 75 IU in Group II, and at 150–225 IU in Groups I and III, IV and V (Table 4).

**Table 3** Follicle stimulating hormone pharmacokinetics after a single intravenous, intramuscular (i.m.) or subcutaneous (s.c.) dose of 300 IU Puregon in healthy female volunteers (mean ± SD)

| *Parameter* | *Intravenous* ($n = 5$) | *Intramuscular* ($n = 5$) | *Subcutaneous* ($n = 5$) | *Bioequivalence i.m. vs. s.c.* |
|---|---|---|---|---|
| $C_{max}$ (IU/l) | 42.99 ± 3.89 | 6.86 ± 0.90 | 5.41 ± 0.72 | not proven |
| $t_{max}$ (h) | n.a. | 18.15 ± 10.15 | 17.38 ± 7.68 | not proven |
| $AUC_{0-\infty}$(IU h/l) | 587.8 ± 202.7 | 445.7 ± 135.7 | 455.6 ± 141.4 | proven |
| Absolute bioavailability (%) (95% CI) | n.a. | 76.4 (69.7–83.8) | 77.8 (70.9–85.2) | — |

n.a., not applicable

**Table 4** Disposition of female subjects participating in the pilot IVF efficacy study[24]

| | *Treatment group* | | | | |
|---|---|---|---|---|---|
| *Variable* | *I* (*n* = 9) | *II* (*n* = 9) | *III* (*n* = 11) | *IV* (*n* = 11) | *V* (*n* = 10) |
| GnRH agonist | none | buserelin | buserelin | triptorelin | triptorelin |
| Protocol | — | short | long | long | long |
| Dose | — | 4 × 150 μg/day | 4 × 150 μg/day | 3.75 mg | 100 μg |
| Route | — | intranasal | intranasal | intramuscular | subcutaneous |
| Start Puregon (day) | 3 | 3 | > 15 | > 15 | > 15 |

GnRH, gonadotrophin releasing hormone

In total, 51 healthy females of infertile couples started one treatment cycle with Puregon. One subject was cancelled because of a premature LH surge. The pharmacodynamics and clinical outcome could be assessed in 50 subjects.

At the start of Puregon treatment, the concentrations of endogenous FSH and LH were lower in subjects treated with buserelin or triptorelin in a long protocol (groups III, IV and V) than in groups I and II (Table 5). In the former groups, endogenous LH concentrations were further decreased at the day of hCG administration, suggesting a progressive pituitary suppression during treatment.

Regardless of the concentration of serum LH, Puregon treatment resulted in all groups in normal rises of oestradiol. At the day of hCG administration, serum concentrations of oestradiol were within the normal preovulatory range. They correlated well with the degree of multiple follicular development. The median number of oocytes recovered per group varied from seven to 11 and all but two cumulus–corona complexes were classified as mature. The median fertilization rate between the groups ranged from 40 to 73%, the median cleavage rate from 73 to 100%. In total, 43 women had an embryo transfer; clinical pregnancies were established in ten women, eight of whom had an ongoing pregnancy (19%).

The results from this study indicated that Puregon, alone or in conjunction with different GnRH agonist regimens, is effective in the induction of controlled ovarian hyperstimulation. Stimulation leads to adequate preovulatory oestradiol concentrations, irrespective of the degree of pituitary (LH) suppression.

A pivotal IVF study (European Puregon Collaborative IVF Study) was set up to compare the efficacy and safety of Puregon and Metrodin in infertile pituitary-suppressed women undergoing controlled ovarian hyperstimulation followed by IVF/ET[25]. The study was designed as a randomized (Puregon : Metrodin = 3 : 2), assessor-blind, group-comparative, multicentre study with 981 subjects. Both groups received buserelin (Suprecur, Hoechst; 4 × 150 μg/day intranasally), starting on day 1 of the cycle. Treatment with Puregon or Metrodin started only after confirmation of down-regulation of the pituitary. From treatment days 1 to 4, subjects received an intramuscular dose of 150 or 225 IU Puregon or Metrodin, once daily. Thereafter, the dose and treatment duration were individualized, guided by ovarian response. Stimulation was continued until there was ultrasonic evidence of adequate multiple follicular development, i.e. at least three follicles ≥ 17 mm. When this criterion was met, hCG was administered, and follicle puncture and oocyte pick-up were carried out.

In each of the 18 centres, one of the main efficacy parameters, i.e. the mean number of oocytes per aspiration, was higher in the Puregon group (Figure 2). This resulted in a significantly greater overall mean number

**Table 5** Mean results of pharmacodynamic parameters in the pilot efficacy study[24] (range in parentheses)

| *Parameter* | *Treatment group* *I* ($n$ = 9) | *II* ($n$ = 9) | *III* ($n$ = 11) | *IV* ($n$ = 11) | *V* ($n$ = 10) |
|---|---|---|---|---|---|
| Serum concentrations before start of Puregon treatment, median (range) | | | | | |
| FSH (IU/l) | 9 (6–14) | 6 (3–9)† | 4 (1.7–10) | 3 (1–11) | 4.4 (< 0.9–7) |
| LH (IU/l) | 6.7 (5.6–12.0) | 4.9 (2.4–7.3) | 3.2 (0.1–4.6) | 2.8 (2.3–4.9) | 2.4 (1.5–4.5) |
| $E_2$ (ng/l) | 39 (17–59) | 33 (21–38) | 33 (14–65) | 27 (< 15–34) | 24 (< 20–266) |
| Serum concentrations at the day of hCG administration, median (range) | | | | | |
| FSH (IU/l) | 21 (14–26) | 13 (4–17) | 15 (4–24) | 17 (9–27) | 17 (8–30) |
| LH (IU/l) | 5.1 (1.2–20.0) | 2.3 (< 0.5–12.0) | 1.3 (< 0.5–7.1) | 1.2 (0.8–3.5) | 1.6 (< 0.5–2.7) |
| $E_2$ (ng/l) | 1101 (684–2467) | 1899 (948–2640) | 1773 (711–2958) | 1768 (781–2952) | 1531 (893–3350) |

†Measured at the start of GnRH agonist treatment; FSH, follicle stimulating hormone; LH, luteinizing hormone; $E_2$, oestradiol; hCG, human chorionic gonadotrophin

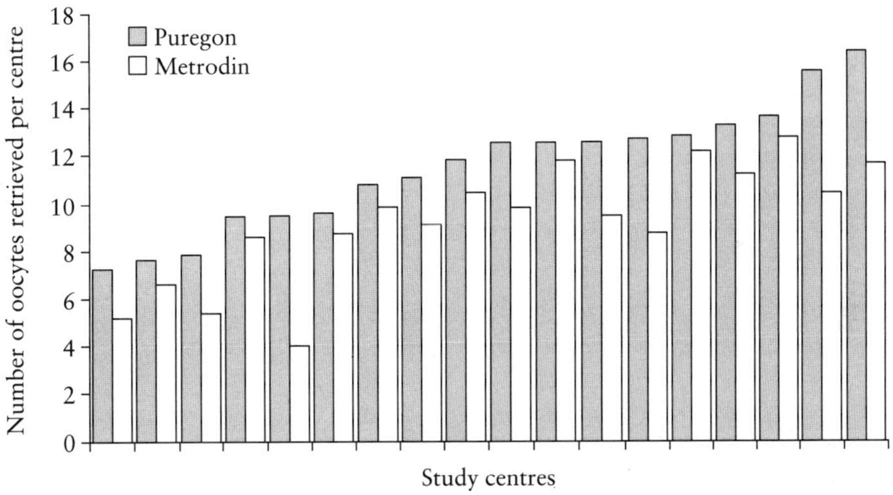


**Figure 2** Mean number of oocytes retrieved with Puregon and Metrodin in 18 study centres (number of subjects = 981)

of oocytes per aspiration (10.8 vs. 9.0, $p < 0.0001$; Table 6). This is reflected in significantly greater mean numbers of mature oocytes and high-quality (type 1 and type 2) embryos found in the Puregon group ($p = 0.003$). Although the number of embryos transferred was standardized in both groups (i.e. a maximum of three embryos was transferred), a slight (4%), though not statistically significant, difference in ongoing pregnancy rate was found in favour of the Puregon group (Table 6).

For the subjects with oocyte retrieval, the efficiency parameters, viz. the total FSH dose and the mean number of treatment days necessary to reach the criteria for hCG administration, were statistically significantly lower ($p < 0.0001$) in the Puregon group compared to

**Table 6** Results of Puregon vs. Metrodin in *in vitro* fertilization/embryo transfer using buserelin intranasally as gonadotrophin releasing hormone agonist[25]

| *Parameter* | *Puregon* ($n$ = 585) | *Metrodin* ($n$ = 396) | *p value* |
|---|---|---|---|
| *Efficiency* | | | |
| Total FSH dose (IU) | 2138 | 2385 | < 0.0001 |
| Duration of treatment (days) | 10.7 | 11.3 | < 0.0001 |
| *Efficacy* | | | |
| Maximum serum oestradiol (pmol/l) | 6084 | 5179 | < 0.0001 |
| Total number of oocytes retrieved | 10.8 | 9.0 | < 0.0001 |
| Number of mature oocytes retrieved | 8.6 | 6.8 | < 0.0001 |
| Number of follicles ≥ 15 mm | 7.5 | 6.7 | 0.0002 |
| Number of follicles ≥ 17 mm | 4.6 | 4.4 | 0.09 |
| Number of high-quality embryos | 3.1 | 2.6 | 0.003 |
| Ongoing pregnancy rate per cycle | 22.2% | 18.2% | 0.13 |
| Ongoing pregnancy rate per cycle including frozen embryo cycles | 25.7% | 20.4% | 0.05 |

FSH, follicle stimulating hormone

Metrodin (i.e. 2138 vs. 2385 IU and 10.7 vs. 11.3 days, respectively). Next to the fact that Puregon treatment required a lower total dose of FSH and a shorter treatment period, a number of other parameters differed in favour of Puregon. There was a statistically significant difference for the number of follicles ≥ 15 mm (7.5 vs. 6.7 for Puregon and Metrodin, respectively, $p = 0.0002$). The mean maximal serum oestradiol concentration was also significantly higher in the Puregon group (6084 vs. 5179 pmol/l, $p < 0.0001$). In 11 out of the 18 centres, immunoreactive FSH in serum was measured. The mean immunoreactive FSH concentration just before or on the day of hCG administration was significantly higher in the Metrodin group than in the Puregon group (12.1 vs. 11.5 IU/l, $p = 0.03$).

When the results of the frozen embryo cycles are included (143 cycles with Puregon and 88 with Metrodin), the cumulative ongoing pregnancy rate per cycle was 25.7% with Puregon and 20.4% with Metrodin. Statistical analysis of the difference in cumulative pregnancy rate after the FSH treatment cycle, including frozen embryo cycles, showed that the difference of 5.3% in favour of the Puregon-treated women was statistically significant ($p = 0.05$).

A total of 19.3% of subjects in the Puregon group and 15.6% of subjects in the Metrodin group experienced at least one adverse experience, of whom 9.3% with Puregon were considered drug-related as compared to 6.8% in the Metrodin group. In both treatment groups the most frequently reported adverse experiences were classified as 'reproductive disorders' (10.7% vs. 9.5%). Ovarian hyperstimulation syndrome (OHSS) leading to hospitalization occurred in 3.2% with Puregon and in 2.9% with Metrodin. Statistical analysis of the total incidence of OHSS (5.2% vs. 4.3%) revealed no statistically significant difference between the Puregon and the Metrodin groups. Neither anti-FSH antibodies nor anti-CHO cell-derived protein antibodies were found in any of the subjects for whom serum was available, even after three treatment cycles. From this study, it was concluded that Puregon was more efficacious than Metrodin in controlled ovarian hyperstimulation in infertile pituitary-suppressed women who were undergoing IVF/ET, as assessed by the number and the degree of maturity of oocytes retrieved and the number of type 1 and 2 embryos after the first treatment cycle. Furthermore, Puregon was more efficient because oocyte retrieval was achieved using a lower total dose in a shorter treatment period. The pregnancy rate (including frozen embryo cycles) was significantly higher in the Puregon group compared to Metrodin. There was no difference between Puregon and Metrodin with respect to safety.

An additional study was performed using another GnRH agonist. The experimental design of this study was analogous to the design of the pivotal IVF study[25], except for the fact that triptorelin instead of buserelin was used for pituitary suppression[26]. Treatment with Puregon or Metrodin started only after confirmation of down-regulation of the pituitary, and from treatment days 1 to 4 subjects received a daily intramuscular dose of 150 or 225 IU Puregon or Metrodin. Thereafter, the dose and duration were individualized, guided by ovarian response.

In total, 60 subjects were randomized to Puregon and 39 to Metrodin (randomization 3 : 2). The two treatment groups were similar with respect to infertility, demographic and menstrual cycle characteristics. The main cause of infertility was of tubal origin. The main efficacy parameter, i.e. the total number of oocytes, was comparable for both groups. After standardization of the total number of embryos transferred (2.9 for the Puregon group and 2.5 for the Metrodin group), higher pregnancy rates (though not statistically significant) were seen in the Puregon group; the ongoing pregnancy rates per attempt and per transfer were 30.2% vs. 17.4% and 34.0% vs. 18.8% for the Puregon and Metrodin groups, respectively. The efficiency parameters, viz. total FSH dose and the duration of treatment, were not different in the Puregon and Metrodin treatment groups (Table 7).

A total of 15.8% of subjects experienced at least one adverse experience (including subjects with subjective adverse experiences) in the Puregon group as compared to 12.1% in the Metrodin group. In the Puregon group, 12.3% of subjects and in the Metrodin group, 6.1% had drug-related adverse experiences. Adverse experiences leading to hospitalization were reported in three subjects in the Puregon group (5.3%; all with OHSS) and in one subject in the Metrodin group (3.0%; abdominal pain). Neither anti-FSH antibodies nor anti-CHO cell-derived protein antibodies were found in any of the subjects for whom serum was available. It was concluded that there was no significant difference in efficacy and safety between Puregon and Metrodin treatment in controlled ovarian hyperstimulation in infertile women

**Table 7** Results of Puregon vs. Metrodin in *in vitro* fertilization/embryo transfer using triptorelin subcutaneously as gonadotrophin releasing hormone agonist[26]

| *Parameter* | *Puregon* ($n$ = 57) | *Metrodin* ($n$ = 33) | *p value* |
|---|---|---|---|
| *Efficiency* | | | |
| Total FSH dose | 2265 | 2213 | n.s. |
| Duration of treatment (days) | 10.2 | 10.3 | n.s. |
| *Efficacy* | | | |
| Maximum serum oestradiol (pmol/l) | 7551 | 5514 | n.s. |
| Total number of oocytes retrieved | 9.7 | 8.9 | n.s. |
| Number of mature oocytes retrieved | 8.1 | 6.9 | n.s. |
| Number of follicles ≥ 15 mm | 7.3 | 7.2 | n.s. |
| Number of follicles ≥ 17 mm | 5.4 | 5.5 | n.s. |
| Number of high-quality embryos | 3.7 | 4.0 | n.s. |
| Ongoing pregnancy rate per transfer | 34.0% | 18.8% | n.s. |
| Ongoing pregnancy rate per cycle | 30.2% | 17.4% | n.s. |

FSH, follicle stimulating hormone; n.s., not significant

undergoing IVF/ET whose pituitaries were triptorelin-suppressed.

In order to investigate local safety aspects associated with subcutaneous administration of Puregon, one pivotal study was performed[27]. This phase III study was primarily designed to assess the local tolerance and safety, and, secondarily, to compare the efficacy of Puregon administered either intramuscularly or subcutaneously in infertile women undergoing IVF. The study was designed as a randomized (2 : 3 ratio between the intramuscular and subcutaneous groups), open, group-comparative, multicentre study. Local tolerance parameters (bruising, redness, itching, pain and swelling) were scored by the subject as either none, mild, moderate or severe. Both groups received buserelin (Suprecur, Hoechst; 4 × 150 μg/day intranasally) for pituitary down-regulation, starting on day 1 of the cycle. Treatment with Puregon started after confirmation of down-regulation. From treatment days 1 to 4, subjects received daily 150 or 225 IU Puregon intramuscularly or subcutaneously. Thereafter, the dose and duration were individualized, as guided by ovarian response. After intramuscular injection, the incidences of overall local symptoms, bruising, pain, redness, swelling and itching were 63.6%, 37.7%, 31.2%, 13.0%, 7.8% and 6.5%, respectively; after subcutaneous injection, the corresponding figures were 68.6%, 54.2%, 28.0%, 16.1%, 5.9% and 3.4%. Only bruising was significantly lower in the intramuscular group (95% confidence interval −29.7% to −2.6%; $p = 0.019$), most likely because, after subcutaneous administration, bruising is more easily visible due to the more superficial injection site. The results regarding the efficacy after intramuscular or subcutaneous Puregon treatment were similar (Table 8), and also very similar to the results reported by others[25,26]. This is in accordance with the expectations based on the bioequivalence reported between the two routes.

In total, 6.5% of subjects in the intramuscular group and 12.7% in the subcutaneous group experienced adverse experiences. A total of 3.6% of subjects had drug-related adverse experiences, two subjects in the Puregon intramuscular group (2.6%) and five subjects in the Puregon subcutaneous group (4.2%). One subject treated in the intramuscular group (1.3%) and six subjects in the subcutaneous group (5.1%) experienced subjective adverse experiences. Most frequently reported adverse experiences were OHSS (intramuscular: 2.6%; subcutaneous: 5.9%) and ectopic pregnancy

**Table 8** Results of Puregon intramuscular vs. subcutaneous administration in *in vitro* fertilization/embryo transfer using buserelin intranasally as gonadotrophin releasing hormone agonist[27]

| *Parameter* | *Intramuscular* ($n = 77$) | *Subcutaneous* ($n = 118$) | *p value* |
|---|---|---|---|
| *Efficiency* | | | |
| Total no. of ampoules/vials used | 29.8 | 28.2 | n.s. |
| Duration of treatment (days) | 9.9 | 9.7 | n.s. |
| *Efficacy* | | | |
| Mean serum oestradiol on day of hCG (pmol/l) | 5509 | 7109 | n.d. |
| Total number of oocytes retrieved | 9.8 | 10.4 | n.s. |
| Number of mature oocytes retrieved | 8.2 | 8.6 | n.s. |
| Number of follicles ≥ 15 mm | 8.1 | 8.5 | n.s. |
| Number of follicles ≥ 17 mm | 4.3 | 5.0 | n.s. |
| Number of high-quality embryos | 4.3 | 3.8 | n.s. |
| Ongoing pregnancy rate per transfer | 30.1% | 29.3% | n.s. |
| Ongoing pregnancy rate per cycle | 27.1% | 26.1% | n.s. |

hCG, human chorionic gonadotrophin; n.s., not significant; n.d., not determined (intramuscular: 1.3%; subcutaneous: 1.7%). Serum anti-FSH antibodies were not found in any of the subjects for whom serum was available.

There were no statistically significant differences in the occurrence of most local tolerance symptoms (pain, redness, swelling and itching) and safety parameters between intramuscular and subcutaneous administration of Puregon in infertile women. Bruising was seen significantly more often in subjects receiving Puregon subcutaneously, most likely because this is more easily visible due to the more superficial injection. Overall local tolerance, however, was not statistically significantly different. No clinically relevant differences in efficacy between intramuscularly or subcutaneously administered Puregon were found.

*Ovulation induction*

A phase III study was designed to compare the efficacy and safety of Puregon and Metrodin for the induction of ovulation in patients with chronic anovulation (World Health Organization (WHO) group II) who failed to ovulate and/or conceive during clomiphene citrate treatment. The study was designed as a randomized (Puregon : Metrodin = 3 : 2), assessor-blind, group-comparative, multicentre study. The study period covered a maximum of three treatment cycles. When significant follicular development was observed, during the course of treatment, the daily FSH dose was not increased. This dose was maintained until a follicle diameter ≥ 18 mm was observed or two or three follicles had reached a diameter of ≥ 15 mm. Ovulation was then induced by administration of 10 000 IU of hCG. The two treatment groups were similar with respect to demographic and menstrual cycle characteristics. The main preovulatory criteria were two or three follicles ≥ 15 mm or a dominant follicle ≥ 18 mm.

With Puregon, a statistically significantly greater number of follicles ≥ 12 mm was found in the first treatment cycle and mean preovulatory oestradiol levels were higher. These results were obtained using significantly fewer ampoules in a significantly shorter treatment period. Statistical significance was proven for the efficiency parameters in the first treatment cycle. No statistically significant differences were found regarding the distribution of first-time ovulations, even in the most conservative statistical approach, in which dropouts are considered as subjects who did not achieve ovulation in the subsequent cycles. Cumulative ovulation rates after three cycles were also not different for Puregon and Metrodin (Table 9).

**Table 9** Results of Puregon vs. Metrodin in ovulation induction (WHO group II) (Out *et al.*, manuscript in preparation)

| *Parameter* | *Puregon* ($n$ = 105) | *Metrodin* ($n$ = 67) | *p value* |
|---|---|---|---|
| *Efficiency* | | | |
| Median total dose (IU)† | 750 | 1035 | < 0.001 |
| Median duration of treatment (days)† | 10.0 | 13.0 | < 0.001 |
| *Efficacy* | | | |
| Median maximum oestradiol (pmol/l)†* | 1400 | 1000 | n.s. |
| Number of follicles ≥ 12 mm†* | 3.6 | 2.6 | < 0.001 |
| Number of follicles ≥ 15 mm†* | 2.0 | 1.7 | n.s. |
| Cancellations | 11.4% | 10.4% | n.s. |
| Cumulative ovulation rate | 95% | 96% | n.s. |
| Cumulative pregnancy rate | 27% | 24% | n.s. |

†In the first cycle; *on day of hCG administration; hCG, human chorionic gonadotrophin

Adverse experiences were reported in 29.5% of subjects in the Puregon group and in 34.3% in the Metrodin group. For seven subjects on Puregon and five on Metrodin, the adverse experiences were serious. There were eight subjects on Puregon (7.6%) and three on Metrodin (4.5%) with OHSS and one of these in the Puregon group was reported as a subjective adverse experience. The difference is not statistically significant. In each treatment group, about 18% of adverse experiences were considered as drug-related. Serum anti-FSH antibodies were not found in any of the subjects for whom serum was available, even after three treatment cycles. Based on the data obtained, it is concluded that there are no significant differences in the efficacy and safety of Puregon and Metrodin for induction of ovulation in subjects with chronic anovulation (WHO group II) who failed to ovulate and/or conceive during clomiphene citrate treatment. With Puregon, however, ovulation was obtained with significantly fewer ampoules in a significantly shorter treatment period, indicating a higher efficiency in ovulation induction. The higher efficiency of Puregon, and the fact that a greater number of follicles ≥ 12 mm were stimulated, suggest that Puregon treatment may be started at a lower dose than Metrodin and maintained at this lower dose for a longer period of time.

*Male hypogonadotrophic hypogonadism*

Fertility in men depends on both LH and FSH to induce androgen production and spermatogenesis. In hypogonadotrophic hypogonadal men with GnRH deficiency or hypopituitarism, administration of exogenous urinary gonadotrophins stimulates both androgen and sperm production[28]. A pharmacokinetic study indicated that serum FSH increases in a dose-proportional fashion after intramuscular administration in hypogonadotrophic hypogonadal men[16]. Recently, the first case of successful induction of spermatogenesis with Puregon in a postpubertal hypogonadotrophic hypogonadal male was reported[29]. After 18 weeks of treatment, the first sperm was observed in the ejaculate of this patient, reaching normal levels in the course of further treatment. Puregon was well tolerated and without side-effects.

## CONCLUSIONS

In controlled ovarian hyperstimulation programmes followed by IVF/ET, Puregon proved to be more efficacious than Metrodin. Puregon treatment resulted in a significantly greater number of oocytes. The ongoing pregnancy rate with Puregon was significantly higher than that with Metrodin in the European Puregon Collaborative IVF Study after the inclusion of frozen embryo cycles. Furthermore, these results were achieved with a lower total dose within a shorter treatment period. This indicates a higher efficiency of Puregon in IVF.

In ovulation induction, ongoing pregnancy rates (per attempt and per transfer) were not statistically different for the Puregon and Metrodin groups. Puregon treatment, however, required a 30% lower total follicle stimulating hormone dose and a shorter treatment period to achieve the same result. This indicates a higher efficiency of Puregon also in ovulation induction.

Subcutaneous and intramuscular administration of Puregon were equally efficacious, as expected because there are no significant pharmacokinetic differences regarding bioavailability and extent of absorption.

Puregon is efficacious when used without and with different gonadotrophin releasing hormone agonists.

Intramuscular and subcutaneous administrations of Puregon were well tolerated and the safety pattern is similar to that of intramuscular Metrodin. With respect to the most common adverse experience, ovarian hyperstimulation syndrome, statistically significant differences were reached in none of the studies. In none of the Puregon-treated subjects analysed, was specific antibody formation against either follicle stimulating hormone or Chinese hamster ovary cell-derived proteins found, even after three treatment cycles. These results indicate that this biotechnologically manufactured gonadotrophin preparation is safe and effective in controlled ovarian hyperstimulation and ovulation induction, using both the intramuscular and subcutaneous routes.

## ACKNOWLEDGEMENT

The text above is an edited version of a review published in *Drugs of Today* (1996, **32**, 239–58) and is reproduced with permission of the publishers.

## REFERENCES

1. Healy, D. L., Trounson, A. O. and Andersen, A. N. (1994). Female infertility: causes and treatment. *Lancet*, **343**, 1539–44
2. van Wezenbeek, P., Draaijer, J., van Meel, F. and Olijve, W. (1990). Recombinant follicle-stimulating hormone. I. Construction, selection and characterization of a cell line. In Crommelin, D. J. A. and Schellekens, H. (eds.) *From Clone to Clinic*, pp. 245–51. (Dordrecht: Kluwer Academic Publishers)
3. Krasnow, J. (1991). Advances in understanding ovarian physiology: regulation of steroidogenic enzymes in ovarian follicular differentiation. *Semin. Reprod. Endocrinol.*, **9**, 283–302
4. Heindel, J. J. and Treinen, K. A. (1989). Physiology of the male reproductive system: endocrine, paracrine and autocrine regulation. *Toxicol. Pathol.*, **17**, 411–45
5. Mannaerts, B., de Leeuw, R., Geelen, J., van Ravenstein, A., van Wezenbeek, P., Schuurs, A. *et al.* (1991). Comparative *in vitro* and *in vivo* studies on the biological characteristics of recombinant human follicle-stimulating hormone. *Endocrinology*, **129**, 2623–30
6. Mannaerts, M. J. L., Kloosterboer, H. J. K. and Schuurs, A. H. W. M. (1987). Applications of *in vitro* bioassays for gonadotropins. In Rolland, R. *et al.* (eds.) *Neuroendocrinology of Reproduction*, pp. 49–58. (Amsterdam: Elsevier Science Publishers)
7. Overes, H. W. T. M., De Leeuw, R. and Kloosterboer, H. J. (1992). Regulation of aromatase activity in FSH-primed rat granulosa cells *in vitro* by follicle-stimulating hormone and various amounts of human chorionic gonadotropin. *Hum. Reprod.*, **7**, 191–6
8. Odell, W. D. and Griffin, J. (1989). Pulsatile secretion of chorionic gonadotropin during the normal menstrual cycle. *J. Clin. Endocrinol. Metab.*, **69**, 528–32
9. Wide, L. (1992). Les facteurs intrinsèques et extrinsèques qui influencent la stimulation des gonades et la réceptivité des tissus génitaux féminins formes circulantes des gonadotrophines et leur variabilité. Les gonadotrophines chez l'homme. *Contracept. Fertil. Sex.* **20**, 455–62
10. Stokman, P. G. W., de Leeuw, R., van der Wijngaard, H. A. G. W., Kloosterboer, H. J., Vemer, H. M. and Sanders, A. L. M. (1993). Human chorionic gonadotropin in commercial human menopausal gonadotropin preparations. *Fertil. Steril.*, **60**, 175–8
11. Moore, S. and Stein, W. H. (1951). Chromatography of amino acids on polystyrene resins. *J. Biol. Chem.*, **192**, 663–81
12. Mannaerts, B., Uilenbroek, J., Schot, P. and de Leeuw, R. (1994). Folliculogenesis in hypophysectomized rats after treatment with recombinant human FSH. *Biol. Reprod.*, **51**, 72–81
13. Mannaerts, B. and de Leeuw, R. (1993). Gonadotrophins and follicular growth. In Shaw, R. W. (ed.) *The Control and Stimulation of Follicular Growth*, pp. 1–11. (Carnforth, UK: Parthenon Publishing)
14. Porchet, H. C., Le Cotonnec, J.-Y., Canali, S. and Zanolo, G. (1993). Pharmacokinetics of recombinant human follicle stimulating hormone after intravenous, intramuscular, and subcutaneous administration in monkeys, and comparisons with intravenous administration of urinary follicle stimulating hormone. *Drug Metab. Dispos.*, **21**, 144–50
15. Drickamer, K. (1991). Clearing up glycoprotein hormones. *Cell*, **67**, 1029–32
16. Mannaerts, B., Shoham, Z., Schoot, D., Bouchard, P., Harlin, J., Fauser, B., Jacobs, H., Rombout, F. and Coelingh Bennink, H. (1993). Single-dose pharmacokinetics and pharmacodynamics of recombinant human follicle-stimulating hormone (Org 32489) in gonadotropin-deficient volunteers. *Fertil. Steril.*, **59**, 108–14
17. Zuidema, J., Pieters, F. A. J. M. and Duchateau, G. S. M. J. E. (1988). Release and absorption rate aspects in intramuscularly injected pharmaceuticals. *Int. J. Pharm.*, **47**, 1–12
18. Schoot, D. C., Harlin, J., Shoham, Z., Mannaerts, B. M. J. L., Lahlou, N., Bouchard, P., Coelingh Bennink, H. J. T. and Fauser,

B. C. J. M. (1994). Recombinant human follicle-stimulating hormone and ovarian response in gonadotrophin-deficient women. *Hum. Reprod.*, **9**, 1237–42
19. Mannaerts, B., Fauser, B., Lahlou, N., Harlin, J., Shoham, Z., Coelingh Bennink, H. and Bouchard, P. (1995). Serum hormone concentrations during treatment with multiple rising doses of recombinant follicle stimulating hormone (Puregon) in men with hypogonadotropic hypogonadism. *Fertil. Steril.*, **65**, 406–10
20. Devroey, P., Van Steirteghem, A., Mannaerts, B. and Coelingh Bennink, H. (1992). Successful *in vitro* fertilisation and embryo transfer after treatment with recombinant human FSH. *Lancet*, **339**, 1170–1
21. Devroey, P., Van Steirteghem, A., Mannaerts, B. and Coelingh Bennink, H. (1992). First singleton term birth after ovarian superovulation with rhFSH. *Lancet*, **340**, 1108–9
22. Donderwinkel, P. F. J., Schoot, D. C., Coelingh Bennink, H. J. T. and Fauser, B. C. J. M. (1992). Pregnancy after induction of ovulation with recombinant human FSH in polycystic ovary syndrome. *Lancet*, **340**, 983–4
23. van Dessel, H. J. H. M., Donderwinkel, P. F. J., Coelingh Bennink, H. J. T. and Fauser, B. C. J. M. (1994). First established pregnancy and birth after induction of ovulation with recombinant human follicle-stimulating hormone in polycystic ovary syndrome. *Hum. Reprod.*, **9**, 55–6
24. Devroey, P., Mannaerts, B., Smitz, J., Coelingh Bennink, H. and Van Steirteghem, A. (1994). Clinical outcome of a pilot efficacy study on recombinant human follicle-stimulating hormone (Org 32489) combined with various gonadotrophin-releasing hormone agonist regimens. *Hum. Reprod.*, **9**, 1064–9
25. Out, H. J., Mannaerts, B. M. J. L., Driessen, S. G. A. J. and Coelingh Bennink, H. J. T. (1995). A prospective, randomized, assessor-blind, multicentre study comparing recombinant and urinary follicle stimulating hormone (Puregon versus Metrodin) in *in vitro* fertilization. *Hum. Reprod.*, **10**, 2534–40
26. Hedon, B., Out, H. J., Hugues, J. N., Camier, B., Cohen, J., Lopes, P., Zorn, J. R., Van der Heijden, B. and Coelingh Bennink, H. J. T. (1995). Efficacy and safety of recombinant FSH (Puregon) in infertile women pituitary-suppressed with triptorelin undergoing *in vitro* fertilisation: a prospective, randomised, assessor-blind, multicentre trial. *Hum. Reprod.*, **10**, 3102–6
27. Out, H. J., Reimitz, P. E. and Coelingh Bennink, J. H. T. (1995). A prospective, randomized, multicentre study comparing recombinant FSH (Puregon) either given intramuscularly or subcutaneously in subjects undergoing IVF. *Hum. Reprod.*, **10** (abstract book 1), 6
28. Kliesch, S., Behre, H. M. and Nieschlag, E. (1994). High efficacy of gonadotropin or pulsatile GnRH treatment in hypogonadotropic hypogonadal men. *Eur. J. Endocrinol.*, **131**, 347–54
29. Kliesch, S., Behre, H. and Nieschlag, E. (1995). Recombinant human follicle-stimulating hormone and human chorionic gonadotropin for induction of spermatogenesis in a hypogonadotropic male. *Fertil. Steril.*, **63**, 1326–8

# Computer applications in reproductive medicine

# 30

*David A. Viniker*

## INTRODUCTION

We have witnessed the arrival of the age of information technology. Computers are involved in almost every aspect of our lives. Our newspapers are formatted on desktop publishing computer programs. In communications, whether at the telephone exchange or in satellites transmitting the news instantaneously across the world, computers are involved. Financial institutions, such as the banks, record all transactions on computer. Illustrations in books and magazines are more likely to have been designed on computer than by an artist with a paintbrush. The professional photographer can use a computer to enhance his pictures. Computers can make calculations on numerical data at unimaginable speed. Data are information held on computer in contrast to programs which manipulate the data. Enormous volumes of text can be stored on small computer disks and sections of text can be moved within a document at the touch of a button. The objective of this chapter is to show how a computer can be of practical assistance to the clinician with a special interest in reproductive endocrinology. Other clinicians may also find these applications helpful.

Perhaps only those clinicians who once kept card-index systems of medical papers or those who wrote or rewrote, typed or retyped draft documents, can fully appreciate from personal experience the enormous benefits that computers have brought. The author uses computers regularly for several hours each day in clinics to document clinical data and also to prepare papers, lectures and artwork for teaching purposes. No doubt, many readers of this book will know a great deal more about computers and computer science than the author. Many colleagues, juniors and students show a keen interest in how I use a computer and have suggested that this chapter be written. A brief overview of computer systems will be presented followed by the applications that are most frequently used. It is not my intention to cover the subject from a detailed technical point of view.

In 1982, the author submitted his MD Thesis to the University of London. It was almost exactly at that time that personal computers were beginning to become available in high street shops. Computers were no longer confined to major companies and university departments but were to find their place within the home.

Our juniors today, find it difficult to believe that in the early 1980s medical literature searches were conducted by trawling through enormous volumes of *Index Medicus* or that each draft of a chapter or paper had to be rewritten or retyped. After the thesis was submitted, the author spent a couple of months learning the basics of computing before purchasing a BBC computer. The professor expressed his disappointment in the resulting delay of producing the next paper. Within 3 weeks of purchasing the 'BBC', a draft paper was completed and professorial editing was provided the same day. During that evening, the amendments were made on the computer word processor and the following morning the updated paper was carefully placed on the professor's desk exactly where the first draft had been the evening before. Later that morning, the professor initially expressed his disappointment that I had not yet looked through the first draft but he enjoyed the jest when he realized that, with the benefit of a computer, an updated draft had been turned round so quickly. Never slow to accept the benefits of technological advance, the professor invited me to look at maternity computer systems and computers have been a hobby ever since. Combining hobbies, such as computing and reproductive medicine, enhances enjoyment.

## HARDWARE

### The personal computer

*Hardware* is an electronic component or unit of a computer system and it includes the computer itself, monitor (screen) and the keyboard. Early computers were enormous and in industry these *mainframes* may still be occasionally found. As transistors and silicon chips have in succession replaced valves, computer components have become smaller. An early popular *personal computer* (PC), the BBC computer, was more powerful than the earliest 'Enigma' computers developed in the UK in the 1940s to break military codes. The 'BBC' was small enough to fit into a medium-sized case.

The *motherboard* of a PC is the printed circuitboard to which all components within the main housing of the computer are connected directly or indirectly. If the motherboard is regarded as the spinal column and cord, then the *central processing unit* (*CPU*) is the heart and brain combined. The CPU keeps everything functioning and controls all communications. The speed at which the processor functions is described in Megahertz (millions of actions per second – MHz). Most early PCs, such as the 'BBC' had processors called '8088's. As faster, more powerful processors have been required to meet ever increasing demands, new generations of processors have been developed. The '8088's were successively replaced by the '286', '386' and '486'. Newer processors seem to arrive at 2-year intervals and standard PCs would currently have a 586 (*Pentium*) processor. Early 486 machines were rated at 25 MHz to be followed by 33 MHz, 50 MHz, 66 MHz and eventually 100 MHz. Pentiums start at 75 MHz (P75) and there are now some rated at 200 MHz. A P100 processor is several times faster than a 486 100 MHz processor.

The computer *monitor* is the computer screen which, on a desktop computer, is essentially a cathode ray tube similar to a television. The smallest addressable dot on the screen is a pixel. The resolution of a monitor is expressed in pixels with horizontal and vertical figures. A standard VGA (*video graphics array*) monitor would be 640 × 480. Larger monitors require higher resolution (SVGA – super VGA) such as 1024 × 768 on a 15″ screen or 1152 × 882 on a 17″ screen. Modern monitors are likely to emit less radiation than their predecessors. Liquid crystal display (LCD) panels, used in notebook computers can be used as full screen monitors but they remain expensive. The cursor is a marker on the screen indicating where text or numbers or a graphics shape will be entered next. It may be a 'blinking' line in a text document or an arrow in a graphics picture.

The keyboard is the most frequently used device for entering data onto the computer. The standard typewriter configuration of character keys is called QWERTY which is the order of the first six character keys. WYSIWYG is an acronym for 'What You See Is What You Get'. In other words what you see on the monitor is what the printer will output.

The computer requires an operating system which allows the CPU to communicate with other hardware. The operating system provides utilities for activities, such as loading data into memory and saving data from the computer onto a back-up system. The two operating systems most frequently used by PCs have been developed by 'Microsoft' and 'Apple'. The early Microsoft operating system for the PC was called DOS (Disk Operating System). The other main computer operating system is the 'Macintosh' which is produced by Apple. IBM-compatible PCs use operating systems released by 'Microsoft' – it is these computers that are now referred to as PCs. DOS was superseded by Windows (see below) and in 1995 by Windows 95. Previews of Windows 97 are appearing in the journals at the time of writing. 'IBM-compatible' originally referred to a PC that used DOS but has become expanded to include PCs with Intel or equivalent processors using DOS, Windows or Windows 95. Although a computer may be running Windows or Windows 95, there is still provision for access to DOS.

The binary digit (*Bit*) is the basic unit in computing and can be either '1' or '0'. A *byte* (binary digit eight) is a group of eight bits (e.g. 10011101). A *kilobyte* (kb) is $2^{10}$ (1024) bytes. A *megabyte* (Mb) is 1024 kb and a *gigabyte* (Gb) is 1024 Mb. Text must be converted into binary for a computer to process it. ASCII (American Standard Code for Information Interchange) assigns binary format to text characters. ASCII is essentially plain text without formatting (italics, underlining or bold).

## Memory

There are two basic types of chip memory, RAM (random access memory) and ROM (read only memory). RAM has been compared to a desktop. It is the space to which the computer has direct and immediate access. My original BBC computer had 32 kb of RAM. This space was sufficient for a word processing program and a document of about six pages. The six-page document could be saved onto an audio-cassette (it took 5 minutes). Operating systems and computer programs require ever greater memory resources as their sophistication increases. The speed of memory chips is measured in nanoseconds. A nanosecond is one thousand millionth of a second. When the computer is switched off, everything in RAM is lost. Although there are different sorts of memory, the term, when used alone, refers to RAM.

ROM allows programs or data to be transferred (read) into RAM but one cannot transfer (write) to ROM. When the computer is switched on (cold start), it goes through a process (boot) in which it loads the operating system into memory from ROM. The advantage of ROM chips are that their contents are permanent and are not lost when the power is switched off. ROM may be in the form of memory chips or, more recently, disks identical to CDs used in audio systems (see below).

Few PCs today have less than 4 Mb of memory as standard and most have 8 Mb. Additional RAM chips can usually be introduced later although this is limited by the motherboard capacity. Every program that is running, however, needs some access to the first 640 kb of conventional memory. The operating system needs some and so do device drivers (utility programs that drive hardware such as printers) and the conventional memory is a limited resource. The way that the computer utilizes the conventional memory significantly affects the way the computer functions. The upper memory is between 640 kb and 1 Mb and has been traditionally reserved for ROM programs including the BIOS (Basic Input/Output System), and the hard disk controller. The BIOS is a set of fundamental software routines that allow the computer to address devices including the monitor, keyboard and disk drives. There was a need for more memory and several leading computer companies agreed on a new standard called the Expanded Memory System (EMS) which is a portion of the upper memory. Only a 64 kb block can be guaranteed but this is utilized by many games programs. Expanded memory managers are available but these are probably best left to experts to use.

*Cashe memory* is temporary and is set aside by the computer for information that is being most frequently accessed, thus speeding up this activity. The Pentium processor has 8 Kb of cache and additional, *secondary cashe* increases performance further.

## Printers

Printers output a hard copy (paper print-out) of formatted data from the computer. The word 'font' is derived from the Latin word *fount* which is a complete set of type faces of one sort, with all that is necessary for printing in that kind of letter. Fonts can be applied to screen or printed text. *True type* fonts are stored as shape descriptors that can be scaled to required size. Recently, I purchased an upgrade to a graphics package (Coreldraw 6) for £260. It included a selection of 1000 fonts and each can be printed at different sizes and in any colour. These fonts can be used interchangeably with any Windows application.

My first printer, 14 years ago, used a daisywheel and was capable of printing 16 characters per second, which is fractionally faster than a typist. For about £20, additional daisywheels with different fonts could be purchased. With three daisywheels and a choice of 10 or 12 cpi (characters per inch) the variety of formats seemed incredible. To begin with, I could print in any colour I wanted (provided it was black). Different colour ribbon cartridges gradually became available. My current printer will print up to six pages each minute and high quality colour pictures are simple to produce.

Dot-matrix printers have print-heads with at least nine pins. These pins create text characters and graphics as the print-head moves across the paper. The dots are clearly apparent. Inkjet printers produce better quality output although not at photographic quality and bubble jet technology has improved quality further. A cartridge with the three primary colours allows an almost infinite number of colours and black was produced by a combination of the colours. Most colour bubble jets now have a separate black cartridge. Laser printers provide better quality print and they are faster but colour laser printers still cost £2000–£3000. Thermal wax printers are slow but are capable of near-photorealism.

*Ports* are sockets around the PC to which leads from *peripheral devices*, such as printers, can be connected. *Serial ports* allow information to pass one piece at a time and are commonly used for transferring data between computers. *Parallel ports* have a set of lines allowing faster communication. Printers usually use parallel ports.

### Storing data and programs

Data and program files developed on computer must be saved from RAM as they would otherwise be lost when the computer is switched off. Nothing can be more frustrating than losing data. One of the advantages of data held on computer is that it can be backed-up (copied) so quickly. About 20 years ago and well before PCs, someone had their MD manuscripts stolen; there were no copies! Paper documents can be copied but this is laborious. Computer data files up to 1.5 Mb can easily be backed-up onto floppy disks. It is tempting to back-up everything on a computer but provided one has a personal copy of the program packages there really is little advantage in storing several copies. Even if a computer is 'lost', it is usually technically essential to load programs from the original rather than a back-up copy onto the replacement computer. My original BBC used an audio cassette recorder. A six-page document (3000 words or 20 000 characters) would take 5 minutes to record or load back into RAM.

*Floppy disks* are inserted into drives which are able to transfer data from RAM (write) or into RAM (read). These disks were initially $5^1/4''$ and could store about 100 kb. The six-page document would now take just 10 seconds to save and files could be much longer. For extra security, more than one copy of a file could be stored. With twin floppy disks, a program could be in one drive and the data file on the other. The computer would refer to the appropriate floppy disk for more program or data information as required. Files larger than the 32 kb RAM could be processed by transferring data backwards and forwards between the floppy disks and RAM. Furthermore, programs could be more complex. For the last 10 years, the most popular floppy disks have been $3^1/2''$. These are more rigid and typically store about 1.5 Mb. Being more robust and also compact they have been reliable.

*Hard disks* are sealed units, usually housed within the computer, and have relatively large storage capacity. An Amstrad 1640 purchased 12 years ago had a hard disk capacity of 20 Mb. At that time it sounded like infinity. My current notebook computer has a 200 Mb hard disk (top of the range just 3 years ago). The operating system has a *compression program* which effectively increases the capacity to 360 Mb. Saving a 52 000 word document file (300 kb) with this system takes 20 seconds. The average PC will now have a 1 Gb hard disk.

Ten years ago the choice for back-up was between the $5^1/_4''$ or $3^1/_2''$ floppy disks. The floppy disk is still extremely useful. Most computers have $3^1/_2''$ drives so that the only additional purchase is the floppy disks. These disks will typically store more than 1 Mb of data which is likely to be more than adequate for the majority of text or database files. Most computer users will have several, and perhaps many, files that need to be regularly backed-up. Inevitably, at some unexpected and typically most inconvenient moment, disaster strikes – the computer fails or 'disappears' and, without back-up, all is lost. We have all paid the price for not heeding the advice to back-up regularly and frequently.

A *CD-ROM drive* reads from a CD-ROM which is identical to an audio CD except the digital information it holds may represent computer programs and data rather than just sound. A CD-ROM can hold up to 680 Mb of data, which is equivalent to 485 high-density floppy disks. In 1993 standard speed CD-ROM drives transferred data at 150 kb/s. In 1996 10 speed drives are available with theoretical transfer speeds of 1500 kb/s (1.5 Mb/s). It is only possible to write once onto a laser CD and these are now available for the home-market. They are ideal for archiving. A floppy drive is standard on most computers and CD-ROM drives are becoming popular. The CD-ROM drive should now be considered as essential hardware. Many computer programs are entered onto computer from a CD-ROM which is a rapid process particularly when compared to loading a program from perhaps 40 or more floppy disks. CD-ROMs can hold video and sound files as well as text and graphics and these can be used on-line. My colleague, Dr Tim Appleton, has produced a CD-ROM utilizing all these features. His CD has skilled explanations for couples seeking advice about infertility and stories for children conceived by assisted conception.

The choice of back-up systems has become almost bewildering. Interestingly, the early tape recorder concept used for data storage has been modified to allow rapid digital data recording for back-up. A *tape streamer* is a magnetic tape recorder designed for backing up large volumes of data on special data storage tapes. There are a range of easy-to-use internal or external (connects to the parallel port) back-up drives. A capacity of 100 Mb (Figure 1) was novel a year or two ago but 1 Gb and 3.2 Gb drives are now available at prices below £500. Two-in-one CD-ROM drives with optical CD rewritable disks (650 Mb) have been introduced. These can record 650 Mb on the optical system and also read conventional CD-ROMs.

The computer transports data along a *data highway* or *bus* to whatever it is communicating with. There are different types of bus including local bus, ISA (Industry Standard Architecture) and EISA (Extended ISA). These are being replaced by PCI. Macintosh PCs have used SCSI which is used for connecting devices such as hard disk drives and CD-ROM drives and this type of bus has been adopted in some IBM compatibles.

The time taken for a device to be accessed, the *access time*, is measured in milliseconds (ms) for hard disks and nanoseconds (ns) for memory. Better performance is indicated by lower access times. The fastest access time for the computer is with RAM.

### Desktop, notebook and palmtop computers

The terms 'desktop computer' and 'notebook computer' are self-explanatory. *Laptop* computers were the first to be portable but were still cumbersome and were replaced by the notebook computer. Notebook computer manufacturers are continuing their quest to squeeze greater functionality into smaller spaces.

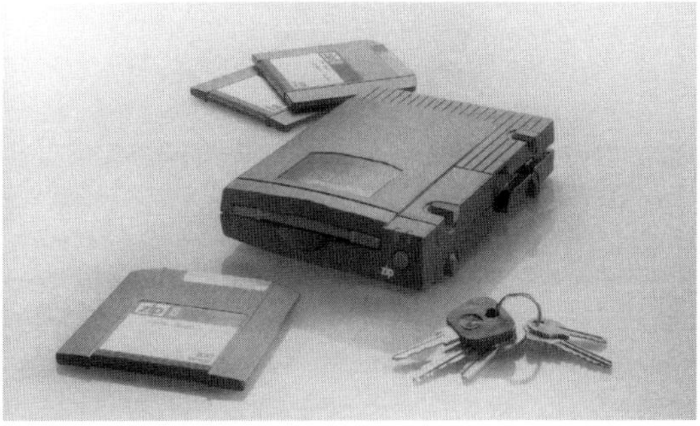

**Figure 1** Iomega ZIP back-up drive

Battery-life technology is improving and is just about keeping pace with ever increasing demands. Lithium ion and nickel metal hydride batteries are lighter than the older Nicad (nickel cadmium) batteries. Battery lives of over 6 h are quoted. Most notebooks have programs allowing shutdown of devices after user-defined times to save the battery.

An *expansion card* is a circuit board that fits into an expansion slot in a desktop computer and provides extra or enhanced function. A sound card will provide high-quality sound when the computer is connected to appropriate speakers. One or two slots available in a notebook computer for PCMCIA cards are invaluable. A card can act for example as a modem link allowing a fax facility or connection to Medline or the Internet.

*Palmtop computers* are small enough to fit into a jacket pocket and at the time of writing have memory capacity of up to 4 Mb (Figure 2). Small *flashcards* with additional memory are available.

### Scanners

Text documents, drawings and photographs can be scanned into the computer. Hand-held scanners are portable and seem attractive but in practice they are not easy to use (Figure 3). The author has a small scanner which is adequate for scanning-in black and white documents. Flat-bed scanners occupy more space which could be justified if scanning is frequently employed. The quality of images scanned into a computer is defined in terms of dots per inch (dpi). Higher resolution images have more dots per inch. Colour scanners are a little more expensive.

A colour image scanned in at high resolution can produce an enormous file. A holiday snap in colour, scanned at a resolution of 1200 dpi, will produce a file of 100 Mb. An A4 page in 24-bit colour could take an hour to scan. High resolution is required only if one plans to enlarge the image; most quality magazines print at 200 dpi. Digital imaging cameras are likely to take a significant proportion of photography away from conventional film cameras. The digital image can be edited allowing exciting possibilities. For the clinician with hobbies including photography and computing, these developments will need special consideration when upgrading hardware, but for the majority, colour scanning is not likely to be required. Digital imaging photography with digital cameras has some advantages with medical illustrations[1].

### Computer communications

A *modem* (modulator/demodulator) is hardware (it can be an expansion card) that lets the computer interact with other computers through the telephone line. The *Baud rate* indicates the speed at which data can be sent along a communications channel. Modem speeds are normally measured in bits per second. The maximum speed is determined by the Baud rate of the slower modem.

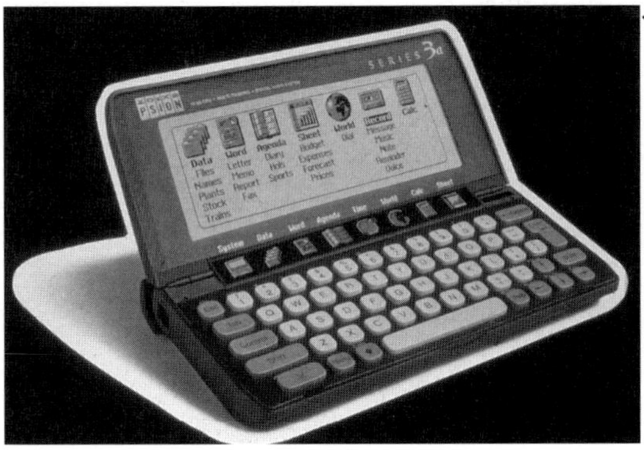


**Figure 2** Psion Series 3a palmtop computer

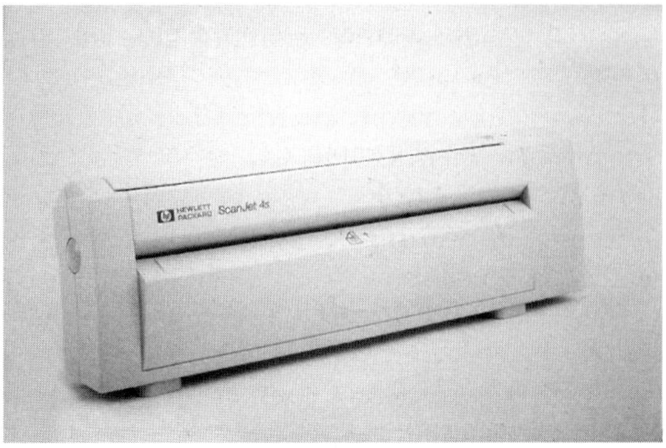


**Figure 3** Hewlett Packard 4S Scanjet scanner

A *network* is a group of computers linked by cable. Resources, such as data and printers are shared. One computer acts as the *server*. Programs suitable for networks were once very specialized but many current packages are compatible with networks and operating systems for networks are available for PCs. A significant degree of expertise for setting up and running a network is still required.

## SOFTWARE

A computer *program* (or *software*) is essentially a set of instructions. Like a recipe or service manual, it tells the computer what actions we want to be taken and the order in which these actions are to be undertaken. Early programs were in *machine code* which is incomprehensible to most users. Programmers are professionals who design programs that are simple (user friendly) to use. Programs have become increasingly sophisticated.

An *application* is one or more programs used for a task such as word processing or graphics. A suite of applications is a group of programs released by a software house in a package; the cost of the suite of programs is usually considerably less than the sum of the individual applications. The suite of programs is usually designed to link quickly. Software houses employ programmers who are highly skilled and who form teams to create and update sophisticated applications. Faults (bugs) must be detected and corrected before release but early versions of programs may still have problems. A program may cost millions of pounds to produce but may be purchased for perhaps a few hundred pounds as the development costs (and profits) are shared by large numbers of purchasers.

There has been a rapid change in the operating systems used by PCs from DOS to Windows and on to Windows 95. Windows and Windows 95 allow multiple programs and files to be open on the desktop (in RAM) simultaneously. When the RAM is full, the computer will move parts of data and programs to and from the hard disk. The Apple Macintosh used a high quality Graphics User Interface (GUI) before IBM compatibles and some still believe that it is superior. The GUI tends to use pictures to help the user point to required actions rather than using text commands required by DOS. Windows was developed by Microsoft as a rival to Apple's Macintosh system. Items are chosen by pointing at them with a pointing device (mouse) and left-clicking (the left mouse button is pressed). Right-clicking conventionally brings up a menu which is a choice of options such as being able to define a font. There is little doubt that Windows has simplified the use of computers.

Program updates are usually signalled by the *version* number. Word 6.0 would suggest that this is the sixth version of the program that has not yet had an upgrade. Sometimes, there is a jump between versions e.g. 3.2 to 6.0 as a software house may be concerned that their program might appear to have had fewer enhancements than that of their competitors. *Backwards compatibility* of software indicates that the new version is capable of accepting data files from earlier productions. Frequently it is a one-way process, that is to say that files created on the new software cannot be processed by earlier versions.

Upgrading to newer operating systems can lead to older equipment becoming obsolete. Most hardware manufacturers work closely with the major software companies. They can usually ensure that updated drivers, which are the programs that allow peripheral hardware such as printers to work with the computer, can be obtained.

Every computer program and all documents and artwork produced on a computer are held in *files*. Each file has a *filename* which is limited to eight characters by DOS or Windows but more characters can be used with Windows 95. Most files have *extensions* of three letters which help the computer select relevant files for particular programs. Document files for *Word for Windows*, a word-processing program (see below), have '.DOC' file extensions. Each file is located by its *path*. The path 'C:\winword\chapters\Chapter1.DOC' tells the computer to look for the file labelled 'Chapter1.DOC' on the C drive (hard disk) with the *directory* (branch) called 'winword' and the *subdirectory* called 'chapters'. Windows 95 calls files with data in them '*documents*'. (Those who use terms like 'hypogonadotrophic hypogonadism, menopause and climacteric' for the 'change of life' are not in a strong position to complain). Floppy disk drives are usually the 'A' or 'B' drive and CD-ROM drives are usually the 'D' drive; an additional CD-ROM is likely to be the 'E' drive.

File *compression* is a self-explanatory term. A double space program allows me to store 360 Mb on to the 200 Mb hard disk of my notebook computer. In some situations, particularly with graphics, 20-fold compression ratios are feasible. As memory capacity has become relatively cheap, there is less reason to utilize compression programs for hard drives as they tend to reduce performance. ZIP is a commly used compression utility. ZIPped files have extensions with '.ZIP'. There are programs allowing compression techniques for RAM but reports suggest that they are probably not as beneficial as they might seem at first glance.

## Databases

The most widely used application amongst all types of computer today is the *database*. A database is a collection of information. It allows the computer to store vast amounts of data in an organized fashion from which the information can be retrieved quickly. Some databases are purchased from an institution or software house for the information they hold. Medline, a database with information from medical journals (see below) is a valuable source of medical literature. Cochrane has produced a database of controlled trials in maternity care. Some database packages hold no data (other than examples) but allow the user to develop a personalized data record system.

### *Patient record systems*

When I consult in the independent sector, I use a database program called 'Access', in addition to conventional written notes. Access is a program with the tools to allow simple personalized database development. Data is entered onto a *form* (Figure 4). As information is written on the form it is stored in two *tables* (Figure 2). The first table holds patient details (*fields*) such as the surname, first name, date of birth, allergies, contraception, smear results and information leaflets that have been given to the patient. The row of fields for each patient in the table represents each patient's record. When a patient attends for follow-up or surgery, I only want to enter the new information and this is entered onto the event's section of the form. This event data is stored on a second 'events' table. The two tables are linked by a key field which, in this case, is the Patient_ID. On the patient record table, the Patient_ID field is a *counter* field – the computer automatically assigns the number '1' to the first record and each additional patient receives the next unique number allocated by the computer. The patient and the events tables are linked (related) through the Patient_ID field which appears in both tables (Figure 5). A relational database has two or more related tables. Databases that do not have related tables are called flat-file or non-relational databases.

It takes just a few seconds to type the data in but it saves time in the long run. Results cross my desk just once. If a bacteriology swab result shows *Candida*, I can see at a glance whether the patient has been treated and if not then a prescription can be written and sent. Results and treatment appear on the computer in sequence and can be quickly reviewed. Similarly, it is readily apparent when the next smear is due. Finally, if a patient calls me during an evening clinic and asks whether I recall the name of the white tablets I gave her 6 months ago, I have no problem. Usually a record is selected on first name and surname, but the date of birth, telephone number or address fields could be used. The size of my patient database file is over 5 Mb, but it takes just 2 seconds to locate a record, and this is with my 3-year-old 486 notebook computer.

With the lessons learned from designing, and modifying, the personal patient information system, the author has developed a database on

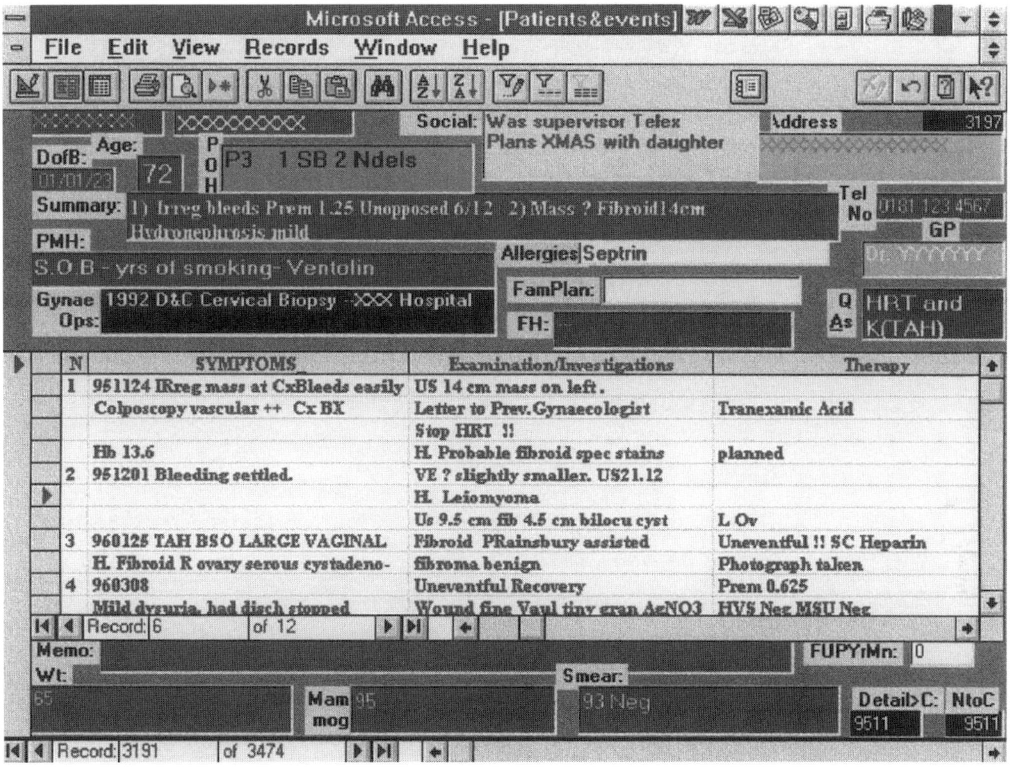


Figure 4 Database – a patient record

Microsoft Access for our fertility units at Whipps Cross Hospital and The BUPA Roding Hospital. In common with the personal patient record described above, data are stored in two tables, a patient details table and an event table. It is possible to select records by looking for matching criteria within one or more fields. We could look for all IVF treatment cycles in 1995 and then determine how many had clinical pregnancies or took home a baby. Most of the fields are specifically named according to Human Fertilisation and Embryology Authority (HFEA) form fields. Data can be entered onto forms, such as the ovulation induction treatment form (Figure 6). The layout of the HFEA form, as it appears on the computer, is shown in Figure 7. The advantage of an in-house system is that we can easily add our own special interest fields. The importance of ensuring absolute security and confidentiality of all information held on patients in general, and for those attending fertility units licenced by the HFEA in particular, cannot be over-emphasized.

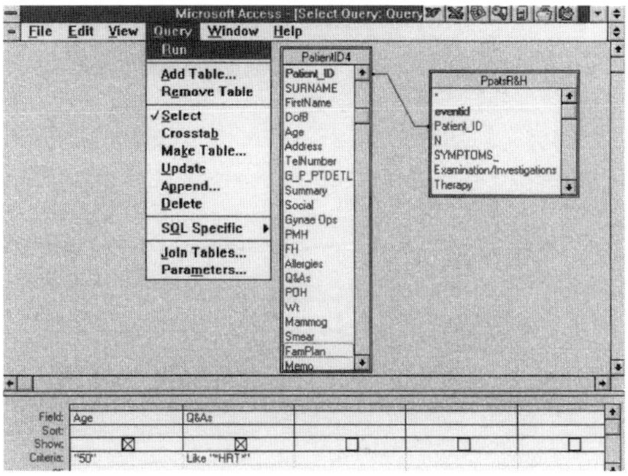


Figure 5 Database showing how two tables are linked

*The 'paperless' office*

Once each month, the author has an outreach clinic with a group practice of general

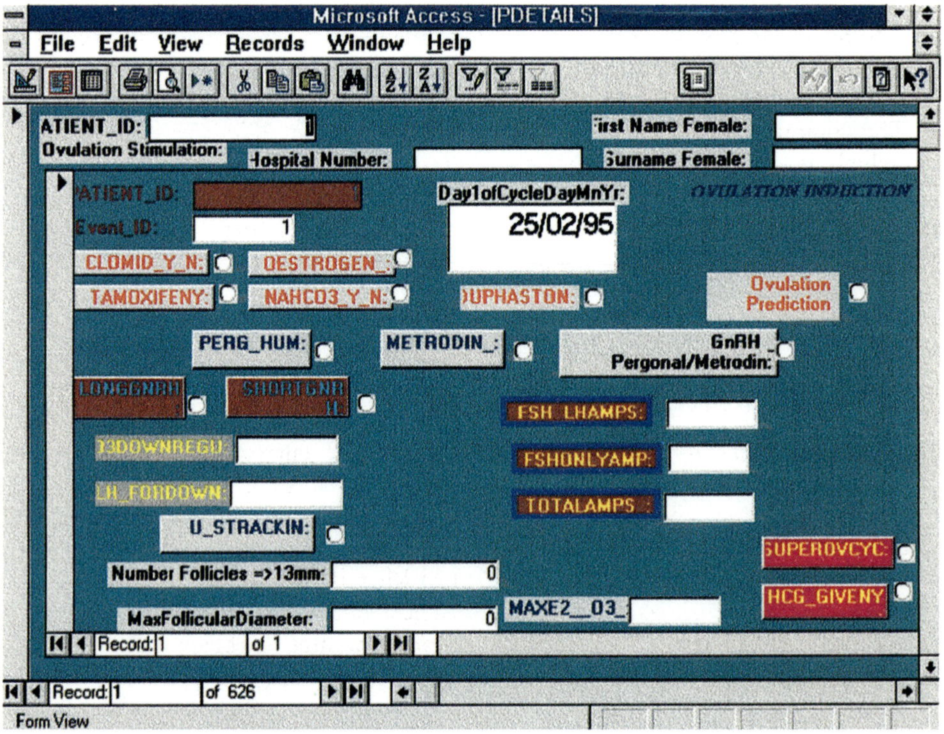


**Figure 6** Database – ovulation induction form

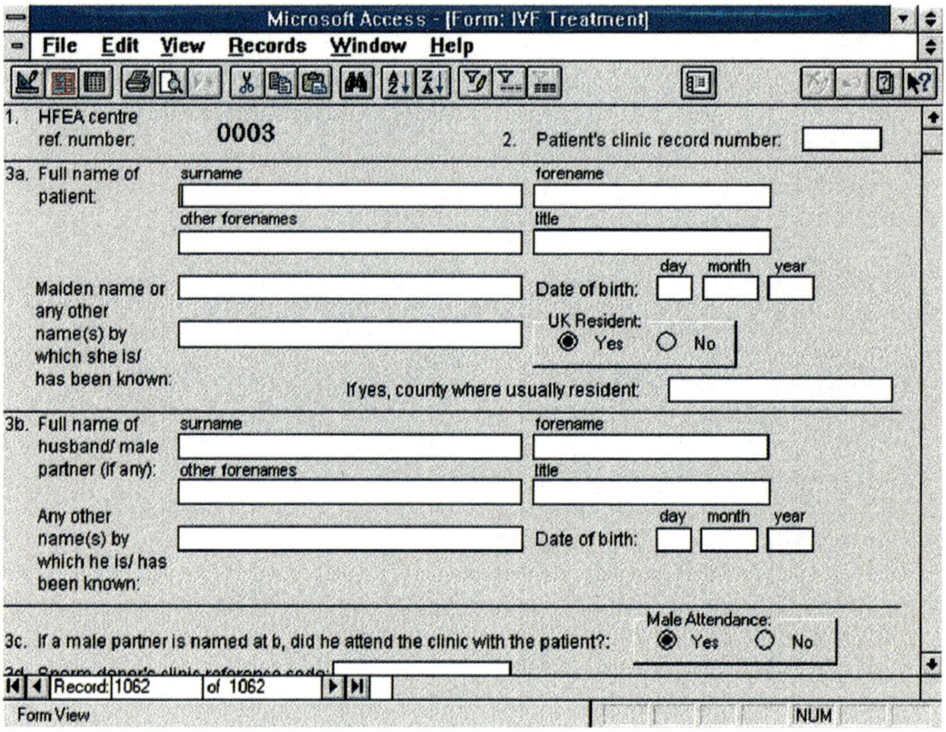


**Figure 7** HFEA form on a database program

practitioners. All consultations are recorded onto their computer database system. When the 'Insert' key is activated, data is stored and cannot be revoked; no hand-written records are required. The computer will provide a patient summary which is attached to the letter of referral. The 'paperless' general practice is becoming popular[2,3]. A 'paperless' hospital would be desirable. Missing notes would no longer be a problem. Laboratory and radiological results could be entered directly and reviewed on screen. Confidentiality could be achieved by various levels of password security.

*Personalized medical paper retrieval systems*
Storing medical papers, information about new treatments and management guidelines in one simple retrievable system is a desirable goal. There are an average of four papers in every journal that I read that I wish to retain. Space is limited and storing every journal is not possible. The papers to be kept are removed from the journal and each paper is given the next available number. A hundred papers is a convenient number for each folder in the filing cabinet. Details of each paper are entered onto a medical papers database, again designed on Access (Figure 8). The underlying table design form appears in Figure 9. Next to the field name is the Data (field) Type. The PAPER_ID is the key field. The cursor has been brought onto the AUTHORS field (arrow). This is a text field. Other field types available include 'numbers' (which would allow numerical calculations) and date/time fields. In the design for this database, the DATE field will automatically allocate the current date and time from the computer's in-built time facility. The 'Review Article' field is a 'Yes/No' type field. The computer assumes that the data in the field is 'No' but when the '*control*' (in this case the 'Review Article' button on the form) is 'clicked' with the mouse pointer, a black fill appears in the 'options box' and the 'No' is replaced by 'Yes'

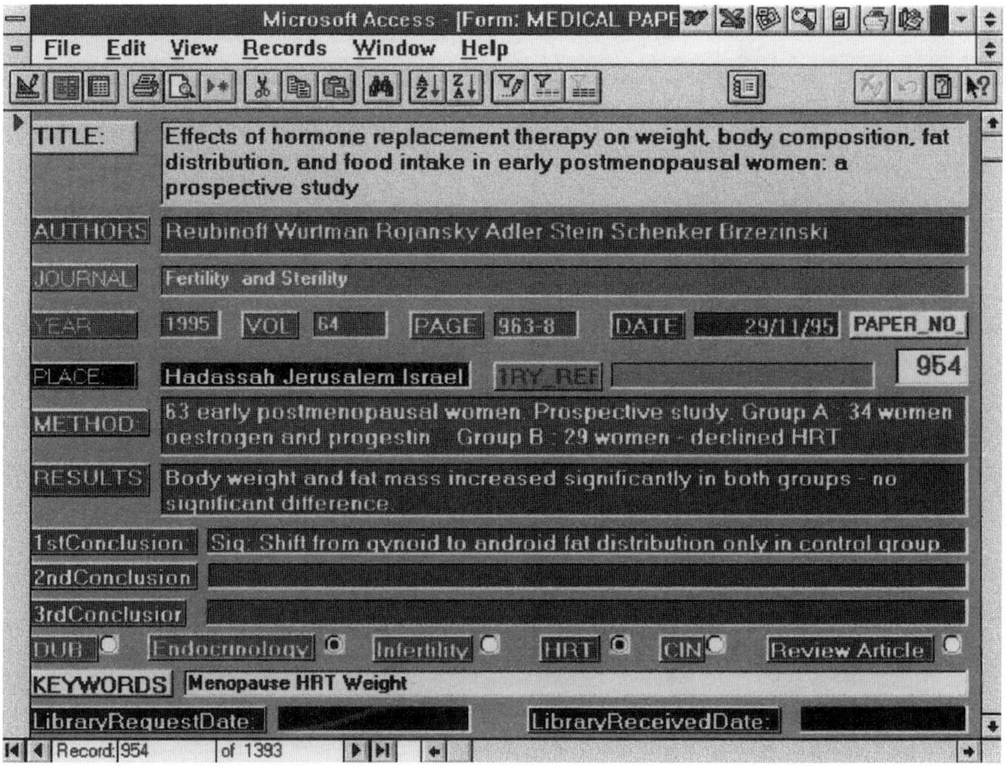


**Figure 8** A database of medical papers showing a typical record

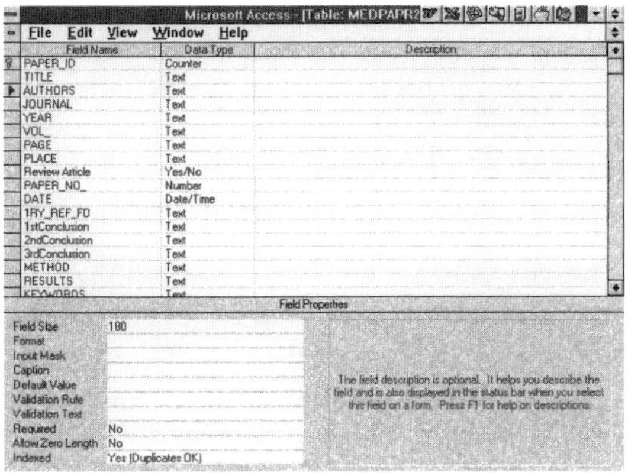


**Figure 9** The Medical Papers Database showing the fields construction

in the table. This facility provides a quick method for recalling records. In Figure 8 the options boxes with the endocrinology and hormone replacement therapy (HRT) controls have been clicked on. A search on either of these fields or for 'HRT', 'Menopause' or 'Weight' from the keywords field would select the 'Reubinoff *et al.*' record together with others matching the search criteria.

Option boxes and option groups provide modern mouse-operated choices. Some older systems still employ bar-codes. Bar-codes have a place when the data they represent changes. An item in a shop, such as a box of cereal, could be represented by a bar-code. The cashier swipes the bar-code reader across the code and the item is entered on the account. If the price is changed, it is altered on the computer and no time is wasted putting new labels on every item. There is little place for bar-codes in clinical situations. Drop-down choice option boxes are easy to develop and use. When the author was comparing maternity computer systems, midwives reported that they did not like bar-code data entry systems.

A paper-free method of storing articles has been chosen by my colleague Paul Rainsbury. Each article is scanned into his computer. A program (Scanning–Watermark Software Inc., 129 Middlesex Turnpike, Burlington MA 01803) produces a file of 1 Mb for a letter-sized page at 300 × 300 dpi. This can be compressed to 35–50 kb. Twenty pages of compressed image still requires 1 Mb. The company advise that even compressed images will soon fill the average hard disk and they recommend use of an optical storage system. The software provides its own database facility to allow retrieval of documents which can be printed when required.

*Medline*

Searching for medical references is a frequent requirement. Many postgraduate medical libraries will have 'Medline' on CD-ROM and the latest version is on Windows. BMA members, with their individual allocated passwords, can dial into the BMA library Medline database for the cost of a normal telephone call. A modem is required for the computer to communicate through the telephone line. The system is available at all times and is capable of serving up to 20 simultaneous searches. In a recent development, the BMA Medline can be assessed through the Internet and is then presented in 'Windows' format.

A Medline search is shown in Figure 10. There were 2363 references found under 'Estrogen Replacement Therapy' (1) and 25 629 references with the word 'weight' in the title (2). Combining these two searches (Control and N keys) looking for papers about HRT and with the word 'weight' in the title, found eight references (3). These eight references were then viewed (Control and K keys) and there were two selected (spacebar key) (4). One of these papers, as it appears on Medline is shown in Figure 11. Medline allows a choice of fields to appear on screen and in the downloaded files. One of these fields is the Medical Subheadings (MeSH). There are 17 500 MeSH headings used by the United States National Library of Medicine which produces Medline.

Searches can be conducted on 'author', 'subject', 'word' or string of words in the title, 'journal', 'year of publication' and numerous other choices. Similarly, the search can be limited to review articles, meta-analyses, experimental clinical trials, language and numerous other options. The author finds it helpful at times to search on the MeSH associated with

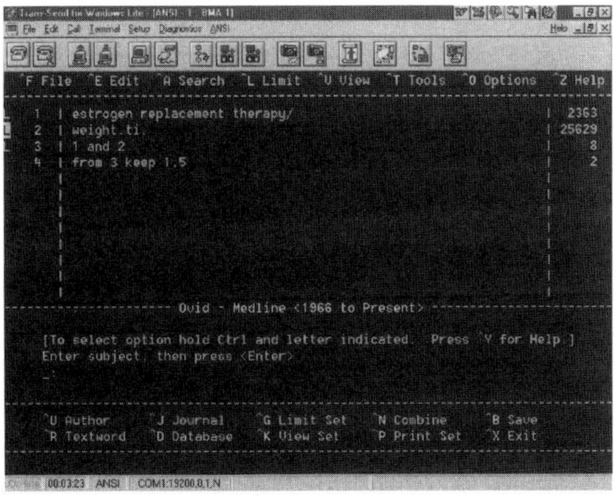


**Figure 10** Medline database showing a typical literature search

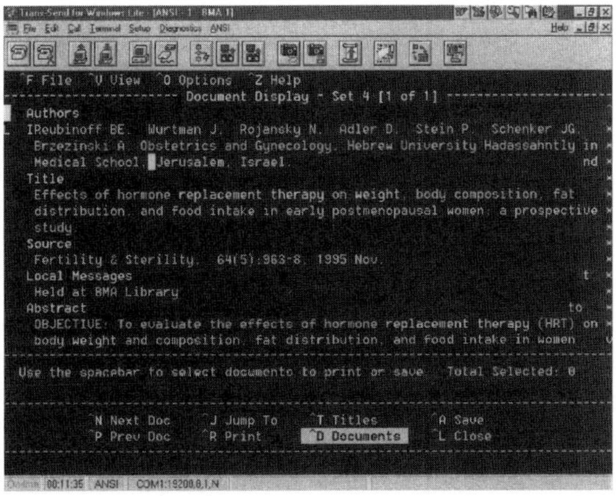


**Figure 11** Medline database showing a typical summary of a paper

one useful reference to find others of a similar nature.

Files downloaded from Medline can be opened into a word processor – the author uses 'Word 6'. With the cursor positioned at the end of one paper, by using the 'control' and 'return' keys together, a 'pagebreak' is introduced after each reference. Each paper, as summarized by Medline, can then be printed out on a separate sheet.

## Word processing

The modern secretary would regard a word processor as a basic necessity. Documents can be saved and amendments quickly made. For the majority of doctors writing a clinical paper, there is a need to introduce additional words or paragraphs and to be able to move whole sections of text about. A word processor is all that is required. A basic familiarity with a word processing program would take no more than an hour to achieve from the accompanying documentation (books that come with the program).

No doctor would aspire to type as professionally as a secretary but typing skills are a tremendous asset. There are several computer typing teacher programs available from most computer shops or mail order companies. These provide typing exercises and encourage building up speed. The computer keyboard has a variety of additional keys including *function keys* which are allocated special functions by each computer program. The 'F1' key conventionally provides *help* – advice on how to achieve a required task.

The author uses 'Word 6' which is a word-processing package produced by Microsoft. A sample of text in preparation for the first chapter of this book appears in Figure 12. The text area has been split allowing the reference section to be seen simultaneously with the main text. In the preparatory stages of an article or chapter, each paper in the text and reference section has its unique identifying number (allocated from the medical paper database – see above). A 'Find' utility appears as a box which appears on the screen by pressing the 'control' and 'F' keys simultaneously. In this example, the computer has quickly located the required first author on a 'String-search'. The split screen facility allows the lifting of one section of text into another area to be observed directly.

At the top of the screen is the *title bar* with the name of the program and the filename. To the right of the filename are a series of icons on buttons. These icons represent the programs available in the Microsoft 'Office Professional Suite'. From the left, these are Word, Excel (a spreadsheet program), Powerpoint (a graphics program ideal for creating slides), and Access. The filing cabinet represents 'File Manager', a Windows program allowing assessment and management of all the files on the computer.

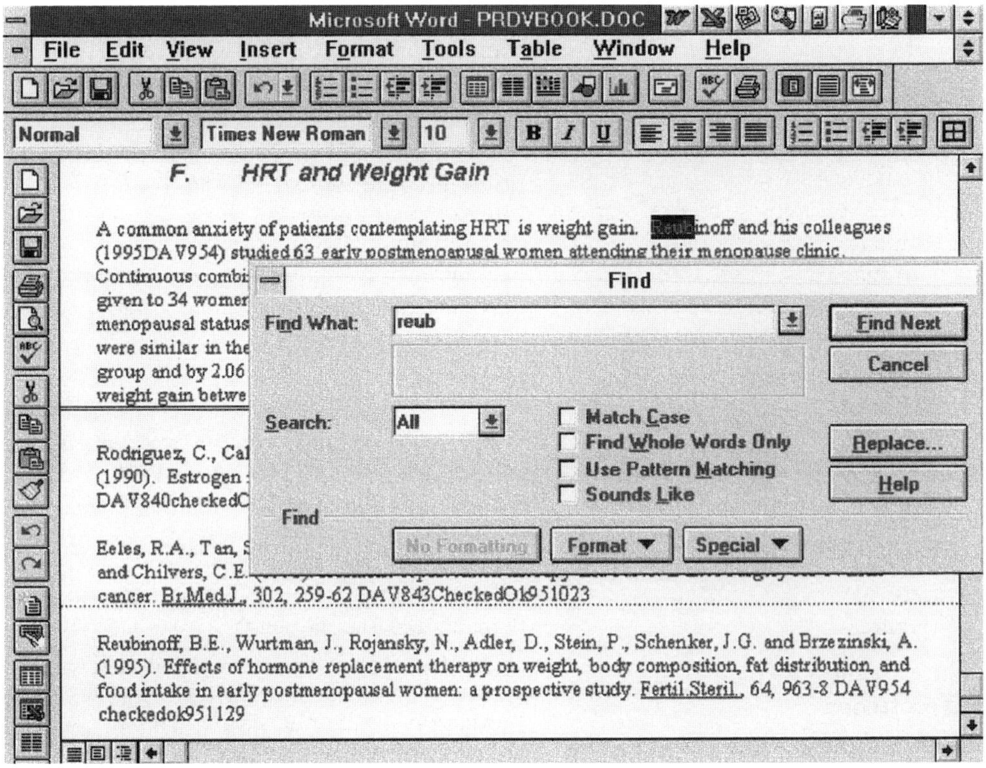


**Figure 12** A document on a word processor (Word 6 for Windows)

The printer icon is self-explanatory. When the mouse pointer is moved to one of these icons and left-clicked, the appropriate program is launched. Windows allows more than one program to be active simultaneously. For example, a text document on 'Word' can be active with Access and my 'medical papers' file open in the background. When the Access icon is activated, the database screen becomes active immediately and exactly as it last appeared.

Below the title bar is the *menu* bar. Click on 'File' and a menu of options drops down. These include facilities to open a new file, save the current file and print. The 'Format' drop down menu provides facilities to change the paragraph format and choose from the selection of fonts. The 'Tools' menu includes a spelling checker, word counter and thesaurus. Below the menu bar, there are two *toolbars*. On the lower toolbar are click buttons for bold text ('**B**'), italics ('*I*') and underline ('U'). On the upper toolbar, the scissors click button is for cutting – select a section of text and click on this button and that section disappears from the screen. The 'cut' section is stored onto the '*clipboard*'. The clipboard will only retain the latest selection entered. To the right of the scissors' icon is the copy button – select a section of text and clicking on this button will copy the selected text onto the clipboard whilst leaving the original *in situ*. The next icon is the paste icon. Moving the cursor to the required position and then clicking on this button results in the contents of the clipboard being pasted into this area. Selected text, graphics, pictures and tables can be stored onto the clipboard.

The contents of the clipboard are retained as long as Windows is active and the 'paste' facility can be used between different Windows programs. For example, when the 'printscreen' key is used whilst a Windows program is active, the entire screen is stored onto the clipboard. This picture of the screen can be pasted onto a graphics program such as Powerpoint and the files used to produce slides or pictures (Figures 1–9).

*Patient information leaflets*

The value of patient information leaflets in reproductive medicine is discussed in Chapter 2. Producing one's own information leaflets allows regular updating. It also avoids providing patients with mass-produced leaflets which may differ in emphasis, if not necessarily content, from the oral information given at consultation. To date the author has developed fifteen leaflets. The 'Format' menu on Word has a columns option. The text is printed in three columns on A4 paper with 'Page Setup' from the File menu set at 'Landscape' (horizontal) rather than 'Portrait' (vertical) printing. Pre-scored colour papers for easy folding are available in a variety of designs and enhance the presentation (Figure 13).

## Security and protection

Doctors must take all reasonable measures to ensure confidentiality of patient information. Computers usually have software utility programs which allow password protection. Back-up disks do not have this protection and appropriate caution is needed. In the UK, the data protection act (1984) requires that all computer systems holding data relating to living people must be registered with the Data Protection Registrar.

The psychopathology of lunacy is outside the scope of reproductive medicine but we must be aware of its existence and take appropriate precautions. There are those who obtain incomprehensible pleasure from developing a program that will destroy the data held on computer by some unsuspecting and unknown individual or institution. The virus can only infect a computer by being read into RAM. New floppy disks, and software purchased from reputable companies are safe. Disks borrowed from others may be 'infected'. For children, the temptation to look at a game 'borrowed' from a friend may be irresistible. When a computer is connected to the Internet, there is a particular danger. The computer is effectively travelling around the world with potentially dangerous contact possibilities. Prevention, by immunization against potential infection is basic medicine. There are some excellent anti-virus toolkits that provide immunity from known viruses; these are highly recommended for any computer put 'at-risk'.

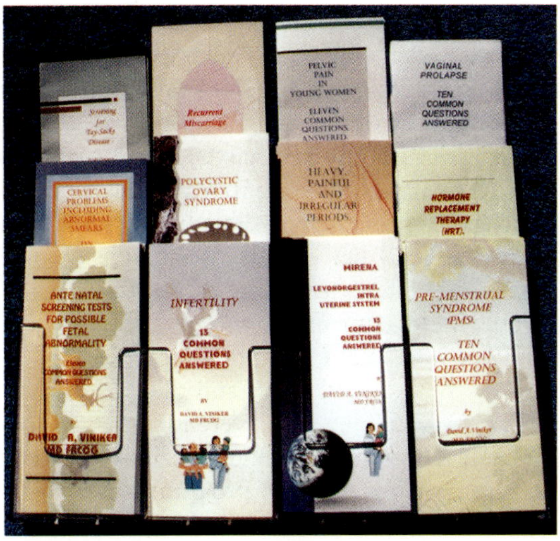


**Figure 13** Patient information leaflets designed on a word processor

## Graphics

Graphics programs include programs for drawings and digital photograph manipulation. Flow chart programs allow the use of shapes which can be moved around. Text can be added to each shape and colours and shadowing are just a couple of 'clicks' away. Arrows can be 'snapped' onto the shapes – when the shape is moved, the arrow remains attached. Examples of flow charts using 'Vision 3' are seen in Chapters 3, 7, 17, 26 and 28.

'Powerpoint' and 'Coreldraw 6' are 'friendly' graphics applications programs with many features. Using the Tab-key in 'Powerpoint' will alter the size of text characters and position of text automatically and logically. An array of backgrounds can be chosen to complete the presentation. The author finds these programs help embellish a few simple words into attractive slides in just a short time

(Figure 14). Drawing programs, included with Coreldraw 6 can be fun to use; three-dimensional shapes and pictures can be created.

### Spreadsheets

A spreadsheet application is useful for performing arithmetical calculations. These applications usually have integrated graphic representation of the data.

### Desktop publishing

Desktop publishing programs, as their name suggests, allow relatively simple integration and movement of words and graphics to design pages like a newspaper. The author has never found a requirement for this type of program.

### Organizer programs

Lotus Organizer is a delightful program to use for anyone who enjoyed using a Filofax but wants to move away from paper. The program appears on the screen like a Filofax with sections including a diary and addresses. In practice it is excellent for someone who is happy to keep their work diary on the computer and keep a separate system when walking around. The program allows pages to be printed out, even in colour but this is very time consuming. These organizers are fine for business use but if you want to integrate all your diary, address book and frequently used notes and keep them ready to hand, they do not seem to work: even notebook PCs cannot be kept in a jacket pocket.

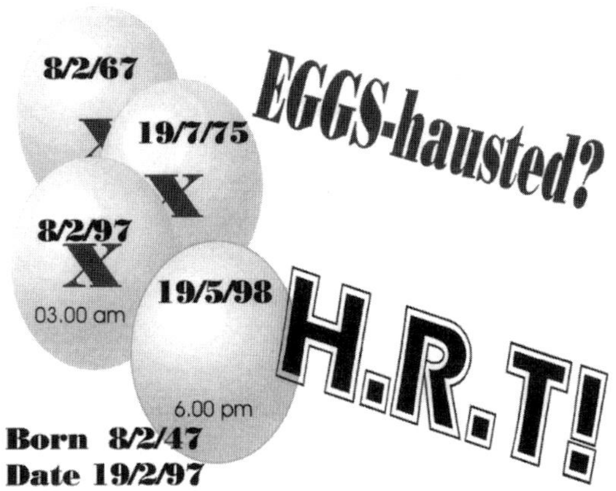


**Figure 14** A 'slide' designed on a graphics program (Coreldraw 6)

### Palmtop computer organizers

The author uses a Psion Series 3A for a number of applications. It is smaller than a Filofax ('Palmtop' size) and can be carried conveniently at all times. The diary can be viewed in a number of formats. The 'repeat' option of a computer diary is a bonus. For example, if there is a clinic that takes place on the second Friday of the calendar month, it takes a few seconds to enter it and use the repeat option. There is a 'to-do list' facility allowing prioritization; the list can be integrated with the diary. Alarms can be set as reminders. Birthdays, anniversaries and other annual events have their own section and these similarly integrate with the diary. The database function can be used for addresses and telephone numbers as well as other applications. There is also a reasonably sophisticated word processor.

Either the database or word processor can be used for keeping brief notes about patients in a research study. In my antenatal clinic, a brief record of patients with a history of infertility treatment and/or multiple pregnancy is entered onto the Psion, facilitating analysis at a later date. Parallel and serial links are available to connect the Psion to a PC or printer. The Psion is available with a choice of internal memory capacities. My Psion has a 1 Mb capacity which has a full diary, 350 addresses and several word processed and database files. Less than half the full capacity has been used to date. The data can be backed up onto a small solid state disk or onto a PC.

### The Internet

HTMP (Hypertext mark-up language) is used in the creation of World Wide Web (WWW) pages which is the latest format used to 'surf the Internet information super highway'. The Internet and WWW have a whole new vocabulary. To enter the Internet, a modem and a contract with an appropriate company are required. There is a monthly charge for the link and all calls are charged at local rates. The company will provide a personal E-mail address at which all incoming messages or files are received. The Internet is expanding exponentially. According to one survey reported in June 1996, there are 9 million people connected to the Internet in the USA. The majority of companies will have WWW pages advertising their wares. 'Clicking' on icons or words in blue launches the next required page. The Medical Education Centre at Whipps Cross Hospital has its own Web site (Figure 15). A map of the local area appears on the 'welcome page'. Details of courses and lectures can be obtained from the site. In the UK, the government has recently launched a scheme to photograph all icons in our art galleries and museums together with appropriate information. These will be accessible on the Internet. Many universities and libraries are accessible on the Internet or through a special academic link 'Janet'.

## PRACTICAL GUIDELINES: PURCHASING HARDWARE AND SOFTWARE

When purchasing hardware or software, one has no option but to accept that the product will be almost instantly outdated. It is advisable to allow for expansion of requirements greater than envisaged and even then within 12 months it is still likely to feel cramped. Usually when an article is purchased, one has a clear objective in mind. If we consider a camera, we know in advance if it is for still or video photography and whether it will be used for family and holiday snaps or more hobby or professional purposes. Computers are different because there is an ever increasing set of unforeseen applications.

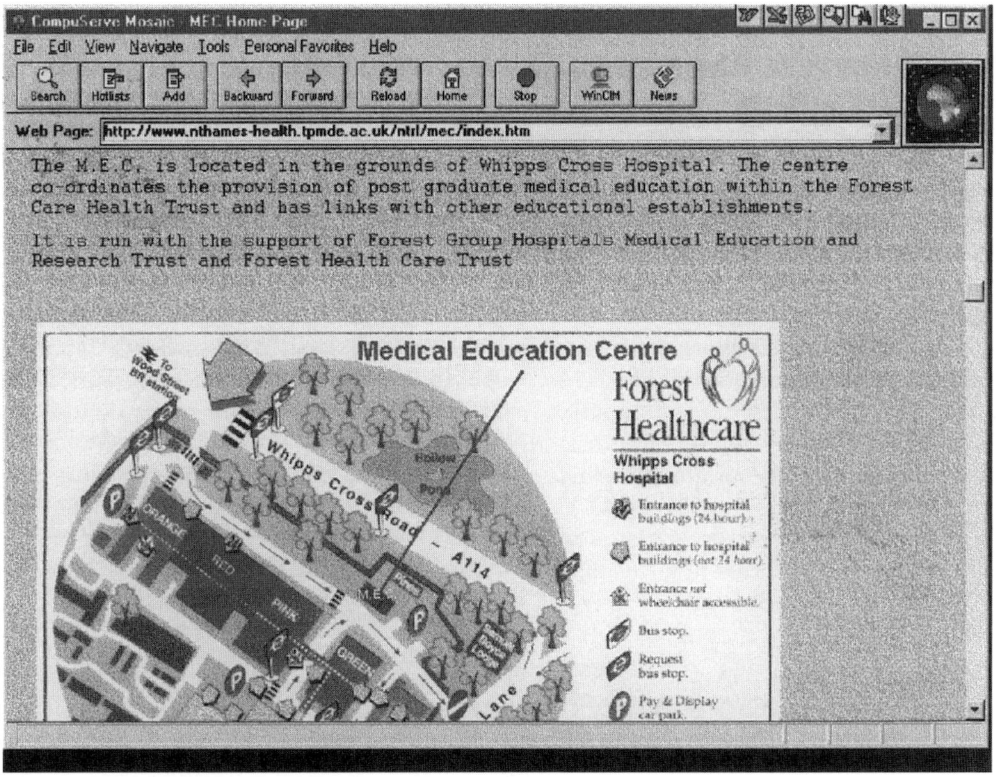


**Figure 15** The Medical Education Centre (Whipps Cross Hospital) showing an example of a 'Welcome Page' at a Web site on the Internet

Computer hardware and software prices follow an undulating pattern. When a new piece of hardware or software application reaches the market, the price is initially high. Competitors soon offer a comparable item and prices quickly tumble. Within a year, the prized 'top-of-the-range' article is out of date and may be available at greatly reduced cost. Over the years, the cost of an average PC has been around £2000. As time goes by, a more powerful computer system is purchased for the same amount of money.

With each development of the operating system, from DOS, to Windows, Windows 95 and soon Windows 97, comes a new round of software enhancements. There does not seem to have been the same quantum leap from DOS to Windows as from Windows to Windows 95. Some have suggested that upgrades in software are driven by economic considerations rather than for user advantage but the author would not wish to comment. It seems wise to consider purchasing a system accepting that it is likely to have a life-expectancy of about 4 years.

Opinion is divided on the benefits of application suites. On the positive side, the layouts of the programs tend to be similar so that learning how to use one program helps with the next. Integration may not necessarily be silky-smooth and not all programs within the suite match the quality of its best facility. If you are buying a set of programs for the first time or upgrading it is usually cheaper to buy a complete suite rather than individual programs. The computer market is volatile with billions of pounds at stake. My first PC database, *Rapidfile*, was produced by Ashton-Tate, the company responsible for the original leading database development program, *D-Base*. Ashton-Tate was taken over by Borland and in 1994 that company was reported to have made a loss of $1.4 million in just 3 months. The typical business suite of programs would include a word processor, database and spreadsheet. Graphics programs and personal organizers may be included.

A variety of books quickly appear following the launch of a new program or version update which may add clarification. The author has found video teaching cassettes to be helpful as an introduction to a new program. They will usually demonstrate the most important tools of the application often with the benefit of accompanying examples on disk. With the computer loaded with the program and example data, the video can be advanced and replayed providing an on-line tutor.

Each individual must decide on the likely requirements of the computer system or software application. Computer journals give ready assessment of the choice currently available. My personal preference is for a notebook rather than a desktop computer. My notebook weighs less than 3 kg and can be carried around with ease. Batteries allow about 2 h of use but I rarely use the computer in places where it cannot be connected to the mains. For academics flying around the world, battery life, and weight of extra batteries might be a consideration. Transformers are getting lighter and this is an advantage.

It is probably wise to purchase a brand-name notebook. No company is completely safe in the computer world but established companies at least have a track-record. It is worth spending time getting the feel of a notebook, preferably at a venue where a variety can be tested. Specifications are important; keyboards react differently; the *trackball* (the notebook equivalent of the mouse), connects to a port on the side of the Texas Travelmate 4000E notebook computer. Later models integrate the trackball below the keyboard. The trackball is being replaced by trackpads and some notebooks have a stick, which is like the eraser on top of a pencil.

Notebook screens can be mono (two-tone), dual scan colour (256 colours) or TFT (64 000 colours). The cost differential between mono and dual scan, and also between dual scan and TFT varies between £300 and £500 depending on manufacturer. Mono is probably adequate for many applications including word processing but, as with television and photography, colour is more pleasing to use. Dual scan screens have improved and are worth considering allowing funds to be used elsewhere in the system.

Older notebook computers were relatively difficult or impossible to upgrade. More recent notebook computers have upgradable RAM and hard disks. Trackballs, which are the notebook equivalent of the mouse, were disconnectable but now they can be integral, retractable, or replaced by a pad. Some notebooks feature replaceable screens which can be upgraded. A docking station is often available allowing the portable notebook computer to become part of a desktop system with all additional facilities for the office or home. The docking station incorporates a larger screen monitor, bays for additional hard drives or a CD-ROM drive and usually IBM-compatible expansion slots.

The advantage of portability is apparent. Unless it is certain that the computer is to be used in one place only, a notebook has much to commend it. There is a slight tendency for notebook components to lag behind desktop specifications by just a few months and there is usually a small extra premium to pay. The differential is not enormous. At the time of writing, a notebook computer with a P100 CPU, 1 Gb hard disk and a six-speed CD-ROM drive would be sensible. A colour bubble jet printer would provide excellent hard copies of data.

When buying a computer system for the first time, floppy disks are probably all that are required in the fist instance to back-up files. The author would again emphasize the fact that there is little point in backing up purchased programs as these are best loaded onto a computer from the original disks. Graphics files down-loaded from the internet or from a colour scanner will occupy large volumes of storage. Optical CD-ROM drives or tape streamers would then need consideration. My tape-streamer, now 3 years old, will back-up 300 Mb from my notebook in 20 min (with a 486 CPU) so that I could not justify up-grading (yet). At this time, modular notebooks have conventional CD-ROM drives without optical CD. A tapestreamer in addition, should more than suffice. One company has released an expansion card with accompanying software at a most competitive price that allows back-up of several Gb onto a video cassette with a conventional video recorder.

Computers can be linked to projector systems for presentations and lectures. Very large monitors are available in some lecture theatres. Projectors and transparent LCD screens that sit on overhead projectors are available but they are expensive. Hundreds of photographs (or slides) can be stored on a single CD-ROM. Within a few years, lecturers will only need to carry a CD-ROM rather than boxes or magazines of 35 mm slides.

Before purchasing, determine your probable requirements and perhaps choose a medium-priced system towards the upper end of the range rather than from a more expensive selection towards the lower end of the range. Unlike classic cars, out-dated computers have little value and there is, therefore, little merit in purchasing an expensive system in anticipation of it lasting more than a few years. When upgrading the operating system, for example from Windows to Windows 95 great caution is required. Important files should be backed up in advance and it is best to choose a time when a failure would not be catastrophic. Most newsagents sell a selection of computer magazines and these will have critical comparative reviews of current hardware and software applications. For the enthusiast, there is a computer TV channel on cable (JCN).

A personal computer will not release time for leisure activities. It allows the user to undertake more activities in a given time than would have otherwise been possible. The back-up facility provides reassurance that irreplaceable data need not be lost. Finally, the palmtop computer is really a computerized diary/address book/memo/Filofax system to be considered separately from mainstream computing.

## REFERENCES


1. Meire, H. B., Darzi, A. and Lee, N. (1995) Digital imaging. *Br. Med. J.*, **311**, 1218–21
2. Millman, A., Lee, N. and Brook, A., (1995). Computers in general practice – I. *Br. Med. J.*, **311**, 800–2
3. Purves, I. N. (1996). The paperless general practice. *Br. Med. J.*, **312**, 1112–13

# Index